# Online Access to the NCLEX-RN® Prep Course!

Dear Customer,

Thank you for your purchase of this NCLEX-RN Study Guide. Included with your purchase is **full 60-day access to our online NCLEX-RN Prep Course.**

We have structured our online course to perfectly complement the printed study guide. The NCLEX-RN Prep Course contains **in-depth lessons** that cover all the most important topics, **over 100 video reviews** that explain difficult concepts, more than **1,800 practice questions** to ensure you feel prepared, and over **1,000 digital flashcards**, so you can fit in some studying while you're on the go.

***Online NCLEX-RN Prep Course***

**Topics Covered:**

- Management of Care
- Safety and Infection Prevention and Control
- Health Promotion and Maintenance
- Psychosocial Integrity
- Basic Care and Comfort
- Pharmacological and Parenteral Therapies
- Reduction of Risk Potential
- Physiological Adaptation

**Course Features:**

- NCLEX-RN Study Guide
  - Get content that complements our best-selling study guide.
- 12 Full-Length Practice Tests
  - With over 1,800 practice questions, you can test yourself again and again.
- Mobile Friendly
  - If you need to study on the go, the course is easily accessible from your mobile device.
- NCLEX-RN Flashcards
  - Our course includes a flashcard mode consisting of over 1,000 content cards to help you study.

To validate your purchase and begin your 60-day free access, simply scan this QR code with your smartphone or go to **pv.mometrix.com** and enter SKU: **nclexrn-31183**

If you have any questions, please contact us at support@mometrix.com.

Sincerely,

**Mometrix**
TEST PREPARATION

# ACCESS YOUR ONLINE RESOURCES

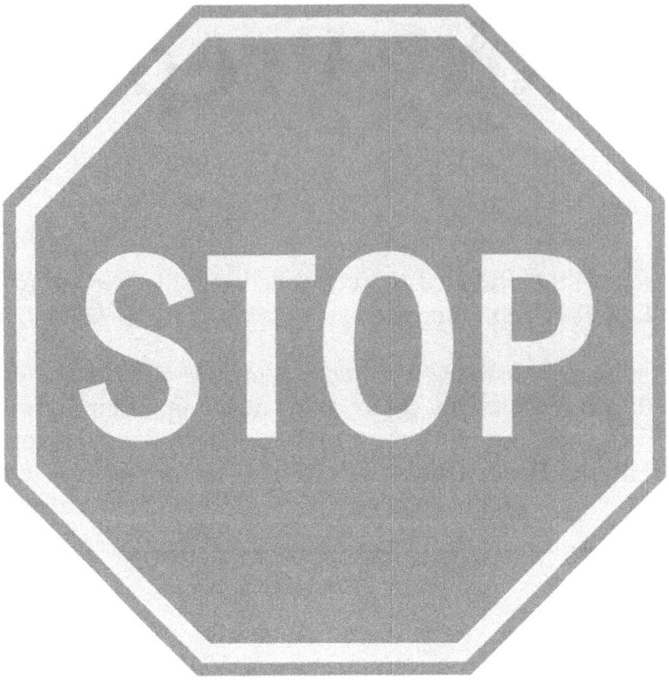


**DON'T MISS OUT ON THE ONLINE RESOURCES INCLUDED WITH YOUR PURCHASE!**

Your purchase of this product unlocks access to our Online Resources page. Elevate your study experience with our **interactive practice test interface**, along with all of the additional resources that we couldn't include in this book.

**Flip to the Online Resources section at the end of this book to find the link and a QR code to get started!**

Mometrix
TEST PREPARATION

Mometrix
TEST PREPARATION

# NCLEX RN®

# Prep Book + Online Course

## NCLEX RN® Examination Secrets Study Guide 2026-2027 with Practice Tests and Video Tutorials

Updated for the 2026 Test Plan

Written and edited by Matthew Bowling

This paper meets the requirements of ANSI/NISO Z39.48-1992 (Permanence of Paper).



Paperback
ISBN 978-1-5167-3118-3
ISBN 10: 1-5167-3118-2

# Dear Future Exam Success Story

First of all, **THANK YOU** for purchasing Mometrix study materials!

Second, congratulations! You are one of the few determined test-takers who are committed to doing whatever it takes to excel on your exam. **You have come to the right place.** We developed these study materials with one goal in mind: to deliver you the information you need in a format that's concise and easy to use.

In addition to optimizing your guide for the content of the test, we've outlined our recommended steps for breaking down the preparation process into small, attainable goals so you can make sure you stay on track.

We've also analyzed the entire test-taking process, identifying the most common pitfalls and showing how you can overcome them and be ready for any curveball the test throws you.

Standardized testing is one of the biggest obstacles on your road to success, which only increases the importance of doing well in the high-pressure, high-stakes environment of test day. Your results on this test could have a significant impact on your future, and this guide provides the information and practical advice to help you achieve your full potential on test day.

**Your success is our success**

**We would love to hear from you!** If you would like to share the story of your exam success or if you have any questions or comments in regard to our products, please contact us at **800-673-8175** or **support@mometrix.com**.

Thanks again for your business and we wish you continued success!

Sincerely,
The Mometrix Test Preparation Team

**Need more help? Check out our flashcards at:**
**http://mometrixflashcards.com/NCLEX**

# TABLE OF CONTENTS

# Introduction

**Thank you for purchasing this resource!** You have made the choice to prepare yourself for a test that could have a huge impact on your future, and this guide is designed to help you be fully ready for test day. Obviously, it's important to have a solid understanding of the test material, but you also need to be prepared for the unique environment and stressors of the test, so that you can perform to the best of your abilities.

For this purpose, the first section that appears in this guide is the **Secret Keys**. We've devoted countless hours to meticulously researching what works and what doesn't, and we've boiled down our findings to the five most impactful steps you can take to improve your performance on the test. We start at the beginning with study planning and move through the preparation process, all the way to the testing strategies that will help you get the most out of what you know when you're finally sitting in front of the test.

We recommend that you start preparing for your test as far in advance as possible. However, if you've bought this guide as a last-minute study resource and only have a few days before your test, we recommend that you skip over the first two Secret Keys since they address a long-term study plan.

If you struggle with **test anxiety**, we strongly encourage you to check out our recommendations for how you can overcome it. Test anxiety is a formidable foe, but it can be beaten, and we want to make sure you have the tools you need to defeat it.

## Review Video Directory

As you work your way through this guide, you will see numerous review video links interspersed with the written content. If you would like to access all of these review videos in one place, click on the video directory link found on the online resources page: **mometrix.com/resources719/nclexrn-31183**

## Chapter Quizzes

Transform passive reading into active learning! After immersing yourself in each chapter, put your comprehension to the test by taking a quiz. The insights you gained will stay with you longer this way. Scan this QR code to go directly to the chapter quiz interface for this study guide. If you're using a computer, simply visit the online resources page at **mometrix.com/resources719/nclexrn-31183** and click the Chapter Quizzes link.

# Secret Key #1 – Plan Big, Study Small

There's a lot riding on your performance. If you want to ace this test, you're going to need to keep your skills sharp and the material fresh in your mind. You need a plan that lets you review everything you need to know while still fitting in your schedule. We'll break this strategy down into three categories.

## Information Organization

Start with the information you already have: the official test outline. From this, you can make a complete list of all the concepts you need to cover before the test. Organize these concepts into groups that can be studied together, and create a list of any related vocabulary you need to learn so you can brush up on any difficult terms. You'll want to keep this vocabulary list handy once you actually start studying since you may need to add to it along the way.

## Time Management

Once you have your set of study concepts, decide how to spread them out over the time you have left before the test. Break your study plan into small, clear goals so you have a manageable task for each day and know exactly what you're doing. Then just focus on one small step at a time. When you manage your time this way, you don't need to spend hours at a time studying. Studying a small block of content for a short period each day helps you retain information better and avoid stressing over how much you have left to do. You can relax knowing that you have a plan to cover everything in time. In order for this strategy to be effective though, you have to start studying early and stick to your schedule. Avoid the exhaustion and futility that comes from last-minute cramming!

## Study Environment

The environment you study in has a big impact on your learning. Studying in a coffee shop, while probably more enjoyable, is not likely to be as fruitful as studying in a quiet room. It's important to keep distractions to a minimum. You're only planning to study for a short block of time, so make the most of it. Don't pause to check your phone or get up to find a snack. It's also important to **avoid multitasking**. Research has consistently shown that multitasking will make your studying dramatically less effective. Your study area should also be comfortable and well-lit so you don't have the distraction of straining your eyes or sitting on an uncomfortable chair.

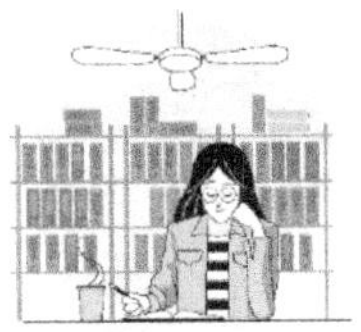

The time of day you study is also important. You want to be rested and alert. Don't wait until just before bedtime. Study when you'll be most likely to comprehend and remember. Even better, if you know what time of day your test will be, set that time aside for study. That way your brain will be used to working on that subject at that specific time and you'll have a better chance of recalling information.

Finally, it can be helpful to team up with others who are studying for the same test. Your actual studying should be done in as isolated an environment as possible, but the work of organizing the information and setting up the study plan can be divided up. In between study sessions, you can discuss with your teammates the concepts that you're all studying and quiz each other on the details. Just be sure that your teammates are as serious about the test as you are. If you find that your study time is being replaced with social time, you might need to find a new team.

# Secret Key #2 – Make Your Studying Count

You're devoting a lot of time and effort to preparing for this test, so you want to be absolutely certain it will pay off. This means doing more than just reading the content and hoping you can remember it on test day. It's important to make every minute of study count. There are two main areas you can focus on to make your studying count.

## Retention

It doesn't matter how much time you study if you can't remember the material. You need to make sure you are retaining the concepts. To check your retention of the information you're learning, try recalling it at later times with minimal prompting. Try carrying around flashcards and glance at one or two from time to time or ask a friend who's also studying for the test to quiz you.

To enhance your retention, look for ways to put the information into practice so that you can apply it rather than simply recalling it. If you're using the information in practical ways, it will be much easier to remember. Similarly, it helps to solidify a concept in your mind if you're not only reading it to yourself but also explaining it to someone else. Ask a friend to let you teach them about a concept you're a little shaky on (or speak aloud to an imaginary audience if necessary). As you try to summarize, define, give examples, and answer your friend's questions, you'll understand the concepts better and they will stay with you longer. Finally, step back for a big picture view and ask yourself how each piece of information fits with the whole subject. When you link the different concepts together and see them working together as a whole, it's easier to remember the individual components.

Finally, practice showing your work on any multi-step problems, even if you're just studying. Writing out each step you take to solve a problem will help solidify the process in your mind, and you'll be more likely to remember it during the test.

## Modality

*Modality* simply refers to the means or method by which you study. Choosing a study modality that fits your own individual learning style is crucial. No two people learn best in exactly the same way, so it's important to know your strengths and use them to your advantage.

For example, if you learn best by visualization, focus on visualizing a concept in your mind and draw an image or a diagram. Try color-coding your notes, illustrating them, or creating symbols that will trigger your mind to recall a learned concept. If you learn best by hearing or discussing information, find a study partner who learns the same way or read aloud to yourself. Think about how to put the information in your own words. Imagine that you are giving a lecture on the topic and record yourself so you can listen to it later.

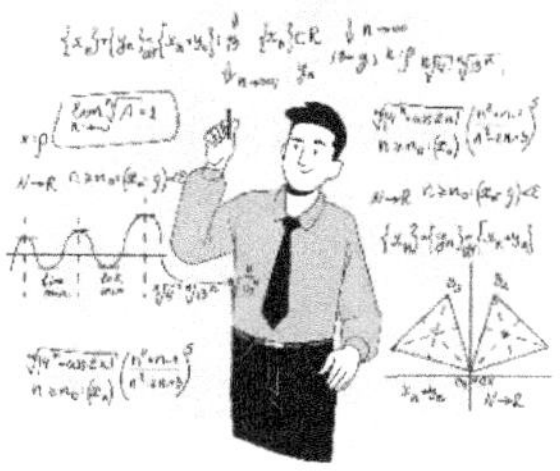

For any learning style, flashcards can be helpful. Organize the information so you can take advantage of spare moments to review. Underline key words or phrases. Use different colors for different categories. Mnemonic devices (such as creating a short list in which every item starts with the same letter) can also help with retention. Find what works best for you and use it to store the information in your mind most effectively and easily.

# Secret Key #3 – Practice the Right Way

Your success on test day depends not only on how many hours you put into preparing, but also on whether you prepared the right way. It's good to check along the way to see if your studying is paying off. One of the most effective ways to do this is by taking practice tests to evaluate your progress. Practice tests are useful because they show exactly where you need to improve. Every time you take a practice test, pay special attention to these three groups of questions:

- The questions you got wrong
- The questions you had to guess on, even if you guessed right
- The questions you found difficult or slow to work through

This will show you exactly what your weak areas are, and where you need to devote more study time. Ask yourself why each of these questions gave you trouble. Was it because you didn't understand the material? Was it because you didn't remember the vocabulary? Do you need more repetitions on this type of question to build speed and confidence? Dig into those questions and figure out how you can strengthen your weak areas as you go back to review the material.

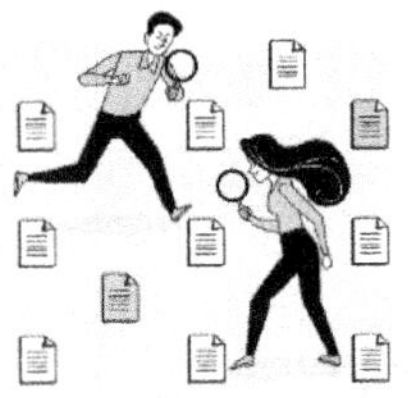

Additionally, many practice tests have a section explaining the answer choices. It can be tempting to read the explanation and think that you now have a good understanding of the concept. However, an explanation likely only covers part of the question's broader context. Even if the explanation makes perfect sense, **go back and investigate** every concept related to the question until you're positive you have a thorough understanding.

As you go along, keep in mind that the practice test is just that: practice. Memorizing these questions and answers will not be very helpful on the actual test because it is unlikely to have any of the same exact questions. If you only know the right answers to the sample questions, you won't be prepared for the real thing. **Study the concepts** until you understand them fully, and then you'll be able to answer any question that shows up on the test.

It's important to wait on the practice tests until you're ready. If you take a test on your first day of study, you may be overwhelmed by the amount of material covered and how much you need to learn. Work up to it gradually.

On test day, you'll need to be prepared for answering questions, managing your time, and using the test-taking strategies you've learned. It's a lot to balance, like a mental marathon that will have a big impact on your future. Like training for a marathon, you'll need to start slowly and work your way up. When test day arrives, you'll be ready.

Start with the strategies you've read in the first two Secret Keys—plan your course and study in the way that works best for you. If you have time, consider using multiple study resources to get different approaches to the same concepts. It can be helpful to see difficult concepts from more than one angle. Then find a good source for practice tests. Many times, the test website will suggest potential study resources or provide sample tests.

## Practice Test Strategy

If you're able to find at least three practice tests, we recommend this strategy:

### Untimed and Open-Book Practice

Take the first test with no time constraints and with your notes and study guide handy. Take your time and focus on applying the strategies you've learned.

### Timed and Open-Book Practice

Take the second practice test open-book as well, but set a timer and practice pacing yourself to finish in time.

### Timed and Closed-Book Practice

Take any other practice tests as if it were test day. Set a timer and put away your study materials. Sit at a table or desk in a quiet room, imagine yourself at the testing center, and answer questions as quickly and accurately as possible.

Keep repeating timed and closed-book tests on a regular basis until you run out of practice tests or it's time for the actual test. Your mind will be ready for the schedule and stress of test day, and you'll be able to focus on recalling the material you've learned.

# Secret Key #4 – Pace Yourself

Once you're fully prepared for the material on the test, your biggest challenge on test day will be managing your time. Just knowing that the clock is ticking can make you panic even if you have plenty of time left. Work on pacing yourself so you can build confidence against the time constraints of the exam. Pacing is a difficult skill to master, especially in a high-pressure environment, so **practice is vital**.

Set time expectations for your pace based on how much time is available. For example, if a section has 60 questions and the time limit is 30 minutes, you know you have to average 30 seconds or less per question in order to answer them all. Although 30 seconds is the hard limit, set 25 seconds per question as your goal, so you reserve extra time to spend on harder questions. When you budget extra time for the harder questions, you no longer have any reason to stress when those questions take longer to answer.

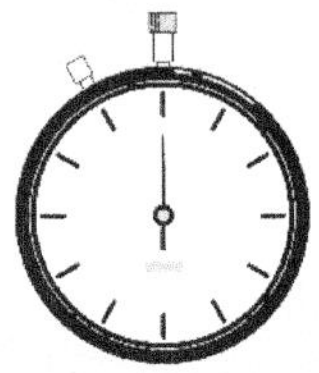

Don't let this time expectation distract you from working through the test at a calm, steady pace, but keep it in mind so you don't spend too much time on any one question. Recognize that taking extra time on one question you don't understand may keep you from answering two that you do understand later in the test. If your time limit for a question is up and you're still not sure of the answer, mark it and move on, and come back to it later if the time and the test format allow. If the testing format doesn't allow you to return to earlier questions, just make an educated guess; then put it out of your mind and move on.

On the easier questions, be careful not to rush. It may seem wise to hurry through them so you have more time for the challenging ones, but it's not worth missing one if you know the concept and just didn't take the time to read the question fully. Work efficiently but make sure you understand the question and have looked at all of the answer choices, since more than one may seem right at first.

Even if you're paying attention to the time, you may find yourself a little behind at some point. You should speed up to get back on track, but do so wisely. Don't panic; just take a few seconds less on each question until you're caught up. Don't guess without thinking, but do look through the answer choices and eliminate any you know are wrong. If you can get down to two choices, it is often worthwhile to guess from those. Once you've chosen an answer, move on and don't dwell on any that you skipped or had to hurry through. If a question was taking too long, chances are it was one of the harder ones, so you weren't as likely to get it right anyway.

On the other hand, if you find yourself getting ahead of schedule, it may be beneficial to slow down a little. The more quickly you work, the more likely you are to make a careless mistake that will affect your score. You've budgeted time for each question, so don't be afraid to spend that time. Practice an efficient but careful pace to get the most out of the time you have.

# Secret Key #5 – Have a Plan for Guessing

When you're taking the test, you may find yourself stuck on a question. Some of the answer choices seem better than others, but you don't see the one answer choice that is obviously correct. What do you do?

The scenario described above is very common, yet most test takers have not effectively prepared for it. Developing and practicing a plan for guessing may be one of the single most effective uses of your time as you get ready for the exam.

In developing your plan for guessing, there are three questions to address:

- When should you start the guessing process?
- How should you narrow down the choices?
- Which answer should you choose?

## When to Start the Guessing Process

Unless your plan for guessing is to select C every time (which, despite its merits, is not what we recommend), you need to leave yourself enough time to apply your answer elimination strategies. Since you have a limited amount of time for each question, that means that if you're going to give yourself the best shot at guessing correctly, you have to decide quickly whether or not you will guess.

Of course, the best-case scenario is that you don't have to guess at all, so first, see if you can answer the question based on your knowledge of the subject and basic reasoning skills. Focus on the key words in the question and try to jog your memory of related topics. Give yourself a chance to bring the knowledge to mind, but once you realize that you don't have (or you can't access) the knowledge you need to answer the question, it's time to start the guessing process.

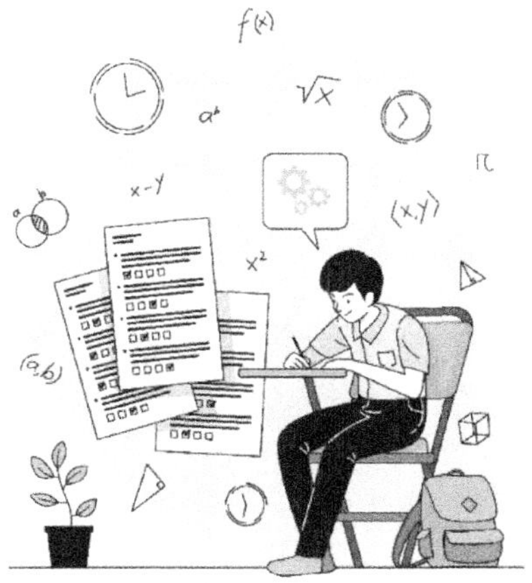

It's almost always better to start the guessing process too early than too late. It only takes a few seconds to remember something and answer the question from knowledge. Carefully eliminating wrong answer choices takes longer. Plus, going through the process of eliminating answer choices can actually help jog your memory.

**Summary**: Start the guessing process as soon as you decide that you can't answer the question based on your knowledge.

## How to Narrow Down the Choices

The next chapter in this book (**Test-Taking Strategies**) includes a wide range of strategies for how to approach questions and how to look for answer choices to eliminate. You will definitely want to read those carefully, practice them, and figure out which ones work best for you. Here though, we're going to address a mindset rather than a particular strategy.

Your odds of guessing an answer correctly depend on how many options you are choosing from.

| **Number of options left** | 5 | 4 | 3 | 2 | 1 |
|---|---|---|---|---|---|
| **Odds of guessing correctly** | 20% | 25% | 33% | 50% | 100% |

You can see from this chart just how valuable it is to be able to eliminate incorrect answers and make an educated guess, but there are two things that many test takers do that cause them to miss out on the benefits of guessing:

- Accidentally eliminating the correct answer
- Selecting an answer based on an impression

We'll look at the first one here, and the second one in the next section.

To avoid accidentally eliminating the correct answer, we recommend a thought exercise called **the $5 challenge**. In this challenge, you only eliminate an answer choice from contention if you are willing to bet $5 on it being wrong. Why $5? Five dollars is a small but not insignificant amount of money. It's an amount you could afford to lose but wouldn't want to throw away. And while losing $5 once might not hurt too much, doing it twenty times will set you back $100. In the same way, each small decision you make—eliminating a choice here, guessing on a question there—won't by itself impact your score very much, but when you put them all together, they can make a big difference. By holding each answer choice elimination decision to a higher standard, you can reduce the risk of accidentally eliminating the correct answer.

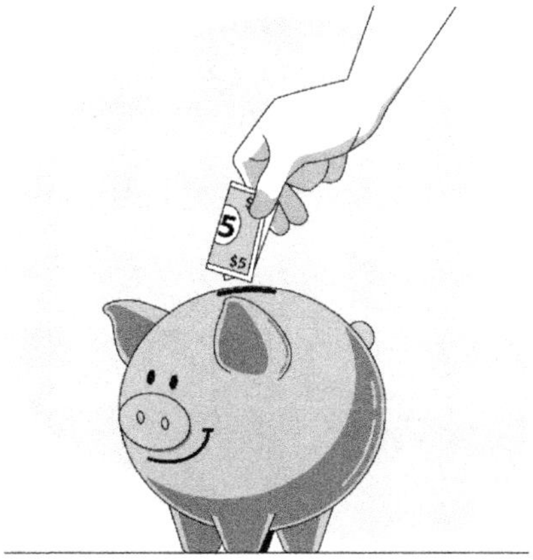

The $5 challenge can also be applied in a positive sense: If you are willing to bet $5 that an answer choice *is* correct, go ahead and mark it as correct.

**Summary**: Only eliminate an answer choice if you are willing to bet $5 that it is wrong.

## Which Answer to Choose

You're taking the test. You've run into a hard question and decided you'll have to guess. You've eliminated all the answer choices you're willing to bet $5 on. Now you have to pick an answer. Why do we even need to talk about this? Why can't you just pick whichever one you feel like when the time comes?

The answer to these questions is that if you don't come into the test with a plan, you'll rely on your impression to select an answer choice, and if you do that, you risk falling into a trap. The test writers know that everyone who takes their test will be guessing on some of the questions, so they intentionally write wrong answer choices to seem plausible. You still have to pick an answer though, and if the wrong answer choices are designed to look right, how can you ever be sure that you're not falling for their trap? The best solution we've found to this dilemma is to take the decision out of your hands entirely. Here is the process we recommend:

**Once you've eliminated any choices that you are confident (willing to bet $5) are wrong, select the first remaining choice as your answer.**

Whether you choose to select the first remaining choice, the second, or the last, the important thing is that you use some preselected standard. Using this approach guarantees that you will not be enticed into selecting an answer choice that looks right, because you are not basing your decision on how the answer choices look.

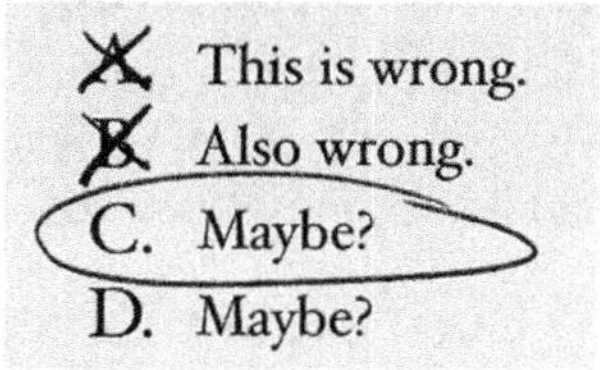


This is not meant to make you question your knowledge. Instead, it is to help you recognize the difference between your knowledge and your impressions. There's a huge difference between thinking an answer is right because of what you know, and thinking an answer is right because it looks or sounds like it should be right.

**Summary**: To ensure that your selection is appropriately random, make a predetermined selection from among all answer choices you have not eliminated.

# Test-Taking Strategies

This section contains a list of test-taking strategies that you may find helpful as you work through the test. By taking what you know and applying logical thought, you can maximize your chances of answering any question correctly!

It is very important to realize that every question is different and every person is different: no single strategy will work on every question, and no single strategy will work for every person. That's why we've included all of them here, so you can try them out and determine which ones work best for different types of questions and which ones work best for you.

## Question Strategies

### ✓ Read Carefully

Read the question and the answer choices carefully. Don't miss the question because you misread the terms. You have plenty of time to read each question thoroughly and make sure you understand what is being asked. Yet a happy medium must be attained, so don't waste too much time. You must read carefully and efficiently.

### ✓ Contextual Clues

Look for contextual clues. If the question includes a word you are not familiar with, look at the immediate context for some indication of what the word might mean. Contextual clues can often give you all the information you need to decipher the meaning of an unfamiliar word. Even if you can't determine the meaning, you may be able to narrow down the possibilities enough to make a solid guess at the answer to the question.

### ✓ Prefixes

If you're having trouble with a word in the question or answer choices, try dissecting it. Take advantage of every clue that the word might include. Prefixes can be a huge help. Usually, they allow you to determine a basic meaning. *Pre-* means before, *post-* means after, *pro-* is positive, *de-* is negative. From prefixes, you can get an idea of the general meaning of the word and try to put it into context.

### ✓ Hedge Words

Watch out for critical hedge words, such as *likely, may, can, often, almost, mostly, usually, generally, rarely,* and *sometimes.* Question writers insert these hedge phrases to cover every possibility. Often an answer choice will be wrong simply because it leaves no room for exception. Be on guard for answer choices that have definitive words such as *exactly* and *always.*

### ✓ Switchback Words

Stay alert for *switchbacks.* These are the words and phrases frequently used to alert you to shifts in thought. The most common switchback words are *but, although,* and *however.* Others include *nevertheless, on the other hand, even though, while, in spite of, despite,* and *regardless of.* Switchback words are important to catch because they can change the direction of the question or an answer choice.

### ✓ Face Value

When in doubt, use common sense. Accept the situation in the problem at face value. Don't read too much into it. These problems will not require you to make wild assumptions. If you have to go beyond creativity and warp time or space in order to have an answer choice fit the question, then you should move on and consider the other answer choices. These are normal problems rooted in reality. The applicable relationship or explanation may not be readily apparent, but it is there for you to figure out. Use your common sense to interpret anything that isn't clear.

# Answer Choice Strategies

## ✓ Answer Selection

The most thorough way to pick an answer choice is to identify and eliminate wrong answers until only one is left, then confirm it is the correct answer. Sometimes an answer choice may immediately seem right, but be careful. The test writers will usually put more than one reasonable answer choice on each question, so take a second to read all of them and make sure that the other choices are not equally obvious. As long as you have time left, it is better to read every answer choice than to pick the first one that looks right without checking the others.

## ✓ Answer Choice Families

An answer choice family consists of two (in rare cases, three) answer choices that are very similar in construction and cannot all be true at the same time. If you see two answer choices that are direct opposites or parallels, one of them is usually the correct answer. For instance, if one answer choice says that quantity *x* increases and another either says that quantity *x* decreases (opposite) or says that quantity *y* increases (parallel), then those answer choices would fall into the same family. An answer choice that doesn't match the construction of the answer choice family is more likely to be incorrect. Most questions will not have answer choice families, but when they do appear, you should be prepared to recognize them.

## ✓ Eliminate Answers

Eliminate answer choices as soon as you realize they are wrong, but make sure you consider all possibilities. If you are eliminating answer choices and realize that the last one you are left with is also wrong, don't panic. Start over and consider each choice again. There may be something you missed the first time that you will realize on the second pass.

## ✓ Avoid Fact Traps

Don't be distracted by an answer choice that is factually true but doesn't answer the question. You are looking for the choice that answers the question. Stay focused on what the question is asking for so you don't accidentally pick an answer that is true but incorrect. Always go back to the question and make sure the answer choice you've selected actually answers the question and is not merely a true statement.

## ✓ Extreme Statements

In general, you should avoid answers that put forth extreme actions as standard practice or proclaim controversial ideas as established fact. An answer choice that states the "process should be used in certain situations, if…" is much more likely to be correct than one that states the "process should be discontinued completely." The first is a calm rational statement and doesn't even make a definitive, uncompromising stance, using a hedge word *if* to provide wiggle room, whereas the second choice is far more extreme.

## ✓ Benchmark

As you read through the answer choices and you come across one that seems to answer the question well, mentally select that answer choice. This is not your final answer, but it's the one that will help you evaluate the other answer choices. The one that you selected is your benchmark or standard for judging each of the other answer choices. Every other answer choice must be compared to your benchmark. That choice is correct until proven otherwise by another answer choice beating it. If you find a better answer, then that one becomes your new benchmark. Once you've decided that no other choice answers the question as well as your benchmark, you have your final answer.

### ✓ Predict the Answer

Before you even start looking at the answer choices, it is often best to try to predict the answer. When you come up with the answer on your own, it is easier to avoid distractions and traps because you will know exactly what to look for. The right answer choice is unlikely to be word-for-word what you came up with, but it should be a close match. Even if you are confident that you have the right answer, you should still take the time to read each option before moving on.

## General Strategies

### ✓ Tough Questions

If you are stumped on a problem or it appears too hard or too difficult, don't waste time. Move on! Remember though, if you can quickly check for obviously incorrect answer choices, your chances of guessing correctly are greatly improved. Before you completely give up, at least try to knock out a couple of possible answers. Eliminate what you can and then guess at the remaining answer choices before moving on.

### ✓ Check Your Work

Since you will probably not know every term listed and the answer to every question, it is important that you get credit for the ones that you do know. Don't miss any questions through careless mistakes. If at all possible, try to take a second to look back over your answer selection and make sure you've selected the correct answer choice and haven't made a costly careless mistake (such as marking an answer choice that you didn't mean to mark). This quick double check should more than pay for itself in caught mistakes for the time it costs.

### ✓ Pace Yourself

It's easy to be overwhelmed when you're looking at a page full of questions; your mind is confused and full of random thoughts, and the clock is ticking down faster than you would like. Calm down and maintain the pace that you have set for yourself. Especially as you get down to the last few minutes of the test, don't let the small numbers on the clock make you panic. As long as you are on track by monitoring your pace, you are guaranteed to have time for each question.

### ✓ Don't Rush

It is very easy to make errors when you are in a hurry. Maintaining a fast pace in answering questions is pointless if it makes you miss questions that you would have gotten right otherwise. Test writers like to include distracting information and wrong answers that seem right. Taking a little extra time to avoid careless mistakes can make all the difference in your test score. Find a pace that allows you to be confident in the answers that you select.

### ✓ Keep Moving

Panicking will not help you pass the test, so do your best to stay calm and keep moving. Taking deep breaths and going through the answer elimination steps you practiced can help to break through a stress barrier and keep your pace.

# Final Notes

The combination of a solid foundation of content knowledge and the confidence that comes from practicing your plan for applying that knowledge is the key to maximizing your performance on test day. As your foundation of content knowledge is built up and strengthened, you'll find that the strategies included in this chapter become more and more effective in helping you quickly sift through the distractions and traps of the test to isolate the correct answer.

Now that you're preparing to move forward into the test content chapters of this book, be sure to keep your goal in mind. As you read, think about how you will be able to apply this information on the test. If you've already seen sample questions for the test and you have an idea of the question format and style, try to come up with questions of your own that you can answer based on what you're reading. This will give you valuable practice applying your knowledge in the same ways you can expect to on test day.

**Good luck and good studying!**

# Five-Week NCLEX RN Study Plan

On the next few pages, we've provided an optional study plan to help you use this study guide to its fullest potential over the course of five weeks. If you have ten weeks available and want to spread it out more, spend two weeks on each section of the plan.

Below is a quick summary of the subjects covered in each week of the plan.

- Week 1: Management of Care & Safety and Infection Control
- Week 2: Health Promotion and Maintenance & Psychosocial Integrity
- Week 3: Basic Care and Comfort & Pharmacological and Parenteral Therapies
- Week 4: Reduction of Risk Potential & Physiological Adaptation
- Week 5: Practice Tests

Please note that not all subjects will take the same amount of time to work through.

Three full-length practice tests are included in this study guide. We recommend saving the third test any additional tests for after you've completed the study plan. Take these practice tests without any reference materials a day or two before the real thing as practice runs to get you in the mode of answering questions at a good pace.

# Week 1: Management of Care & Safety and Infection Prevention and Control

## Instructional Content

First, read carefully through the Management of Care & Safety and Infection Control chapters in this book, checking off your progress as you go:

- ❑ Client Rights, Client Advocacy, and Delegation of Care
- ❑ Case Management
- ❑ Collaborative Care Management
- ❑ Ethical Practice
- ❑ Information Technology
- ❑ Legal Issues and Performance Improvement
- ❑ Referrals
- ❑ Accident, Error, and Injury Prevention
- ❑ Emergency Response
- ❑ Handling Hazardous Materials
- ❑ Infectious Diseases and Infection Control
- ❑ Body Mechanics and Home Safety
- ❑ Incident Reporting
- ❑ Client Safety

As you read, do the following:

- Highlight any sections, terms, or concepts you think are important
- Draw an asterisk (*) next to any areas you are struggling with
- Watch the review videos to gain more understanding of a particular topic
- Take notes in your notebook or in the margins of this book

After you've read through everything, go back and review any sections that you highlighted or that you drew an asterisk next to, referencing your notes along the way.

# Week 2: Health Promotion and Maintenance & Psychosocial Integrity

## Instructional Content

First, read carefully through the Health Promotion and Maintenance & Psychosocial Integrity chapters in this book, checking off your progress as you go:

- ❑ Ante/Intra/Postpartum and Newborn Care
- ❑ Developmental Stages and Transitions
- ❑ Health Promotion and Disease Prevention
- ❑ Nutrition Screening
- ❑ Health Screening
- ❑ High Risk Behaviors
- ❑ Techniques of Physical Assessment
- ❑ Abuse
- ❑ Behavioral Interventions
- ❑ Crisis Intervention
- ❑ Cultural Awareness
- ❑ End-of-Life Care
- ❑ Mental Health Concepts
- ❑ Stress Management
- ❑ Support and Therapeutic Communication

As you read, do the following:

- Highlight any sections, terms, or concepts you think are important
- Draw an asterisk (*) next to any areas you are struggling with
- Watch the review videos to gain more understanding of a particular topic
- Take notes in your notebook or in the margins of this book

After you've read through everything, go back and review any sections that you highlighted or that you drew an asterisk next to, referencing your notes along the way.

# Week 3: Basic Care and Comfort & Pharmacological and Parenteral Therapies

## Instructional Content

First, read carefully through the Basic Care and Comfort & Pharmacological and Parenteral Therapies chapters in this book, checking off your progress as you go:

- ❑ Elimination
- ❑ Mobility/Immobility
- ❑ Non-Pharmacological Comfort Interventions
- ❑ Nutrition, Hydration, Hygiene, and Rest
- ❑ Principles of Pharmacology
- ❑ Pharmacologic Interventions
- ❑ Blood Transfusions
- ❑ Intravenous Infusions
- ❑ Pain Management
- ❑ Intravenous Nutrition

As you read, do the following:

- Highlight any sections, terms, or concepts you think are important
- Draw an asterisk (*) next to any areas you are struggling with
- Watch the review videos to gain more understanding of a particular topic
- Take notes in your notebook or in the margins of this book

After you've read through everything, go back and review any sections that you highlighted or that you drew an asterisk next to, referencing your notes along the way.

# Week 4: Reduction of Risk Potential & Physiological Adaptation

## Instructional Content

First, read carefully through the Reduction of Risk Potential & Physiological Adaptation chapters in this book, checking off your progress as you go:

- ❑ Abnormal Vital Signs
- ❑ Diagnostic Procedures
- ❑ Laboratory Values and Samples
- ❑ Potential Risks and Complications
- ❑ System-Specific Assessments
- ❑ Therapeutic Procedures
- ❑ Alterations in Body Systems
- ❑ Fluid and Electrolyte Imbalances
- ❑ Hemodynamics
- ❑ Illness Management
- ❑ Medical Emergencies
- ❑ Pathophysiology

As you read, do the following:

- Highlight any sections, terms, or concepts you think are important
- Draw an asterisk (*) next to any areas you are struggling with
- Watch the review videos to gain more understanding of a particular topic
- Take notes in your notebook or in the margins of this book

After you've read through everything, go back and review any sections that you highlighted or that you drew an asterisk next to, referencing your notes along the way.

# Week 5: Practice Tests

Your success on test day depends not only on how many hours you put into preparing, but also on whether you prepared the right way. It's good to check along the way to see if your studying is paying off. One of the most effective ways to do this is by taking practice tests to evaluate your progress. Practice tests are useful because they show exactly where you need to improve. Every time you take a practice test, pay special attention to these three groups of questions:

- The questions you got wrong
- The questions you had to guess on, even if you guessed right
- The questions you found difficult or slow to work through

This will show you exactly what your weak areas are, and where you need to devote more study time. Ask yourself why each of these questions gave you trouble. Was it because you didn't understand the material? Was it because you didn't remember the vocabulary? Do you need more repetitions on this type of question to build speed and confidence? Dig into those questions and figure out how you can strengthen your weak areas as you go back to review the material.

## Practice Test #1

Now that you've read over the instructional content, it's time to take a practice test. Complete Practice Test #1. Take this test with **no time constraints**, and feel free to reference the applicable sections of this guide as you go. Once you've finished, check your answers against the provided answer key. For any questions you answered incorrectly, review the answer rationale, and then **go back and review** the applicable sections of the book. The goal in this stage is to understand why you answered the question incorrectly, and make sure that the next time you see a similar question, you will get it right.

## Practice Test #2

Next, complete Practice Test #2. This time, give yourself **5 hours** to complete all of the questions. Note that this is the total time allotted for the exam and includes instructional time, optional breaks and a possible total of 150 questions. You should again feel free to reference the guide and your notes, but be mindful of the clock. If you run out of time before you finish all of the questions, mark where you were when time expired, but go ahead and finish taking the practice test. Once you've finished, check your answers against the provided answer key, and as before, review the answer rationale for any that you answered incorrectly and then go back and review the associated instructional content. Your goal is still to increase understanding of the content but also to get used to the time constraints you will face on the test.

As you go along, keep in mind that the practice test is just that: practice. Memorizing these questions and answers will not be very helpful on the actual test because it is unlikely to have any of the same exact questions. If you only know the right answers to the sample questions, you won't be prepared for the real thing. **Study the concepts** until you understand them fully, and then you'll be able to answer any question that shows up on the test.

# Management of Care

## Patient Rights

### Patient Rights and Responsibilities

Empowering patients and families to act as their own advocates requires that they have a clear understanding of their **rights and responsibilities.** These should be given (in print form) and/or presented (audio/video) to patients and families on admission or as soon as possible:

- **Rights** include competent, non-discriminatory medical care that respects privacy and allows participation in decisions about care and the right to refuse care. They should have clear understandable explanations of treatments, options, and conditions, including outcomes. They should be apprised of transfers, changes in care plan, and advance directives. They should have access to medical records and billing information.
- **Responsibilities** include providing honest and thorough information about health issues and medical history. They should ask for clarification if they don't understand information that is provided to them, and they should follow the plan of care that is outlined or explain why that is not possible. They should treat staff and other patients with respect.

**Review Video: Patient Advocacy**
Visit mometrix.com/academy and enter code: 202160

### Informed Consent

The patient or their legal guardian must provide informed consent for all treatment the patient receives. This includes a thorough explanation of all procedures and treatment and associated risks. Patients/guardians should be apprised of all options and allowed to have input on the decision-making process. They should be apprised of all reasonable risks and any complications that might be life threatening or increase morbidity. The American Medical Association has established **guidelines for obtaining informed consent:**

- Explanation of the diagnosis
- Nature and reason for the treatment or procedure
- Risks and benefits of the treatment or procedure
- Alternative options (regardless of cost or insurance coverage)
- Risks and benefits of alternative options, including no treatment

Obtaining informed consent is a requirement in all states; however, a patient may waive their right to informed consent. If this is the case, the nurse should document the patient's waiving of this right and proceed with the procedure. Informed consent is not necessary for procedures performed to save life or limb in which the patient or guardian is unable to consent.

### Confidentiality

Confidentiality is the obligation that is present in a professional-patient relationship. Nurses are under an obligation to protect the information they possess concerning the patient and family. Care should be taken to safeguard that information and provide the privacy that the family deserves. This is accomplished through the use of required passwords when family calls for information about the patient and through the limitation of who is allowed to visit. There may be times when confidentiality must be broken to save the life of a patient, but those circumstances are rare. The nurse must make all efforts to safeguard patient records and identification. Computerized record keeping should be done in such a way that the screen is not visible to others, and paper records must be secured.

# Ethics

## Ethical Principles

**Autonomy** is the ethical principle that the individual has the right to make decisions about his or her own care. In the case of children or patients with dementia who cannot make autonomous decisions, parents or family members may serve as the legal decision maker. The nurse must keep the patient and/or family fully informed so that they can exercise their autonomy in informed decision-making.

**Justice** is the ethical principle that relates to the distribution of the limited resources of healthcare benefits to the members of society. These resources must be distributed fairly. This issue may arise if there is only one bed left and two sick patients. Justice comes into play in deciding which patient should stay and which should be transported or otherwise cared for. The decision should be made according to what is best or most just for the patients and not colored by personal bias.

**Beneficence** is an ethical principle that involves performing actions that are for the purpose of benefitting another person. In the care of a patient, any procedure or treatment should be done with the ultimate goal of benefitting the patient, and any actions that are not beneficial should be reconsidered. As conditions change, procedures need to be continually reevaluated to determine if they are still of benefit.

**Nonmaleficence** is an ethical principle that means healthcare workers should provide care in a manner that does not cause direct intentional harm to the patient:

- The actual act must be good or morally neutral.
- The intent must be only for a good effect.
- A bad effect cannot serve as the means to get to a good effect.
- A good effect must have more benefit than a bad effect has harm.

## Nursing Code of Ethics

There is more interest in the **ethics** involved in healthcare due to technological advances that have made the prolongation of life, organ transplants, prenatal manipulation, and saving of premature infants possible, sometimes with poor outcomes. Couple these with healthcare's limited resources, and **ethical dilemmas** abound. Ethics is the study of **morality** as the value that controls actions. The American Nurses Association Code of Ethics contains nine statements defining **principles** the nurse can use when faced with moral and ethical problems. Nurses must be knowledgeable about the many ethical issues in healthcare and about the field of ethics in general. The nurse must help a patient to reveal their values and morals to the health care team so that the patient, family, and team can resolve moral issues pertaining to the patient's care. As part of the healthcare team, the nurse has a right to express personal values and moral concerns about medical issues.

## Bioethics

Bioethics is a branch of ethics that involves making sure that the medical treatment given is the most morally correct choice given the different options that might be available and the differences inherent in the varied levels of treatment. In the health care unit, if the patients, family members, and the staff are in agreement when it comes to values and decision-making, then no ethical dilemma exists; however, when there is a difference in value beliefs between the patients/family members and the staff, there is a bioethical dilemma that must be resolved. Sometimes, discussion and explanation can resolve differences, but at times the institution's ethics committee must be brought in to resolve the conflict. The primary goal of bioethics is to determine the most morally correct action using the set of circumstances given.

## Ethical Decision-Making Model

There are many ethical decision-making models. Some general guidelines to apply in using ethical decision-making models could be the following:

- Gather information about the identified problem
- State reasonable alternatives and solutions to the problem
- Utilize ethical resources (for example, clergy or ethics committees) to help determine the ethically important elements of each solution or alternative
- Suggest and attempt possible solutions
- Choose a solution to the problem

It is important to always consider the **ethical principles** of autonomy, beneficence, nonmaleficence, justice, and fidelity when attempting to facilitate ethical decision-making with family members, caregivers, and the healthcare team.

## Professional Boundaries

### *Gifts*

Over time, patients may develop a bond with nurses they trust and may feel grateful to the nurse for the care provided and want to express thanks, but the nurse must make sure to maintain professional boundaries. Patients often offer **gifts** to nurses to show their appreciation, but some adults, especially those who are weak and ill or have cognitive impairment, may be taken advantage of easily. Patients may offer valuables and may sometimes be easily manipulated into giving large sums of money. Small tokens of appreciation that can be shared with other staff, such as a box of chocolates, are usually acceptable (depending upon the policy of the institution), but almost any other gifts (jewelry, money, clothes) should be declined: "I'm sorry, that's so kind of you, but nurses are not allowed to accept gifts from patients." Declining may relieve the patient of the feeling of obligation.

### *Sexual Relations*

When the boundary between the role of the professional nurse and the vulnerability of the patient is breached, a boundary violation occurs. Because the nurse is in the position of authority, the responsibility to maintain the boundary rests with the nurse; however, the line separating them is a continuum and sometimes not easily defined. It is inappropriate for nurses to engage in **sexual relations** with patients, and if the sexual behavior is coerced or the patient is cognitively impaired, it is **illegal**. However, more common violations with adults, particularly elderly patients, include exposing a patient unnecessarily, using sexually demeaning gestures or language (including off-color jokes), harassment, or inappropriate touching. Touching should be used with care, such as touching a hand or shoulder. Hugging may be misconstrued.

### *Attention*

Nursing is a giving profession, but the nurse must temper giving with recognition of professional boundaries. Patients have many needs. As acts of kindness, nurses (especially those involved in home care) often give certain patients extra attention and may offer to do **favors**, such as cooking or shopping. They may become overly invested in the patients' lives. While this may benefit a patient in the short term, it can establish a relationship of increasing **dependency** and **obligation** that does not resolve the long-term needs of the patient. Making referrals to the appropriate agencies or collaborating with family to find ways to provide services is more effective. Becoming overly invested may be evident by the nurse showing favoritism or spending too much time with the patient while neglecting other duties. On the other end of the spectrum are nurses who are disinterested and fail to provide adequate attention to the patient's detriment. Lack of adequate attention may lead to outright neglect.

### Coercion

Power issues are inherent in matters associated with professional boundaries. Physical abuse is both unprofessional and illegal, but behavior can easily border on abusive without the patient being physically injured. Nurses can easily **intimidate** older adults and sick patients into having procedures or treatments they do not want. Regardless of age, patients have the right to choose and the right to refuse treatment. Difficulties arise with cognitive impairment, and in that case, another responsible adult (often the patient's child or spouse) is designated to make decisions, but every effort should be made to gain patient cooperation. Forcing the patient to do something against his or her will borders on abuse and can sometimes degenerate into actual abuse if physical coercion is involved.

### Personal Information

When pre-existing personal or business relationships exist, other nurses should be assigned care of the patient whenever possible, but this may be difficult in small communities. However, the nurse should strive to maintain a professional role separate from the personal role and respect professional boundaries. The nurse must respect and maintain the confidentiality of the patient and family members, but the nurse must also be very careful about **disclosing personal information** about him or herself because this establishes a social relationship that interferes with the professional role of the nurse and the boundary between the patient and the nurse. The nurse and patient should never share secrets. When the nurse divulges personal information, he or she may become vulnerable to the patient, a reversal of roles.

## Skills Needed for Collaboration

Nurses must learn the set of skills needed for collaboration in order to move nursing forward. Nurses must take an active role in gathering data for evidence-based practice to support nursing's role in health care, and they must share this information with other nurses and health professionals in order to plan staffing levels and to provide optimal care to patients. Increased and adequate staffing has consistently been shown to reduce adverse outcomes, but there is a well-documented shortage of nurses in the United States, and more than half currently work outside the hospital setting. Increased patient loads not only increase adverse outcomes but also increase job dissatisfaction and burnout. In order to manage the challenges facing nursing, nurses must develop the following skills needed for collaboration:

- Be willing to compromise
- Communicate clearly
- Identify specific challenges and problems
- Focus on the task
- Work with teams

## Communication Skills

Collaboration requires a number of communication skills that differ from those involved in communication between nurse and patient. These skills include:

- **Using an assertive approach**: It's important for the nurse to honestly express opinions and to state them clearly and with confidence, but the nurse must do so in a calm, non-threatening manner.
- **Making casual conversation**: It's easier to communicate with people with whom one has a personal connection. Asking open-ended questions, asking about others' work, or commenting on someone's contributions helps to establish a relationship. The time before meetings, during breaks, and after meetings presents an opportunity for this type of conversation.
- **Being competent in public speaking**: Collaboration requires that a nurse be comfortable speaking and presenting ideas to groups of people. Speaking and presenting ideas competently also helps the nurse to gain credibility. Public speaking is a skill that must be practiced.
- **Communicating in writing**: The written word remains a critical component of communication, and the nurse should be able to communicate clearly and grammatically.

### *Communication and Handoffs*

The nurse is usually the primary staff member responsible for **external and internal handoff transitions of care**, and should ensure that communication is thorough and covers all essential information. The best method is to use a standardized format:

- **DRAW**: Diagnosis, recent changes, anticipated changes, and what to watch for.
- **I PASS the BATON**: Introduction, patient, assessment, situation, safety concerns, background, actions, timing, ownership, and next.
- **ANTICipate**: Administrative data, new clinical information, tasks, illness severity, contingency plans.
- **5 Rs**: Record, review, round together, relay to team, and receive feedback.

A reporting **form** or checklist may be utilized to ensure that no aspect is overlooked.

For external transitions, the nurse must ensure that the type of transport team and monitoring is appropriate for patient needs, and provide insight when determining the most appropriate mode of transportation: ground transfer for short distance, helicopter for medium to long distance, and fixed-wing aircraft for long distances.

### *SBAR Technique*

The SBAR technique is used to hand-off a patient from one caregiver to another to provide a systematic method so that important information is conveyed:

- **(S) Situation**: Overview of current situation and important issues
- **(B) Background**: Important history and issues leading to current situation
- **(A) Assessment**: Summary of important facts and condition
- **(R) Recommendation**: Actions needed

## Care Coordination and Collaboration

### *Shift Reporting*

Shift reporting should include bedside handoff when possible with oncoming staff members. The nurse handing off the patient should follow a specific format for handoff (such as I PASS the BATON) so that handoff is done in the same manner every time, as this reduces the chance of omitting important information. The shift report should include introduction of the oncoming staff to the patient, the triage category or acuity level of the patient, diagnosis (potential or confirmed), current status, laboratory and imaging (completed or pending) and results if available, and medications or treatments administered and pending. Any monitoring equipment (pulse oximetry, telemetry) should be examined. Any invasive treatments (Foley catheter, IV) should be discussed and equipment examined. The nurse should report any plans for admission, transfer, or discharge. It is essential that all staff be trained in shift reporting and the importance of consistency.

### Collaboration Between Nurse and Patient/Family

One of the most important forms of collaboration is that between the nurse and the patient/family, but this type of collaboration is often overlooked. Nurses and others in the healthcare team must always remember that the point of collaboration is to improve patient care, and this means that the patient and patient's family must remain central to all planning. For example, including family in planning for a patient takes time initially, but sitting down and asking the patient and family, "What do you want?" and using the Synergy model to evaluate patient's (and family's) characteristics can provide valuable information that saves time in the long run and facilitates planning and expenditure of resources. Families, and even young children, often want to participate in care and planning and feel validated and more positive toward the medical system when they are included.

## Collaboration with External Agencies

The nurse must initiate and facilitate collaboration with external agencies because many have direct impacts on patient care and needs:

- **Industry** can include other facilities sharing interests in patient care or pharmaceutical companies. It's important for nursing to have a dialog with drug companies about their products and how they are used in specific populations because many medications are prescribed to women, children, or the aged without validating studies for dose or efficacy.
- **Payers** have a vested interest in containing health care costs, so providing information and representing the interests of the patient is important.
- **Community groups** may provide resources for patients and families, both in terms of information and financial or other assistance.
- **Political agencies** are increasingly important as new laws are considered about nurse-patient ratios and infection control in many states.
- **Public health agencies** are partners in health care with other facilities and must be included, especially in issues related to communicable disease.

## Interdisciplinary Teams

There are a number of skills that are needed to lead and facilitate coordination of **intra- and inter-disciplinary teams**:

- Communicating openly is essential. All members must be encouraged to participate as valued members of a cooperative team.
- Avoiding interrupting or interpreting the point another is trying to make allows free flow of ideas.
- Avoiding jumping to conclusions, which can effectively shut off communication.
- Active listening requires paying attention and asking questions for clarification rather than to challenge other's ideas.
- Respecting others' opinions and ideas, even when opposed to one's own, is absolutely essential.
- Reacting and responding to facts rather than feelings allows one to avoid angry confrontations and diffuse anger.
- Clarifying information or opinions stated can help avoid misunderstandings.
- Keeping unsolicited advice out of the conversation shows respect for others and allows them to solicit advice without feeling pressured.

## Leadership Styles

Leadership styles often influence the perception of leadership values and commitment to collaboration. There are a number of different leadership styles:

- **Charismatic**: Relies on personal charisma to influence people, and may be very persuasive, but this type leader may engage followers and relate to one group rather than the organization at large, limiting effectiveness.
- **Bureaucratic**: Follows organization rules exactly and expects everyone else to do so. This is most effective in handling cash flow or managing work in dangerous work environments. This type of leadership may engender respect but may not be conducive to change.
- **Autocratic**: Makes decisions independently and strictly enforces rules. Team members often feel left out of process and may not be supportive of the decisions that are made. This type of leadership is most effective in crisis situations, but may have difficulty gaining the commitment of staff.
- **Consultative**: Presents a decision and welcomes input and questions, although decisions rarely change. This type of leadership is most effective when gaining the support of staff is critical to the success of proposed changes.

- **Participatory**: Presents a potential decision and then makes final decision based on input from staff or teams. This type of leadership is time-consuming and may result in compromises that are not entirely satisfactory to management or staff, but this process is motivating to staff who feel their expertise is valued.
- **Democratic**: Presents a problem and asks staff or teams to arrive at a solution, although the leader usually makes the final decision. This type of leadership may delay decision-making, but staff and teams are often more committed to the solutions because of their input.
- **Laissez-faire ("free reign")**: Exerts little direct control but allows employees/teams to make decisions with little interference. This may be effective leadership if teams are highly skilled and motivated, but in many cases, this type of leadership is the product of poor management skills and little is accomplished because of this lack of leadership.

## Facilitating Change

Performance improvement processes cannot occur without organizational change, and resistance to change is common for many people, so coordinating collaborative processes requires anticipating resistance and taking steps to achieve cooperation. Resistance often relates to concerns about job loss, increased responsibilities, and general denial or lack of understanding and frustration. Leaders can prepare others involved in the process of change by taking these steps:

- Be honest, informative, and tactful, giving people thorough information about anticipated changes and how the changes will affect them, including positives.
- Be patient in allowing people the time they need to contemplate changes and express anger or disagreement.
- Be empathetic in listening carefully to the concerns of others.
- Encourage participation, allowing staff to propose methods of implementing change, so they feel some sense of ownership.
- Establish a climate in which all staff members are encouraged to identify the need for change on an ongoing basis.
- Present further ideas for change to management.

## Conflict Resolution

Conflict is an almost inevitable product of teamwork, and the leader must assume responsibility for conflict resolution. While conflicts can be disruptive, they can produce positive outcomes by opening dialogue and forcing team members to listen to different perspectives. The team should make a plan for dealing with conflict. The best time for conflict resolution is when differences emerge but before open conflict and hardening of positions occur. The leader must pay close attention to the people and problems involved, listen carefully, and reassure those involved that their points of view are understood. Steps to conflict resolution include:

- Allow both sides to present their side of conflict without bias, maintaining a focus on opinions rather than individuals.
- Encourage cooperation through negotiation and compromise.
- Maintain the focus, providing guidance to keep the discussions on track and avoid arguments.
- Evaluate the need for re-negotiation, formal resolution process, or third-party involvement.
- Utilize humor and empathy to diffuse escalating tensions.
- Summarize the issues, outlining key arguments.
- Avoid forcing resolution if possible.

## Healthcare Team Members

### *Role of Nursing Care to Support Therapies Provided by Other Disciplines*

Nursing care often involves providing support to therapies provided by other disciplines. The nurse works as a team member with physicians, occupational and physical therapists, respiratory therapists, social workers, and discharge planners. Floor nurses may work with nurses in other specializations, such as critical care or psychiatric nurses. As a primary coordinator of the care plan, the nurse ensures that the necessary therapies from all disciplines are administered as ordered, and maintains clear communication with all members of the patient's healthcare team. Nurses also support nutritional services by assuring that the patient receives the proper diet for the particular medical or surgical condition, and they communicate with housekeeping to ensure that the patient's environment is appropriate.

### *Occupational Therapy*

The function of occupational therapy is to enable the patient to attain functional outcomes that enhance health, prevent further injury or impairment, and sustain or improve the highest attainable level of independence. The occupational therapist's role is to **facilitate interventions** that aid the patient in improving basic motor and cognitive skills and to **introduce strategies** for meeting challenges at work or at home. In cases of permanent disability or loss of mobility, the occupational therapist works with the patient on adaptive measures to improve function and the ability to perform daily living tasks. Occupational therapists may use physical exercises to improve muscle strength, balance, and dexterity, or cognitive exercises and strategies to improve problem-solving and memory. They help patients with disabilities or cognitive impairments adapt to particular environments, such as a private home or workplace, and teach patients how to use adaptive equipment like wheelchairs, orthotic devices, or computer programs.

### *Respiratory Therapy*

The function of respiratory therapy is to provide care to patients with respiratory and cardiopulmonary disorders. The role of the respiratory therapist is to diagnose, evaluate, and treat patients with these disorders, and manage their therapeutic care. The respiratory therapist administers aerosolized medications and provides bronchopulmonary hygiene and postural drainage therapy. The role of the respiratory therapist is also to provide support for mechanically-ventilated patients and to maintain an artificial or natural airway. Many respiratory therapists perform pulmonary function testing as well as hemodynamic monitoring. Some respiratory therapists obtain arterial blood gases and other blood samples, as well as assemble and maintain respiratory equipment. They also teach patients how to self-administer aerosol medications and use life-support respiratory equipment in the home environment.

### *Case Manager*

The case manager is an RN that works for a healthcare insurer as a **manager of the provision of healthcare services** to the people the company insures. One manager or a group of managers are given a caseload of patients with the same range of diagnoses. The case manager is an expert in the range of diagnoses and coordinates services to fulfill the healthcare needs of that particular group of patients. The patient is followed throughout the continuum of care to ensure quality and cost-effectiveness of treatments and care. Complications are prevented and the incidence of repeat hospitalization is decreased. The case manager utilizes evidence-based pathways, clinical pathways, or other plans to track the care and progress of the patient. They are the ones who precertify care, negotiate for payment, and authorize treatment. Patient progress reports from the hospital utilization review or other liaison to the case manager are required at periodic intervals during the hospital stay.

## Identifying the Need for Patient Referral

Issues to consider when making patient referrals include:

- **Necessity**: The referral may be needed if the patient's needs are outside of the provider's scope or practice or field of expertise and if the provider cannot provide adequate assessment and treatment for the patient's condition.
- **Insurance requirements**: The provider should determine whether the patient's carrier requires preauthorization or other steps to make sure the patient's referral is covered.
- **Selection of specialist/therapist**: The specialist, in many cases, must be selected from a group of physicians who are participating in an insurance plan if the service is to be covered completely or at all by the insurance company. When possible, the patient should be given choice of referrals.
- **Submission**: The referral should be sent along with appropriate records and releases. The provider may need to make personal contact if specialists are selective, have waiting lists, and may not approve a referral.

## Five Rights of Delegation

Prior to delegating tasks, the nurse should assess the needs of the patients and determine the task that needs to be completed, assure that he/she can remain accountable and can supervise the task appropriately, and evaluate effective completion. The **5 rights of delegation** include:

- **Right task**: The nurse should determine an appropriate task to delegate for a specific patient. This would not include tasks that require assessment or planning.
- **Right circumstance**: The nurse has considered the setting, resources, time factors, safety factors, and all other relevant information to determine the appropriateness of delegation. A task that is usually in one's scope (such as feeding a patient) may require assessment that makes it inappropriate to delegate (feeding a new stroke patient).
- **Right person**: The nurse is in the right position to choose the right person (by virtue of education/skills) to perform a task for the right patient.
- **Right direction**: The nurse provides a clear description of the task, the purpose, any limits, and expected outcomes.
- **Right supervision**: The nurse is able to supervise, intervene as needed, and evaluate performance of the task.

## Delegation of Tasks in Teams

On major responsibility of leadership and management in performance improvement teams is using delegation effectively. The purpose of having a team is so that the work is shared, and leaders can cripple themselves by taking on too much of the workload. Additionally, failure to delegate shows an inherent distrust in team members. Delegation includes:

- Assessing the skills and available time of the team members, determining if a task is suitable for an individual
- Assigning tasks, with clear instructions that include explanation of objectives and expectations, including a timeline
- Ensuring that the tasks are completed properly and on time by monitoring progress but not micromanaging
- Reviewing the final results and recording outcomes

Because the leader is ultimately responsible for the delegated work, mentoring, monitoring, and providing feedback and intervention as necessary during this process is a necessary component of leadership. Even when delegated tasks are not completed successfully, they represent an opportunity for learning.

# Models of Care and Health Care Delivery Systems

## Primary Nursing Model

The primary nursing model of care is an individualized and comprehensive model in which the same nurse gives care during the entire period of care. This method stresses care continuity and allows the nurse to provide direct patient care. The primary nurse has total 24-hour care responsibility for the patient. Such nursing care is oriented toward the goal of meeting the individualized needs of the patient. This model of primary nursing also utilizes the primary nurse to communicate with other members of the healthcare team regarding the patient's needs and total health care. Many institutions have rejected this care model as being cost prohibitive.

## Case Management Model

The case management model of care originated in the 1990s. At that time, the model of nursing care was changed from a focus on the quality of care to a focus on the quality of care plus the cost of care. This model of care was used extensively in social work and in outpatient psychiatry. The core of the case management model of care is the case management team. The case management team is an interdisciplinary group that convenes on a regular schedule to discuss and monitor a patient's health care and progress. Many consider this model to be cost effective in the current healthcare system.

## Public Health Nursing Model

The public health nursing model of care is based upon the idea that public health care is population based. This model of care primarily focuses on an entire population that has similar health issues. The public health model of care also focuses on the broad scope of the determinants of health. Public health care targets all levels of prevention, with its primary focus being that of primary prevention. Secondary prevention is an additional focus in the public healthcare model, and it tries to detect and treat healthcare problems in earlier stages. This model also focuses on tertiary prevention to hopefully prevent existing healthcare issues from worsening.

## Family-Centered Model

The family-centered model of care gained prominence in the healthcare field at the end of the twentieth century. The family-centered model recognized that the family is usually the center of a patient's life and that the family often has the most insight about a patient's abilities and needs. This model enables the family to collaborate with the healthcare providers in helping the patient make informed decisions about healthcare services and supports. Strengths and weaknesses of all the family members are often also considered in this model of care. This model of care has resulted in increased patient satisfaction.

## Integrative Model

The integrative model of care is sometimes referred to as the **interdisciplinary model of care**. This model of care involves cooperation and communication between a team of healthcare professionals. Information sharing among such professionals allows for the development of a comprehensive treatment plan that encompasses the medical, psychological, and social needs of a patient. The integrative health team may include physicians, nurses, social workers, psychologists, and occupational/physical therapists. Such a coordinated model of care can improve quality of life, decrease healthcare costs, and provide a positive benefit to patients over their lifespan. This model of care may also include a focus on the holistic or "whole-person" aspects of a patient's care.

## Medical Home Model

The medical home model is a healthcare approach to providing care (primary and comprehensive) to patients. This healthcare model serves to coordinate and improve relationships between patients, their families, and their personal physicians. In March 2007, the American Academy of Family Physicians, American Academy of Pediatrics, American College of Physicians, and American Osteopathic Association developed **joint principles** for the medical home model. The characteristics of these principles are a personal physician, physician-directed medical practice, focus on the whole person, coordinated care, focus on quality and safety of medical care, enhanced patient access, and payment.

## Chronic Care Model

According to the CDC about 133 million Americans are impacted by chronic disease, and approximately 40 million are limited in their usual activities due to chronic disease. The chronic care model was developed to manage patients with chronic medical conditions in a proactive manner as opposed to the traditional reactive manner. This model integrates the basic components for improving medical care in health systems at numerous levels. These levels of health systems are the **community**, the **organization**, the **provider practice**, and the **patient**. There are three basic themes in the chronic care model. The model is **evidence-based**, **population-based**, and **patient-centered**. The theme of evidence-based stresses the importance of evidence and excellence as opposed to autonomy.

## Health Care Delivery Systems

In the United States, healthcare delivery systems are traditionally fragmented, unique, and quite complex in nature. In contrast to the United States, most other countries in developed nations have national health insurance systems, which are commonly referred to as **universal access systems**. Such universal access systems are managed by the government and are funded by taxes. Healthcare delivery systems in the United States consist of subcategories such as managed care, military, vulnerable populations, and integrated service delivery. **Managed care healthcare delivery systems** are the predominant systems for the delivery of health care in the United States.

### *Managed Care Healthcare Delivery System*

The managed care healthcare delivery system promotes efficiency by integrating all the basic functions of healthcare delivery and using management strategies to control healthcare service usage. Managed healthcare delivery systems also determine the **prices** of services and provider reimbursement. The government and employers primarily provide the financing for managed care systems. Managed care delivery systems act like insurance companies in that they use a contract health plan that is an agreement between the managed care system and the subscriber. Subscribers under a managed care delivery system are usually required to use selected healthcare providers.

### *Levels of Health Care*

- **Acute care** is short-term medical treatment, usually in a hospital, for episodic illness or injury.
- **Long-term care** applies to major trauma patients or those with chronic and multiple medical, mental, and social problems who cannot take care of themselves.
- **Custodial care** is mainly for the purpose of assisting clients with their home personal care and does not necessarily require the provider to have specialized skills or training.
- **Intermediate care** applies to patients requiring more than custodial care and might require nursing supervision. Unless true skilled care is required, insurance companies group intermediate and custodial care under the same benefit guidelines.
- **Sub-acute care** is used for patients who are medically stable but still require active care from trained medical professionals. Treatments in this level include frequent or complex wound care, rehabilitation, complex intravenous therapy, and combination therapies. Patients are usually in an extended care facility (ECF), such as a nursing home or a **skilled nursing facility**.

### *Transitional Hospitals*

Transitional hospitals are acute care facilities for patients that are medically stable and whose rehabilitation plan is too complex for an **extended care facility (ECF)**. Transitional hospitals that specialize in medically complex care do so at a lower cost than a traditional hospital because of their specialization. Some transitional hospitals supply only basic patient care, also at a lower cost than a traditional hospital. Examples of transitional hospitals are: burn or extensive wound care, hemodialysis, hospice, infectious disease management, intravenous (IV) medication therapies, neurobehavioral rehabilitation, pain control therapies, rehabilitation, total parenteral nutrition, and ventilator care/weaning from ventilators.

### *TELEHEALTH*

Telehealth refers to the delivery of healthcare services to patients who are not physically present with the healthcare professional, usually due to remote location, disability, or pandemic (such as the recent outbreak of COVID-19). Telehealth can be delivered over a telephone, via email, or by video conference. The primary benefits of telehealth are that it allows for the extension of precious healthcare resources, lowers the overall cost of healthcare, and allows patients to receive healthcare who would not normally have access to it.

There are a number of **ways in which telehealth is useful** to healthcare professionals:

- Consultation with colleagues
- Patient interviews
- Monitor a patient's biometric values and assess their condition
- Evaluate diagnostic images which allows physicians to remotely view and evaluate these images even if they are located overseas (e.g., India)
- Evaluation of microscope slides and laboratory reports

### *COMMUNITY-BASED NURSING*

Community-based nurses strive to promote health, screen for and prevent disease, contain infectious diseases, prevent trauma, manage chronic diseases, rehabilitate, and help maintain function. These nurses work in schools, workplaces, government agencies, county programs, public health agencies, ambulatory care clinics, mental and student health centers, physician offices, home health/hospice agencies, and religious parishes. They give direct care, act as managers and supervisors, do screening exams, and offer health programs. They teach people how to care for themselves and how to prevent injury and disease. They provide referrals to other community resources, working with those resources to provide a smooth transition that results in continuous care. Nurses work with others to write grants to obtain services for specific populations. **Community resources** used to meet healthcare needs include church programs such as food pantries, transportation programs, or visiting programs. Federal programs, mental health, domestic abuse services, senior citizen groups and services, and programs in workplaces and schools are other resources.

# Nursing Process

## PURPOSE OF NURSING ASSESSMENT

**Nursing assessment** evaluates patient data to help in diagnosis and treatment. The nurse assesses baseline health and medical history to be sure the patient will be safe. The nurse also determines what limitations the patient may have in terms of understanding or cooperation. Nursing assessment is an ongoing process, which includes baseline information, information on the patient's response and recovery to the intervention, and continued efforts to maintain the patient's health. The nurse can collaborate with other team members to help in this assessment.

## PURPOSE OF NURSING DIAGNOSIS AND PLANNING

**Nursing diagnosis** is directed at patient comfort and outcome. With a diagnosis, nurses establish nursing interventions that are needed for the patient to be safe and comfortable. The nurse uses the diagnosis to direct therapies and to anticipate potentially needed interventions.

**Planning** allows the nurse to outline the methods needed to achieve patient goals. This accounts for alternative therapies that may be needed, setting priorities, satisfactory outcomes to be achieved, and expectations for discharge. The nurse needs to document the plan. The plan outlines nursing responsibilities, possible interventions, and expected outcomes.

### Implementation of Nursing Plan

**Implementing** the nursing plan requires a measure of fluidity. The original plan is based on initial data. As new data is accumulated, however, the original plan may be modified. There is a need to incorporate individual needs of the patient as the plan proceeds. Different interventions may be called for depending on individual responses or limitations. The nurse needs to continually monitor the patient's response and status to be able to offer appropriate nursing interventions. Documentation is essential at every step of the way. The information can be useful in further treatment of the individual. It can also be used to assess the process so that improvements or adjustments can be made. The documentation may also be used for research purposes to further the knowledge of nursing practice. The record may become necessary for legal purposes as well.

### Evaluation Process

In order to provide the best care for the patient, the nurse must **evaluate** the process in effect. This entails reviewing procedures and interventions in relation to standards of care, quality of care, and patient outcomes. Critical evaluation of the nursing process can lead to changes that may improve the quality of care for patients and/or identify personnel issues that need to be addressed. Modifying care plans is important to maintaining effective patient care. Deficiencies may be noted and can, therefore, be addressed. This underscores the importance of adequate documentation. In order to evaluate the process, the nurse must have access to the documentation to assess the present process. This evaluation may lead to changes that improve the quality of care in the nursing unit.

## Nursing Care Planning

### Planning of Nursing Care for Patients

The patient's needs as defined by the **nursing diagnoses** are first prioritized with the help of the patient and family:

- **Critical needs** are met immediately and then other needs are ranked according to the patient's priorities and Maslow's Hierarchy of Needs.
- When diagnoses are prioritized, **desirable outcomes** for each diagnosis are defined. Outcomes include desirable changes in patient behavior and are the backbone of the care plan. Outcomes are used to determine whether the nursing care has met its objectives.
- **Goals** for each nursing diagnosis are devised with patient and family input. Immediate, intermediate, and long-term goals that combine to meet the desired outcome are defined along with a timetable. Intermediate and long-term goals usually pertain to the prevention of complications and patient and family teaching concerning self-care and rehabilitation needs.

Each goal is then completed by a list of specific **actions** needed to achieve the goal. These actions include nursing interventions and may also include coordination of actions by other healthcare personnel.

**Review Video: Plan of Care**
Visit mometrix.com/academy and enter code: 300570

## Resources for Care Planning

Various resources provide lists of nursing diagnoses, interventions, and expected outcomes to help guide the nurse care planning process:

- The **North American Nursing Diagnosis Association (NANDA)** compiles a list of the most commonly used nursing diagnoses and refines them so that they are acceptable for study and nursing research. This list is updated biannually and is useful when developing care plans.
- **Nursing-Sensitive Outcomes Classification (NOC)** lists nursing outcomes for specific needs. Each outcome has an associated scale of achievement and can be used to evaluate patient progress in achieving the outcome desired.
- **Nursing Interventions Classification (NIC)** consists of interventions appropriate for specific nursing needs. These interventions can be individualized for each patient's needs.

NANDA, NIC, and NOC utilize the **Taxonomy of Nursing Practice** to classify nursing diagnoses, outcomes, and interventions. The Taxonomy of Nursing Practice divides patient problems into four domains:

- **The functional domain** includes classes consisting of patient movement, relief of symptoms, developmental status, nutrition, ADLs, sexuality, belief systems, and sleep.
- **The physiological domain** consists of bodily needs for proper functioning divided into classes concerning the cardiovascular, respiratory, gastrointestinal, genitourinary, neurological, metabolic, immune, reproductive, musculoskeletal, and integumentary systems. The effects of medications and other substances on system functioning are included.
- **The psychosocial domain** contains classes concerning emotional health (coping mechanisms, mental state, self-image, and self-esteem), mental health (knowledge and behaviors), and social status (communication with others, relationships, and support network).
- **The environmental domain** is concerned with patient populations, public and individual health and safety in the environment, healthcare delivery, and management of risks.

By using the taxonomy, all three tools describe the same problems in the same way in language that is specific and refined, yet universal.

## Utilizing Clinical Pathways in Care Planning

**Clinical pathways** are written tools that direct the treatment of a specific group of patients according to diagnosis. They provide a way to standardize medical and nursing care according to evidence-based practice guidelines, predict the cost of the care, and ensure quality, timeliness, and cost-effectiveness of care. Each plan consists of the DRG or group that it addresses, time segments with specific activities, and desired outcomes for each time segment. They include a place to record activities that deviate from the pathway. Nursing care is charted according to the pathway, which serves as the patient's plan of care. Nurses are responsible for helping to formulate and change clinical pathways. They initiate the pathways when the patient presents for treatment and ensure that the care is given for each time segment. They also use the pathways to monitor patients as case managers for hospitals or insurance companies. The patient may receive a copy that the nurse then discusses to make the patient aware of the treatment course and desired goals.

## Incorporating Patient and Family Rights into Plan of Care

In order for patient and family rights to be incorporated into the plan of care, the care plan needs to be designed as a **collaborative effort** that encourages participation of patients and family members. There are a number of different programs that can be useful, such as including patients and families on advisory committees. Additionally, assessment tools, such as surveys for patients and families, can be utilized to gain insight in the issues that are important to them. While infants and small children and sometimes the elderly cannot speak for themselves, the "patient" is generally understood to include not only the immediate family but also other groups or communities who have an interest in the care of the individual. Because many hospital stays are now short-term, programs that include follow-up interviews and assessments are especially valuable in determining if the needs of the patient were addressed in the care plan.

## Psychosocial Factors That Affect Care Planning

There are many psychosocial factors that affect patient care. A patient's **psychological state** influences how that patient interacts with others, including nurses and hospital staff, and can also affect compliance and positive health outcomes. For instance, anxiety or depression can make a patient incapable of performing the instructions necessary for completing a full recovery; the psychological problem would need to be addressed in the patient's care plan.

Social and culture factors also shape a patient's **perception** of health and disease, communication style, and decision-making methods. It is important to understand that differences in ethnicity, race, sex, gender, religion, age, socioeconomic status, family dynamics, sexual orientation, and life experiences mean that patients experience illness and healing differently. Being sensitive to these differences can lead to more effective patient care across the spectrum.

## Consideration of Comorbidities in Care Planning

**Comorbidity**, also known as multimorbidity, refers to the coexistence of multiple chronic or acute medical diseases within one patient. Comorbid conditions are associated with poorer outcomes, the need for more complex medical or surgical management, and elevated healthcare costs. It is now the norm, as opposed to the exception, that patients have multiple comorbid medical conditions. Some examples would be an obese patient with concomitant diabetes, heart disease, and osteoarthritis; a multi-system trauma patient with diabetes, chronic obstructive pulmonary disease, and cardiovascular disease; or a cancer patient with anxiety, depression, and multiple pulmonary emboli.

## Implementation of a Nursing Plan

The patient's nursing care plan is implemented as soon as the patient has been stabilized. During stabilization, nursing care is guided by standards of practice and logarithms that define care for life-threatening situations. Once the patient is stabilized, **interventions** are guided by the patient's individualized plan of care:

- The nurse has the responsibility of performing the planned nursing interventions and of delegating and coordinating care given by others to meet the patient's needs.
- All care is documented along with patient response.
- Additional patient information, changes in condition, patient priorities, and needs guide the nurse in continuously modifying the care plan.
- Orders are analyzed, clarified, and questioned as needed to meet collaborative patient needs.
- Patient input is necessary to the evaluation of nursing care and revision of the care plan as needed. Patient response to interventions, treatments, and procedures is assessed and care is given accordingly.
- The results of labs and tests are also used to determine actions according to the care plan.

# Medical Terminology and Transcription

## Common Nursing Abbreviations

The following abbreviations are important for the nurse to know when communicating with health care team members regarding the health status of the client:

| Abbreviation | Meaning | Abbreviation | Meaning |
|---|---|---|---|
| ADL | activities of daily living | N/V/D | nausea, vomiting, and diarrhea |
| BMP | basic metabolic panel | ORIF | open reduction internal fixation |
| BP | blood pressure | RBC | red blood cell |
| CBC | complete blood count | ROM | range of motion |
| CNS | central nervous system | RR | respiratory rate |
| ESRD | end-stage renal disease | S&S | signs and symptoms |
| GI | gastrointestinal | SOB | shortness of breath |
| h | hours | URI | upper respiratory infection |
| HR | heart rate | US | ultrasound |
| IV | Intravenous | UTI | urinary tract infection |
| MI | myocardial infarction | VS | vital signs |
| MOA | mechanism of action | WBC | white blood cells |

## Verbal Orders

Telephone and direct verbal orders both pose a risk of misinterpretation and error because they rely on the nurse correctly understanding and remembering the orders, especially if there are multiple orders. According to the Joint Commission, telephone and verbal orders should be written in their entirety, read back, and confirmed before the orders are carried out. If the ordering physician is present, the physician should write the orders rather than giving verbal orders.

## Recording and Communicating Client Information

Documents used to record and communicate client information include:

- **Medical records**: Include demographic information, history and physical, progress notes, lists of allergies, treatment plan, physician's orders, and various reports as well as the discharge planning form. Medical records may be in paper form or electronic.
- **Referral forms**: Include client's name, birthdate, contact information, address, and insurance information. The reason for the consultation, the diagnosis and ICD-10-CM code, and information about the referring physician/therapist are included.
- **Transfer forms**: May vary but include the client's name, date of birth, gender, contact person, physicians name and telephone number, any code status (such as DNR), the date and time of transfer and the reason for transfer as well as vital signs, report of pain, client diagnosis, use of restraints, respiratory needs, allergies, sensory status, skin condition, diet, list of personal items, risk alert, mobility/weight-bearing status, mental status, functional ability, immunization record, bowel and bladder status, and list of medication as well as any attached documents, such as operative reports, advance directives, and medication reconciliation.
- **Various report forms**: May include laboratory and imaging reports, consultation reports, and therapy reports.

# Legal Regulations

## Regulation of Nursing by States' Nurse Practice Act

Each state's **nurse practice act** seeks to regulate nursing within the state. It specifies the amount and type of education required to become an RN or LPN/LVN. It defines the nurse's role and responsibilities in healthcare settings. It directs the actions that the nurse may take based on standards of care and defines advanced practice education, experience, responsibilities, and limitations. It gives nurses the authorization to perform within their scope. It also regulates delegation and supervision responsibilities of the nurse. Nurse practice acts are administrated by the state board of nursing, which is responsible for issuing and renewing nurse licenses as well as discipline and censure of nurses. Most state boards of nursing now have a website that provides state-specific information about licensure and nursing rights and responsibilities.

## Nurse's Accountability for Nursing Care

Nurses are part of an interdisciplinary team responsible for patient outcomes. Nurses have the responsibility for the outcomes of nursing care as a professional group. This responsibility is outlined in each state's nurse practice act, the American Nurses Association (ANA) Code of Ethics, and the nurse's job description. Tools, such as the nursing care plan that includes standardized nursing diagnoses, interventions, and expected outcomes, enable the nurse to fulfill this responsibility. Empowerment to act as the patient advocate allows the nurse to point out factors in the patient's individual situation that can be addressed to further improve outcome. Critical thinking during decision-making and detailed documentation are also important. The nurse is held accountable for delegation as well as supervising care by others and evaluation of the outcomes of that care as well. The nurse has personal **accountability** in terms of being responsible for their own ethical and moral conduct and the consequences of that conduct. Since clinical knowledge is crucial to critical thinking, the nurse must strive to increase knowledge continuously through professional development throughout his or her career.

## Advance Directives

In accordance to Federal and state laws, individuals have the right to self-determination in health care, including the right to make decisions about end of life care through **advance directives** such as living wills and the right to assign an individual to make healthcare-related decisions through a medical power of attorney in the case that they are incapacitated in any way that impacts their ability to advocate for their own wishes. Patients should routinely be questioned about an advance directive as they may present at a healthcare provider without the document. Patients who have indicated that they desire a do-not-resuscitate (DNR) order should not receive resuscitative measures (CPR, manual ventilation, intubation, vasopressor support, etc.) in the case that they experience cardiac or respiratory arrest. Patients and families of those with terminal illnesses should be questioned as to whether the patients are Hospice patients. For those with DNR requests or those withdrawing life support, staff should provide the patient palliative rather than curative measures, such as pain control and/or oxygen, and emotional support to the patient and family. Religious traditions and beliefs about death should be treated with respect.

## HIPAA

The Health Insurance Portability and Accountability Act (HIPAA) and state laws govern **who may receive healthcare information** about a person, how permission is to be obtained, how the information may be shared, and patients' rights concerning personal information. HIPAA strives to protect the **privacy** of an individual's healthcare information. Facilities must prevent this information from being accessed by unauthorized personnel. Healthcare information is required to be protected on the **administrative**, **physical**, and **technical** levels. The patient must sign a release form to allow sharing of patient information outside of that necessary for the treatment. There are tiered penalties for violation of these laws (updated annually), ranging from $141 for an unintentional violation to $71,162 for a willful violation (as of 2025). Facilities that violate HIPAA may also be subject to corrective actions. Penalties are governed by the Department of Health and Human Services' Office for Civil Rights and the state attorneys general.

### *Application of HIPAA to Practice*

As an integral member of the health care team, the nurse must always be aware of HIPAA regulations and apply this knowledge to practice. The nurse is responsible for the following efforts to protect and maintain patient privacy:

- The nurse must read and follow facility policies regarding the transfer of patient data.
- Communication between health care personnel about a patient should always be in a private place so that this information is not overheard by those who do not have the right to share the information.
- Access to charts must be restricted to only those health care team members involved in that patient's care.
- Patient healthcare information should not be posted in place of public view and all efforts should be made to maintain patient privacy.
- The nurse must not give information casually to anyone (e.g., visitors or family members) unless it is confirmed that they have the right to have that information.
- Family members must not be relied upon to interpret for the patient; a qualified medical interpreter must be offered whenever possible to protect patient privacy.
- Computers with patient information must have passwords and safeguards to prevent unauthorized access of patient information.
- The nurse should leave limited voicemail messages, providing basic details of the facility and a call back number (unless approved to do otherwise).

**Review Video: HIPAA**
Visit mometrix.com/academy and enter code: 412009

## OSHA

The **Occupational Safety and Health Administration (OSHA)** seeks to keep workers safe and healthy while on the job. OSHA mandates that employers maintain a safe environment, assists employers to ensure that workers are made fully aware of any hazards, assists in educating employees in workplace safety, and ensures that access to personal protective gear is made available to workers who come into contact with hazardous or infectious materials. By following these regulations, an employer keeps injury and illness of workers to an absolute minimum. This fosters productivity, since workers are not absent due to illness or injury, employee health costs are contained, and the turnover rate is decreased, saving money spent on hiring and training new employees. OSHA is concerned about healthcare employee exposure to radiation, as well as chemical and biological agents, when caring for patients. Information is available to help hospitals and other facilities write plans that comply with best practices to deal with this and other threats to employees. Cleaning procedures, decontamination, and hazardous waste disposal are all covered by OSHA and apply to everyday hospital operation as well as disaster situations.

**Review Video: Intro to OSHA**
Visit mometrix.com/academy and enter code: 913559

## CMS

The **Centers for Medicare and Medicaid Services (CMS)**, part of the US Department of Health and Human Services, see to it that healthcare regulations are observed by healthcare facilities that receive federal reimbursement. Through an indirect process that includes contractors and state agencies, CMS reimburses facilities for care given to Medicare, Medicaid, and the state Children's Health Insurance Program (CHIP) recipients. They also monitor adherence to HIPAA Administration Simplification standards. CMS examines documentation of patient care when deciding to reimburse for care given. CMS has regulations for all types of medical facilities, and these regulations have profoundly impacted nursing practice because nurses must ensure that they comply with regulations related to the quality of patient care and concerns regarding cost-containment. Each facility should provide guidelines to assist nursing staff in meeting the specific documentation requirements of CMS.

## OBRA 1987

The **Omnibus Budget Reconciliation Act of 1987 (OBRA 1987)**, also known as the Nursing Home Reform Act, instituted requirements for nursing homes with the purpose of strengthening and protecting patient rights. These requirements are as follows: "a facility must provide each patient with a level of care that enables him or her to attain or maintain the highest practicable physical, mental, and psychosocial wellbeing." OBRA 1987 required that all nursing home patients receive an initial evaluation with yearly follow-ups. Every patient is required to have a comprehensive assessment within 14 days of admission and a comprehensive care plan within 7 days of completion of the assessment. Patients were ensured the right to medical care and the right to be informed about and refuse medical treatment. OBRA 1987 requires each state to establish, monitor, and enforce nursing facility requirements through education, routine surveys, and creating standards for investigating grievances and complaints. Each state is also required to fund, staff, and maintain investigative and Ombudsman units.

## OBRA 1990 (PSDA)

The Omnibus Budget Reconciliation Act of 1990 included the amendment called the **Patient Self Determination Act (PSDA)**. The PSDA required healthcare facilities that participate in Medicaid to provide written information about advanced healthcare directives to adult patients and to educate patients on the right to accept or reject medical or surgical treatments. Patients who make an advanced directive are leaving instructions about what medical interventions they authorize or refuse if they are incapacitated by illness or injury. They can also nominate another person to make these decisions for them in this situation. The PSDA also protected the right of patients to accept or refuse medical treatments. Healthcare facilities and hospitals are legally required to communicate these rights to all patients, to respect these rights, and to educate staff and personnel about these rights.

## EMTALA

The **Emergency Medical Treatment and Active Labor Act (EMTALA)** is designed to prevent patient "dumping" from emergency departments (ED) and is an issue of concern for risk management that requires staff training for compliance:

- Transfers from the ED may be intrahospital or to another facility.
- Initial medical screening must be done prior to inquiring about insurance or ability to pay.
- All possible efforts towards stabilization of the patient with emergency conditions or active labor must be done in the ED prior to transfer. Stabilization of the patient in active labor is considered to be after the delivery of both child and placenta. If stabilization in the ED is not possible, transfer to the appropriate facility or admission to the appropriate unit should be done.
- Stabilization requires treatment for emergency conditions and reasonable belief that, although the emergency condition may not be completely resolved, the patient's condition will not deteriorate during transfer.
- Women in the ED in active labor should deliver both the child and placenta before transfer.
- The receiving department or facility should be capable of treating the patient and dealing with complications that might occur.
- Transfer to another facility is indicated if the patient requires specialized services not available intrahospital, such as to burn centers.

## AHRQ

The **Agency for Healthcare Research and Quality (AHRQ)** is part of the US Department of Health and Human Services. This agency is concerned about healthcare and primarily promotes scientific research into the safety, effectiveness, and quality of healthcare. It encourages evidence-based healthcare that produces the best possible outcome while containing healthcare costs. It makes contracts with institutions to review any published evidence on healthcare in order to produce reports used by other organizations to write guidelines. AHRQ also funds evidence-based practice centers (EPCs) to assist with these initiatives and to guide recommendations put forth by the United States Preventative Services Task Force (USPSTF).

# Nursing Research

## Elements of Research

The following are elements of research:

- **Variable**: An entity that can be different within a population
- **Independent variable**: The variable that the researchers hypothesize will impact the outcome and therefore is controlled by the researchers to evaluate its effect
- **Dependent variable**: The variable that is measured based on the impact of the independent variable
- **Hypothesis**: The proposed explanation to describe an expected outcome in a study
- **Sample**: The selected group to be studied that is meant to represent the larger population to which the study will be applied
- **Experimental group**: The subset within the sample that undergoes the treatment or intervention
- **Control group**: The subset within the sample that is not exposed to the treatment or intervention being evaluated (placebo)

The nurse must be taught and must understand the process of critical analysis and know how to conduct a survey of the literature. **Basic research concepts** include:

- **Survey of valid sources**: Information from a juried journal and an anonymous website or personal website are very different sources, and evaluating what constitutes a valid source of data is critical.
- **Evaluation of internal and external validity**: Internal validity shows a cause-and-effect relationship between two variables, with the cause occurring before the effect and no intervening variable. External validity occurs when results hold true in different environments and circumstances with different populations.
- **Sample selection and sample size**: Selection and size can have a large impact on the results, but a sample that is too small may lack both internal and external validity, depending on the population it is meant to represent. Selection may be so narrowly focused that the results can't be generalized to other groups.

## Validity, Generalizability, and Replicability

Many research studies are most concerned with **internal validity** (adequate unbiased data properly collected and analyzed within the population studied), but studies that determine the efficacy of procedures or treatments, for example, should have **external validity** as well; that is, the results should be **generalizable** (applicable) for the population that was targeted by the study. **Replication** of the study under different circumstances and with different subjects and researchers should produce similar results. For various reasons, some people may be excluded from a study so that instead of randomized subjects, the subjects may be highly selected (a non-probability sample) so when data is compared with another population in which there is less or more selection, results may be different. The selection of subjects, in this case, would interfere with external validity. Part of the design of a study should include considerations of whether or not it should have external validity or whether there is value for the institution based solely on internal validation, which would then determine the sampling technique utilized.

## HYPOTHESIS

A hypothesis should be generated about the probable cause of the disease/infection based on the information available in laboratory and medical records, epidemiologic study, literature review, and expert opinion. For example, a hypothesis should include the infective agent, the likely source, and the mode of transmission: "Wound infections with *Staphylococcus aureus* were caused by the reuse of single-use irrigation syringes used during wound care in the ICU." Population, setting, and time frame may also be added.

**Hypothesis testing** includes data analysis, laboratory findings, and outcomes of environmental testing. It usually includes case-control studies, with 2-4 controls picked for each case of infection. They may be matched according to age, sex, or other characteristics, but they are not infected at the time they are picked for the study. Cohort studies, whose particpants are defined by exposure rather than utilizing controls, may also be instituted. If the hypothesis cannot be supported, then a new hypothesis or different testing methods may be necessary.

## CRITICAL READING

There are several steps to critical reading to evaluate research:

- **Consider the source** of the material. If it is in the popular press, it may have less validity compared to something published in a peer-reviewed journal.
- **Review the author's credentials** to determine if a person is an expert in the field of study.
- **Determine the hypothesis**, or the central claim of the research. It should be clearly stated.
- **Examine the organization** of the article, whether it is based on a particular theory, and the type of methodology used.
- **Review the evidence** to determine how it is used to support the main points. Look for statistical evidence and sample size to determine if the findings have wide applicability.
- **Evaluate** the overall article to determine if the information seems credible and useful and should be communicated to administration and/or staff.

## MAJOR STUDY TYPES UTILIZED IN STATISTICAL ANALYSIS

When conducting research, the nurse should be aware of the **types of studies** available and when each type of study is appropriate and most reliable:

- **Case-control studies** are simple. They review pre-existing cases of individuals with the disorder of interest and controls (individuals without the disorder) to assess prior exposures that may have contributed to the disorder. For example, case-control studies may be done with mesothelioma and exposure to possible pleural irritants. These are good for rare diseases to determine possible association.
- **Cross-sectional studies** utilize a cross-section of data from the population and analyze variables at one time point. They are not good for determining cause and effect, but they are useful for estimating exposure prevalence and disease burden.
- **Cohort studies** follow a cohort of a population for a period of time and attempt to make a link with diseases. As in the previous example, researchers could follow a group exposed to asbestos and study the incidence of mesothelioma.
- **Randomized controlled trial** is the gold standard, with patients assigned to the control or experimental group. This is a difficult type of test to design and implement but very useful, as the data is often well-controlled. It is the most expensive type of study.

### Bias in Research

**Selection bias** occurs when the method of selecting subjects results in a cohort that is not representative of the target population because of inherent error in design. For example, if all patients who develop urinary infections are supposed to be evaluated with urine culture and sensitivities for microbial resistance, but only those patients with clinically-evident infections are included, a number of patients with sub-clinical infections or no symptoms may be missed, skewing the results. Selection bias can occur in a variety of study designs.

**Information bias** occurs when there are errors in classification, so an estimate of association is incorrect. Non-differential misclassification occurs unrelated to the disease or exposure status (often related to equipment/instruments or random error). Differential misclassification occurs when there is a misclassification of disease or exposure that is dependent on outcome or exposure (often related to recall bias).

### Qualitative and Quantitative Data

Both qualitative and quantitative data are used for analysis, but the focus is quite different:

- **Qualitative data**: Data are described verbally or graphically, and the results require reporting or observation. Interviews may be used as a tool to gather information, and the researcher's interpretation of data is important. Gathering this type of data can be time-intensive, and is not intended for generalization to a larger population.
- **Quantitative data**: Data are described in terms of numbers within a statistical format. This type of information gathering is done after the design of data collection is outlined. Tools may include surveys, questionnaires, or other methods of obtaining numerical data.

## Evidence-Based Practice

### Classes of Evidence-Based Practice

**Evidence-based practice** is treatment based on the best possible evidence, including a study of current research. Literature is searched to find evidence of the most effective treatments for specific diseases or injuries, and those treatments are then utilized to create clinical pathways that outline specific multi-departmental treatment protocols, including medications, treatments, and timelines. Evidence-based guidelines are often produced by specialty organizations that undertake the task of searching and analyzing literature to produce policies, procedures, and guidelines that become the standard of care for the disease. These guidelines are then used when a patient fits the disease criteria for that guideline. **Evidence-based nursing** aims to improve the quality of nursing care by integrating evidence-based research into nursing practice. This can be done on the individual level or the systems level, in which facilities incorporate evidence-based research into the development of clinical pathways and guidelines.

### Evidence-Based Practice Guidelines

The creation of evidence-based practice guidelines is usually facility-driven as a means of ensuring these practices are implemented across the system. The process of guideline creation usually includes the following components:

- **Focus on the topic/methodology:** This includes outlining possible interventions and treatments for review, choosing patient populations and settings, and determining significant outcomes. Search boundaries (such as types of databases, types of studies, dates of studies) should be determined.
- **Evidence review:** This includes review of literature, critical analysis of studies, and summarizing of results, including pooled meta-analysis.
- **Expert judgment:** Recommendations based on personal experience from a number of experts may be utilized, especially if there is inadequate evidence based on review, but this subjective evidence should be explicitly acknowledged.

- **Engage stakeholders and patients:** Survey relevant key stakeholders (physicians, nurses, etc.) and patients who would be implementing or subjected to the care outlined in the guideline for feedback.
- **Policy considerations:** This includes cost-effectiveness, access to care, insurance coverage, availability of qualified staff, and legal implications.
- **Policy:** A written policy must be completed with recommendations. Common practice is to utilize letter guidelines, with "A" being the most highly recommended, usually based on the quality of supporting evidence.
- **Review:** The completed policy should be submitted to peers for review and comments before instituting the policy.

## Clinical Pathways

Clinical pathway development is done by those involved in direct patient care. The pathway should cover the entire scope of an illness. Steps include:

1. Selection of patient group and diagnosis, procedures, or conditions, based on analysis of data and observations of wide variance in approach to treatment and prioritizing organization and patient needs; consider inclusion/exclusion criteria
2. Creation of interdisciplinary team of those involved in the process of care, including physicians to develop pathway
3. Analysis of data including literature review and study of best practices to identify opportunities for quality improvement
4. Identification of all categories of care, such as nutrition, medications, and nursing
5. Discussion and reaching consensus
6. Identifying the levels of care and number of days to be covered by the pathway (with flexibility to accommodate various possible lengths of stay)
7. Pilot testing and redesigning steps as indicated
8. Educating staff about standards
9. Monitoring and tracking variances in order to improve pathways

## HICPAC Categories of Evidence-Based Practice

Levels of evidence are categorized according to the scientific evidence available to support the recommendations, as well as existing state and federal laws. While recommendations are voluntary, they are often used as a basis for state and federal regulations.

- **Category IA** is well supported by evidence from experimental, clinical, or epidemiologic studies and is strongly recommended for implementation.
- **Category IB** has supporting evidence from some studies, has a good theoretical basis, and is strongly recommended for implementation.
- **Category IC** is currently required by state or federal regulations.
- **Category II** is supported by suggestive clinical or epidemiologic studies, has a theoretical basis, and is suggested for implementation.
- **Unresolved** means there is no recommendation because of a lack of consensus or evidence.

### PROCESS MONITORING AND OUTCOME EVALUATION

Process monitoring and outcome evaluation are important components of evidence-based practice, which incorporate both internal and external research with subject matter expert opinion and patient preferences. All treatments are subjected to review to determine if they produce positive outcomes, and policies and protocols for outcome evaluation should be in place. **Process monitoring** over the course of treatment involves careful observation and record-keeping that notes progress, with supporting laboratory and radiographic evidence as indicated by condition and treatment **Outcome evaluation** includes the following:

- **Evaluating** results includes reviewing records as well as current research to determine if outcomes are within acceptable parameters.
- **Sustaining** involves maintaining treatment that has proven effective and continuing to monitor and evaluate.
- **Improving** means to continue the treatment but with additions or modifications in order to improve outcomes.
- **Replacing** the treatment with a different treatment must be done if outcome evaluation indicates that current treatment is ineffective.

## Quality Improvement and Risk Assessment

### CONTINUOUS QUALITY IMPROVEMENT

Continuous quality improvement is a multidisciplinary management philosophy that can be applied to all aspects of an organization, whether related to such varied areas as the cardiac unit, purchasing, or human resources. The skills used for epidemiologic research (data collection, analysis, outcomes, action plans) are all applicable to the analysis of multiple types of events, because they are based on solid scientific methods. Multi-disciplinary planning can bring valuable insights from various perspectives, and strategies used in one context can often be applied to another. All staff, from housekeeping to supervising, must be alert to not only problems but also opportunities for improvement. Increasingly, departments must be concerned with cost-effectiveness as the costs of medical care continue to rise, so the quality professional in the cardiovascular unit is not in an isolated position in an institution but is just one part of the whole, facing similar concerns as those in other disciplines. Disciplines are often interrelated in their functions.

### NURSE'S INVOLVEMENT IN QUALITY IMPROVEMENT

The following are ways in which nurses can be involved in quality improvement in their facility:

- **Identify situations** in the nursing unit that require improvement and might benefit patient outcomes (cost containment, incident reporting, etc.) if changed.
- **Identify potential items** that can be measured to be able to test the problem or to be able to monitor patient outcomes.
- **Collect data** on those measurements and determine current patient outcomes.
- **Analyze the data** and identify procedures, methods, etc., that can be utilized to potentially make positive changes in patient outcomes, doing research if necessary.
- **Make recommendations for changes** to be implemented to determine the effect on patient outcomes.
- **Implement recommendations** after approval from administrative personnel.
- **Collect data** using the same measurements and determine if the changes improved patient outcomes or not.

### Risk Management

Risk management attempts to prevent harm and legal liability by being proactive and by identifying a patient's **risk factors**. The patient is educated about these factors and ways that they can modify their behavior to decrease their risk. Treatments and interventions must be considered in terms of risk to the patient, and the patient must always know these risks in order to make healthcare decisions. Much can be done to avoid mistakes that put patients at risk. Patients should note medications and other aspects of their care so that they can help prevent mistakes. They should feel free to question care and to have their concerns heard and addressed. When mistakes are made, the actions taken to remedy the situation are very important. The physician should be made aware of the error immediately, and the patient notified according to hospital policy. Errors must be evaluated to determine how the process failed. Honesty and caring can help mitigate many errors.

### Nursing Malpractice, Negligence, Unintentional Torts, and Intentional Torts

- **Malpractice** is unethical or improper actions or lack of proper action by the nurse that may or may not be related to a lack of skills that nurses should possess.
- **Negligence** is the failure to act as any other diligent nurse would have acted in the same situation.
- Negligence can lead to an **unintentional tort**. In this case, the patient must prove that the nurse had a duty to act, a duty proven via standards of care, and that the nurse failed in this duty and harm occurred to the patient as a result of this failure.
- **Intentional torts** differ in that the duty is assumed and the nurse breached this duty via assault and battery, invasion of privacy, slander, or false imprisonment of the patient.

**Review Video: Medical Negligence**
Visit mometrix.com/academy and enter code: 928405

## Health Care Policy and Delivery

### Health Policy

Health policy is the legal effort to make positive change in systemic health care and health care outcomes through a compilation of decisions, plans and actions made by representatives of the health care community in combination with local, state, and federal government representatives. Often, the first step in health care policy efforts is to identify the goals and desired outcomes of new policy, then working backwards to formulate a plan and collect relevant needs that must be met in order for those goals to be attained.

Due to the inherently political nature of health policy, it is important that health care representatives commit to contributing to policy changes in the arenas they have deemed necessary from their work experience. Local politicians rely heavily on the expertise and knowledge of health care professionals to inform and guide policy change. The nurse has the unique skill set of working as a nurse, and also working as a clinical leader, which provides a critical dichotomy of insight that can be extremely valuable in addressing health policy change. Nurses have the opportunity to provide both hands on patient care and administrative duties, and often it is the miscommunication between these two entities that present challenges in policy formation. As a nurse it is a responsibility to contribute not only to change on the unit, but change in systemic policy to the benefit of patients and patient safety nationwide.

## Impact of Social, Political, Regulatory, and Economic Forces

The delivery of care is impacted by numerous forces:

- **Social forces** are increasing demand for access to treatment and medical services, both traditional and complementary. As society views equitable medical care as a right, then delivery of care must be available to all.
- **Political forces** affect medical care as the Federal and state governments increasingly become purchasers of medical care, imposing their guidelines and limitations on the medical system.
- **Regulatory forces** may be local, state, or Federal and can have a profound effect of delivery of care and services, differing from one state or region to another.
- **Economic forces**, such as managed care or cost-containment committees, try to contain costs to insurers and facilities by controlling access to and duration of treatment, and limiting products. Economic pressure is working to prevent duplication of services in a geographical area, and providers are creating networks to purchase supplies and equipment directly.

## Nursing's Agenda for Health Care Reform from ANA (1991)

Nursing's Agenda for Health Care Reform encourages the development of health care that provides patients the ability to get to receive medical attention and help without excessive costs, and it encourages continual primary care. It fundamentally asks for **vital medical attention** to be accessible to everyone and for there to be a **reorganized health care system** that centers on patients' wellbeing and conditions so that they may get medical help in familiar and local places. It advocates providing for ongoing medical needs and insurance changes so that patients can use their coverage more easily. It asks for organizational assessment on public and private sectors regarding the use of resources, lowering expenses, and getting balanced and even reimbursement for each provider.

# Billing and Reimbursement Concepts

## Medicare

Medicare, a federally directed program, was introduced by the Title XIX Social Security Act in 1965. It provides health insurance to elderly patients and to patients with disabilities. The patient who is covered will receive hospital, doctor, and further medical care as needed. The patient's income is not a factor for eligibility. **Original Medicare** consists of **Part A** and **Part B**, and covers the majority of medical care when the patient seeks care at a facility that accepts Medicare. If the patient requires prescription drug assistance, they may opt into **Part D**, which is the Medicare drug plan, or they may opt into the **Medicare Advantage Plan (Part C)**, which bundles Parts A, B and D.

### *Medicare Part A*

Medicare Part A covers hospital care (inpatient), care at a skilled nursing facility or nursing home, hospice care, and home health care. Anyone 65 years of age or older that is eligible to receive **Social Security** is automatically enrolled even if still working. Patients are also able to receive Social Security if they or their spouse put money into the system by way of working for at least 40 quarters. If the patient has less than 40 quarters of work, Medicare Part A requires a payment each month. If the patient is not yet 65 but has a complete disability that will remain for the rest of their life, Medicare Part A can be used after receiving Social Security benefits for 2 years. A patient with ongoing renal disease who needs either dialysis or transplant can become eligible for Part A without waiting for 2 years.

### *Medicare Part B*

Medicare Part B covers both medically necessary services and preventive services such as doctor visits, physical therapy, occupational therapy, speech therapy, medical equipment, assessments, clinical research, mental health support and wellness visits. The patient has to **pay a monthly premium for Medicare Part B,** which is either directly billed to the patient or deducted from their Social Security or other benefit payment.

The program covers 80% of the authorized expense for any medical attention that is required (following a yearly deductible).

## Medicaid

1965 Title XIX Social Security Act introduced **Medicaid** as a federal/state matching plan for low-income individuals supervised by the federal government. Funding comes from federal and state taxes, with no less than 50%, but no more than 83% being funded federally. Each state is able to add optional eligibility criteria on the list, and they may also put restrictions (to a point) on federally directed aid. Patients who receive Medicaid cannot get a bill for the aid, but states are able to require small copayments or deductibles for particular types of help.

Federal regulations require that states support certain individuals or groups of individuals through Medicaid, although not everyone who falls below the federal poverty rate is eligible. **Mandatory eligibility groups** include the following:

- Patients deemed categorically needy by their state, and receive financial support from various federal assistance programs.
- Individuals receiving Federal Supplemental Security income (SSI).
- Patients that are older than 65 that are blind or have complete disability.
- Pregnant women and children younger than 6 years of age who live in families that are up to 133% of the federal poverty level (some states allow for a higher income to meet eligibility in this class).
- Adults under the age of 65 that make less than or equal to 133% of the federal poverty level and are not receiving Medicare.

**Review Video: Medicare & Medicaid**
Visit mometrix.com/academy and enter code: 507454

## Third Parties That Give Compensation

Other than Medicare and Medicaid, the following are some **third parties** that give compensation for medical care:

- **Private insurance**: Will reimburse according to contract; particular for each state insurance commission.
- **TRICARE**: Used by patients in the armed forces, their dependents that may be living beyond a time when they have died, their families, or retirees.
- **Federal Employees Health Benefit Program** (FEHBP): Provided to non-military federal employees and their family.

## Billing and Coding for Reimbursement in the Pediatric Office Setting

### *International Classification of Diseases*

**International Classification of Diseases, 10th revision, Clinical Modifications (ICD-10-CM)** is a coding system used to code diagnoses. While the World Health Organization (WHO) has released the 11th revision of the ICD (ICD-11), the United States has not begun implementation of this version. ICD-10-CM codes are used for billing purposes to ensure that procedure codes match appropriate diagnoses. The codes all have at least 3 characters but may have up to 4 additional sub-categories. The first character must be alpha, the second and third, numeric, and the remaining alpha or numeric. A decimal point is placed after the first 3 characters. Diagnoses are classified by type of disease or system involved. For example, main categories include neoplasms and diseases of the respiratory systems. With ICD-10-CM, injuries are grouped by body part rather than category of injury. Thus, all injuries to the thorax (S20-S29) are grouped together. The chapter dealing with injuries, poisoning and other consequences of external causes are divided by two letters, S and T. The S-coded injuries are grouped by single body regions; however, some injuries are not localized, such as poisonings, and these are T-coded injuries.

### CPT Codes

**Current procedural terminology (CPT)** codes were developed by the American Medical Association (AMA) and used to define those licensed to provide services and to describe medical and surgical treatments, diagnostics, and procedures. CPT 2012 codes specific procedures as well as typical times required for treatment. CPT codes are usually updated each October with revisions (additions, deletions) to coding. The use of CPT codes is mandated by both CMS and HIPAA to provide a uniform language and to aid research. These codes are used primarily for billing purposes for insurances (public and private). Under HIPAA, HHS has designed CPT codes as part of the national standard for electronic healthcare transactions:

- Category I codes are used to identify a procedure or service.
- Category II codes are used to identify performance measures, including diagnostic procedures.
- Category III codes identify temporary codes for technology and data collection.

### HCPCS Level II Codes

**Healthcare Common Procedure Coding Systems (HCPCS Level II) codes** are used when filing claims for equipment, supplies and services that are not covered by CPT codes (Level I codes), including non-physician products such as durable medical equipment, ambulance services, laboratory service, orthotics, and prosthetics. HCPCS codes are also used for outpatient hospital care, chemotherapeutic drugs, and Medicaid:

- D codes are used for dental procedures.
- E codes are used for durable medical equipment, such as bedside commodes.
- L codes are used for orthotic and prosthetic procedures and devices, such as orthopedic shoes.
- P codes are used for pathology and laboratory services.

HCPCS Level II codes are comprised of 5 alphanumeric characters, beginning with a letter that indicates the grouping. For example, metal underarm crutches would be coded as E0114. The letter E indicates the item is durable medical equipment. The codes are updated on a quarterly basis.

### Diagnostic-Related Groups

Diagnostic-related groups (**DRGs**) were instituted in 1982 as a way to classify patients who shared similar diseases and treatments for billing purposes, under the assumption that patients who shared symptoms and/or diseases use the same amount of resources and should be **billed the same amount**. There are approximately 500 different DRGs, and patients are placed into specific DRGs using **International Classification of Disease (ICD) codes**, along with specific patient information such as sex, age, and the presence of comorbidities. By placing patients into DRGs, Medicare is able to determine how much the hospital should be reimbursed for patient care. The institution of DRGs has changed the health care system from one that was provider-driven (meaning the individual clinician determined the billable amount) into one that is payer-driven (meaning that Medicare determines reimbursement).

## Chapter Quiz

Ready to see how well you retained what you just read? Scan the QR code to go directly to the chapter quiz interface for this study guide. If you're using a computer, simply visit the online resources page at **mometrix.com/resources719/nclexrn-31183** and click the Chapter Quizzes link.

# Safety and Infection Prevention and Control

## Patient Safety and Injury Prevention in the Hospital

### Joint Commission's Patient Safety Goals

The Joint Commission has a set of **goals that impact patient safety** for each type of healthcare facility. Within the hospital environment, there are several goals that pertain:

- Each facility must have a way to identify patients that will avoid errors of identification.
- Caregivers are to give careful, accurate communications about patients and their care so that mistakes are not made.
- A system to avoid medication errors must be in place.
- Medications must be reconciled when the patient moves from place to place within the hospital or is discharged to other caregivers.
- The risk of infection must be decreased so that patients are at less risk for hospital-related infections.
- The facility must have a fall prevention program and evaluate its effectiveness.

All patients and family must be encouraged to be active in their own care to help to avoid errors. They must also know how to make sure their concerns for safety of care are heard and acted upon.

### Environmental Aspects of Patient Safety in the Hospital

Deliberate decisions by the health care providers/facility can help create an environment conducive for patient safety. Some of those aspects include:

- **Educating the patient on signaling staff**: The patient must be educated about the use of the call light, and the call light placed within easy reach. If the patient is unable to use the call light, then an alternative means of calling for help, such as a handheld bell, should be available. If the patient is unable to manage any type of signaling system, then the nurse should check on the patient at least every hour.
- **Protecting from falls and electrical hazards**: All clutter should be removed from floors and cords secured away from walkways. All electrical appliances should be checked to ensure they are working properly and have no frayed cords. Patients should be provided assistive devices, such as walkers, if necessary, to improve stability.
- **Making appropriate room assignments**: Patients with the greatest need for supervision should be placed closest to the nursing desk and within the line of sight whenever possible. In environments such as critical care, each nurse should be able to visualize their patient assignment from their nursing station.

### Medication Errors

There are about 7,000 deaths yearly in the United States attributed to **medication errors.** Studies indicate that there are errors in 1 in 5 doses of medication given to patients in hospitals. Patient safety must be ensured with proper handling and administering of medications:

- **Avoid error-prone abbreviations or symbols.** The Joint Commission has established a list of abbreviations to avoid, but mistakes are frequent with other abbreviations as well. In many cases, abbreviations and symbols should be avoided altogether or restricted to a limited approved list.
- **Prevent errors due to illegible handwriting or unclear verbal orders.** Handwritten orders should be block printed to reduce chance of error; verbal orders should be repeated back to the physician.
- **Institute barcoding and scanners** that allow the patient's wristband and medications to be scanned for verification.

- **Provide lists of similarly-named medications** to educate staff.
- Establish an **institutional policy** for the administration of medications that includes protocols for verification of drug, dosage, and patient, as well as educating the patient about the medications.

## Assessing Patients for Non-Drug Allergies

When assessing patients for **allergies** it's important to determine the type of symptoms they have, when the initial reaction occurred, and what type of treatment they have used in the past to manage this complication (including antihistamines). Allergies of particular interest include:

- **Food**: Ask patients about any specific foods that cause an adverse reaction as some foods may have cross-reactivity to latex (such as kiwi, papaya, avocado, and bananas), so patients may be at risk of developing latex allergy and should avoid contact with latex. Some medications may contain substances derived from food, such as eggs, fish, gelatin, lactose, and soy.
- **Latex**: Sensitivity to latex can result in mild reactions, such as itching and rash, to severe anaphylactic reactions, and is common among those with repeated contact with healthcare environments, such as those with spina bifida or multiple surgeries, so it should be suspected with these clients. While non-latex options are more readily available in most hospitals (non-latex gloves and Foley catheters, for instance), latex continues to be used in hospital materials, therefore this allergy must be assessed immediately upon arrival so that appropriate materials can be substituted if necessary.
- **Environmental**: The most common environmental allergies include pollens, dust mites, animals, cigarette smoke, cockroaches, and mold/mildew, so the nurse should be sure to ask about these as well as any other environmental allergies. Some patients are sensitive to strong colognes and perfumes, so the use of these is often regulated by hospital dress codes on units with immunocompromised patients.

## Non-Pharmacologic Prescription Precautions

Some non-pharmacologic prescriptions may contribute to accident or injury, including the following:

- **Oxygen supplies**: Oxygen may be administered at the wrong level of liters (too much or too little), and the oxygen supply may be inadvertently obstructed or disconnected. Oxygen concentrators may not have backup batteries and may fail to function if electricity goes off. If people smoke around oxygen, this increases the risk of fires. Nasal cannulas and face masks that delivery oxygen, when used over prolonged periods of time, can cause pressure injuries, therefore appropriate assessment and skin care is also necessary.
- **Assistive devices**: If equipment, such as canes and walkers, are improperly fitted, they may increase risk of falls.
- **Dialysis equipment**: Contamination of equipment is always a concern and can result in peritonitis (peritoneal dialysis) and sepsis (hemodialysis). If the lines become separated, the client may exsanguinate.
- **Hot/cold compresses**: If cold compresses are placed directly on the skin, they may damage the tissue, especially if left in place for too long. Hot compresses may cause burns if temperature is too high and may damage wounds if placed directly over them.

## Seizure Precautions

Seizure disorders are broadly categorized as partial seizures (which begin locally) or generalized seizures (which are bilateral and symmetrical and may be convulsive or non-convulsive):

- **Partial seizures** include *simple partial* (with motor, sensory, and/or autonomic symptoms but without impaired consciousness), *complex partial* (with cognitive, affective, psychosensory, and/or psychomotor symptoms, as well as impaired consciousness), or *partial secondarily generalized.*
- **Generalized seizures** include seizures that are bilateral and symmetric without local onset and may be convulsive or non-convulsive. These seizures include *tonic-clonic, tonic, clonic, absence* (petit mal), *atonic*, and *myoclonic seizures*, as well as *unclassified seizures*.

**Seizure precautions** are a standard set of safety protocol that ensure patient safety in those patients with a high risk or history of seizures. Generally, these precautions include padding the siderails, keeping the bed at the lowest position, and maintaining suctioning at the bedside. Precautions also include ensuring privacy and providing supportive care in the event of a seizure, such as easing the patient to the floor and providing padding to protect the head. Side rails should be raised and pillow removed if the patient is in bed. The patient should be placed on one side with the head flexed so the tongue does not block the airway. The patient should *not* be restrained or a padded tongue-blade inserted between the teeth. Seizure start and stop time should be noted.

## PATIENT DEFICITS THAT IMPEDE CLIENT SAFETY

Certain patient deficits can inherently impede client safety, including the following:

- **Visual impairment**: Patients are at risk of trips, slips, falls, burn injuries, poisoning (mistaken containers, ingredients), and medication errors because of taking the wrong medication or wrong dosage.
- **Hearing impairment**: Patients are at increased risk of falls and may not hear danger signals, such as fire alarms, smoke detectors, police/fire sirens, and tornado warning sirens, and may, therefore, not be aware that they are in danger. Most smoke detectors emit a high-frequency alarm that cannot always be detected by those with high-frequency hearing loss.
- **Sensory/perceptual impairment**: Patients (such as those with stroke or brain injury) may exhibit a wide variety of impairments so safety concerns may vary. For example, those with one-sided neglect may have injuries to the neglected side, such as from running into doors or other things. Those with face blindness may easily get lost if away from familiar places or people.



## R.A.C.E. ACRONYM FOR FIRE SAFETY

RACE is an acronym used for fire safety on the hospital unit:

- **R**escue: Remove all patients from area of danger
- **A**ctivate alarm: Pull fire alarm/call 911
- **C**onfine the fire: Close doors to unit/place
- **E**vacuate/Extinguish (NFPA/OSHA fire safety): Use **PASS** for fire extinguisher
  - **P**ull
  - **A**im at the base of the flames
  - **S**queeze the trigger
  - **S**weep: Use a sweeping motion across the flames

## ERGONOMICS

Ergonomics is the study of preventing workplace injury and stress. In nursing, it refers to the way in which a nurse can prevent injury to self and others due to the stressors and strains required in the nursing field. Some important **ergonomic principles** include:

- **Body mechanics:** The body should be kept in proper alignment during tasks, with a wide base of support and center of gravity low. Use larger muscles (buttocks, thighs, shoulders) for activities rather than smaller when possible. Avoid twisting or jerking movements. Maintain 90° angle in elbows and knees when sitting, elbows at the side, with back straight and looking straight ahead.
- **Lifting:** Use appropriate transfer devices; use as many people as necessary. Manual lifting should be avoided. Bend at the knees, tighten core, and keep weights close to the body - *never* bend or twist when lifting.
- **Repetition**: Avoid repetitive movements/stressors and use proper safety equipment when needed (earplugs for loud noises, etc.).

# Disaster Management and Emergency Response

## Disaster

A disaster is an event where many people are exposed to hazards that result in injury, death, and damage to property. There are a number of hazards that have the potential to lead to a disaster situation. In general, they can be **classified** as natural, technological, or caused by human conflict. Some specific examples of each are as follows:

- **Natural**: Firestorms, flood, land shift, tornado, epidemic, earthquake, volcano, hurricane, high winds, blizzard, heat wave
- **Technological**: Hazmat spills, explosions, utility failure, building collapse, transportation accident, power outage, nuclear accident, dam failure, fire, water loss, ruptured gas main
- **Human conflict**: Riots, strikes, suicide bombings, bomb threat, employee violence, mass shootings, equipment sabotage, hostage events, transportation disruption, weapons of mass destruction, computer viruses/worms

## Disaster Management Plan

### *Development*

There are many different types of disaster management plans. Regardless of the type, there are several basic steps for its **development**. To begin with, a **planning team** must be established that includes representatives from all levels within the organization. The planning team is responsible for creating a timeline for completion of the plan as well as an estimation of the costs, fees, and resources necessary to complete the plan. Once this is done, an **analysis of potential disasters** can begin. In this step, potential hazards are identified and vulnerability of the organization to disasters is assessed. A **disaster response plan** is established that includes the reduction/removal of hazardous situations. The final steps are **plan implementation and review**. The plan can be tested for efficacy through drills and mock disaster situations. It is critical to review and update the plan yearly.

### *Types*

There are several different **types of disaster management plans**, some more specific than others. They are listed and briefly described below:

- **Emergency action plan**: OSHA required, evacuation plans and emergency drills
- **Business continuity plan**: Business operation-specific, aimed at reducing losses and resuming productivity
- **Risk management plan**: Off-site effects of chemical exposures
- **Emergency response plan**: Immediate response to disasters
- **Contingency plan**: General, designed to handle events not covered in other plans
- **Federal response plan**: Coordinates federal resources
- **Spill prevention, control, and countermeasures plan**: Deals with the prevention, control, and clean-up of oil spills
- **Mutual aid plan**: Plan for shared resources between other companies/firms
- **Recovery plan**: Deals with repair and rebuilding post-disaster
- **Emergency management plan**: Plan for healthcare facilities
- **All-hazard disaster management plan**: General plan that is not hazard-specific

## Emergency Response Plans

Emergency response plans must include plans for communication, resources and assets available, safety and security measures, responsibilities of staff, utilities, and measure to support clinical activities.

### *Bomb Threats*

The response to a **bomb threat** depends on the type of bomb threat and the information gleaned from the threat. The first response is to notify the police and designated staff via landlines (avoiding cell phones, which can trigger some devices) or overhead paging. An initial search may be carried out by staff in each area to try to locate possible bombs. Administration should make the decision about evacuation, and plans for evacuation should be in place. With terrorist bombing and improvised explosive devices (IEDs), situational awareness is critical because multiple explosive devices (some undetonated) may be at the scene. IEDs may be inside backpacks, suitcases, and packages left unattended. Additionally, people wearing suicide vests or belts may mix in with other victims or people escaping the blast area.

### *Active Shooters*

Medical facilities can be targets of active shooters given their accessibility to a large number of people combined with the possibility of trauma experienced within a medical facility that may motivate a shooter. Every medical facility, particularly hospitals, must have a plan for responding to an active shooter due to the amount of damage that may be done in the small amount of time before local law enforcement can respond to the distress call. Plans should begin with education to all employees of the facility, often using the Run (evacuate the space, helping others if possible), Hide (if unable to evacuate, find a spot to hide that is out of view and ideally can be locked or blocked), Fight (if unable to evacuate or hide, take action against the shooter) method. The Department of Homeland Security also recommends the formation of an Emergency Action Plan (EAP) for active shooters, which include the preferred method(s) for reporting a shooter to authorities, evacuation plans, training, and prevention/monitoring measures.



### *Natural Disasters*

Plans vary according to type of **natural disaster**. If anticipated, extra food, clothing, and supplies should be stockpiled for both clients and staff (who may be required to stay at the facility for extended periods). A command structure should be in place. With a hurricane or tornado, clients may need to be moved away from windows and to more secure areas, such as interior hallways, during the storm. The hospital must prepare plans to evacuate clients if necessary (such as with flooding, earthquakes, or storm damage) and transfer them to other facilities and must also be prepared for an influx of clients.

### *Community Planning*

Healthcare providers, such as hospitals, should work closely with the community to identify community resources that are available for emergency response and the needs that may arise in response to disasters, including the number of people who may depend on the hospital for care.

**Review Video: Emergency Response, Business Continuity, and Disaster Planning**
Visit mometrix.com/academy and enter code: 678024

## ICS

The **Incident Command System** (ICS) was developed by the Department of Homeland Security as a part of the **National Incident Management System**. It is a highly organized, hierarchical disaster management system that focuses on planning and organization, communication and delegation of responsibility, as well as response evaluation so that any disaster or emergency response effort runs as smoothly as possible. An **Incident Commander (IC)** is established as the person in charge. Safety officers, operations section officers, planning officers, and logistics officers are all appointed. These different officer positions are responsible for reporting back to the IC.

## Multiple-Casualty Incidents Versus Mass-Casualty Incidents

**Multiple-casualty incidents** involve more than one person, but different jurisdictions may quantify the total number of persons differently. It usually refers to the following:

- An incident involving at least three patients
- An incident involving only one jurisdiction and only one to three agencies (ambulance, fire department, and police)
- An incident requiring triage, but generally only primary triage
- Standards of care are maintained, and all patients not coded black (deceased) are transported for care

**Mass-casualty incidents** also involve more than one person, but may involve much larger numbers—dozens, if not hundreds to thousands.

- Often involves multiple jurisdictions and agencies
- Requires triage but may also involve separate waiting areas for color-coded individuals and secondary triage
- Standards of care may be modified, and patients coded black (expectant) and not expected to live may be left in the field and/or receive delayed care if they are still living after the red- and yellow-coded individuals are transported

## Principles of Triage During Mass Casualty Events

**Primary triage** is a rapid method (30-60 seconds) of prioritizing clients based on severity of condition and carried out at the scene of multiple casualty incidents. All clients are triaged and tagged according to international color-coding priority (P) guidelines on foot or wrist (not clothing):

- **P1—Red**: Immediate care needed for urgent systemic life-threatening conditions, such as airway/breathing problems, severe bleeding, severe burns (especially with breathing problems), decreased mental status, shock, and severe medical problems, Glasgow Coma Score ≤13.
- **P2—Yellow**: Delayed care and able to wait 45-60 minutes for treatment. Conditions include burns (without breathing problems), multiple bone/joint injuries, back and/or spinal cord injuries (unless in respiratory distress).
- **P3—Green**: Hold, able to wait hours for treatment of minor injuries.
- **P4—Black**: Deceased or with injuries so extensive that they are not survivable.

Resource management involves identifying a triage officer, who remains at the scene during the event, and identifying the need for additional personnel and equipment and providing those to the clients with the highest priority.

## Identifying Clients to Discharge in Disaster Situations

In the event of a **disaster situation**, the surge capacity of a hospital may need to increase markedly with a large influx of clients in need of emergency care and hospitalization, so appropriate clients must be quickly identified for possible discharge. All elective admissions and procedures should be cancelled and non-critical clients, such as those with non-life-threatening conditions or those near discharge, should be discharged or transferred to other facilities if possible. Generally, hospitalists, charge nurses, or team leaders may be in the best position to identify clients for discharge as well as the person tasked with monitoring length of stay. If an acuity-based model of client care is utilized, then those already categorized as the least acute should be quickly assessed for discharge. Ideally, each unit should have plans in place for rapid discharge so that assessment and discharge can be carried out quickly and safely.

## Terrorism

Terrorism is defined as the use of violence (or threat of violence) to frighten and coerce governments or societies into accepting the instigator's (terrorists) **demands**. The demands and goals of terrorists are often extreme and focused on areas with high population densities. This means that large companies can become potential targets of a terrorist attack. For this reason, when developing an emergency preparedness/disaster management plan, terrorist attacks should be included as a potential disaster. There are many different possible ways that terrorists can strike. Some examples are weapons of mass destruction, biological agents (i.e., bacteria, viruses, or toxins), nuclear and radiological incidents, incendiary devices, chemicals, and explosive devices.

## Organizational Plan for Bioterrorism

The ICP and the infection control team should develop specific plans for dealing with different **bioterrorism** agents, and training should be provided to staff. An organized approach should include the following:

- Be on the alert for possible bioterrorism-related infections, based on clusters of patients or symptoms.
- Use personal protection equipment, including respirators when indicated.
- Complete thorough assessment of patient, including medical history, physical examination, immunization record, and travel history.
- Provide a probable diagnosis based on symptoms and lab findings, including cultures.
- Provide treatment, including prophylaxis, while waiting for laboratory findings.
- Use transmission precautions as well as isolation for suspected biologic agents.
- Notify local, state, and federal authorities per established protocol.
- Conduct surveillance and epidemiological studies to identify at-risk populations.
- Develop plans to accommodate large numbers of patients:
    - Restricting elective admissions
    - Transferring patients to other facilities



## B-NICE Hazardous Material Incidents Associated with Terrorist Attacks

| Category | Response |
|---|---|
| **B—Biological (bacteria, viruses, fungi, toxins)** | Inhalation type—evacuate for 80 feet, shut down air-handling systems, wear appropriate PPE and SCBA, and avoid contamination.<br>Visible agent—decontaminate with soap and water. Symptoms may vary but are usually delayed. |
| **N—Nuclear/ Radiological** | Inhalation type (most common)—Isolate/Secure the area, avoid smoke/fumes, stay upwind, and use PPE and SCBA. Isolate victims and decontaminate as appropriate. Symptoms are usually delayed. |
| **I—Incendiary** | Be on alert for multiple devices and sabotaged fire suppression equipment. Symptoms include burns, pain, and trauma. |
| **C—Chemical** | Isolate/Secure the area, decontaminate victims with soap and water, and be on alert for chemical dispersal devices. Approach toward uphill and upwind. Isolate symptomatic patients from others. Symptoms vary but may include burns, blistering, vomiting, breathing difficulty, and neurological damage. |
| **E—Explosives** | Be alert for secondary devices, undetonated devices, and secondary hazards (unstable buildings and debris). Remove victims from the area, secure the perimeter, and stage away from the incident area. Decontaminate as necessary. Symptoms include burns, amputations, cuts, and penetrating and blunt trauma. |

## All-Hazards Safety Approach to Mass-Casualty Incidents

The all-hazards safety approach to mass-casualty incidents aims to provide plans that can be used to deal with all types of hazards (natural disasters, terrorist attacks, and mass-casualty incidents) as well as encompassing the four components of emergency management: mitigation, preparedness, response, and recovery. Organizations in an area coordinate to develop joint action plans that can be activated in response to incidents, with the chain of command clearly outlined. This approach lowers costs to individual organizations and provides for faster and more effective response. However, although the basic structure may be the same for responding to all hazards, there are inevitable differences between (for example) a terrorist attack with active shooters and a natural disaster, such as a hurricane, which can be anticipated and mitigated to some degree. For this reason, modifying existing incident action plans to meet the needs of a situation is essential.

## Disaster Recovery Aspect of Disaster Planning and Management

Disaster recovery is the final stage of any disaster response and deals with the actions necessary to return the disaster site to normal. The recovery effort can be divided into **two different periods**:

- The **restoration period** is an immediate recovery step in which the area is made safe, utilities repaired, wreckage removed, and evacuees are allowed to return.
- The **reconstruction/replacement period** is a longer process where the disaster area is rebuilt and returned to its pre-disaster condition, both physically and economically. The reconstruction period can take many years, and is dependent on the degree of damage and availability of resources for reconstruction efforts.

As a part of the disaster recovery process, steps should be taken to prevent a recurrence of the disaster in the future.

## Security Plan

A security plan is a plan that is set in place to help guide the actions of employees in case of a breach in security at a healthcare facility. All employees must be educated and comfortable with their facilities plan, in order to facilitate the safety of staff and patients alike. The security plan usually has several components:

- **Security workers**: Most facilities have securities guards who patrol the campus and help maintain patient and visitor safety. If a patient/visitor threatens violence or becomes combative, security should be called immediately.
- **Silent alarms**: Most units have "silent alarms," which are usually buttons or switches underneath the secretary's desk or in some other discreet location. These are pushed in the case of a threat to security in which a call cannot safely be made.
- **Locked units**: Certain units in the hospital (such as mother/baby, critical care units, psychiatric floors, etc.) are locked and require an access code to enter.
- **Do not acknowledge**: Certain patients may be deemed as "do not acknowledge," meaning that the nurse cannot give out any information regarding these patients, including acknowledging the patients' presence in the facility. Examples include psychiatric patients, victims of crime, celebrities, and others. If someone calls asking about the patient, it is appropriate and ethical for the nurse to state, "I do not have any information regarding a patient with that name."
- **Overhead announcements**: Many facilities have different codes that they may call overhead to alert staff of emergences/safety threats without overt language.
- **Newborn nursery security**: Measures include matching ID bands for infant and parents/caregivers, foot-printing and photographing the infant after birth, transporting infants in bassinets rather than carrying them, utilizing a tracking and security alarm system that can trigger automatic lockdown, limiting access to obstetrics and nursery areas, having staff wear easily-identifiable ID badges, and utilizing video surveillance.
- **Violence prevention**: Measures include educating staff about de-escalation techniques, having an alarm system in place, providing adequate security, utilizing video surveillance, limiting access, identifying clients who may be at risk for behaving violently, and requiring visitors' badges.
- **Controlled access**: Measures include locked areas that require a password, biologic ID (fingerprint, eye scan), access card for entry, turnstiles at entry and/or metal detectors, security personal stationed at entry points, and video surveillance of entries, exits, stairwells, hallways, elevators, and storage areas.

### *Principles of Evacuation in a Security Plan*

Principles of evacuation in a security plan, according to OSHA, should include:

- Conditions that would trigger an evacuation
- Chain of command for decision making
- Procedures for evacuation, including methods of evacuation and preferred routes. Exits should be clearly identified
- Procedures for assisting clients who are disabled and those who do not speak English
- Procedures for determining who are responsible for terminating critical operations
- Procedures for tracking personnel and clients
- Transportation plans for transferal of clients to other facilities

The path of least resistance is an important concept to understand for evacuation, especially if they involve fire and any products of combustion (smoke, heat, gas). Fire's path of least resistance is usually vertical, although fire also spreads horizontally, especially if a vertical path is not available. Water, on the other hand, also flows vertically, but downward and then horizontally if the downward flow is blocked. Clients should be evacuated according to the path of least resistance; that is, the route that is the easiest and safest.



# Hazardous Materials

## Hazardous Materials

Hazardous materials, those that are ignitable, corrosive, reactive, or toxic, are any that are harmful to humans or the environment and may be solids, liquids, solid gases, or sludges. Hazardous wastes are generally transported by hazardous waste transporters in special hazardous waste containers to Treatment Storage and Disposal Facilities (TSDFs) where they are stored, inactivated, and/or recycled. Each facility should have a plan in place for appropriate **handling of hazardous materials**:

- Staff must be trained in safe handling of hazardous materials with training repeated at least annually.
- Appropriate personal protective equipment (PPE) should be available for staff members handling hazardous materials.
- Hazardous materials should be clearly labeled for easy identification.
- All hazardous materials must be safely and securely stored in appropriate environmental temperatures and conditions.
- Safety Data Sheets (SDS) must be readily available for all hazardous materials.
- Decontamination procedures must be reviewed and appropriate decontamination facilities (such as eyewash stations and showers) must be available.
- Records must be maintained for any accidental exposures (with or without injury) and reported to the appropriate authorities.

### *Biohazard Symbol*

### Biological/Biohazardous Waste

Biological wastes are those that contain or are contaminated with pathogens (human, plant, animal); rDNA; and blood, cell, or tissue products; and cultures. Biological wastes that are, or may, be infectious or rDNA contaminated (biohazardous waste) must be inactivated before disposal in hazardous waste containers. Typically, inactivation is carried out with autoclaving or treating with hypochlorite solution (bleach). Contaminated sharps must be maintained in special sharps containers to avoid injury to handlers, and inactivated before disposal. Non-infectious biological wastes, such as uncontaminated gloves, do not require deactivation and are disposed of in biological waste containers.

### Routes Biological Hazards May Take to Enter the Body

Biological hazards may **enter the body** through the following avenues:

- Airborne (through the nasal passage into the lungs)
- Ingestion (eating/drinking)
- Subcutaneous (broken skin/open wounds)
- Percutaneous (through intact skin)
- Mucosal (through the lining of the mouth and nose)

### Cleaning up Small Blood Spills

The best way to clean a small blood spill is to absorb the blood with a paper towel or gauze pad. Then disinfect the area with a disinfectant. Soap and water are not considered a disinfectant nor is alcohol. Never scrape a dry spill; this may cause an aerosol of infectious organisms. If blood is dried, use the disinfectant to moisten the dried blood.

### Internal Radiation Therapy

Internal radiation therapy **(brachytherapy)** may be utilized to treat a variety of cancers, including prostate, breast, and cervical cancer. Radiation implants may be permanent or temporary. Temporary implants may have high-dose radiation (HDR) or low-dose radiation (LDR). Systemic brachytherapy may be administered per IV with radioactive isotopes; intraluminal and intracavity, per catheters or tubes; and interstitial, per seeds, needles, small implants, or wires. Symptoms relate to the area being irradiated, but the skin and GI tract are usually the most sensitive. Bone marrow suppression may occur if the source of radiation is near bone marrow, and patients may experience fatigue and weakness. Because patients emit radiation during therapy, safeguards include:

- Specific limitations and safeguards posted at room by x-ray department outlining requirements, such as time limits for contact time
- Visitors limited to non-pregnant adults who must be 6 feet from the patient and remain in room no longer than 30 minutes each day
- Staff, limited to those who are non-pregnant, wear dosimeters for contact with patient
- Patient placed in private room
- Staff limit time in room to only that necessary to carry out care (in accordance with posted guidelines)

# Infection Control

## Nosocomial Infections

Nosocomial infections are those that are hospital-acquired and present after 48 hours in the hospital. The following is a list of pathogenic agents that cause the most common nosocomial infections.

- *Enterococci* infections include urinary infections, bacteremia, endocarditis as well as infections in wounds and the abdominal and pelvic areas.
- *Enterobacteriaceae* cause about half of the urinary tract infections and a quarter of the postoperative infections.
- *Escherichia coli* primarily causes urinary tract infections (especially related to catheters), diarrhea, and neonatal meningitis but it can also lead to pneumonia, and bacteremia (usually secondary to urinary infection).
- Group B β-hemolytic *Streptococci* (GBS) has increasingly been a cause of infections in neonatal units, causing pneumonia, meningitis, and sepsis. GBS infections may occur as wound infections after Cesarean sections, especially in those immunocompromised.
- *Staphylococcus aureus* is a major cause of nosocomial post-operative infections, both localized and systemic, and from indwelling tubes and devices.
- Methicillin-resistant *Staphylococcus aureus (MRSA)* is a common cause of surgical infections.
- *Clostridioides difficile* causes more nosocomial diarrhea cases than any other microorganism.
- *Candida*, a yeast fungal pathogen, can overgrow and lead to mucocutaneous or cutaneous lesions and sepsis.
- *Aspergillus* spp., filamentous fungi, produce spores that become airborne and can invade the respiratory tract, causing pneumonia.
- *Pseudomonas aeruginosa* is a common causative agent of ventilator-associated pneumonia (VAP), catheter-associated UTIs (CAUTIs), and multidrug resistance.

## Catheter-Related Infections

Intravenous catheter-related infections are a significant cause of morbidity and mortality in the hospital setting. Usually, these infections are due to *Staphylococcus aureus*, *enterococcus*, or fungal infection such as *Candida*. These infections are important because they may progress and eventually lead to bacteremia, infective endocarditis, septic pulmonary emboli, septic shock, osteomyelitis, or superficial thrombophlebitis. Therefore, vigilance should be maintained to prevent these infections. The patient may exhibit fevers, chills, and discomfort around the catheter site. The site itself may show purulence or erythema. The subclavian vein is the preferred intravenous site and the femoral is the least-preferred site due to high infection rates. Infections are diagnosed with blood cultures and catheter tip cultures. Initial treatment generally includes removal of the catheter and antibiotic treatment. Antibiotics should be empiric at first, then directed toward culture results. Treatment duration is dependent on the causative agent and the severity of infection.

## Infection Control Measures

**Standard infection control** measures are designed to prevent transmission of microbial substances between patients and/or medical providers. These measures are indicated for everyone and include frequent handwashing, gloves whenever bodily fluids are involved, and face shields and gowns when splashes are anticipated. For more advanced control with tuberculosis, SARS, vesicular rash disorders (such as VZV), and most recently COVID-19, **airborne precautions** should be instituted to prevent the spread of tiny droplets that can remain suspended in the air for days and travel throughout a hospital environment. Therefore, negative pressure rooms are essential, and providers should wear high-efficiency N95 masks and be fitted in advance. Patients should wear surgical masks when transported. For disorders such as influenza or other infections spread by droplets (spread by cough or sneeze) basic surgical masks should be worn (**droplet precautions**) with eye protection when in close range to the patient or when splashes may be possible. For **contact precautions** in the setting of fecally transmitted infection or vesicular rash diseases (which require both airborne and contact precautions), gowns and gloves should be used and contact limited. White coats are not a substitute for proper gowning. In the case of a *Clostridioides difficile* infection, contact precautions should be used in addition to washing hands with soap and water (rather than alcohol-based hand sanitizer) after patient contact.

## Infection Control and Surveillance Plan

The purpose of an infection control/surveillance plan should be clearly outlined and may be multifaceted, including the following elements:

- **Decreasing rates of infection**: The primary purpose of a surveillance plan is to identify a means to decrease healthcare-associated infections, including a notification system and laboratory surveillance.
- **Evaluating infection control measures**: Surveillance can evaluate effectiveness of infection control measures. (Surgical checklists, hand hygiene, housekeeping, ventilation).
- **Establishing endemic threshold rates**: Establishing threshold rates can help to enact control measures to reduce rates.
- **Identifying outbreaks**: About 5–10% of infections occur in outbreaks, and comparing data with established endemic threshold rates can help to identify these outbreaks if analysis is done in a regular and timely manner.
- **Achieving staff compliance**: Objective evidence may convince staff to cooperate with infection control measures.
- **Meeting accreditation standards**: Some accreditation agencies require reports of infection rates.
- **Providing defense for malpractice suits**: Providing evidence that a facility is proactive in combating infections can decrease liability.
- **Comparing infection rates with other facilities**: Comparing data helps focus attention and resources.

## Protocol for Needlestick Injury and Postexposure Prophylaxis

If the healthcare provider experiences a **needlestick injury**, the individual's initial response should be to irrigate the wound with soap and water. As soon as possible, the incident must be reported to a supervisor and steps taken according to established protocol. This may include testing and/or prophylaxis, depending on the patient's health history, the exposure type, and the fluid involved. In some cases, the patient may also be tested for communicable diseases, such as HIV, in order to determine the risk to the healthcare provider. PEP (post-exposure prophylaxis) is available for exposure to HIV (human immunodeficiency virus) and hepatitis B virus (hepatis B immune globulin and HBV vaccination if needed). However, no PEP is available for HCV (hepatitis C virus) although the CDC does provide a plan for management. PEP should be initiated within 72 hours of exposure. All testing and treatments associated with the needlestick injury must be provided free of cost at a hospital or medical facility.

# Infectious Diseases

## Viral Infections

### *Herpes Simplex Virus Infections*

There are 2 types of the herpes simplex virus (HSV), human herpesvirus 1 and 2. **HSV-1** usually causes a **gingivostomatitis** (often referred to as "cold sores" or "fever blisters") and is transmitted through **close contact**. **HSV-2** usually causes painful **genital lesions** through **sexual contact**. Either may be found in other areas of the body.

- **Incubation** period is around 2–12 days.
- The primary infection is usually more severe (causes systemic **symptoms**) than the reactivated infection, but it may be asymptomatic. After the primary infection, the virus remains dormant in the nerve ganglia, and can be reactivated especially during times of stress, illness, immunosuppression, or sun exposure. While patients are most contagious during times of active lesions, the disease may be spread while asymptomatic. The frequency of the outbreaks usually decreases over time.
- HSV **lesions** are grouped vesicles with an erythematous base. They are usually painful, and a prodrome of tingling, pain, or burning sensations may be felt hours to a couple days before the eruption. Lesions last for approximately 2–3 weeks in primary infection (up to 4 weeks with genital HSV), and 1–2 weeks in recurrent infections.
- HSV is **diagnosed** clinically and confirmed with a + culture, a PCR test, or both.
- Symptomatic **treatment**, proper wound care, and antivirals (acyclovir, valacyclovir, or famciclovir) may be given.
- **Complications** include perinatal infection, keratitis, herpetic whitlow, herpes gladiatorum, secondary infections, and encephalitis.

### *Epstein-Barr Infection*

Epstein-Barr virus (EBV) is a **herpesvirus** (human herpesvirus 4) and is responsible for causing **infectious mononucleosis**. After the initial infection, it remains latent in B cells and epithelial cells. It has been linked to certain epithelial and lymphatic neoplasms (e.g., nasopharyngeal carcinoma, Burkitt lymphoma, Hodgkin lymphoma).

- EBV is **transmitted** through **body fluids** like saliva, so it is sometimes referred to as the kissing disease. It is most common in teenagers and college-age young adults
- **Incubation** period is typically 30–50 days.
- **Symptoms** of EBV infection range from being asymptomatic to swollen painful lymph nodes, pharyngitis (can mimic strep pharyngitis), extreme fatigue, fever, and possibly hepatosplenomegaly. The WBC count is elevated (~10,000–20,000 cells/mL) with 10–30% atypical lymphocytes in the differential.
- Confirm **diagnosis** with a Mono Spot test or EBV antibody serology tests.
- **Treatment** is supportive, and antibiotics are not helpful in treating this viral infection. Therefore, avoid unnecessary antibiotics in those with EBV, especially since administration of ampicillin or amoxicillin is often associated with a pruritic, maculopapular rash. Analgesics, warm salt water gargles, increased fluid intake, and rest will help to relieve some of the symptoms. Symptoms may last for several weeks and fatigue may last even longer. Patients should avoid contact sports for up to 2 months.
- **Complications** include hepatitis, cytopenias (e.g., thrombocytopenia), Guillain Barré syndrome, and splenic rupture.

### *Measles, Mumps, and Rubella*

**Measles (rubeola) virus** is highly contagious, is spread through **respiratory secretions** (incubation is 7–14 days), and peaks in late winter to spring. It causes a prodrome of high fever (4–7 days), cough, congestion, conjunctivitis; then Koplik spots (pathognomonic), and finally a maculopapular rash (spreads cephalocaudally). Report suspected cases immediately to the health dept. **Diagnose** with a + IgM antibody test (collected after 3 days of rash), viral culture, or PCR. **Treatment** is supportive.

**Mumps (parotitis)** is a viral infection that is spread via **saliva** (incubation is 12–24 days), and often occurs during winter and spring. It causes painful swelling of the salivary glands (parotid). Report to health dept. Supportive **treatment**. Complications include orchitis (infertility), pancreatitis, and meningitis.

**Rubella (German measles)** is a virus that spreads via **respiratory droplets** (incubation is 2–3 weeks), and peaks in the spring. There is a mild prodrome (fever, aches, sore throat, conjunctivitis, swollen nodes [esp. suboccipital, postauricular, & posterior cervical]), then a maculopapular rash (face first, then down). Report to health dept. Confirm with rubella antibodies IgM or IgG. Symptomatic care.

### *Influenza*

Influenza is a highly contagious viral infection that affects the entire **respiratory system** from the nose to the lungs. There are 3 types of **influenza virus**: **A** (causes epidemics), **B** (only in humans), and **C**. Types A and B are seen most often and are the strains that the annual flu vaccine is most effective against; and type C is not as common and much less severe.

- Prevention is key and annual, age-appropriate influenza **vaccines** should be given to those ≥6 months; 2 vaccines are required in first-time vaccine patients if 6 mo. through 8-year-olds (separated by 28 days).
- **Incubation** period is 1–4 days and it is spread via respiratory droplets.
- Though **symptoms** can be very similar, the flu and the common cold differ in that the flu has a very sudden onset. Symptoms of influenza include a high fever (may last up to 5 days), headache, myalgias, dry cough, rhinorrhea, and fatigue. There may also be vomiting and diarrhea, although children are more prone to this.
- Clinical judgment, community patterns, and rapid influenza tests (high specificity, but lower sensitivity) aid in **diagnosis**, but RT-PCR or viral culture definitively confirm the diagnosis; pulse oximetry and CXR as needed for pulmonary issues.
- Antibiotic **treatment** is not effective unless there is a secondary bacterial infection (e.g., pneumonia). Look for signs of secondary infections (e.g., dyspnea, cyanosis, fever that goes away and returns, confusion/lethargy). Supportive treatment with rest, fluids, and analgesics. Antivirals should be considered in those who are at high risk (<5 years old, elderly, pregnant, chronic conditions). These are most effective if initiated within 24–48 hours of symptom onset. The neuraminidase inhibitors (oseltamivir, zanamivir) treat type A, type B, and avian H5N1. There is extensive resistance to the adamantanes (amantadine, rimantadine) so they are rarely used.
- **Complications** include pneumonia, ARDS, and death.

### *Coronavirus*

A coronavirus is a common virus that causes cold-like symptoms, including a cough, runny nose, sore throat, and congestion. Most cases of coronavirus are not dangerous and are often given little attention or go entirely unnoticed. However, specific coronavirus strains have led to two worldwide pandemics. The first, **severe acute respiratory syndrome (SARS)**, appeared in China in 2002 and quickly spread worldwide. Presenting symptoms of SARS were fever, cough, dyspnea, and general malaise. It was extremely virulent, spreading easily from person to person through close contact by way of contaminated droplets produced by coughing or sneezing. SARS was also very deadly, with a case fatality rate of nearly 10%. High rates of infection occurred in health care workers and others in contact with infected patients, so prompt diagnosis and proper isolation were essential. By 2004, there were no longer any documented active cases of SARS.

The most recent coronavirus outbreak was the **COVID-19** strain, which first appeared in China in 2019 and quickly became a global pandemic. Presentation of COVID-19 was similar to that of SARS, with the notable additional symptom of acute loss of taste/smell as a unique identifier.

**Precautions** to take when treating patients with COVID-19 include the following:

- Contact and droplet precautions, including eye protection and appropriate personal protection equipment.
- Airborne precautions (recommended by the CDC), especially with aerosol-producing procedures (ventilators, nebulizers, intubation).
- Activity restrictions of exposed health care workers planned in coordination with public health officials.



### *Cytomegalovirus*

Cytomegalovirus (CMV) is a herpes virus, occurring in most people by the time they are adults.

- **Transmission** can occur through secretions during personal contact and from mother to baby before, during or after birth.
- Most cases have no **symptoms**, although a few infants will have fetal damage, such as jaundice, hepatitis, brain damage, or growth retardation.
- **Treatment** for those with severe infections is with ganciclovir, an antiviral drug.

### *Respiratory Syncytial Virus*

Respiratory syncytial virus (RSV) is a virus that infects the respiratory tract, causing symptoms of nasal congestion, cough, sore throat, and headache. Severe cases can lead to high fever, breathing difficulties, severe cough, and cyanosis.

- Respiratory syncytial virus may **manifest** as a cold in adults and older children; however, there are some children who are more at risk of developing complications.
- **Transmission** is through contact with droplets from an infected person's nose or throat, generally through coughing and sneezing.
- Infants born prematurely, children with chronic lung disease, children with cystic fibrosis, and children who are in an immunocompromised state because of surgery or illness are at **high risk** of breathing difficulties, poor oxygenation, and even death from RSV.

Vaccination for RSV is now recommended for at-risk populations, including pregnant women, infants who are less than 8 months old and entering into season of high RSV spread (fall to spring), adults ages 60–74 with increased risk for complications, and all adults ages 75 and older. Vaccination may not prevent the disease, but will lessen its severity.

### *Fifth Disease*

Fifth disease, or **erythema infectiosum**, is a viral illness caused by parvovirus B19. It is most prevalent in the spring, with outbreaks in preschools, daycares, and elementary schools.

- The **incubation** period is 4-20 days, and it may be communicable for several days before the rash appears.
- **Transmission** occurs through oral and nasal secretions and possibly blood.
- **Symptoms** are possible fever, headache, nasal congestion, general unwell feeling, and rash starting on the cheeks (slapped cheek appearance). The rash typically spreads to the rest of the body as a lacy red rash that may come and go for up to a month.

- Use over-the-counter fever medications as needed and provide **supportive care**.
- The virus can cause fetal death if contracted during pregnancy. There is no vaccine for fifth disease, and because it is a viral infection, it is not treated with antibiotics.

### *Chickenpox*

Chickenpox (Varicella) is a viral infection, most prevalent in the late winter and early spring in children under 10 years of age.

- It has an **incubation** period of 10-21 days and is communicable from 1-2 days before the rash appears to after all lesions have dried up.
- **Transmission** is through direct contact and contact with respiratory droplets.
- **Symptoms** are low fever and feeling unwell, followed by the itchy rash (raised red bumps that develop vesicles which then ooze and crust over).
- The patient should be isolated until all lesions are dry. Aveeno baths and Benadryl help with the itching. Ibuprofen or acetaminophen can be used for the fever, and acyclovir is indicated in some cases. Encourage the patient not to scratch the lesions to prevent secondary infections. Provide supportive care as indicated.

### *Roseola*

Roseola is a viral illness, most prevalent in children 6-24 months of age.

- The **incubation** period is about 9 days.
- **Transmission** may be through oral and nasal.
- The illness begins with a high fever for 3-5 days; the patient appears well otherwise. The fever drops and then the rash appears. The rash is a light pink maculopapular rash which lasts 1-2 days.
- Parents should **treat the fever** as needed with anti-inflammatory medications.

### *Poliomyelitis*

Poliomyelitis (commonly referred to as **polio**) is caused by an enterovirus and occurs most often in babies and young children.

- The **incubation** period is 3-14 days, and transmission occurs through direct contact with respiratory secretions and the oral-fecal route.
- The **symptoms** are slight fever, sore throat, general malaise, nausea and vomiting, headache, stomach ache, and constipation, but there can be severe pain, muscular weakness, and then paralysis.
- There are no drug therapies for polio. Observe for respiratory distress, provide general support measures, and provide for physical therapy.

### *Rotavirus*

Rotavirus is a viral illness that causes diarrhea, fever, and vomiting in children.

- It can be extremely **contagious** within groups where large numbers of children are present, such as in daycare centers, preschools, pediatric offices, clinics, and children's units in hospitals.
- Rotavirus can be prevented through **immunization** with a vaccine, as recommended by the American Academy of Pediatrics. Immunization can prevent up to 98% of severe cases of the illness.
- Children should wash their hands before eating and after using the bathroom to avoid spreading the disease. Caregivers should wash their hands before preparing food, after changing diapers, and after using the bathroom; they should avoid letting small children place toys or other items in their mouths and should disinfect surfaces after use.

## Bacterial Infections

### Diphtheria

Diphtheria, caused by ***Corynebacterium diphtheriae***, is most prevalent in fall and winter.

- The **incubation** period is 2–7 days, possibly longer, and transmission is through direct contact with nasal, eye, and oral secretions.
- The **symptoms** are slight fever, nasal discharge, sore throat, feeling unwell, poor appetite, and swelling of the airway.
- If the disease is severe, death can result. The patient requires isolation, bed rest, fluids, antibiotics, medication for fever, and an antitoxin. The patient may also require oxygen therapy and tracheostomy if the airway is obstructed.

### Tetanus

Tetanus, caused by ***Clostridium tetani***, occurs all over the world. The spores formed by the bacillus are present in soil, dust, and the GI tracts of animals and humans.

- The **incubation** period is 3–21 days.
- **Symptoms** start with headache, irritability, jaw muscle spasms, and inability to open the mouth. This is followed by severe back muscle spasms, seizures, incontinence, and fever.
- **Treatment** requires human tetanus immune globulin, penicillin G, Valium, and placement on a ventilator. The environment should be kept quiet because the spasms are initiated by stimuli.

### Scarlet Fever

Scarlet fever, caused by **group A beta-hemolytic streptococci**, is most prevalent in school-age children during the fall, winter, and spring.

- The **incubation** period is 1-7 days, and transmission occurs through direct or indirect contact with oral and nasal secretions.
- The illness begins with a high fever, very sore throat, headache, malaise, chills and possibly vomiting and stomach pain. A rash appears in about 12 hours as sandpapery red pinpoints in creases of the skin, flushed face and then a strawberry tongue.
- Antibiotics will be prescribed, but patients should be isolated until taking the antibiotic for 24 hours. Analgesics are needed to bring down the fever and the patient should be encouraged to drink plenty of fluids.

### Whooping Cough

Whooping cough, caused by ***Bordetella pertussis* bacillus**, is most prevalent in infants and children who were not immunized.

- The **incubation** period is 6-20 days, and transmission occurs through direct contact with oral and nasal secretions.
- The **symptoms** are cold symptoms for 1-2 weeks, when the cough will worsen and progress to a whoop sound, usually occurring at night. Vomiting will usually follow an episode of intense coughing. As the patient recovers, the coughing will subside. In babies, a mucus plug or apnea can result in death by respiratory arrest. Hospitalization is usually required for infants less than 6 months of age and those with a severe case of pertussis.
- The patient needs isolation and bed rest, with a calm, quiet environment to limit coughing spells. Fluid intake needs to be monitored and humidified air will help.
- Watch for signs of respiratory distress and give antibiotic and pertussis immune globulin as prescribed.

### *Impetigo*

Impetigo is a skin infection that is most commonly seen in preschool children or those in young childhood.

- Impetigo causes blister-like sores on skin areas that may already be compromised, such as under the nose, on the hands or neck, or in the diaper area. It is caused by a bacterial infection, most commonly *Staphylococcus aureus* or group A *Streptococcus*. The sores may itch or the patient may already have irritation at the site, such as a diaper rash.
- To **prevent the spread of infection**, children and caregivers should wash their hands frequently and avoid scratching the sores and then touching items. Isolation by staying home from school or daycare may be necessary until the sores have crusted over. Treating skin irritations, such as poison ivy or eczema, can also prevent infection from spreading to impetigo.

## Fungal Infections

### *Cryptococcosis*

Cryptococcosis is an infection resulting from inhaling the **fungus** *Cryptococcus neoformans,* which is found worldwide in soil (can be associated with bird droppings), or *Cryptococcus gattii,* which is associated with certain trees in the Northwest.

- Cryptococcosis is most often due to *C. neoformans*. It is often found among those with compromised immune systems and is an **AIDS-defining opportunistic infection**.
- Healthy patients may be asymptomatic and the only finding may be pulmonary lesions on CXR that resolve spontaneously. The fungus can disseminate and cause meningitis, encephalitis, cutaneous lesions, and affect long bones and other tissues. **Symptoms** are based on the area of involvement. Patients may experience cough, pleuritic chest pain, weight loss, and fever if there is pulmonary involvement; headache, double vision, light sensitivity, N/V, and confusion if CNS involvement; cutaneous lesions (papules, pustules, nodules, ulcers) if the skin is involved.
- **Diagnosis** includes microscopic analysis, culture (gold standard), or an antigen test (highly sensitive; good for detecting early infection) for *Cryptococcus* using CSF, tissue, sputum, blood, or urine. Check CSF by India ink (limited sensitivity) or culture so meningitis can be ruled out. Confirm that no mass lesion is present by CT or MRI before LP is performed.
- Mild cases may only require monitoring to ensure that the infection does not spread. In more advanced cases, the infection is treated with different antifungal medications (e.g., fluconazole for pulmonary infections, amphotericin B ± flucytosine for meningitis). The patient should also be monitored for CNS infection and medication side effects. AIDS patients may need lifelong antifungals.
- **Complications** include cryptococcal meningitis, neural deficits, optic nerve damage, and hydrocephalus.

### *Histoplasmosis*

Histoplasmosis is an infection caused by inhalation of **spores** from the fungus *Histoplasma capsulatum* that is found in soil and is associated with bird and bat droppings (e.g., chicken coops, caves).

- Healthy patients are usually asymptomatic and those with symptoms are typically immunocompromised or those who've had a heavy exposure to spores. The primary **pulmonary infection** occurs 3–17 days after exposure and can present with flu-like symptoms. It is typically self-limited but may become chronic. Histoplasmosis can also spread through the **blood** and can cause progressive disseminated disease in the immunocompromised (high mortality rate); this is an **AIDS-defining illness**.
- **Diagnose** through antigen tests (urine, serum), histopathology, or cultures; order a CXR. Mild and even moderate acute pulmonary histoplasmosis may resolve on its own.
- If needed, **treat** mild to moderate infections with itraconazole and severe illness with amphotericin B.

### *Pneumocystis*

Pneumocystis jiroveci is a **fungus** (previously known as *Pneumocystis* carinii) that causes **pneumonia** (PJP, previously PCP) in the immunocompromised. Most people have been exposed to this by the age of 3 or 4.

- **Symptoms** of PJP include a dry nonproductive cough, fever, dyspnea, and weight loss.
- CXR may show diffuse bilateral infiltrates or it may be normal; and pulse oximetry may be low, especially on exertion. **Diagnosis** is confirmed with sputum histopathology using sputum induction or bronchoalveolar lavage.
- **Treat** immediately with TMP-SMX (trimethoprim/sulfamethoxazole) for 21 days if HIV + and for 14 days in other cases. Steroids may be added for HIV patients with severe PJP. HIV/AIDS patients with CD4 counts <200/µL should receive PJP prophylaxis with TMP-SMX. Dapsone and pentamidine are alternatives.
- **Complications** include ARDS and death.



### *Candidal Infections*

*Candida* is a type of yeast that may cause a variety of infections:

- **Oral thrush** is commonly seen in diabetic patients and those who are immunosuppressed (HIV or underlying neoplasm). Patients often complain of burning on the tongue or in the mouth, associated with "curd-like" white patches that can be scraped away leaving reddish tissue underneath. Diagnosis is with KOH prep. Treatment is with oral or topical antifungals, including nystatin (swish and swallow or troches).
- **Candida esophagitis** also occurs in the immunosuppressed population, and patients may complain of dysphasia, odynophagia, and chest pain. This is diagnosed on EGD and may be treated with oral or IV antifungals (ketoconazole).
- **Candidal intertrigo**, or diaper rash, presents with beefy-red lesions at skin fold areas as well as satellite lesions. Treatment is with topical antifungals.
- **Candidemia** is diagnosed with fungal blood cultures and may lead to osteomyelitis, endocarditis, and other complications. Treatment is with IV antifungals.

### *Ringworm*

Ringworm is caused by an infection from the ***Tinea* fungus**, which produces patches on the skin that have normal centers, giving the appearance of a ring.

- The fungus can cause hair loss and patches of scaly skin that may develop blisters that ooze or crust.
- It is **transmitted** by touching the affected skin or through objects that have touched the affected skin.
- Ringworm may be **diagnosed** by viewing the skin section under a Wood's lamp. Skin cultures may also be taken for examination to identify the fungus. A potassium hydroxide (KOH) exam involves scraping the affected skin and placing the skin sample in KOH to test for the presence of the fungus.

## Vector-Borne and Parasitic Infections

### *Malaria*

Malaria is a **blood-borne disease** caused by a **parasite** from the genus *Plasmodium and* found in tropical areas. There are 4 known to cause disease in humans (*P. malariae, P. vivax, P. ovale,* and *P. falciparum*). These protozoa are transmitted by the **female *Anopheles* mosquito**. They travel to the **liver** where they multiply, are released, and then infect the RBCs, where they continue to multiply. Incubation time can be as little as 9 days or as much as multiple years depending on the species of the infecting parasite.

- **Signs/symptoms** include headache, high fever with shaking chills and sweating (rigors; occurs when merozoites, an immature form of the parasite, are released from RBCs), jaundice, anemia, and hepatosplenomegaly. Take a thorough history including recent travel.

- **Diagnose** with thin and thick blood smears (gold standard) stained with Giemsa (preferred). When smears are negative but infection is suspected, additional smears may be tested. Labs typically show elevated LDH, thrombocytopenia, and atypical lymphocytes. Rapid antigen tests are also available as well as PCR.
- **Treat** with chloroquine. If travelling, chemoprophylaxis depends on the area of travel due to species and resistance patterns, and may include chloroquine, primaquine, mefloquine, Malarone, or doxycycline. Report infections to your local or state health department.
- **Complications** include severe anemia and hemolysis, organ failure (liver, spleen, kidneys), cerebral malaria, ARDS, and death.

### *LYME DISEASE*

Lyme disease occurs from a bite from a **deer tick** (blacklegged tick) infected with the **spirochete bacterium** *Borrelia burgdorferi*. It is the most common tick-borne disease in the U.S. and is more prevalent in heavily wooded areas. Adult ticks are more active during colder times whereas the nymphs (<2 mm in size) are more active in the warm, spring or summer months. Once the tick bites, it stays attached; however, it takes about 36–48 hours for nymphs and about 48–72 hours for adult ticks before the spirochete is transmitted to the person. **Incubation** period is 3–30 days. There are 3 stages to this disease: early localized, early disseminated, and chronic disseminated.

- At **Stage 1**, 75% have the characteristic expanding red rash (erythema migrans; can be large, ~30cm) which can progress to have central clearing (bull's eye), headache, fever, chills, myalgias, and fatigue.
- **Stage 2** occurs weeks to months after initial infection and involves systemic symptoms (flu-like), neck stiffness, headaches, migrating pain in muscles and joints, rashes, paresthesias, Bell's palsy, confusion, fatigue, myocarditis, and heart palpitations.
- **Stage 3** occurs months to years after initial infection and involves neurologic (e.g., encephalitis) and rheumatologic issues, especially arthritis of large joints (e.g., knee).

**Review Video: Lyme Disease**
Visit mometrix.com/academy and enter code: 505529

#### DIAGNOSIS AND TREATMENT OF LYME DISEASE

Diagnose Lyme disease using 2-tiered testing: antibodies (IgM, IgG), then Western blot. Antibiotic treatment for localized Lyme disease involves 2–3 weeks of doxycycline, amoxicillin, or cefuroxime axetil is started immediately after diagnosis. IV antibiotics may be needed for severe disease (e.g., IV ceftriaxone). Prevention is key by wearing clothes covering the skin, using tick repellents, showering soon after being outdoors in tick-prone areas, and thoroughly checking for ticks (especially in hard to see areas by using a mirror). The Lyme vaccine is no longer available and previous vaccine recipients are still at risk of contracting the disease as protection decreases over time. Complications are prevalent with untreated Lyme disease and include chronic arthritis, fatigue, chronic musculoskeletal issues, acrodermatitis chronica atrophicans, and memory and concentration issues. Report cases to the local health dept.

### *ROCKY MOUNTAIN SPOTTED FEVER*

Rocky Mountain spotted fever is a tick-borne illness caused by **Rickettsia rickettsii**. It tends to occur in spring and summer throughout the United States.

- **Incubation** period is about one week.
- **Symptoms** include headache, fever, nausea, vomiting, loss of appetite, muscle pain, and rash on the ankles and wrists.
- **Treatment** requires an antibiotic, usually doxycycline.

### *ZIKA VIRUS IN PREGNANT WOMEN*

Zika virus is a **flavivirus** that is transmitted by the *Aedes* mosquito and through sexual contact. This virus can be passed on to an unborn baby causing severe congenital defects while causing mild or no disease in the mother. It is advised that all pregnant women avoid traveling to areas with the Zika virus (e.g., Central and South America, Mexico, Caribbean, Africa).

- **Incubation** period is 3–14 days and symptoms may last 4–7 days. The virus has been found to remain longer in semen than in other body fluids.
- If **symptoms** are present, they may include fever, headache, myalgias, arthralgias, a maculopapular rash, and conjunctivitis. Congenital defects include severe microcephaly, severe brain abnormalities, macular scarring, hearing loss, motor disabilities (e.g., hypertonia), and contractures. Women should be screened for Zika exposure at each prenatal visit.
- **Diagnostic** testing is recommended for all asymptomatic pregnant women who have continued exposure to Zika and for all symptomatic pregnant women who have possibly been exposed to the Zika virus. Testing includes RNA NAT testing on serum and urine, and serum IgM Zika antibody testing. Prenatal ultrasound helps determine if the effects of Zika are present. Report cases to the state health department; and the CDC can be consulted.
- There is **no treatment** or cure for the Zika virus.



### *HELMINTH INFESTATIONS*

Helminth infestations (worms) include **roundworms** [nematodes: *Ascaris*, hookworms (cause anemia), **filariae** (cause elephantiasis)] and **flatworms** [tapeworms (cause weight loss); **flukes** (intestinal or liver)]. **Pinworms** are a type of roundworm that cause enterobiasis and is the most common helminth infestation. Pinworms are more prevalent in warmer areas of the country and infestations occur more frequently in children. The worms lay eggs within the digestive tract and then travel to the anal area where they are usually found. Pinworms are highly contagious. As a patient itches the anal area where the eggs are located, the eggs cling to the fingers and can easily be transmitted to other people either directly or through food or surfaces. The eggs can survive for 2–3 weeks on inanimate objects.

- Patients may be asymptomatic or have intense anal itching that is usually worse at night and can cause insomnia. Abdominal pain, nausea, and vomiting can also occur.
- **Diagnose** with the "tape test" which involves pressing cellophane tape over the perianal area to pick up eggs or worms and examine under the microscope. Most other helminth infestations can be diagnosed with a stool sample for ova and parasites; filariasis requires a blood smear or antigen test.
- Anthelmintic medications are given in a single dose and repeated in 2 weeks to kill the pinworms and their larvae (mebendazole, albendazole, or pyrantel pamoate). The entire family and close contacts should be treated simultaneously since pinworms are so contagious.

### *GIARDIA LAMBLIA*

*Giardia lamblia* is a **protozoan** that infects water supplies and spreads to children through the fecal-oral route. It is the most common cause of non-bacterial diarrhea in the United States, causing about 20,000 cases of infection each year in all ages.

- Children often become infected after swallowing recreational waters (pools, lakes) while swimming or putting contaminated items into the mouth. *Giardia* live and multiply within the small intestine where cysts develop.
- **Symptoms** occur 7–14 days after ingestion of 1 or more cysts and include diarrhea with greasy floating stools (rarely bloody), stomach cramps, nausea, and flatulence, lasting 2–6 weeks. A chronic infection may develop that can last for months or years.
- **Treatment** includes furazolidone 5–8 mg/kg/day in 4 doses for 7–10 days or metronidazole 40 mg/kg/day in 3 doses for 7–10 days. Chronic infections are often very resistant to treatment.

### *Toxoplasmosis*

Toxoplasmosis is an infection caused by the **parasite *Toxoplasma gondii***, which is commonly found in soil. It is widespread and transmitted through cat feces; however, it also may be contracted by eating undercooked meat (especially pork, lamb, or venison) or poorly washed vegetables. Toxoplasmosis can cause serious disease and can affect various organs; and immunocompromised and pregnant women and their unborn babies are especially likely to have side effects of the disease (the "T" in congenital TORCH infections).

- Healthy patients are usually asymptomatic; however, once infected the parasite can remain latent until the patient becomes immunocompromised and the parasite is reactivated causing **symptoms**. The disease can cause a flu-like illness with fever, myalgias, and lymphadenopathy. More serious effects include retinochoroiditis, brain lesions, and encephalitis. Congenital toxoplasmosis may cause retinochoroiditis, microcephaly, hydrocephalus, intellectual disability, and possibly miscarriage or stillbirth.
- **Diagnose** with serology for *Toxoplasma* antibodies IgM and IgG. Also, PCR may be used to test amniotic fluid, CSF, or tissue.
- **Treat** with pyrimethamine (preferred) plus folinic acid or sulfadiazine plus folinic acid. Pregnant women should avoid high-risk practices like changing the cat litter and should avoid sand boxes.

## Chapter Quiz

Ready to see how well you retained what you just read? Scan the QR code to go directly to the chapter quiz interface for this study guide. If you're using a computer, simply visit the online resources page at **mometrix.com/resources719/nclexrn-31183** and click the Chapter Quizzes link.

# Health Promotion and Maintenance

## Immunizations

### Immunization vs. Vaccination

**Immunization** refers to the body's buildup of defenses (antibodies) against specific diseases. It has an important role in preventing the spread of infection. Immunization prevents the individual from contracting a disease or lessens the severity of the disease, and can also prevent the complications (encephalitis, hearing loss, paralysis) associated with the infectious diseases. **Vaccination** is one method of creating immunity through the introduction of a small amount of the virus's or bacteria's antigen to the body, which then stimulates the body's creation of antibodies against that disease. Vaccination prevents the spread of infection to infants who are too young to have developed immunity and to those who are immunocompromised (cancer patients, transplantation recipients). Herd immunity results from a majority of the population being immune to a disease, therefore minimizing transmission. It is defined in terms of the percentage of the population that must be immunized in order to prevent outbreaks. This percentage may range from 80-85% for some disorders, but those that are highly contagious, such as measles, may require a herd immunity of 93-95%. Herd immunity can be obtained via widespread vaccination or widespread infection, though it is not recommended that individuals avoid immunization and rely on herd immunity for protection, as rates of immunization vary from one community to another.

### Types of Vaccines

There are a number of different types of vaccines:

- **Conjugated forms**: An organism is altered and then joined (conjugated) with another substance, such as a protein, to potentiate immune response (such as conjugated Hib).
- **Killed virus vaccines**: The virus has been killed but can still cause an immune response (such as inactivated poliovirus).
- **Live virus vaccines**: The virus is live but in a weakened (attenuated) form so that it doesn't cause the disease but confers immunity (such as measles vaccine).
- **Recombinant forms**: The organism is genetically altered and, for example, may use proteins rather than the whole cell to stimulate immunity (such as Hepatitis B and acellular pertussis vaccine).
- **Toxoid**: A toxin (antigen) that has been weakened by the use of heat or chemicals so it is too weak to cause disease but stimulates antibodies.

Some vaccines are given shortly after birth; others begin at 2 months, 12 months, or 2 years and some later in childhood.

### DTaP and Tdap Vaccines

Diphtheria and pertussis (whooping cough) are highly contagious bacterial diseases of the upper respiratory tract. Cases of diphtheria are now rare in the United States, although they still occur in some developing countries. There have, however, been recent outbreaks of pertussis in the United States. Tetanus is a bacterial infection contracted through cuts, wounds, and scratches. The **diphtheria, tetanus, and pertussis (DTaP) vaccine** is recommended for all children. DTaP is a newer and safer version of the older DTP vaccine, which is no longer used in the United States. **Tdap** is the DTaP booster shot meant to continue immunity to these diseases through adulthood, given every 10 years starting at age 11.

DTaP requires 5 doses:

- 2 months
- 4 months
- 6 months
- 5-18 months
- 4-6 years (or at 11-12 years if booster missed between 4-6)

According to recent ACIP recommendations, DTaP may now also be administered to children ages 7-9 as part of a catch-up series, but children will then require their routine Tdap dose at age 11-12. If DTaP is administered to children ages 10-18 it can be counted as their adolescent Tdap booster. Adverse reactions can occur, but they are usually mild soreness, fever, and/or nausea. About 1 in 100 children will have high fever (>105 °F) and may develop seizures. Severe allergic responses can occur.

## HPV Vaccine

**Human papillomavirus (HPV)** comprises >100 viruses. About 40 are sexually transmitted and invade mucosal tissue, causing genital warts, which are low risk for cancer, or changes in the mucosa, which can lead to cervical cancer. Most HPVs cause little or no symptoms, but they are very common, especially in those 15-25. Over 99% of cervical cancers are caused by HPV and 70% are related to HPVs 16 and 18. The HPV vaccine, Gardasil, protects against HPVs 6 and 11 (which cause genital warts), along with 16 and 18, which can cause cancer. Protection is only conveyed if the female has not yet been infected with these strains. The vaccine is currently recommended for females under 26 but studies have determined that those not adequately covered over the age of 26 and up to 45 can benefit. A series of 3 injections is required over a 6-month period:

- Initial dose 11-12 years (but may be given as young as 9 or ≥18)
- 2 months after first dose
- 6 months after first dose

## PPV

**Pneumococcal polysaccharide-23 vaccine** (PPV) (Pneumovax and Pnu-Immune) is a vaccine that has been available since 1977 to protect against 23 types of pneumococcal bacteria. It is given to adults ≥65 and children ≥2 years in high-risk groups that include:

- Children with chronic heart, lung, sickle cell disease, diabetes, cirrhosis, alcoholism, and leaks of cerebrospinal fluid
- Children with lowered immunity from Hodgkin's disease, lymphoma, leukemia, kidney failure, multiple myeloma, nephrotic syndrome, HIV/AIDS, damaged or missing spleen, and organ transplant

Children ≤2 may not respond to this vaccine and should take PCV-7. Administration is as follows:

- One dose is usually all that is required although a second dose may be advised for children with some conditions, such as cancer or organ/bone marrow transplantations.
- If needed, a second dose is given 3 years after the first for children ≤10 and 5 years after the first for those ≥10.

## Hepatitis A Vaccine

Hepatitis A is a contagious virus that causes liver disease and can cause serious morbidity and death. It is spread through the feces of a person who is infected and often causes contamination of food and water. The **Hep A vaccine** is now recommended for all children at one year of age. It is not licensed for use in younger infants. Two doses are needed:

- 12 months (12-23 months)
- 18 months (or 6 months after previous dose)

Older children and teenagers may receive the two-injection series if they are considered at risk, depending upon lifestyle, such as young males having sex with other males or those using illegal drugs. It is also recommended if outbreaks occur. Adverse reactions are mild and include soreness, headache, anorexia, and malaise although severe allergic reactions can occur as with all vaccines.

## Hepatitis B Vaccine

Hepatitis B is transmitted through blood and body fluids, including during birth; therefore, it is now recommended for all newborns as well as all those <18 and those in high-risk groups >18. Hepatitis B can cause serious liver disease leading to liver cancer. Three injections of **monovalent HepB** are required to confer immunity:

- Birth (within 12 hours)
- At 1-2 months
- ≥24 weeks

Note: If combination vaccines are given after the birth dose, then a dose at 4 months can be given.

If the mother is Hepatitis B positive, the child should be given both the monovalent HepB vaccination as well as HepB immune globulin within 12 hours of birth. Adolescents (11-15) who have not been vaccinated require 2 doses, 4-6 months apart. Adverse reactions include local irritation and fever. Severe allergic reactions can occur to those allergic to baker's yeast.



## Rotavirus Vaccine

Rotavirus is a cause of significant morbidity and mortality in children, especially in developing countries. Most children, without vaccination, will suffer from severe diarrhea caused by rotavirus within the first 5 years of life. There are two rotavirus vaccines available in the US, neither being preferred over the other. RV5 (RotaTeq) requires three oral doses at 2, 4, and 6 months of age. RV1 (Rotarix) requires two doses at 2 and 4 months of age.

## Inactivated Poliovirus Vaccine

**Poliomyelitis** is a serious viral infection that can cause paralysis and death. Prior to introduction of a vaccine in 1955, there were >20,000 cases of polio in the United States each year. There have been no cases of polio caused by the poliovirus for >20 years in the United States, but it still occurs in some third world countries, so continuing vaccinations is very important. Oral polio vaccine (OPV) is no longer recommended in the United States because it carries a very slight risk of causing the disease (1:2.4 million). Children require 4 doses of injectable polio vaccine (IPV):

- 2 months
- 4 months
- 6-18 months
- 4-6 years (booster dose)

IPV is contraindicated for those who have had a severe reaction to neomycin, streptomycin, or polymyxin B. Rare allergic reactions can occur, but there are almost no serious problems caused by this vaccine.

## Varicella Vaccine

**Varicella (chickenpox)** is a common infectious childhood disease caused by the varicella zoster virus, resulting in fever, rash, and itching, and it can also cause skin infections, pneumonia, and neurological damage. After infection, the virus retreats to the nerves by the spinal cord and can reactivate years later, causing herpes zoster (shingles), a significant cause of morbidity in adults. Infection with varicella conveys immunity, but because of associated problems, it is recommended that all children receive varicella vaccine. Two doses are needed:

- 12-15 months
- 4-6 years (or at least 3 months after first dose)

Children ≥13 years and adults who have never had chickenpox or previously received the vaccine should receive 2 doses at least 28 days apart. Children should not receive the vaccine if they have had a serious allergic reaction to gelatin or neomycin. Most reactions are mild and include soreness, fever, and rash. About 1:1000 may experience febrile seizures. Pneumonia is a very rare reaction.

## MMR Vaccine

Measles is a viral disease characterized by fever and rash but can cause pneumonia, seizures, severe neurological damage, and death. Mumps is a viral disease that causes fever and swollen glands but can cause deafness, meningitis, and swelling of the testicles. Rubella, also known as German measles) is also a viral disease that can cause rash, fever, and arthritis, but the biggest danger is that it can cause a woman who is pregnant to miscarry or deliver a child with serious birth defects. The **measles, mumps, and rubella (MMR) vaccine** is given in 2 doses:

- 12-15 months
- 4-6 years

Children can get the injections at any age if they have missed them, but there must be at least 28 days between injections. Children with severe allergic reactions to gelatin or neomycin should not get the injection. Severe adverse reactions are rare, but fever and mild rash are common. Teenagers may have pain and stiffness in joints. Occasional seizures (1:3000) and thrombocytopenia (1:30,000) occur.

## PCV-7

**Heptavalent pneumococcal conjugate vaccine (PCV-7)** (Prevnar) was released for use in the United States in 2001 for treatment of children under 2 years old. It provides immunity to 7 serotypes of *Streptococcus pneumoniae* to protect against invasive pneumococcal disease, such as pneumonia, otitis media, bacteremia, and meningitis. Because children are most at risk ≤1, vaccinations begin early:

Administration is in 4 doses:

- 6-8 weeks
- 4 months
- 6 months
- 12-18 months

Although less effective for older children, PCV-7 has been approved for children between 2 and 5 years of age who are at high risk because of the following conditions:

- Chronic diseases: sickle cell disease, heart disease, lung disease, liver disease
- Damaged or missing spleen
- Immunosuppressive disorders: diabetes, cancer
- Drug therapy: chemotherapy, steroids

PCV-7 may also be considered for all children ≤ 5, especially those ≤3 and in group day care and in some ethnic groups (Native American, Alaska Natives, and African Americans).

## Meningococcal Vaccine

**Meningitis** is severe bacterial meningitis that can result in severe neurological compromise or death. A number of different serotypes of *meningococci* can cause meningitis and current vaccines protect against 4 types although not against subtype B, which causes about 65% of meningitis cases in children. However, the vaccines provide 85-100% protection against sub-types A, C, Y, and W-135. There are 2 types of vaccine:

- **Meningococcal polysaccharide vaccine (MPSV4)** is made from the outer capsule of the bacteria and is used for children 2-10.
  - One dose is given at 2 years, although those at high risk may receive 2 doses, 3 months apart.
  - Under special circumstances, children 3-24 months may receive 2 doses, 3 months apart.
- **Meningococcal conjugate vaccine (MCV4)** is used for children ≥11 (who have not received MPSV4). One dose is required:
  - Ages 11-12, all children should receive the vaccine.
  - If not previously vaccinated, high school and college freshmen should be vaccinated.
- Side effects are usually only local tenderness.

## Hib Vaccine

***Haemophilus influenzae* type b (Hib) vaccine** (HibTITER and PedvaxHIB) protects against infection with *Haemophilus influenzae,* which can cause serious respiratory infections, pneumonia, meningitis, bacteremia, and pericarditis in children ≤5 years old. *Administration* is as follows:

- 2 months
- 4 months
- 6 months (may be required, depending upon the brand of vaccine)
- 12-15 months (this booster dose must be given at least 2 months after the earlier doses for those who start at a later age than 2 months)

Children over age 6 usually do not require Hib, but it is recommended for older children and adults. Here are some conditions that place them at risk:

- Sickle cell disease
- HIV/AIDS
- Bone marrow transplant
- Chemotherapy for cancer
- Damaged or missing spleen

Some chemotherapy drugs, corticosteroids, and other immunosuppressive drugs may interact with the vaccine.

## Infant Immunization, Screening, and Prophylaxis Schedule Summary

The recommended schedule for immunizations and screening/prophylaxis for the infant is summarized below:

- All newborns receive **ophthalmic drops or ointment**, to prevent blindness from possible gonorrhea infection, and an injection of vitamin K to prevent hemorrhagic disease.
- Before discharge, newborns are tested for **phenylketonuria** and **hypothyroidism**, and will possibly have their **hematocrit** and **hemoglobin** checked.
- **Hepatitis B vaccine** is given at birth, 1-2 months, and 6-18 months.
- **Diphtheria/tetanus/pertussis vaccine** is administered at 2 months, 4 months, 6 months, and 15-18 months.
- **Hib (Haemophilus influenza type b) vaccine** is given at 2 months, 4 months, and 12 months or later.
- **Poliovirus vaccine** is given at 2 months, 4 months, and 6-18 months.
- **MMR vaccine** is given at 12-18 months.
- **Varicella (chickenpox) vaccine** can be given at 12 months.

**Review Video: Child Immunizations and Schedule**
Visit mometrix.com/academy and enter code: 167190

## Required Immunization History for Children up to 6 Years of Age

According to the Centers for Disease Control and Prevention, by 6 years of age, children in the United States should receive a three-part series of hepatitis B, three doses of rotavirus prevention; four injections protecting against diphtheria, tetanus, and pertussis; four doses of *Haemophilus influenzae* type b; four doses of pneumococcal vaccine; four doses of polio vaccine; two injections that protect against measles, mumps, and rubella; two varicella vaccinations; one hepatitis A vaccination; and a yearly influenza prevention injection.

## Vaccination of Children with Uncertain Immunization Histories

Children who have uncertain immunization histories may need vaccinations to meet guidelines. The number of vaccinations needed depends on the child's history. For children who are not up-to-date on immunizations, the necessary injections must be determined. These vaccinations can then be given on a schedule so that the child can catch up. For children with no immunization history or uncertain status, such as refugees or internationally adopted children, restarting the immunization series may be necessary to ensure adequate coverage with all vaccines, particularly measles, mumps, and rubella; varicella; hepatitis B; *Haemophilus influenzae* type b; and polio.

## Possible Side Effects

Common reactions to immunizations include irritability, decrease in appetite, fever less than 102 °F, and swelling, redness and tenderness at injection site. These may last for the first 1-2 days and can be treated with acetaminophen every 4-6 hours for the first day if severe, although risks of muting the antibody response and thereby decreasing the effectiveness of the vaccine have been associated with acetaminophen administration before or soon after immunization. If more severe reactions occur, such as fever greater than 102 °F, severe prolonged irritability, or high-pitched crying, or the symptoms last more than 2 days, the parents should call the healthcare provider immediately.

## Important Considerations When Giving Immunizations

Every time a child comes into contact with the healthcare system, his **immunization status** should be assessed. Children are required, by all states, to be immunized before entering a licensed school or day care. Specific requirements will vary from state to state. Vaccines must be handled and stored according the manufacturers guidelines. Immunizations must be documented according to specific guidelines and parents must sign a consent form every time a vaccine is administered. Common illnesses such as colds, ear infections and diarrhea will not usually preclude giving vaccines. The MMR and varicella vaccines should not be given during pregnancy. There are two situations in which immunizations are contraindicated: a previous severe allergic reaction to a vaccine or one of its components and encephalopathy occurring within 7 days of giving a DTP or DTaP vaccine.

### The Anti-Vaccination Movement

While **opposition to vaccination** is not a new concept, it is a movement that has gained momentum with the power of information sharing via social media. Opposers to vaccination, often referred to as "Anti-Vaxxers," believe that vaccinations can cause complications such as autism and SIDS, especially when administered in infancy and early childhood, and believe that these risks far outweigh the benefits. There are also those who oppose such medical interventions due to religious beliefs.

While the therapeutic effects of vaccinations have been supported by evidence for both individuals and communities, it is important that healthcare professionals be equipped to respectfully inform and care for those that oppose vaccinations. Individuals should be educated regarding the evidence supporting vaccinations and the vaccinations required by law. The CDC offers a wealth of resources for healthcare workers and for individuals regarding vaccinations. The most notable resource is the CDC's Vaccine Information Statement, a living document that outlines the benefits and risks of vaccines, that healthcare workers can use to inform individuals and parents. If, despite efforts to educate, the individual or caregiver still refuses vaccination, there are ICD codes that providers are required to use to document this refusal (for example, ICD-10-CM: Z28.82: Immunization not carried out because of caregiver refusal). The healthcare worker must also document that preventive medical counseling was provided.

## Education Theory

### Bandura's Theory of Social Learning

In the 1970s, Bandura proposed the theory of social learning, in which he posited that learning develops from observing, organizing, and rehearsing behavior that has been modeled. Bandura believed that people are more likely to adopt the behavior if they value the outcomes, if the outcomes have functional value, and if the person modeling the behavior is similar to the learner and is admired because of status. Behavior is the result of observation of behavioral, environmental, and cognitive interactions. There are **four conditions** required for modeling:

- **Attention**: The degree of attention paid to modeling can depend on many variables (physical, social, and environmental).
- **Retention**: People's ability to retain models depends on symbolic coding, creating mental images, organizing thoughts, and rehearsing (mentally or physically).
- **Reproduction**: The ability to reproduce a model depends on physical and mental capabilities.
- **Motivation**: Motivation may derive from past performances, rewards, or vicarious modeling.

## Transtheoretical Model of Change

The transtheoretical model of change puts forth concepts applicable to the process of educating patients and their family members. The **stages** of the transtheoretical model of change include the following:

- The first stage is **precontemplation**. At this point, the patient is not aware of any need for a change in the health behavior.
- In the next stage, **contemplation**, the patient begins to realize why the change may be necessary after recognizing that the health behavior in question is unhealthy and weighing the consequences of continuing this behavior.
- During the stage of **preparation**, the patient imagines making the change at a future time and starts to formulate a plan to do so.
- The **action** stage occurs when the patient makes specific modifications in health behavior and begins to note the resulting positive changes.
- During the **maintenance** stage, the patient is able to implement the change over time by utilizing strategies to prevent a return to previously unhealthy behaviors.
- **Termination** is the stage at which a patient has incorporated the changed behavior into daily functioning, and the patient will not resume the previous unhealthy behavior.

## Kurt Lewin

### *Force Field Analysis*

Force field analysis was designed by Kurt Lewin, a social psychologist, to analyze both the driving forces and the restraining forces for change:

- **Driving forces** instigate and promote change, such as leaders, incentives, and competition.
- **Restraining forces** resist change, such as poor attitudes, hostility, inadequate equipment, or insufficient funds.

The educator can use this force field analysis diagram to discuss variables related to a proposed change in process:

- Write the proposed change in the center column.
- Brainstorm and list driving forces and opposed restraining forces. Score the forces. (When driving and restraining forces are in balance, this is a state of equilibrium or the status quo.)
- Discuss the value of the proposed change.
- Develop a plan to diminish or eliminate restraining forces.

### *Lewin's Model of Change Theory*

Lewin's model of change theory may be used to help some patients make decisions for change. Patients can be educated about the need for change and can be assisted with making alterations in behavior or thoughts in order to better facilitate change; however, only the patient can truly implement the change permanently. Lewin's concept of change theory involves a three-part process:

- **Unfreezing** is the part of the model in which the patient becomes open to change, sees a need for it, and removes the boundaries inhibiting change.
- The patient then makes the **actual change** according to expected outcomes and goals.
- Finally, **refreezing** is the process of maintaining the change so that it becomes a habit, and one that the patient is likely to uphold for a long period of time.

Lewin's theory also involves either driving forces or restraining forces. Driving forces are those outside measures that support the change, while restraining forces inhibit success in implementing the change.

# Principles of Education

## Principles of Adult Learning

Adults have a wealth of life and/or employment experiences. Their attitudes toward education may vary considerably. There are, however, some **principles of adult learning** and typical characteristics of adult learners that an instructor should consider when planning strategies for teaching parents, families, or staff.

- Practical and goal-oriented:
  - Provide overviews or summaries and examples.
  - Use collaborative discussions with problem-solving exercises.
  - Remain organized with the goal in mind.
- Self-directed:
  - Provide active involvement, asking for input.
  - Allow different options toward achieving the goal.
  - Give them responsibilities.
- Knowledgeable:
  - Show respect for their life experiences/education.
  - Validate their knowledge and ask for feedback.
  - Relate new material to information with which they are familiar.
- Relevancy-oriented:
  - Explain how information will be applied.
  - Clearly identify objectives.
- Motivated:
  - Provide certificates of professional advancement and/or continuing education credit for staff when possible.

**Review Video: Adult Learning Processes and Theories**
Visit mometrix.com/academy and enter code: 638453



## Learning Styles

Every individual learns differently, some better through listening and talking, others through seeing, and others through interacting. More commonly, learners are most enriched when a combination of teaching styles are utilized to ensure maximum retention across all learning types. A range of teaching materials and methods that relate to all three major learning preferences (visual, auditory, and kinesthetic) and that are appropriate for different ages should be available. Below are various methods through which education can be provided to ensure it is accessible to diverse learning preferences.

- Provide written directions or picture guides, or demonstrate procedures.
- Use charts and diagrams, and provide photos/videos when useful.
- Explain procedures while demonstrating them.
- Plan extra time to discuss and answer questions when possible.
- Provide audio recordings when relevant to the education being provided.
- Provide hands-on experience throughout teaching.
- Encourage handling of supplies and equipment when educating specific skills.
- Allow the learner to demonstrate/practice the skill.

## Approaches to Teaching

There are many approaches to teaching, and the educator must prepare, present, and coordinate a wide range of educational workshops, lectures, discussions, and one-on-one instructions on any chosen topic. All types of classes will be needed, depending upon the purpose and material:

- **Educational workshops** are usually conducted with small groups, allowing for maximal participation. They are especially good for demonstrations and practice sessions.
- **Lectures** are often used for more academic or detailed information that may include questions and answers but limits discussion. An effective lecture should include some audiovisual support.
- **Discussions** are best with small groups so that people can actively participate. This is a good method for problem solving.
- **One-on-one instruction** is especially helpful for targeted instruction in procedures for individuals.
- **Online learning modules** are good for independent learners.

Participants should be asked to evaluate the presentations in the forms of surveys or suggestions, but ultimately the program is evaluated in terms of patient outcomes.

## Readiness to Learn

The patient/family's readiness to learn should be assessed because if they are not ready, instruction is of little value. Often, readiness is indicated when the patient/family asks questions or shows an interest in procedures. There are a number of factors related to readiness to learn:

- **Physical factors:** There are a number of physical factors that can affect ability. Manual dexterity may be required to complete a task, and this varies by age and condition. Hearing or vision deficits may impact a person's ability to learn. Complex tasks may be too difficult for some because of weakness or cognitive impairment, and modifications of the environment may be needed. Health status, age, and gender may all impact the ability to learn.
- **Experience:** People's experience with learning can vary widely and is affected by their ability to cope with changes, their personal goals, motivation to learn, and cultural background. People may have widely divergent ideas about what constitutes illness and/or treatment. Lack of English skills may make learning difficult and prevent people from asking questions.
- **Mental/emotional status:** The external support system and internal motivation may impact readiness. Anxiety, fear, or depression about one's condition can make learning very difficult because the patient/family cannot focus on learning, so the nurse must spend time to reassure the patient/family and wait until they are emotionally more receptive.
- **Knowledge/education:** The knowledge base of the patient/family, their cognitive ability, and their learning styles all affect their readiness to learn. The nurse should always begin by assessing what knowledge the patient/family already has about their disease, condition, or treatment and then build from that base. People with little medical experience may lack knowledge of basic medical terminology, interfering with their ability and readiness to learn.

## Teaching Elderly Patients

The elderly patient's level of functioning must be assessed before teaching. Cognitive abilities and mental functioning may be affected by illness and aging:

- Short-term memory loss can affect the amount of material retained.
- Concentration may be decreased.
- Reaction time is delayed.
- Color discrimination, general vision, and hearing may be decreased.

The nurse should **pace** the teaching accordingly and **tailor** materials for any deficits. Family should be present for teaching if possible, to help the patient to remember key points after discharge. Large print on non-glare paper that is easy to read should be used. The nurse should use color-coding cues only if colors are easily perceived. The learning environment must be quiet and comfortable with no distractions or interruptions.

- Repeat information numerous times and allow the patient as much practice time as needed.
- Use audio-visual aids to reinforce information given verbally.
- Face the patient when speaking and encourage him/her to use hearing devices if used.
- Make sure the lighting in the room is adequate.

## Teaching Patients with Learning Disabilities

Determine the type of learning disability in order to design teaching:

- When a patient has a **visual problem**, the nurse should use **verbal teaching**, repeated several times as needed and record the session for the patient to hear later if possible or use prepared audiotapes or CDs containing the information. The patient should verbalize learning to show attainment of the learning goal.
- When **auditory perception** is a problem, learning materials should be **visual** with as few words as possible. Demonstration, role-playing, and practicing the procedure will be useful to the patient. Printed materials should employ pictures, and computer use can be useful.
- If the patient has an **expressive problem**, he/she needs time to process the input and to ask questions. **Hand gestures, demonstrations, and the senses** should be utilized for teaching when appropriate.

A developmental disability will require information presented in a format that is appropriate for the person's developmental level. The nurse should keep explanations simple, and use gestures, demonstrations, activities, and repetition to teach.

## Teaching to Disabled Patients and Families

The teaching of disabled patients and their families begins with an assessment of the family's willingness and preparation for the heavy duty of care that will be required. The nurse must teach information about diseases or disabilities as well as medications, procedures, diet, and physical therapies. The patients must be taught to perform ADLs as well as possible and caregivers taught how to assist when needed:

- Give patients enough information to understand and manage the disabilities and to empower them with a sense of control and coping.
- Don't overwhelm them with information.
- Plan the teaching to provide information according to learning readiness and priorities but be flexible and change the plan if needed.
- Utilize checklists of skills to help keep track of all that has been learned.
- Give praise, continued feedback, support, and empathy with every teaching session.
- Provide resources that patients and family can use after discharge and refer to home health for continuing support and teaching.

### Importance of Patient's Culture in Design of Teaching Plan

The nurse must always assess the individual's cultural beliefs and values and not assume that they are the same as the culture on a whole. These beliefs determine what information the patient feels that they can pursue. Teaching that conflicts with these beliefs will be rejected. The patient's perception of health and the healthcare system must be determined because a lack of confidence in the teacher can impair motivation to learn. The nurse must **assess the patient's beliefs** about the following to develop a personalized teaching plan:

- Body image, self-esteem
- Abilities and level of knowledge
- Principles of living
- Diet, activity, health practices
- Involvement of family and support persons
- Physical and mental health and disease
- Causes of disease
- Aging
- Gender issues
- Spirituality, customs, rituals, religious precepts

## Theories of Human Growth and Development

### Issues of Human Development

Several issues of human development that are addressed by theory are described below:

- **Universality vs. context specificity**: Universality implies that all individuals will develop in the same way, no matter what culture they live in. Context specificity implies that development will be influenced by the culture in which the individual lives.
- **Assumptions about human nature** (3 doctrines: original sin, innate purity, and tabula rasa):
  - Original sin says that children are inherently bad and must be taught to be good.
  - Innate purity says that children are inherently good.
  - Tabula rasa says that children are born without good or bad tendencies and can be taught right vs. wrong.
- **Behavioral consistency**: Children either behave in the same manner no matter what the situation or setting, or they change their behavior depending on the setting and who is interacting with them.
- **Nature vs. nurture**: Nature is the genetic influences on development. Nurture is the environment and social influences on development.
- **Continuity vs. discontinuity**: Continuity states that development progresses at a steady rate and the effects of change are cumulative. Discontinuity states that development progresses in a stair-step fashion and the effects of early development have no bearing on later development.
- **Passivity vs. activity**: Passivity refers to development being influenced by outside forces. Activity refers to development influenced by the child himself and how he responds to external forces.
- **Critical vs. sensitive period**: The critical period is that window of time when the child will be able to acquire new skills and behaviors. The sensitive period refers to a flexible time period when a child will be receptive to learning new skills, even if it is later than the norm.

## Developmental Tasks According to Erikson

The developmental tasks according to Erik Erikson:

- **Trust vs. mistrust (Birth to 1 year)**: Trust, faith, and optimism develop if the needs of warmth, food, and love are met. If not, this can result in mistrust.
- **Autonomy vs. shame/doubt (Ages 1-3)**: The child desires independence in basic self-care tasks and wants choice. If independence is not encouraged, this can lead to doubt and shame. Independence develops self-control and willpower.
- **Initiative vs. guilt (Ages 3-6)**: The child engages in self-directed play and starts activities without outside influence. Imaginative play and competition are introduced. This can lead to guilt or direction and purpose based on how this initiative is supportive.
- **Industry vs. inferiority (Ages 6-12)**: The child values feeling capable and competent and develops a sense of pride and self-worth. They desire to do what is right and good. Social interactions between peers become more important, and comparing achievements can result in feelings of pride or feelings of inferiority if not properly guided.
- **Identity vs. role confusion (Ages 12-18)**: Parents, teachers, peers, family members, church, culture, and ethnicity all role model and pressure youth to adopt certain behaviors. The task of adolescents is to discover their own identity.
- **Intimacy vs. isolation (Ages 18-40)**: Young people learn to commit to another person in a love or family relationship. They learn the behavior required to maintain this relationship.
- **Generativity vs. stagnation (Ages 40-65)**: Adults have many tasks when they try to find their own interests and niche in the work world. Family, community, and work roles are defined.
- **Integrity vs. despair (Ages 65+)**: Older people ponder their life experiences to put them into perspective. They learn to accept the aging process and begin to think about their own death.

## Sigmund Freud's Stages of Psychosexual Development

Sigmund Freud's stages of psychosexual development are listed and described below:

- **Oral stage (Birth to 1 year)**: obsessed with oral activities and must have these needs met for proper psychosocial development, very attached to mother.
- **Anal stage (Ages 1-3)**: masters toilet training.
- **Phallic stage (Ages 3-6)**: child focuses on childbirth and differences between the sexes, develops sexual obsession with parent of opposite sex (Oedipal complex-boy drawn to mother, Electra complex-girl drawn to father).
- **Latency stage (Ages 6-11)**: Oedipal or Electra complex wanes, focus is now socialization, begins to gravitate toward the same-sex parent to learn appropriate gender roles.
- **Genital stage (Ages 12 and older)**: puberty, attracted to opposite sex, learns to relate to opposite gender and control sexual drive.

## Piaget's Theory of Cognitive Development

Piaget believed that development was progressive and followed a set pattern. He believed the child's environment, his interactions with others in that environment, and how the environment responds help to shape his cognitive development. There are **four stages to Piaget's theory:**

- The **sensorimotor stage (birth to age 2)** is when the child learns to work toward a goal, the relationship between cause and effect, that objects still exist even though they cannot see them, and a sense of self.
- In the **preoperational stage (ages 2-7)**, language skills develop, the child only sees his point of view, he does not think abstractly, and has a difficult time telling fact from fantasy.

- The **concrete operations stage (ages 7-11)** is when children begin to understand relationships between objects and events, learn to classify and use patterns, understand that some occurrences are reversible, and see others' points of view.
- The **formal operations stage (ages 12 years and older)** is the stage of abstract thinking, better reasoning skills, and forward-thinking.

**Review Video:** Piaget's Cognitive Development Theory
Visit mometrix.com/academy and enter code: 100376

## Maslow's Hierarchy of Needs

Maslow defined human motivation in terms of needs and wants. His **hierarchy of needs** is classically portrayed as a pyramid sitting on its base divided into horizontal layers. He theorized that, as humans fulfill the needs of one layer, their motivation turns to the layer above. The layers consist of (from bottom to top):

- **Physiological**: The need for air, fluid, food, shelter, warmth, and sleep.
- **Safety**: A safe place to live, a steady job, a society with rules and laws, protection from harm, and insurance or savings for the future.
- **Love/Belonging**: A network consisting of a significant other, family, friends, co-workers, religion, and community.
- **Esteem or self-respect**: The knowledge that you are a person who is successful and worthy of esteem, attention, status, and admiration.
- **Self-actualization**: The acceptance of your life, choices, and situation in life and the empathetic acceptance of others, as well as the feeling of independence and the joy of being able to express yourself freely and competently.

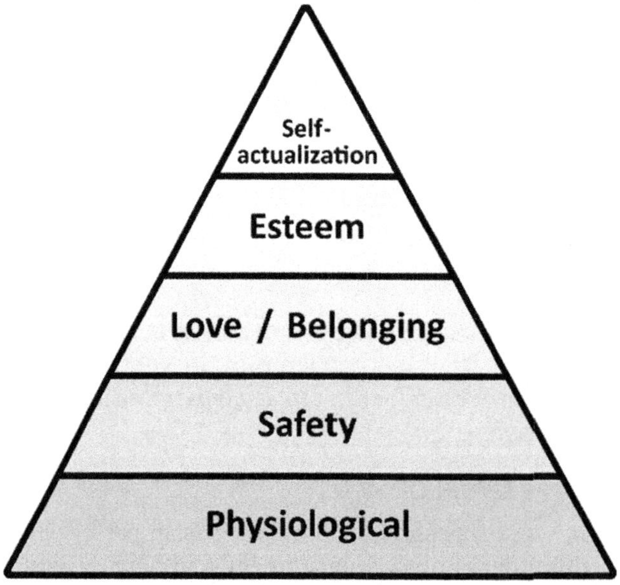


**Review Video:** Maslow's Hierarchy of Needs
Visit mometrix.com/academy and enter code: 461825

## Behavioral Theories

**Pavlov** demonstrated **classical conditioning** when he found that a dog that would salivate when presented with food would also salivate when the person who normally fed him was present. He paired a bell ringing with the feeding and found that after a time, the dog would also salivate to the ringing of the bell. Consequently, his theory was that learning takes place when a behavior can be produced in response to something totally unrelated to that behavior.

**Skinner** demonstrated **operant conditioning** when he found that behavior can be changed depending on the response given to the behavior. If the response to the behavior was positive (praise, a hug), then the behavior would continue or increase in frequency. If the response was negative (a frown, words of criticism), then the behavior would decrease in frequency or cease altogether.

## Biopsychosocial Theory of Patient Care

The biopsychosocial theory of patient care recognizes that **biology, psychology, and social circumstances** all interact in the development of an illness, the patient's perception of the illness, and the patient's ability to make a good recovery. In the biopsychosocial care model, a multidisciplinary healthcare team, including nurses, mental health professionals, social workers, and physicians, work together to address all aspects of a patient's health issue—the medical problem, psychological state, and social, cultural, and economic situation—in order to find an integrated solution. For example, adding stress-reduction, exercise, and nutritional programs to the standard medical treatment protocol for cardiovascular disease patients has been shown to be more effective. Many patients with chronic diseases or conditions may benefit from support groups that provide social and psychological benefits that may enhance the effects of drug therapy and surgery.



## Biological Theories of Aging

There are a number of biological theories of aging:

- **Wearing down**: The body is compared to a machine that begins to wear down over time because of the damage caused by years of use.
- **Autoimmune reaction**: The body develops an autoimmune reaction against itself with aging, causing damage and destruction to tissues.
- **Free radical accumulation**: Chemicals that bring about aging accumulate in the body.
- **Cellular programming**: The cells of every organism have a predetermined programmed life expectancy beyond which one cannot survive.
- **Mutation**: Mutations within the organism occur over time, and these eventually make changes that are incompatible with life.
- **Homeostasis**: Over time, the body is unable to maintain stable levels of necessary chemicals in the body.

## Selye's Theory of Adaptation

Selye developed a theory of adaptation concerning a person's physiologic response to stress called the general adaptation syndrome. This syndrome starts with the classic "fight or flight" response of the body to physiologic stress. Catecholamines are released and the adrenal cortical response begins. This is called the **alarm response** and is short-lived. This immediate response allows the person to respond quickly to stress. Since the alarm response cannot be sustained without resulting in death, the body next shifts into the **resistance stage**. Some cortisol is still being released as the body begins to adapt to the stressor. If the stressor persists, the body becomes exhausted. Changes then occur to the cardiovascular, gastrointestinal, and immune systems, and death can occur. The **exhaustion stage** does not always occur in response to most life stressors. As the body ages, it loses some of its resistance and ability to adapt to stress. This results in exhaustion and death in the elderly more easily than it does in younger people.

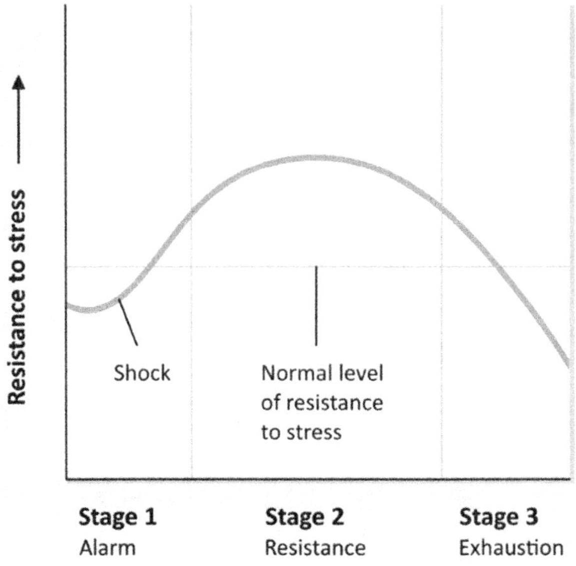


# Health Promotion and Disease Prevention

## Health Promotion

Nurses promote health when they assist individuals to change behavior in ways that help them to attain and maintain the highest level of wellbeing possible. Health promotion is a very popular way to control healthcare costs and reduce illness and early death. Health is increasingly the topic of newscasts and literature. The public is demanding more information pertinent to the maintenance of health and to the ways in which the average person can act independently to do so. Health promotion is centered on ideal personal habits, lifestyles, and environmental control that decrease the risk for disease. The US Public Health Service periodically identifies national health goals and most recently published a program called ***Healthy People 2030***, with measurable goals to increase the general quality and years of life for all and to increase the health status of all groups to an equal level of wellness. Health promotion programs in the community are now offered by workplaces, clinics, schools, and churches, not just by hospitals as in the past.

### *Healthy People 2030*

The 5 **main goals** of *Healthy People 2030* are

- Attaining healthy, thriving lives free of preventable disease, disability, injury, and premature death
- Eliminating health disparities, achieving health equality, and increasing health literacy
- Creating environments conducive to health-promotion
- Improving health in all life stages
- Collaborating with leadership and key stakeholders in policy design that improves the health and well-being of all

*Healthy People 2030* has 62 topic areas with 355 total objectives divided across five sections:

- Health Conditions
- Health Behaviors
- Populations
- Settings and Systems
- Social Determinants of Health

### MAIN COMPONENTS OF HEALTH PROMOTION

Health promotion efforts are concentrated in four areas:

- Individuals must be educated to realize that their **lifestyle and choices** have a large impact on their health. They must then be motivated to choose to modify their personal risk factors and take the responsibility to do so.
- The emphasis on **good nutrition** as the biggest factor that impacts health and the length of life must be brought into general awareness. This is occurring via the media through numerous books and articles educating people about the essential nutrients needed to maintain health.
- **Stress** is a constant in a production-driven society. Individuals must learn ways to manage and decrease stress to achieve and maintain health and to decrease the effects of stress upon chronic illness, risk of infections, and trauma.
- **Physical fitness** helps cardiovascular status, relieves stress, controls weight, delays aging, promotes strength and endurance, and improves appearance and performance. Individuals must have programs that increase activity gradually to prevent injury and are designed to meet individual needs.



## HEALTH SELF-MANAGEMENT

Health self-management includes health maintenance, disease prevention, and health promotion. Health maintenance is defined as strategies that help maintain and/or improve health over time. Health maintenance is dependent on three factors, which include health perception, motivation for behavioral change, and compliance to set goals. Disease prevention is an effort to limit the development or progression of lifestyle-related illness. **Disease prevention** can be categorized into primary, secondary, and tertiary prevention.

- **Primary prevention** measures are employed prior to disease onset and are used in health populations.
- **Secondary prevention** measures are used to screen, detect, and treat disease in earlier stages to prevent further progression or development of other complications.
- **Tertiary prevention** measures are used to prevent the worsening of a disease and the onset of other complications or comorbid conditions secondary to that disease.

Health promotion strategies include risk reduction strategies applied to the general population.

## INFLUENCES ON DECISION TO MODIFY BEHAVIOR TO ACHIEVE AND MAINTAIN HEALTH

Many factors have an influence on people's efforts to change behavior in a way that improves and maintains their health status. These factors include age, ethnicity, gender, lifestyle, level of education, self-esteem, motivation, and self-image. The patient's support network and the availability of health promotion programs and healthcare systems also have an influence on healthcare behaviors. Some people may be prevented from accessing health promotion programs because of lack of medical insurance. Financial status and employment are important as well. The presence of addictions and diseases, the length of illness, and the severity of disabilities are all factors to be considered. The value placed on health, the threat of potential losses, and the perceived benefits of behavior modification are important motivating factors.

### *Strategies to Encourage Smoking Cessation*

The **health impact associated with smoking** varies among smokers and can be affected by the number of cigarettes used daily, exposure to smoking-associated stimuli, and educational level. The presence of stress and depression, psychosocial problems, lack of coping mechanisms, low income, and long-term habitual behavior are problematic for the quitter. Nurses can promote smoking cessation by taking every opportunity to bring up the subject, educating about the dangers of smoking and benefits of quitting, and providing **resources** to help patients quit. Strategies include:

- Educating about the personal effects of smoking upon that individual
- Encouraging patients to set a quit date
- Referring to programs and smoking cessation information
- Educating about the use of nicotine replacements including nicotine gum, lozenges, inhalers, transdermal patches, and nasal sprays
- Educating about the use of medications such as Zyban, Catapres, and Chantix
- Providing support via phone calls or office visits
- Discovering the reason for relapses
- Praising and rewarding any success in the quitting process

## Healthy Nutrition Principles

Healthy nutrition principles include the following:

- Eating a range of different kinds of foods, and eating increased amounts fruits, vegetables, whole grains, poultry, and fish.
- Diets should consist of 55–60% **carbohydrates**, less than 30% **fat**, and the rest should be **protein** (0.8–1.0 g/kg).
- Restrict **saturated fat** to <10%. Restrict **cholesterol** to 300 mg/day.
- Utilize moderate amounts of sugar, salt, and sodium.
- Take a **multivitamin** including folic acid if the patient is female and able to have children. Get 200–800 IU/day of vitamin D in order to absorb calcium.
- **Calcium** intake should be: 1,300 mg/day for women age 13–18 or those who are pregnant/nursing; 1,000 mg/day for women age 19–50 years; 1,500 mg/day for age 51 years and older.
- **Weight loss** may improve diabetes, joint pain, inflammation, cardiovascular disease, hypothyroidism, or renal disease.

## Young Adult Health Screenings

Health screening is encouraged for conditions that are very likely to occur and diseases that are likely to kill if they are not identified early. The assessment should be supported by evidence using standardized techniques and proper follow-up.

**Young adult (ages 20-39 years) screenings,** according to the US Preventive Services Task Force (USPSTF), should include:

- A full head-to-toe physical (every 5-6 years)
- Routine blood pressure screening
- Cholesterol screening (every 5 years; more frequently when total cholesterol is higher than 200 mg/dL)
- PPD test for tuberculosis when patient has had known contact with TB or is at increased risk (health care workers, prisoners, homeless, or immunocompromised)
- Dental check-up (annually)
- Thyroid palpation (every 3 years)
- Depression screening (at every visit)

- Men perform self-testicular exam every month
- Women conduct a self-breast exam every month; should receive a clinical breast exam every 3 years
- Pap smear and pelvic assessments every 3 years (or up to 5 years in conjunction with HPV testing)
- Screening for gonorrhea and chlamydia for all sexually active individuals
- Health education and promotion (every time patient is seen)
- Influenza vaccination (annually)
- Td immunization every 10 years

## Adult Screenings

**Adults (age 40 and older) screenings,** according to the USPSTF, should maintain the same schedule as young adults (unless indicated below) in addition to the following:

- A full head-to-toe physical (annually)
- Blood pressure screening (annually)
- ECG (over 40, annually; only when there are cardiac risks)
- Clinical breast exam (annually in women over 40)
- Mammogram (biennially in women over 40)
- General colorectal cancer screening for risks (annually), and colorectal cancer screening via colonoscopy (every 10 years starting at age 45 until age 75)
- Prostate-specific antigen screening (men over 50 with average risk, or younger if higher risk; upon the patient's informed request only)



## Disease Prevention for the Elderly

Although life spans are longer, **ongoing (chronic) diseases** are still the primary reason patients die. Elderly patients have more of an absolute chance of getting a disease, but they also react well to prevention. Keep good records of the elderly patient's history, including updating every year and following advice for patients over the age of 65 years. Evaluate nutrition, functional ability, alcoholic beverage intake (more than 2 alcoholic beverages a day constitutes abuse), smoking, illegal drugs, misuse of prescriptions, and exercise level.

- **Preventative measures** include a physical, screening assessments, and immunizations.
- Some **routine screenings** include: fasting glucose, papanicolaou smear, dipstick urinalysis, mammography, PPD, fecal occult blood/sigmoidoscopy, electrocardiogram, thyroid function, glaucoma and sight, hearing, and cholesterol.
- **Immunizations** include yearly flu shot, pneumococcal vaccine, and tetanus; respiratory syncytial virus (RSV) vaccination at age 75.

The following screens are controversial: depression for someone with no symptoms, dementia for someone with no symptoms, osteoporosis including bone densitometry for postmenopausal females (counsel females regarding hormone prophylaxis), colon and prostate cancer, and cholesterol for someone with no symptoms.

# Pediatric Illness Prevention

## Risk Analysis as Part of Disease Prevention

Risk analysis is an important part of health promotion and disease prevention because it can help to identify those factors (normed for age and sex) that put a child at risk for current or future disease. Typically, risk analysis uses observations, interviews, and questionnaires to gain information about a child and their family so that interventions and diagnostic testing can be targeted to areas of increased risk. Risk factors may be controllable (diet and exercise) or non-controllable (genetic), but once identified, a plan of care can be formulated. Risk analysis is an important component of cost-containment because early identification and treatment or intervention can reduce future costs of care. **Areas for risk analysis** may include:

- Nutrition
- Exercise
- Cardiovascular
- Diabetes
- Hypertension
- Cancer
- Osteoporosis
- Vision
- Behavior and lifestyle

Results of risk analysis are not diagnostic, but they indicate if the child is at a low, medium, or high risk of developing a disease or health problem.

### *Components of Risk Analysis*

Risk analysis can be used to assess individual risks or to assess the risk and effectiveness of different treatments and programs in a broader sense. Risk analysis should be carried out for all new treatments and procedures to determine if the benefits outweigh the risks and if they are cost-effective. Risk analysis should be an ongoing part of the nurse's role. There are three primary **components** to risk analysis:

- **Assessing** requires gaining information by questioning, observing, or analyzing data, which may be derived from active study or review of the research.
- **Intervening** involves taking information from the assessment and making changes in management, treatments, or procedures to reflect the risk analysis with the aim of providing the most beneficial and cost-effective care.
- **Communicating** requires publishing the results or sharing those with the organization, family, child, or the general public, depending on the scope of the risk analysis.

## Risk Factors for Neonates Associated with Maternal Disease

There are a number of **maternal factors** that put the infant at increased risk:

- **Diabetes mellitus**: Both gestational and pre-existing diabetes put the infant at risk of stillbirth, hypoglycemia, and macrosomia (larger size than normal) as well as birth injury. Maternal pre-existing diabetes is also associated with birth defects, including abnormal development of the cardiovascular and gastrointestinal systems, neurological and spinal cord disorders, and urinary tract abnormalities.
- **HIV/Hepatitis B**: Infectious diseases may be transmitted during pregnancy or delivery.

## Implications of Fetal Drug Exposure

There are many drugs that can profoundly affect the growing fetus. Some are prescribed drugs, such as Accutane, but the greatest numbers are illicit drugs, such as crack, heroin, or cocaine. Increasing numbers of children are born to addicted mothers. While each drug has specific effects, there are many effects that are common with any type of fetal drug exposure:

- Premature weight and low birth weight with infants who are small for gestational age (SGA)
- Failure to thrive often related to poor sucking and dysphagia
- Increased risk of congenital infectious disease (HIV, hepatitis, CMV)
- Increased risk of SIDS
- Withdrawal symptoms typically manifest within 72 hours of birth:
  - Tremors, excitability, seizures
  - Vomiting, diarrhea, diaphoresis
  - Dry, red, irritated skin
- Developmental and cognitive problems that vary with age. Initial problems often subside within the first couple of years, but in a small number of children learning disabilities and behavioral problems persist.

## Implications of Fetal Alcohol Syndrome

**Fetal alcohol syndrome** (FAS) is a syndrome of birth defects that develop as the result of maternal ingestion of alcohol. Despite campaigns to inform the public, women continue to drink during pregnancy, but no safe amount of alcohol ingestion has been determined. FAS results in:

- **Facial abnormalities**: Hypoplastic (underdeveloped) maxilla, micrognathia (undersized jaw), hypoplastic philtrum (groove beneath the nose), and short palpebral fissures (eye slits between upper and lower lids).
- **Neurological deficits**: May include microcephaly, intellectual disability, motor delay, and hearing deficits. Learning disorders may include problems with visual-spatial and verbal learning, attention disorders, and delayed reaction times.
- **Growth retardation**: Prenatal growth deficit persists with slow growth after birth.
- **Behavioral problems**: Irritability and hyperactivity. Poor judgment in behavior may relate to deficit in executive functions.

Indication of brain damage without the associated physical abnormalities is referred to as alcohol-related neurodevelopmental disorder (ARND).

## Infant Withdrawal from Fetal Exposure to Drugs

Fetal exposure to drugs, such as opioids, methadone, cocaine, crack, and other recreational drugs causes **withdrawal symptoms** in about 60% of infants. There are many variables, which include the type of drug, the extent of drug use, and the duration of maternal drug use. For example, children may have withdrawal symptoms within 48 hours for cocaine, heroin, and methamphetamine exposure, but there may be delays of up to 2-3 weeks for methadone. Short hospital stays after birth make it imperative that children who are at risk are identified so that they can receive supportive treatment, particularly since they often feed poorly and can quickly become dehydrated and undernourished. Polydrug use makes it difficult to describe a typical profile of **symptoms**, but they usually include:

- Tremors
- Irritability
- Hypertonicity
- High-pitched crying
- Diarrhea
- Dry skin
- Seizures (in severe cases)

**Treatment** is supportive, but children with opiate exposure may be given decreasing doses of opiates, such as morphine elixir, with close monitoring until the child is weaned off of the medication.

## Fetal Nicotine/Carbon Monoxide Exposure

About 25% of women who smoke regularly before becoming pregnant continue to smoke throughout pregnancy, and others are exposed to second-hand smoke, putting the fetus at risk for a number of abnormalities from **exposure to nicotine and carbon monoxide**:

- Fetal growth retardation with damage to neurotransmitters accompanied by nervous system cell death with concomitant damage to peripheral autonomic nervous system
- Vasoconstriction from nicotine and interference with oxygen transport caused by carbon monoxide can lead to fetal hypoxia
- Vasoconstriction leading to increased risk of spontaneous abortion, prematurity, and low birth weight
- Increased risk for perinatal death and SIDS
- Cognitive deficiency and learning disorders, such as auditory processing defects (Children of mothers who smoke have a 50% increase in idiopathic intellectual disability.)
- Increased cancer risk, especially for acute lymphocytic leukemia and lymphoma

## Cardiovascular Risk Reduction

Some children, specifically those with diabetes mellitus, Kawasaki disease, and familial hypercholesterolemia, are at increased risk of developing **cardiovascular disease**, which can lead to severe coronary artery disease in less than ten years from onset. Screening children who are at risk should begin at age 2 and include cholesterol levels to assess for an elevation of low-density lipoprotein (LDL):

- Total cholesterol <170 and LDL <110: Normal level
- Total cholesterol 170-199 and LDL 110-120: Borderline elevation
- Total cholesterol >200 with LDL >130: Elevated

Early dietary intervention to reduce cholesterol and prevent further increase in LDLs can significantly reduce morbidity and mortality. Dietary recommendations to reduce LDLs include guidelines provided in the *Therapeutic Lifestyle Changes* diet created by the National Institutes of Health for those at risk or with elevated cholesterol.

- 25–30% of diet should be from fat and <7% from saturated fat
- 10–25 g of soluble fiber per day
- <200 mg dietary cholesterol per day
- ≥2 g of plant sterols or stanols per day (found in vegetables, fruits, and nuts)
- 30 minutes of moderate to vigorous exercise per day

# Pediatric Injury Prevention

## Environmental Assessment

### *Environmental Health History*

The environmental health history is important to determine potential hazards in the child's surroundings that may contribute to poor health or injuries. Examples of potential exposures that should be considered when taking a pediatric environmental health history include air pollution, including industrial exposure, cigarette smoke, carbon monoxide from furnaces or machinery; lead exposure through paint or plumbing in older homes; allergen exposure, such as pet dander, pollen, or mold; exposure to ultraviolet radiation during outdoor activities; water quality; and nutrition.

### *Environmental Influences on the Pediatric Patient's Health*

**Safety in the home environment** is a big influence on the health of the child. Accidental injuries in and around the home can include burns from scalding liquids or cooking appliances, drownings in pools or bathtubs, falls from climbing or from bicycles, and motor vehicle accidents or pedestrian-car accidents. Children who spend a great deal of time watching TV or playing video games are at risk for obesity and health issues that accompany obesity. Some children may try to be like characters they see on TV shows or other media, which can lead to aggressive behavior and risk-taking.



### *Consideration of Environmental Factors Prior to a Child's Return Home*

Environmental factors should be assessed within the **actual environment** if at all possible. If not, careful questioning and drawing of diagrams and approximate floor plans with the patient (or the patient's parent)—or asking for a drawing—can be useful, especially when showing the patient needed modifications. Family members may also assist with the assessment, providing useful information. Some patients or their parents, may be reluctant to admit that the home is cluttered or that they are unable to maintain the home environment in a sanitary condition. Brochures and handouts about home safety and assistive devices should be provided to the patient and caretaker as well as contact names and numbers for equipment needed in the home. A checklist should be compiled of all necessary changes or additions, with specific details, such as "Install 18-inch grab bar across from toilet." In some cases, a social worker or occupational therapist should visit the home.

### *General Elements of Environmental Safety*

Some elements of an environmental assessment are not specific to rooms in the house but are **general needs** that must be met in order for individuals, especially the disabled child and their caregivers, to remain safe:

- **Environmental hazards** such as piles of papers or junk on the floors, loose carpet or rugs, and cluttered pathways can cause falls and must be cleared, organized, or repaired.
- **Lighting** should be adequate enough for reading in all rooms and stairways.
- **Heat and air conditioning** must be adequate. The young and the elderly are especially susceptible to heat and cold injury.

- **Sanitation** should ensure that health hazards do not exist, such as from rotting food or infestations of cockroaches or rodents.
- **Animals** should be cared for adequately with access to food, water, toileting, and routine veterinary care.
- **Smoke/chemicals** in the environment may pose a hazard, such as exposure to cigarette smoke or cleaning materials.

## Dangerous Weapons and Toys

Parents should be advised that any guns kept in the home must be secured, with the guns unloaded and with the ammunition separately secured in a different location. All children, from an early age, should be taught to never pick up a gun or point it at anyone, even in play, and to immediately tell a trusted adult if they see anyone with a gun or know of anyone, such as a peer, who is carrying a gun or intends to harm someone with a gun.

Children should be protected from **dangerous toys**, which can include toys with small parts that may cause choking, especially for infants and toddlers. Toys that shoot projectiles, have cords or strings attached, or have sharp edges may pose a risk as well. Some products, such as some types of slime, have been found to contain toxins, so parents should regularly check with the US Consumer Product Safety Commission for alerts and should always read and adhere to warning labels. Smart toys and electronic devices that connect to the internet may provide identifying information about the child to unauthorized individuals.

## Recommendations for Parents and Children Regarding Social Situations

Recommendations for social situations include:

- **Strangers**: Parents should stress the importance of going places and playing outside with a friend or an adult and not being alone. Children should know to run and yell if a stranger asks them to carry something, help get something out of a car, or to help look for or see a puppy or kitten. Parents should stress that children should never get into a car with a stranger or an acquaintance who says that the child's parent has sent the person unless this person uses a password. Children should know to yell what is happening ("This woman is taking me!") and should know their full name, address, and phone number as soon as they are old enough to learn them.
- **Violence**: Parents should limit children's exposure to violent media content (TV, movies, video games) and use blocking tools when appropriate. Parents should encourage children to talk about their feeling if they've experienced or observed violence and to reassure them. If violence is common, children should play only in safe areas and learn safety rules, such as dropping to the ground if they hear gunshots.
- **Bullying**: Parents should recognize the signs that a child is being bullied (depression, withdrawal, dislike of school, change in affect, lack of friends, change of sleep patterns, bruises) and teach children the impact that bullying has on others. Advise parents to teach children to tell an adult if they are being bullied and to respond assertively, act unimpressed, make a joke out of mean comments, and get involved in activities, such as clubs, where they feel safe. If children are cyberbullied, they should block the senders, change passwords, and report it to an adult.
- **Automobile safety/distracted driving**: Children should be seated and secured properly for their age and size and should be taught to avoid yelling, throwing things, and scuffling while in the car as this may distract the driver. Teenage drivers should be taught safe driving (including never driving while drinking), should have clear consequences for unsafe driving (such as a loss of driving privileges), and should have an app on their phones that prevents texting while driving and provides their location to their parents.

## RECOMMENDATIONS FOR SPORTS AND RECREATION

Recommendations regarding sports and recreation include:

- **Concussion risks**: Greatest risks are from sports activities (football, hockey, soccer, lacrosse) and accidents (fall, car/bicycle). Parents should ensure that any sports team a child participates in has adequate safety rules (limits to tackling, for example) and that coaches carefully monitor the children. Children should always wear appropriate safety gear, such as helmets, when engaged in sports activities and should never continue playing if exhibiting any signs of head injury (headache, dizziness, confusion).
- **Helmet use**: Helmets (the appropriate type) should be worn for sports activities that may involve falls or blows to the head (hockey, football, skateboarding, baseball, bicycling). Helmets should fit snuggly so that they don't move if they are rotated, turned, or tilted, and the helmet should be pressed down at the crown to check for fitting of the jaw pads and chin straps. Football helmets may be air/fluid filled or padded.

## VEHICLE SAFETY

### *BOAT SAFETY*

According to the US Coast Guard's recommendations for **boat safety**, infants who are not of the appropriate weight and size to wear approved personal flotation devices (PFDs) should not be taken on recreational boats (rowboats, motorboats, kayaks, sailboats). All other children should wear life jackets that are properly fitted and secured. PFDs do not include swimming aids intended for play, such as water wings or pool noodles. If an infant is on a boat, a caregiver wearing a life jacket should hold the infant at all times and should not place the child in a car seat (which will not float). Infants and young children are more likely to develop hypothermia, so they should be wrapped with a dry blanket or towel if cold and shivering. Children by about age 3 should be taught safety rules, such as keeping hands and feet inside the boat and walking instead of running. All children should take swimming lessons. Older children should take a boat safety course if possible. Adolescents should be cautioned to never engage in drinking or recreational drug use while boating.



### *CAR SEATS*

All infants, regardless of age, must be placed properly in an **infant car seat** during transit. Holding an infant while the car is in motion is not safe. Car seats should be new or in very good condition and fastened according to manufacturer's guidelines to ensure safety:

- Place the car seat in the back seat and away from any side airbags.
- Always securely buckle the child into the seat.
- Face the infant seat toward the rear of the car.
- Recline the seat so that the infant's head does not fall forward.
- Place padding around (not under) the infant if the infant slouches to one side.
- Place blankets OVER the straps and buckles, not under.

The infant/toddler should be placed in the rear-facing seat to the maximum weight and height allowed by the seat (some accommodate up to 65 pounds). Once transitioned to front-facing seats, children should be placed in belt-positioning booster seats until the vehicle's seat/shoulder belts fit properly (usually until 4' 9" and 8-12 years old). Until age 13, children should sit secured in the back seat and not the front.

## LEADING CAUSES OF DEATH BY AGE GROUP

### *BIRTH TO 10-YEAR AGE GROUP*

For the **birth to 10-year** age group, the US Preventive Services Task Force has assembled a list of the **five leading causes of death**. The number one cause of death in this age group is actually a group of conditions that arise in the time period surrounding birth (the "**perinatal period**"). There are a number of conditions that arise surrounding birth that are fatal, including placental problems (premature separation, abruption), umbilical cord problems (cord prolapse, nuchal cord, single umbilical artery), infections (chorioamnionitis, congenital pneumonia), trauma during the birthing process (nerve damage, intracranial hemorrhage), and hemolytic disease of the newborn. The second leading cause of death is attributed to **congenital defects**, including tetralogy of Fallot, transposition of the great arteries, spina bifida, and anencephaly. Other leading causes of death include **sudden infant death syndrome (SIDS)**, **motor vehicle injuries**, and **other unintentional injuries**.

#### Injury Prevention Counseling

Injury prevention counseling is a strong recommendation for the **birth to 10-year** age group, owing to the fact that motor vehicle accidents and other unintentional accidents are leading causes of death for this population. Children and their parents should be advised to use car safety seats until the age of 5 (this is subject to state law, however, as some states require the use of booster seats until a certain height or age is reached). After the age of 5, standard safety belts should always be used. When biking, skating, or skateboarding, a helmet should always be worn; these activities should not take place in the street. Parents should be advised to become CPR certified. They should also be advised to keep drugs, poisons, guns, other weapons, and matches out of the reach of children; to install smoke detectors and plan an escape route in the event of fire; and to make sure that stairs, windows, and pools are safe for children.

### *11- to 24-Year Age Group*

The list of the top five leading causes of death in the **11-24** age population differs significantly from the leading causes of death in the birth to 10-year age population. Leading the list for ages 11-24 are deaths caused by either **motor vehicle accidents or other unintentional accidents**. Second on the list is **homicide**, followed by **suicide**. The fourth leading cause of death in the 11-24 age population is **cancer**. The most common fatal cancers in this age group include leukemia (acute lymphocytic leukemia and acute myeloid leukemia), brain tumors (medulloblastoma, astrocytoma, and brainstem glioma), rhabdomyosarcoma, neuroblastoma, Wilms tumor, Ewing sarcoma, and Hodgkin's lymphoma. The fifth leading cause of death in this age population is due to **general heart diseases**, which may include cardiomyopathies and faulty valves.

## Youth Risk Behavior Surveillance System

The **Youth Risk Behavior Surveillance System** (YRBSS) is a program conducted through the CDC that monitors eight different categories of health-risk behaviors of adolescents:

- Unintentional injuries and violence
- Tobacco use
- Alcohol and other drug use
- Sexual behaviors
- Dietary behaviors
- Physical activity
- Obesity, overweight, and weight control
- Other health topics

The YRBSS gathers data from participating states and local surveys (such as large cities) from grades 9-12 and then compiles the information, assessing for trends. Current results reflect data collected in 2021 and released in 2023. Responses are either weighted (≥60% participation) or unweighted (relates only to those completing survey). Weighted results can be generalized to the teenage population at large in the area of the survey. The data obtained in the YRBSS is used to determine progress in national health objectives for health promotion.

## YRBSS 2021 Results

### *Tobacco Use*

The CDC conducts the Youth Risk Behavior Surveillance System to determine health-risk behaviors that contribute to significant morbidity in adolescents. **Tobacco,** often thought of as an adult issue, is a cause of concern for children and teenagers. Tobacco use is one of the leading preventable causes of death in the United

States, but 2021 results showed that about 6.3% of children (down from 9.5% in 2019) have tried smoking before high school, often beginning by age 12, putting themselves at risk for heart and lung disease as adults. Almost 18% of children have tried smoking in total according to 2021 results, which is a downward trend. A newer trend is the use of electronic vapor products, with 36% of children reporting having tried this product at some point, and 18% reporting current use. Those most at risk are males in low-income families with parents who smoke. Male adolescents may smoke to be rebellious, but females often smoke to lose weight. Other factors include the desire to be part of a group, lack of supervision, and accessibility of tobacco. Intervention includes identifying those smoking, providing information about the dangers of smoking, beginning with children at about 9 years old, and providing programs to help teenagers quit smoking.

### Drug Use

Drug use continues to be a serious problem for children and teenagers, with some starting as young as 9 or 10, using a wide variety of drugs, including marijuana, crack, prescription drugs, cocaine, inhalants (such as glue and lighter fluid), hallucinogens, and steroids. Marijuana is the most reported drug in the high school data, with about 28% of children reporting having used marijuana in their lifetime. Approximately 13% of children reported having used illicit drugs (e.g., cocaine, heroin, inhalants, methamphetamines, ecstasy, or hallucinogens) at least once in their lifetime. Risk factors for drug use include aggressive behavior, poor social skills, and poor academic progress coupled with lack of parental supervision, poverty, and availability of drugs. Small children who use drugs are often reacting to circumstances within the family, while teenagers are more likely to use drugs in response to peer pressure from outside the family. Studies have shown that early intervention to teach children better self-control and coping skills is often more effective than trying to change behavior patterns that are established, so family-based programs often show positive results. Teenagers may need help with basic academic skills and social skills to improve communication. Methods of resisting drugs must be provided and reinforced. Drug recovery programs can be helpful but are often too expensive or not available for those who need them.

### Alcohol Use

Alcohol use is a significant problem in adolescence and even in younger children. It is the most-commonly abused substance. Of high schoolers who responded to the survey question in 2021, about 23% reported having had at least one drink within the past 30 days (down from 30% in 2019). While alcohol can impair development of almost all body systems in a growing child, it is of particular concern for the effects on the neurological system and liver. Additionally, because it interferes with impulse control, adolescents who drink are often involved in violence, abuse, and at-risk sexual behavior. Drinking should be suspected if a child has memory problems, changes in behavior, poor academic progress, emotional lability, and physical changes, such as slurring of speech, general lethargy, or lack of coordination. Intervention includes teaching children from around age 9 about the dangers of drinking, identifying those who are drinking, identifying underlying problems, and providing programs to help teenagers stop drinking, such as counseling or Alcoholics Anonymous.

### High-Risk Sexual Behavior

High-risk sexual behavior in teenagers is often coupled with other health-risk behaviors, such as drinking and drug use. In 2021, about 30% of high school students reported having previously had sex (a significant decline from the 38.4% reported in 2019), with around 3% becoming sexually active before the age of 13. Risk factors include poverty, single-family homes, lack of supervision, and siblings or peers who are sexually active. Those who have sex before age 15 are especially vulnerable, often having multiple partners and unprotected sex, leading to sexually transmitted infections (STIs) and pregnancy. They are often emotionally vulnerable and unable to deal effectively with relationships. Intervention should begin early with age-appropriate honest sex education. Abstinence education, while the ideal, has not been successful in changing the sexual behavior of teenagers, with studies showing that many of those signing pledges to remain virgins are already sexually active. Teenagers who are sexually active should be advised regarding the use of condoms, birth control, and protection from STIs in a non-judgmental manner.

## Prevention of STIs

The **CDC** has developed five strategies to prevent and control the spread of STIs:

- **Educate** those at risk about how to make changes in sexual practices to prevent infection.
- **Identify** symptomatic and asymptomatic infected persons who might not seek diagnosis or treatment.
- **Diagnose** and treat those who are infected.
- **Prevent infection** of sex partners through evaluation, treatment, and counseling.
- Provide pre-exposure **vaccination** for those at risk.

Practitioners are advised to inquire of patients' **sexual histories** and to assess risk. The 5-P approach to questioning is advocated. Practitioners should ask about:

- **Partners**: Gender and number
- **Pregnancy prevention**: Birth control
- **Protection**: Methods used
- **Practices**: Type of sexual practices (oral, anal, vaginal) and use of condoms
- **Past history of STIs**: High-risk behavior (promiscuity, prostitution) and disease risk (human immunodeficiency virus [HIV]/ hepatitis)

The CDC recommends a number of specific preventive methods as part of the clinical guidelines for prevention of sexually transmitted infections:

- **Abstinence or reduction** in number of sex partners.
- Pre-exposure **vaccination**: All those evaluated for STIs should receive hepatitis B vaccination, and men who have sex with men (MSM) and illicit drug users should receive hepatitis A vaccination.
- **Male latex (or polyurethane) condoms** should be used for all sexual encounters with only water-based lubricants used with latex.
- **Female condoms** may be used if a male condom cannot be used properly.
- Condoms and diaphragms should not be used with spermicides containing **nonoxynol-9 (N-9)**, and N-9 should not be used as a lubricant for anal sex.
- **Non-barrier contraceptive measures** provide no protection from STIs and must not be relied on to prevent disease.

## Measures to Prevent Injury/Illness of Toddlers

### *Home and Auto Safety*

Toddlers are curious and very mobile, so accidents can occur easily in and outside the home. **Auto safety** includes using the appropriate size child-safety seat in the back seat, and buckling the child up every time they are in a moving vehicle. Toddlers need to be supervised closely when playing outside, to prevent them from running into the street in front of moving vehicles. Parents can begin to teach them how to stop, look, and listen before crossing a street.

**The home environment** needs to be child-proofed, moving all poisonous substances well away from the toddler's reach (keeping in mind that toddlers will learn to climb). Poisons should be stored in a locked or inaccessible location to the child. Medication should be stored up high and children should not be told that medication is candy when they are taking it.

### *Water, Toy, and Gun Safety, and Burns*

The following are some measures the parents can take to prevent injury and illness of their toddler, focusing on burns and water, toy, and gun safety:

- Never leave a toddler alone in or near water, as they can drown in as little as one inch of water. Toddlers are still unstable and prone to falling, possibly into a puddle or bucket.
- When appropriate, life jackets should be worn by toddlers (in a boat or near a lake, pond, or pool).
- Toddlers should wear helmets when riding tricycles.
- Make sure any toys given to toddlers are appropriate for their age and safe. Balloons, small toys, and plastic bags are potential choking hazards.
- A big concern today is guns kept in the home. Toddlers don't know the difference between a toy gun and a real gun, so all guns kept in the home must be properly secured.
- Teach the toddler the meaning of "hot," while using safety plugs on appliances, keep matches and lighters up high, turn pot handles toward the back of the stove, and don't use tablecloths in the home (toddlers can pull on these and topple hot food/liquids on themselves).

## Measures to Prevent Injury/Illness of Preschoolers

### *Home and Auto Safety*

Preschoolers are aware of potential dangers and can be taught safety rules. Poisonous substances, including medicines, need to have safety caps and be locked up. Watch for unsafe areas at playgrounds. Enforce the wearing of safety equipment when playing sports. Use the appropriate safety seat (booster) in the back seat until the child weighs 80 lb. After 80 lb, use a seat belt in the back seat. Do not leave a child alone in a car or home. Use close supervision when playing outside and near streets. Have the child wear a bike helmet when riding and teach him the rules for safe riding. Parents should have the poison control number saved to their phones or written down somewhere it can be quickly accessed.



### *Auto, Sports, and Water Safety*

**School age children** are especially prone to accidents, due to their mobility and participation in sports and other physical activities. The following rules should be taught to children and enforced by the parents/caregivers:

- Children should always wear a seatbelt, and sit in the backseat, in a moving vehicle.
- When riding anything with wheels, the child should always wear a helmet and elbow and knee pads.
- The child must obey traffic signals when walking on or across streets.
- The school-aged child should participate in swim lessons and be taught to swim with a buddy, wear a life jacket when in a boat, and not dive into shallow water.

## Measures to Prevent Injury/Illness of School Age Children

The following are some measures parents can take to prevent injury/illness of their school age child, focusing on drug, fire, stranger, and gun safety:

- Keep medicine locked and teach children the dangers of taking any medicine without adult supervision.
- Begin teaching the child about illegal drug use and smoking.
- Use sunscreen when playing outside.
- Establish an escape route for each member of the family in case of fire and practice the route monthly.
- Don't allow the child to use the stove without adult supervision.
- Teach the child to stay away from guns. Parents should keep guns unloaded and in a locked location with ammunition stored in a separate location.

- Teach the child to not talk to strangers or approach strange vehicles.
- Make sure the child knows their phone number, their address, and how to call 911.
- Find a neighbor's house that can serve as a safe place for the child if needed.

### Measures to Prevent Injury/Illness of Adolescents

**Adolescents** think they are invincible, which can contribute to risk-taking behaviors.

- Motor vehicle accidents claim many teenagers' lives every year. Teens should take driver's education courses, wear seat belts at all times, obey traffic laws, and refrain from drinking and driving.
- If an adolescent legally uses firearms, they need to be taught safety rules and how to use and store firearms.
- Adolescents should be taught the risks of using drugs, alcohol, and nicotine.
- Sports teams should focus on safety, proper equipment, and appropriate conditioning.
- Adolescents should know proper swimming and water safety and use sunscreen when outside.
- Sexual activity is a high-risk behavior that should be addressed on a family level. If appropriate, the adolescent should be taught sexual responsibility.

### Appropriate Sunscreen Use

While children need some exposure to the sun, sunscreen protects against harmful ultraviolet rays that can cause burns, sun damage, premature aging, and skin cancer. Sunscreen should be generously applied before children go out in the sun, covering the parts of the body that are exposed, including the face, lips, tops of the ears, and back of the neck. It should be reapplied at least every 2 hours, and if children are going to be around water, the sunscreen should be waterproof. The sun protection factor (SPF) should be a minimum of 30 for children older than 6 months, as recommended by the American Academy of Dermatology. The American Academy of Pediatrics recommends that children under the age of 6 months be kept out of direct sunlight. If they must be in direct sunlight, children should be covered by clothing and hats. A small amount of SPF 15 sunscreen is allowed on children under the age of 6 months, but only to small areas such as their face and the backs of their hands.

### Guidelines for Using Insect Repellant

Insect repellant may be used on children to prevent insect bites, but it should be used with caution. Many insect repellants contain N,N-diethyl-meta-toluamide (DEET), which has been shown to be safe for limited use with children over 2 months of age. Repellants used on children should have less than a 30% concentration of DEET and should only be applied once a day. It should be sprayed on a caregiver's hand and then put on the child, rather than spraying the child directly. This decreases the likelihood of the child ingesting the repellant. Insect repellant can also be applied to clothing to provide some protection without applying it directly to the skin.

## Family Education

### Educational Needs of New Mothers

The educational needs of the new mother and family vary depending on age, background, education, experience, and expectations. The needs of the adolescent mother with no experience may be quite different from those of the multiparous mother. Assessing individual needs can be difficult in the short time women are usually hospitalized, so education should cover a wide range of topics. A checklist of topics may be a helpful starting point for the mother to indicate her needs. Because mothers are usually fatigued for the first 24-48 hours, teaching after that time is most effective, but many mothers leave the hospital on the second day. Demonstration with return demonstration is an effective method to ensure that a mother can carry out tasks, but education should anticipate other needs and concerns that may arise. Mothers often have concerns about a variety of issues, such as childcare, contraception, and resuming sexual relations. Pamphlets, website information, or videos that can be sent home with the mother are very helpful.

### SAFE POSITIONING FOR INFANTS

Infants should be placed on their **backs** for sleeping. Sleeping on the stomach increases the risk of **sudden infant death syndrome (SIDS)**.

- Position the infant on the back when unattended or sleeping, but alternate the direction the head faces to prevent one side of the head from flattening (**positional molding**).
- Provide supervised time each day with the infant lying on the abdomen (only on firm surfaces) to strengthen head and neck muscles and to prevent positional molding.
- Hold the infant, rather than leaving them in a carrier.
- Position baby in side-lying position, alternating from one side to the other, using specially designed supports to maintain the position.

### INFANT CAR SEAT

All infants, regardless of age, must be placed properly in an infant car seat during transit. Holding an infant while the car is in motion is not safe. Car seats should be new or in very good condition and fastened according to the manufacturer's guidelines to ensure safety.

- Place the car seat in the back seat and away from any side airbags.
- Always securely buckle the child into the seat.
- Face the infant seat toward the rear of the car.
- Recline the seat so the infant's head does not fall forward.
- Place padding around (not under) the infant if the infant slouches to one side.
- Place blankets over the straps and buckles, not under.

### UMBILICAL CORD CARE

Education surrounding the umbilical cord should include the following information:

- Protect the cord from moisture, with top of diaper folded under the cord instead of covering it.
- If the cord becomes soiled, wash with mild soap and water, rinse, and dry. Swabbing with alcohol is no longer recommended and may increase skin irritation.
- Avoid covering the cord stump with clothing, which may cause irritation.
- Give the infant only sponge baths until the cord falls off in about 10-14 days.
- Report signs of infection, such as erythema, swelling, or purulent discharge.

**Note**: The umbilical cord changes color from grayish-brown to black as it dries and finally falls off.

### FECAL ELIMINATION

The first stool (**meconium**) is usually passed within 24 hours and is black and tarry looking. The stool then transitions to greenish as the baby nurses or takes formula, and by the third day, the stool is usually yellow or yellow-green for breastfed babies and yellow or light brown for formula-fed babies. Typically, babies have 2-3 stools daily by day 3 and ≥4 daily by day 5, but this may vary.

- Report abnormalities, such as bloody stools, watery stools, very hard stools, clay-colored or whitish stools, black stools (after meconium has passed), and "currant jelly" stools.
- Cleanse skin thoroughly after defecation with mild soap and water, plain water, or unscented baby wipes.
- Examine skin carefully for irritation.

## Urinary Elimination

Urination is estimated according to the number of **wet diapers** in a 24-hour period. Typically, the infant has 1 wet diaper the first day, 2 the next, and so on until urination stabilizes at 6-8 wet diapers by about day 6.

- Check diaper frequently. Infants often urinate during or after feeding.
- Change diapers when wet, gently cleansing skin with mild soap and water, plain water, or unscented baby wipes.

## Cradle Cap

Cradle cap may appear as scaly, crusted, or flaky skin on the scalp and other parts of the face. It is not contagious and usually clears by 1 or 2 months. It is not usually a sign of poor hygiene.

- Cleanse scalp or affected areas thoroughly, gently rubbing the area with a terry cloth or brushing to loosen crust or flakes.
- If persistent, try softening the crusts with olive oil. Leave it in for 15 minutes, and then brush or gently comb to loosen crusts or flakes. Finally, wash with baby shampoo.

## Diaper Rash

Diaper rash usually results from leaving the infant in soiled/wet diapers and/or not adequately cleansing the skin, although breastfed infants sometimes react to foods the mother has eaten. A rash may also indicate an allergic response to baby wipes or other products, such as lotions or creams. Antibiotics may cause diaper rash. In some cases, a **fungal infection** may occur, usually characterized by red, weepy open areas. Purulent discharge may indicate infection.

- Change diapers as soon as possible when wet or soiled.
- Cleanse skin gently with water.
- Remove diaper and expose skin to air whenever possible.
- Apply barrier cream or ointment especially formulated for diaper rash to prevent or treat diaper rash.
- Contact physician if rash worsens and does not respond to treatment, as antifungals, cortisone, or topical antibiotics may be indicated.

## Choking or Gagging in Infant

Education regarding chocking/gagging should include the following:

- Ensure small hazardous items, such as pins and cotton balls or materials, such as baby powder are out of reach.
- DO NOT prop bottle for feeding.
- Burp infant regularly during feedings, whether breast or bottle.
- Keep baby in upright position with head elevated during feedings.
- Check nipple of bottle to ensure it is dripping and not running freely.
- If the infant is choking, secure face down on forearm, tilted downward, and use the heel of the hand to thump on the mid-back. Repeat as necessary. If choking does not resolve with evidence of breathing immediately, call 911 and begin CPR.

Note: Prevention is important, as most **choking and gagging episodes** can be avoided.

## Burping the Infant

Both breastfed and bottle-fed babies require **burping** because they swallow air when feeding, although bottle-fed babies tend to require more burping. Infants often show indications (grimacing, squirming, spitting up, and crying) that they are uncomfortable and need to burp.

- Burp the infant routinely after 2 or 3 ounces of formula or after nursing on one breast.
- Position the infant on the shoulder with a burp cloth under the infant's head and gently pat or rub the infant's back.
- Change to a different position if the baby doesn't burp. Try on the opposite shoulder or with the infant sitting on the lap supported by one hand while the other hand pats or rubs the infant's back.

## Bathing the Infant

The infant should receive **sponge baths** until the umbilical cord falls off at 10-14 days, and then a bath in an **infant tub** (NOT in an adult tub). Mild soap/shampoo intended for babies or water alone may be used for the bath.

- Make sure the environmental temperature is warm.
- Fill tub with 2-3 inches of water.
- ALWAYS check water temperature to make sure it is warm and NOT hot.
- Set water heaters ≤120 °F to prevent inadvertent scalding.
- Support the baby during the bath with one arm under upper back to support the neck and head while holding the infant under the axillae.
- Pour water over the child with the free hand and use that hand to wash the hair and the body.
- Lift the baby from the tub and wrap in a towel to dry.
- Dry thoroughly, making sure all skin folds and crevices are dry to prevent irritation and rashes.
- Avoid use of lotions or creams.

## Fontanels

The infant's fontanels (anterior and posterior) are covered by thick membranous tissue and should feel flat but firm.

- Do not be afraid to touch the fontanels or cleanse the scalp.
- Report **bulging** above the level of the skull, as this may indicate increased intracranial pressure.
- Report a **soft fontanel** that sinks below the level of the skull, as this may indicate dehydration.

## Circumcision

Circumcision rates have dropped by 10% over the last 30 years, with about 58% of male infants now being **circumcised** in the United States. The American Academy of Pediatrics has confirmed that the benefits outweigh the risks, though they do not have a formal recommendation for circumcision and instead leave that decision up to the parents. Benefits including decreased risk of prostate cancer, urinary tract infections, and sexually transmitted infections such as HIV. Most parents make their decision based on cultural or religious beliefs or the factor of cost, as some insurance companies and many Medicaid programs do not cover the cost of circumcision. While at one time infants were not thought to experience pain, it is now clear that they do, so circumcision should be done using a local anesthesia or topical EMLA cream.

### Post-Circumcision Care

After circumcision, the end of the foreskin is typically swollen and red, and a small amount of bleeding may persist for 24 hours.

- Change the diaper immediately, because urine may cause pain to the open tissue.
- Cleanse the area gently with water and pat dry.
- Apply petroleum jelly gauze to the incision area as directed by the individual physician.
- Avoid using soap or commercial cleansing products, such as baby wipes, until the circumcision heals.
- Report any change, such as increased swelling, redness, temperature, or purulent discharge.

### Care of the Uncircumcised Penis

The infant's foreskin is different from that of the adult male. It does not **separate and retract** until the child is around 5 years old.

- Do NOT attempt to retract the foreskin.
- Do NOT use cotton swabs to clean.
- Wash the penis with soap and water or just water during the routine bath.

## Shaken Baby Syndrome

Shaken baby syndrome is believed to be the result of vigorous shaking of a neonate, causing acute subdural hematoma with subarachnoid, and retinal hemorrhages. The shaking of the brain may damage vessels and nerves with resultant cerebral edema. Parents should be advised of the importance of always supporting and protecting the neonate's head and avoiding activities that may injure the child, such as throwing and catching a neonate or small child. Parents should be advised that sometimes children may not exhibit obvious neurological symptoms immediately after trauma but have learning disabilities and behavioral disorders that appear in school.

## Neonatal CPR

Most cardiac arrests in newborns are associated with respiratory arrest rather than cardiac arrest, so **cardiopulmonary resuscitation** of newborns follows the ABC protocol rather than the compressions only protocol used for adults. The parent should be advised to take a CPR course, especially if the neonate is at risk and if arrest occurs, immediately call 911 for help or ask someone else to call and begin CPR:

- **Airway:** Tilt the head slightly back and lift the chin to open the airway.
- **Breathing:** If the neonate does not begin breathing, administer 2 puffs to ventilate the lungs. For small neonates, place the mouth to cover the neonate's nose and mouth and ventilate each time for approximately one second, observing the chest to ensure it is rising. For the infant with a heart rate ≥60/minute without normal breathing, administer one breath every 2-3 seconds (20-30 breaths per minute).
- **Compressions:** Infants that require chest compressions should receive two breaths per 30 compressions (30:2) for a single rescuer, and two breaths per 15 compressions for two rescuers (15:2). The chest should be depressed approximately 1.5 inches, using two fingers or two thumbs while encircling the hands around the baby's body. The optimum rate of compressions is approximately 100-120 per minute.

# History and Physical Assessment

## Components of Health History

There are several different components that must be included in a nursing **health history**:

- The **biographic element** of the nursing health history includes the patient's name, age, physical address, sex, marital status, occupational status, religious preference, healthcare financing, and regular physician.
- The **chief complaint** is the next aspect of the history and involves the reason the patient is seeking care.
- Following this, the **history of the present illness** details the current health problem, including date of onset, description of symptoms, and any aggravating factors.
- **Past medical history** entails asking about the patient's usual health status, past medical or surgical problems, immunization status, current medications, allergies (including medication allergies), and family history.
- A detailed **family history** is important as it may reveal risk factors for certain medical conditions such as heart disease, diabetes, arthritis, hypertension, or mental disorders.
- The **review of systems** is used to obtain a full, systematic report by the patient on subjective symptoms. For example, in inquiring about the cardiovascular system, the nurse notes positive or negative answers regarding chest pain and other symptoms or problems that are pertinent to heart function and circulation.

### *Social Determinants of Health*

Social determinants of health refer to the non-medical elements of a person's social environment that have a direct impact on his or her physical health and tendencies. The heavy influence of this component of health is reflected in its being listed as one of the five main sections of *Healthy People 2030,* an initiative of the US Department of Health and Human Services (HHS) that aims to allow people to have longer and healthier lives, to reduce health disparities, to create environments that promote health, and to improve the quality of life and health across all age groups. According to HHS, social determinants of health are "the conditions in the environments where people are born, live, learn, work, play, worship, and age that affect a wide range of health, functioning, and quality-of-life outcomes and risks." For these reasons, a health history should inquire into the patient's social determinants of health also:

- The patient's **lifestyle** is an important component of the nursing health history and includes habits, diet, sleep, hobbies, and the patient's ability to perform the activities of daily living.
- A **social history** is the component of the nursing health history that details family relationships, ethnicity, educational level, economic status, and the condition of the patient's home and environment.
- The nursing health history also includes the patient's **psychological status** and the patient's **usual means of obtaining healthcare.**

## Obtaining a Health History

The health history assessment and review of systems help to identify nursing care needs:

- First, check the patient's chart for information gathered by other health professionals and note any areas that need clarification prior to the patient interview.
- Use the written or electronic template provided by the facility to record the history, customizing it to the patient.
- Record any changes in this information during the patient's hospital stay.
- Plan the time of the interview with the patient when there are not critical care needs that must be met first.
- Take time to alleviate patient's anxiety and establish rapport and trust.

- Approach the patient with an attitude of respect and sincere caring.
- Listen to the patient and use effective therapeutic communication skills during the interview.
- Review all areas of the health history with the patient and then ask for any other information that may be important. The family may be able to fill in missing information if the patient is unable to do so.

## PHYSICAL EXAMINATION TECHNIQUES

The **physical exam** is an important element of nursing assessment. The physical assessment needs to be organized and systematic and should be age- and developmentally-appropriate. The physical exam may be a complete physical exam, a system-specific exam, or an exam of a specific body part. The basic **techniques** of a physical exam are inspection, palpation, auscultation, and percussion. The nurse makes a visual, aural, and olfactory assessment of the patient. This includes paying attention to the patient's skin tone, breathing sounds, and breath odor. Palpation includes techniques for touching the patient's body in order to get physical information such as temperature, skin tone and condition, or swelling in the glands. Auscultation is the examination of sounds within the body, such as heart tones, wheezing or crackling in the lungs, or bowel sounds. Auscultation is usually performed with a stethoscope. Percussion involves making quick taps to parts of the body with the fingers to ascertain the shape and condition of organs, identify areas of tenderness, or assess reflexes.

### *PALPATION*

Use of palpation can provide valuable details during physical assessment of the patient:

- Be sure to wash and warm the hands prior to touching the patient.
- Do not use gloves unless you anticipate contact with bodily fluids.
- Explain the process and how it will feel and instruct the patient to relax the muscles if appropriate. Provide warmth and privacy during palpation.
- Use light palpation to feel the cervical lymph nodes and thyroid glands and to feel the superficial blood vessels for thrills.
- Place your hands on the chest to detect heart vibrations and to feel tactile fremitus during speech.
- Palpate the relaxed abdomen to identify structures and their borders and any masses or nodules on otherwise smooth organ surfaces. Of note, the abdomen should be auscultated prior to palpation since palpation may cause bowel sounds that would not otherwise exist and may be misunderstood.
- Utilize both hands to palpate the female reproductive organs by pushing organs into the reach of the other hand.

Palpation to identify organs and structures takes practice. Each patient is different but after you palpate many patients, the similarities in organ borders and consistency can be determined.

#### PALPATING FOR TACTILE FREMITUS

The act of speaking causes the chest wall to vibrate. This vibration can be felt by placing your hands lightly on the chest wall over a section of the lungs bilaterally while the patient repeats the letter "e" or the numbers "99." The amount of vibration felt depends on the weight of the patient, the muscle mass of the chest and back, gender, deepness of the voice, and condition of the lungs. **Tactile fremitus** is greater over major airways and normal lung tissue. It is less over lungs full of air or with emphysema or a pneumothorax. Lung consolidation will produce increased fremitus. The nurse should not feel for fremitus over the sternum or scapula. The areas above and below the breasts and above, medial to, and below the scapulae should be tested.

### *Percussion*

Percussion is striking part of the body to set the chest or abdominal wall into motion, producing sound that helps to locate underlying organs and reveal whether they are dense or filled with air or fluid. The sounds produced include:

- **Tympany**: Hollow drum sound produced when the organ contains air (stomach, intestines)
- **Resonance**: Hollow, low-pitched sound of normal lungs
- **Hyperresonance**: Low-pitched sound of lungs with emphysema or pneumothorax (louder than resonance)
- **Dullness**: "thud" heard over dense structures such as the liver
- **Flatness**: sound heard over muscles or bones such as in the thigh

Percussion is performed by placing the middle finger of one hand over the area and striking it with the middle finger of the opposite hand. It can be used to find the margins of an organ or area of pathology by repeatedly striking areas near to each other and listening for changes in sound representing the edge of the organ. The extent of lung consolidation can be determined in this manner.

### *Auscultation*

Auscultation is listening to sounds within the body through either the bell or the diaphragm of the stethoscope. These sounds differ in the following ways:

- **Intensity**: The level of sound in terms of loudness
- **Frequency**: Low or high pitch of the sound
- **Quality**: Helps to distinguish between rumbling and musical-type sounds

The **bell** of the stethoscope is best when listening for the lower frequency sounds of heart murmurs or bruit, with the bell placed lightly on the skin. The **diaphragm** is best for high-pitched sounds, such as heart or lung sounds or bowel sounds, with the diaphragm placed firmly on the skin. The nurse should not touch the tubing or place the end of the stethoscope in contact with cloth or hair, or extra sounds will be heard that may obscure the sounds transmitted.



# Pain Assessment

## Pathophysiology of Pain

### *Nociceptors*

Nociceptors are the primary neurons, or **sensory receptors**, responding to stimuli in the skin, muscle, and joints, as well as the stomach, bladder, and uterus. These neurons have specialized responses for mechanical, thermal, or chemical stimuli. The **neuron stimulation** is a direct result of tissue injury and follows four stages: **transduction** where a change occurs, **transmission** where the impulse is transferred along the neural path, **modulation** or translation of the signal, and **perception** by the patient. When injury occurs, the nociceptors initiate the process that begins **depolarization of the peripheral nerve**. Nociceptors may consist of either A-fiber axons or C-fiber axons. The message travels along the neural pathway and creates a perception of pain. A-fiber axons carry these pain messages at a much faster rate than C-fiber axons.

### *Nociceptive Pain*

Nociceptive pain is an umbrella term for pain caused by **stimulation of the neuroreceptor**. This stimulation is a direct result of tissue injury. The severity of pain is proportionate to the extent of the injury. Nociceptive pain can be subdivided into two classifications: somatic and visceral pain. **Somatic pain** is located in the cutaneous tissues, bone joints, and muscle tissues. **Visceral pain** is specific to internal organs protected by a layer of viscera, such as the cardiovascular, respiratory, gastrointestinal, or genitourinary systems. Both types are treatable with opioids.

### Visceral Pain

Visceral pain is associated with the internal organs. It can be very different depending on the affected organ. Not all internal organs are sensitive to pain (some lack **nociceptors**, such as the spleen, kidney, and pancreas), and may withstand a great deal of damage without causing pain. Other internal organs, such as the stomach, bladder, and ureters, can create significant pain from even the slightest damage. Visceral pain generally has a **poorly defined area**. It is also capable of referring pain to other remote locations away from the area of injury. It is described as a squeezing or cramping: a deep ache within the internal organs. The patient may complain of a generalized sick feeling or have nausea and vomiting. Visceral pain generally responds well to treatment with **opioids**.

**Review Video: Visceral Pain**
Visit mometrix.com/academy and enter code: 430402

### Somatic Pain

Somatic pain refers to messages from pain receptors located in the **cutaneous or musculoskeletal tissues**. When the pain occurs within the musculoskeletal tissue, it is referred to as **deep somatic pain**. Metastasizing cancers commonly cause deep somatic pain. **Surface pain** refers to pain concentrated in the **dermis and cutaneous layers** such as that caused by a surgical incision. Deep somatic pain is generally described as a dull, throbbing ache that is well focused on the area of trauma. It responds well to **opioids**. Surface somatic pain is also directly focused on the injury. It is frequently described as sharper than deep somatic pain. It may also present as a burning or pricking sensation.

**Review Video: Somatic Pain**
Visit mometrix.com/academy and enter code: 982772

**Review Video: Somatic Nervous System**
Visit mometrix.com/academy and enter code: 100382

### *Neuropathic Pain*

Neuropathic pain results from injury to the **nervous system**. This can result from cancer cells compressing the nerves or spinal cord, from actual cancerous invasion into the nerves or spinal cord, or from chemical damage to the nerves caused by chemotherapy and radiation. Other causes include diabetes- and alcohol-related damage, trauma, neuralgias, or other illnesses affecting the neural path either centrally or peripherally. When the nerves become damaged, they are unable to carry accurate information. This results in more severe, distinct **pain messages**. The nerves may also relay pain messages long after the original cause of the pain is resolved. It can be described as sharp, burning, shooting, shocking, tingling, or electrical in nature. It may travel the length of the nerve path from the spine to a distal body part such as a hand, or down the buttocks to a foot. NSAIDs and opioids are generally ineffective against neuropathic pain, though adjuvants may enhance the therapeutic effect of opioids. Nerve blocks may also be used.

**Review Video: Neuropathic Pain**
Visit mometrix.com/academy and enter code: 780523

## Adverse Systemic Effects of Pain

Acute pain causes adverse systemic effects that can negatively affect many body systems.

- **Cardiovascular**: Tachycardia and increased blood pressure is a common response to pain, causing increased cardiac output and systemic vascular resistance. In those with pre-existing cardiovascular disease, such as compromised ventricular function, cardiac output may decrease. The increased myocardial need for oxygen may cause or worsen myocardial ischemia.

- **Respiratory**: Increased need for oxygen causes an increase in minute ventilation and splinting due to pain, which may compromise pulmonary function. If the chest wall movement is constrained, tidal volume falls, impairing the ability to cough and clear secretions. Bed rest further compromises ventilation.
- **Gastrointestinal**: Sphincter tone increases and motility decreases, sometimes resulting in ileus. There may be an increased secretion of gastric acids, which irritates the gastric lining and can cause ulcerations. Nausea, vomiting, and constipation may occur. Reflux may result in aspiration pneumonia. Abdominal distension may occur.
- **Urinary**: Increased sphincter tone and decreased motility result in urinary retention.
- **Endocrine**: Hormone levels are affected by pain. Catabolic hormones such as catecholamine, cortisol, and glucagon increase, and anabolic hormones such as insulin and testosterone decrease. Lipolysis increases along with carbohydrate intolerance. Sodium retention can occur because of increased ADH, aldosterone, angiotensin, and cortisol. This in turn causes fluid retention and a shift to extracellular space.
- **Hematologic**: There may be reduced fibrinolysis, increased adhesiveness of platelets, and increased coagulation.
- **Immune**: Leukocytosis and lymphopenia may occur, increasing risk of infection.
- **Emotional**: Patients may experience depression, anxiety, anger, decreased appetite, and sleep deprivation. This type of response is most common in those with chronic pain, who usually have different systemic responses from those with acute pain.

## Core Principles of Pain Assessment and Management

According to the Joint Commission, assessing pain should be a priority in patient care, and organizations must establish **policies** for assessment and treatment of pain and must educate staff members about these policies. The Joint Commission considers a **plan of care** regarding pain control an essential patient right. Hospitals should be consistent in the use of the same assessment tools throughout the organization, specific to different patient populations (for example, pediatrics and geriatrics). The latest standards (2018) of evidence-based practice include the following:

- Organizations must establish a clinical leadership team to oversee pain management and safe prescription of opioids.
- Patients must be involved in planning and setting goals and should receive education regarding safe use of opioid and non-opioid medications.
- Patients should be screened for pain in all assessments, including visits to the emergency department.
- Patients at high risk for opioid misuse or adverse effects must be identified and monitored.
- Healthcare providers should have access to prescription drug monitoring safety databases, such as the prescription databases provided by most states.
- Organizations must provide performance improvement educational programs regarding pain assessment and management and must collect and analyze data on its pain assessment and management.

## Areas Addressed When Assessing Pain

Information concerning a patient's pain can be gathered from a variety of sources, including observations, interviews with the patient and family, medical records, and observations of other health care providers. However, it is important to remember that each patient's pain is **subjective** and **personal**. Pain is defined as whatever the patient says it is. Having the patient give parameters of quality, location, duration, speed of onset, and intensity can all be beneficial in forming a treatment plan based on the patient's needs. Pain is also influenced by psychological, social, and spiritual factors. Behavioral, psychological, and subjective assessment information such as physical demeanor and vital signs can be helpful in further defining a patient's pain parameters.

## Physical Signs of Pain

The best assessment of the patient's pain is **the patient's own report**. All other information is assessed as supporting this report. However, when this method is restricted or unavailable, **physical signs and symptoms** can help the nurse's assessment capabilities. It is important to be familiar with the patient's **baseline** or resting information to give a clear picture of the changes the body may go through when experiencing significant pain. Systolic blood pressure, heart rate, and respirations may all increase above the patient's normal parameters. Tightness or tension may be felt in major muscle groups. Posturing can also occur: the patient may guard areas of the body, curl themselves up into a fetal position, or hold only certain body portions rigid. Calling out, increased volume in speech, and moaning can also be indicators. Facial expressions, such as flat affect or grimacing, and distraction from their surroundings also indicate a significant increase in stressful stimuli.

## Importance of Pain Assessments in Advanced Disease

As many as 90% of all **advanced disease patients** will experience some level of pain. The hospice and palliative care philosophy focuses on the relief of pain and provision for comfort measures for all patients who desire it to improve quality of life. Each patient has the right to accept or refuse treatment for their pain. This becomes difficult when the patient is unable to **communicate** their desires and pain level. It can be assumed that if a patient was experiencing pain when able to communicate, they will continue to experience pain when the ability to communicate has been compromised—pain will be present even in an unconscious state. Changes from previous behavioral, psychological, and subjective and objective assessment data provide the supporting information for continued pain assessments in a nonverbal patient.

## Pain Assessment Tools

### *ABCDE Mnemonic Approach to Pain Assessment*

The Agency for Healthcare Policy and Research recommends use of the **ABCDE method** for assessing and managing pain:

- **Asking** the patient about the extent of pain and assessing systematically.
- **Believing** that the degree of pain the patient reports is accurate.
- **Choosing** the appropriate method of pain control for the patient and circumstances.
- **Delivering** pain interventions appropriately and in a timely, logical manner.
- **Empowering** patients and family by helping them to have control of the course of treatment.

The **5 key elements of pain assessment** include:

- **Quality**: Words are used to describe pain, such as *burning*, *stabbing*, *deep*, *shooting*, and *sharp*. Some may complain of pressure, squeezing, and discomfort rather than pain.
- **Intensity**: Use of a 0–10 scale or other appropriate scale to quantify the degree of pain.
- **Location**: Where does the patient indicate pain?
- **Duration**: Is it constant; does it come and go; is there breakthrough pain?
- **Aggravating/alleviating factors**: What increases the intensity of pain and what relieves the pain?

**Review Video: Assessment Tools for Pain**
Visit mometrix.com/academy and enter code: 634001

**Review Video: How to Accurately Assess Pain**
Visit mometrix.com/academy and enter code: 693250

### *Unidimensional Tools for Pain Assessment*

Unidimensional tools for pain assessment focus on one aspect only: the patient's level of pain. Tools include:

- **Visual analog/numeric rating scale**: A 1–10 rating scale presented visually or verbally from which the patient chooses a number to describe the degree of pain the patient is experiencing. Zero represents no pain, 1 very mild pain, and 10 the most severe pain the patient can imagine.
- **Descriptive**: Pain is described in simple terms that a patient can choose from: mild, moderate, or severe. This may be especially helpful for patients from other countries or cultures where the 1–10 scale is not generally used.
- **FACES**: A chart shows a facial expression scale of simple drawings showing faces with different emotions, such as happiness, fear, and pain. Used primarily for children over age 3 and for nonverbal adults, although both a child's and an adult's version are available. A revised version applies numeric values to expressions so that pain can be assessed according to a numeric rating scale as well.

### *Multidimensional Tools for Pain Assessment*

Multidimensional tools used for pain assessment assess various aspects of pain in addition to its impact on mental health, sleep, and functional status. Tools include:

- **Multidimensional pain inventory**: The patient begins by identifying a significant other and then answering 20 questions (rating scale 0–6) about the current rate of pain, the degree of interference in daily life, the ability to work, satisfaction from social/recreational activities, support level of the significant other, mood, pain during the previous week, changes brought about by pain, concerns of the significant other, ability to deal with pain, irritability, and anxiety.
- **Brief pain inventory**: Patients are assessed on the severity of pain (on a 1–10 scale), location of pain, impact of pain on daily function, pain medication, and amount of pain relief in the past 24 hours or the past week. They are asked if the pain interferes with general activity, walking, normal work, mood, interpersonal relations, sleep, or enjoyment of life.
- **McGill pain questionnaire**: The patient marks areas of internal and external pain on body diagrams and selects appropriate adjectives for 20 different sections regarding sensory, affective, and evaluative perceptions. For example, the questionnaire allows the patient to indicate if the pain is "flickering, quivering, pulsing, throbbing, beating, or pounding." The patient also rates present pain intensity (PPI) from 0 (none) to 5 (excruciating).



### *Assessment Tools for Cognitively Impaired or Nonverbal Patients*

The following are types of assessment tools available for use with cognitively impaired or nonverbal patients:

- **Discomfort Scale for Dementia of the Alzheimer Type (DS-DAT)**: For use with elderly persons experiencing dementia, decreased cognition, and decreased verbalization
- **Assessment of Discomfort in Dementia Protocol (ADD)**: Particularly designed for use with patients exhibiting difficult behaviors
- **Checklist of Nonverbal Pain Indicators (CNPI)**: Pain measurement with cognitive impairment
- **Noncommunicative Patient's Pain Assessment Instrument (NOPPAIN)**: Specifically for use by nursing assistants
- **Pain Assessment for the Dementing Elderly (PADE)**: Assessing physical pain behaviors
- **Pain Assessment Tool in Confused Older Adults (PATCOA)**: Focuses on the observation of nonverbal cues
- **Pain Assessment in Advanced Dementia (PAINAD)**: Adapted from the DS-DAT
- **Pain Assessment Checklist for Seniors with Limited Ability to Communicate (PACSLAC)**: To assess common and subtle symptoms
- **Abbey Pain Scale**: For late-stage dementia in nursing home environments

### PAIN ASSESSMENT OF NEONATES/INFANTS

Pain assessment of neonates and infants depends on careful observation of a number of characteristics. The Neonate/Infant Pain Scale (NIPS) assesses 6 areas with a score >3 indicating pain. Five areas are scored 0-1, depending upon the degree of stress. Crying, which is often the most indicative of pain, is scored 0-2:

| Characteristic | 0 | 1 | 2 |
|---|---|---|---|
| **Expression on face** | Rested, normal | Negative, tightened muscles, grimace | |
| **Crying** | None | Intermittent, moaning, whimper | Loud, shrill continuous crying |
| **Respiratory patterns** | Relaxed, normal | Changes include irregular breathing, tachypnea, holding breath, gagging | |
| **Upper extremities** | Relaxed, random movement | Tense, rigid, or rapid extending and flexing. | |
| **Lower extremities** | Relaxed, random movement | Tense, rigid, or rapid extending and flexing. | |
| **Arousal state** | Quiet, awake or asleep with random leg movements | Restless, fussing, thrashing about. | |

### ASSESSING PAIN IN PEDIATRIC PATIENTS

When assessing the pediatric patient, the nurse must take into consideration the **chronological and developmental age** of the child. These factors help determine which measure the child might use to express pain, as well as treatments that might prove most successful. Assessment parameters must also include the presence of and parameters surrounding chronic illness, as well as neurological impairment. The nurse must identify the underlying cause of the pain, what nonpharmacological measures have been tried for pain control, and what methods can be used to deliver pharmacological interventions. The weight of the child in kilograms determines the appropriate dosages of medications. If the child is able to speak, do the child and the parents speak the same language as the health care provider, and are there any other obvious barriers to communication or pain relief measures?

**Review Video: How to Properly Assess Pediatric Pain**
Visit mometrix.com/academy and enter code: 264352

#### PRETEEN/ADOLESCENT PAIN SCALE

**Pain** is subjective and may be influenced by the individual's pain sensation threshold (the smallest stimulus that produces the sensation of pain) and tolerance threshold (the maximum degree of pain that a person can tolerate). The most common current pain assessment tool for preteens and adolescents is the 1-10 pain scale:

- 0 = no pain
- 1-2 = mild pain
- 3-5 = moderate pain
- 6-7 = severe pain
- 8-9 = very severe pain
- 10 = excruciating pain

However, assessment also includes information about onset, duration, and intensity. Identifying pain triggers and what relieves the pain is essential when developing a pain management plan. Children may show very different behaviors when they are in pain. Some may cry and moan with minor pain, and others may seem indifferent even when they are truly suffering. Thus, judging pain by behavior alone can lead to the wrong conclusions.

### Non-Communicating Children's Pain Checklist

The **Non-Communicating Children's Pain Checklist** (NCCPC) is designed for children ages 3-8 who are cognitively impaired, but a modified version may be used for children recovering from anesthesia. The checklist contains 7 categories with sub-listings that are each scored: 0 (not occurring), 1 (occurring occasionally), 2 (occurring fairly often), 3 (occurring frequently), and NA (not applicable).

- **Vocal**: Moaning, whining, crying, screaming, yelling, or using a specific word for pain
- **Social**: Uncooperative, unhappy, withdrawn, seeking closeness, or can't be distracted
- **Facial**: Furrowed brow, eye changes, not smiling, lips tight or quivering, or clenching or grinding teeth.
- **Activity**: Not moving and quiet or agitated and fidgety.
- **Body and limbs**: Floppy, tense, rigid, spastic, pointing to a part of body that hurts, guarding part of the body, flinching, or positioning body to show pain.
- **Physiological**: Shivering, pallor, increased perspiration, tears, gasping, or holding breath
- **Eating and sleeping**: Eating less or sleeping significantly more or less than usual

The child is usually observed for 2 hours and then scored. All scores are then added together. A score of ≥7 indicates pain.

### QUESTT Pediatric Pain Assessment Tool

QUESTT is designed to focus on assessment, action, and consequent reassessment for results.

- **Question** both the child and parent about the pain experience.
- **Use** assessment tools and rating scales that are appropriate to the developmental stage and situation and understanding of the child.
- **Evaluate** the patient for both behavioral and physiological changes.
- **Secure** the parent's participation in all stages of the pain evaluation and treatment process.
- **Take the cause of the pain into consideration** during the evaluation and choice of treatment methods.
- **Take action** to treat the pain appropriately, and then evaluate the results on a regular basis.



## Barriers to Optimal Pain Assessments

Barriers to optimal pain assessments include:

- **Professional**: Health care providers may lack knowledge about pain assessment and management of different patient populations or may carry out assessments based on personal perceptions rather than validated pain assessment instruments. Some may be concerned about managing adverse effects or the patient's development of tolerance or addiction. In other cases, healthcare providers may lack empathy for patients' suffering. Lack of cultural awareness may affect interpretation of pain. For example, patients in cultures that encourage expression of pain may be assessed as having more pain than patients from cultures that value stoicism.
- **System**: The organization may lack clear policies regarding pain assessment and management, and may not have established clear guidelines for consistent use of pain assessment instruments. Additionally, supervision and accountability may be inadequate, and the organization may be concerned about costs and reimbursement for treatment.
- **Patient**: For personal or cultural reasons, patients may minimize or overstate the degree of pain, interfering with assessment. Some patients may be concerned about addiction or the effects of drugs on cognition (confusion, disorientation, lethargy) or other side effects (constipation, nausea, itching). Some may want to protect family from knowing the extent of pain.

- **Family**: Cultural biases may influence how the family responds to a patient's pain, and this can influence the patient's response as well. Families may lack understanding of the role of pain assessment and management. Some lack understanding about the difference between addiction and pain control at the end of life.
- **Society**: Concerns about drug abuse and addiction often permeate society and influence societal attitudes toward pain control and appropriate drugs to use. Laws and regulations may make access to certain drugs, such as those derived from marijuana, difficult or impossible to obtain.

## Influential Factors in Pain Perception

Factors that can influence the perception of pain include:

- **Emotional state/attitude**: Patients who are extremely upset or anxious may be so overwhelmed they don't feel the pain, or they may experience pain as more severe than those who are relaxed and calm. If patients expect to suffer from pain, they are also more likely to report severe pain than patients who expect that their pain will be controlled.
- **Cultural expectations**: Perception may vary according to cultural beliefs about pain. For example, if a patient believes that pain is punishment, the patient may agonize over past sins. If a patient believes that pain is fate and reflects karma, then the patient may feel that bearing pain is necessary.
- **Pain threshold**: Different patients simply perceive and experience pain to different degrees. What may be a minor pain to one individual may be severe to another.

## Effects of Gender on Pain Experience

Gender can affect pain sensitivity, tolerance, distress, and exaggeration of pain, and the patient's willingness to report pain, as well as displayed nonverbal cues concerning the pain experience. Studies indicate that women generally have **lower pain thresholds** and **less tolerance** for noxious stimuli or pain factors that hinder them from doing things they enjoy. Women seek help for pain-related problems sooner than men and respond better to therapy. Women also experience more **visceral pain** than men. Men are more prone to experience **somatic pain** and show more stoicism regarding pain experiences than women. **Neuropathic pain** seems to be experienced equally between men and women. Nurses need to be careful that biases concerning gender experiences with pain do not skew their assessments of pain. However, they need to be aware that pain experiences are always individual and may differ between the sexes.

## Psychological Factors in Experience of Pain

**Psychological factors** that may influence a patient's experience of pain include:

- **Fear**: The fear of pain and the anticipation of having pain are factors in how much pain a person feels, because the fear stimulates areas of the brain that focus attention on the body so that the patient experiences an increased sensation of pain. Fear also causes muscles to tense, blood pressure to increase, and the heart rate to increase, and all of these can exacerbate the perception of pain. While pain medications may be necessary, practicing relaxation and mindfulness exercises may help to reduce anxiety and have a positive effect.
- **Depression**: The same neurotransmitters that transmit sensations of pain are also those that transmit moods, so many people with depression present first with complaints of pain or discomfort, and this can result in chronic pain if the depression is not resolved. In some cases, pain may lead to depression, but then the depression worsens the pain so it becomes a cycle of worsening discomfort. Patients may benefit from cognitive behavioral therapy or medication such as SSRIs.

## PAIN DOCUMENTATION IN MEDICAL RECORDS

Recommendations for **pain documentation** in the medical record include:

- Describe the time of onset, the location of pain, the character of the pain, and the degree of pain, using a validated pain assessment instrument (either a self-reporting instrument, such as the visual analog scale, or one based on observation, such as PAINAD).
- Document all interventions, both pharmacological (opioids, adjuvants) and nonpharmacological (positioning, massage, relaxation exercises), including the time, the dosage, and the method of administration.
- Assess and document the initial response to the medication based on the expected response time. For example, an IV medication should take effect almost immediately, but oral medications may take up to 20 minutes to take effect.
- Assess and document the duration of response based on the expected duration of the medication. For example, if a medication response is expected to last for 6 hours, the patient's pain level should be assessed at least every 2 hours and more frequently if the rate of pain increases.
- Describe any adverse effects, such as itching or nausea.

**Review Video: Pain Assessment Documentation**
Visit mometrix.com/academy and enter code: 248521

**Review Video: Documentation of Pain Management**
Visit mometrix.com/academy and enter code: 760328

# Cardiovascular Assessment

## ASSESSMENT OF THE CARDIOVASCULAR SYSTEM

**Cardiovascular assessment** includes questioning the patient for any family history of death at a young age or other cardiovascular diseases. Elderly African-American males are at highest risk for cardiovascular problems. One must question the patient about edema, chest pain, dyspnea, fatigue, vertigo, syncope or other changes in consciousness, weight gain, and leg cramps or pain. If chest pain is a symptom, one must ask about the intensity, timing, location, any radiation, quality, meaning to the patient, factors that aggravate or alleviate the pain, nausea, dyspnea, diaphoresis, or any other accompanying symptoms. Physical assessment includes assessment of vital signs, heart and lung sounds, skin assessment, radial, popliteal, and pedal pulses, circulation and sensation of extremities, and auscultation of the aorta, renal, iliac, and femoral arteries for bruits. Blood should be taken for a lipid profile and electrolytes. The patient must be helped to modify risk factors such as hypertension, smoking, diabetes, obesity, hyperlipidemia, inactivity, and stress.

**Review Video: Cardiovascular Assessment**
Visit mometrix.com/academy and enter code: 323076

**Review Video: Functions of the Circulatory System**
Visit mometrix.com/academy and enter code: 376581

**Review Video: Heart Blood Flow**
Visit mometrix.com/academy and enter code: 783139

**Review Video: Mnemonics for Heart Anatomy and Physiology**
Visit mometrix.com/academy and enter code: 849489

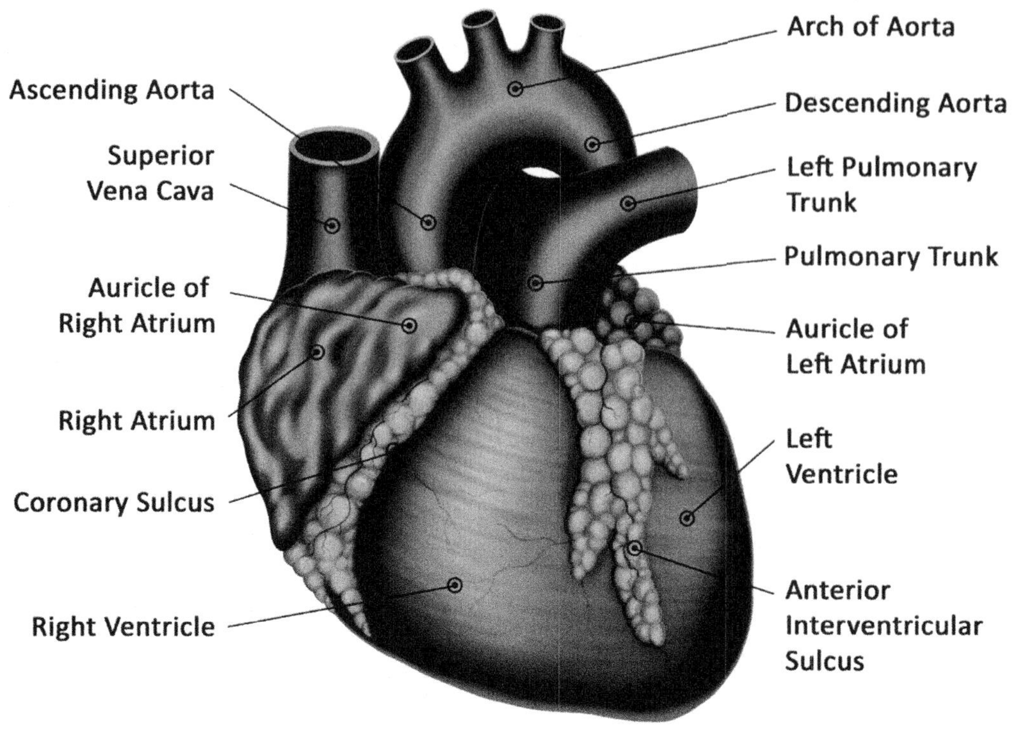


## Assessment of Heart Sounds

Auscultation of heart sounds can help to diagnose different cardiac disorders. Areas to auscultate include the aortic area, pulmonary area, Erb's point, tricuspid area, and the apical area. The **normal heart sounds** represent closing of the valves.

The **first heart sound** (S1) "lub" is closure of the mitral and tricuspid valves (heard at apex/left ventricular area of the heart).

The **second heart sound** (S2) "dub" is closure of the aortic and pulmonic valves (heard at the base of the heart). There may be a slight splitting of the S2.

The time between S1 and S2 is systole and the time between S2 and the next S1 is diastole. Systole and diastole should be silent although ventricular disease can cause gallops, snaps, or clicks and stenosis of the valves or failure of the valves to close can cause murmurs. Pericarditis may cause a friction rub.

**Review Video: Diastolic vs Systolic**
Visit mometrix.com/academy and enter code: 898934

Additional heart sounds:

- **Gallop rhythms**: S3 commonly occurs after S2 in children and young adults but may indicate heart failure or left ventricular failure in older adults (when heard with patient lying on left side). S4 occurs before S1, during the contracting of the atria when there is ventricular hypertrophy, found in coronary artery disease, hypertension, or aortic valve stenosis.
- **Opening snap**: Unusual high-pitched sound occurring after S2 with stenosis of mitral valve from rheumatic heart disease
- **Ejection click**: Brief high-pitched sound after S1; aortic stenosis
- **Friction rub**: Harsh, grating holosystolic sound; pericarditis
- **Murmur**: Sound caused by turbulent blood flow from stenotic or malfunctioning valves, congenital defects, or increased blood flow. Murmurs are characterized by location, timing in the cardiac cycle, intensity (rated from Grade I to Grade VI), pitch (low to high-pitched), quality (rumbling, whistling, blowing) and radiation (to the carotids, axilla, neck, shoulder, or back).

### Cardiac Monitoring

Cardiac monitoring includes the evaluation of different intervals and segments on the electrocardiogram:

- **QT interval**: This is the complete time of ventricular depolarization and repolarization, which begins with the QRS segment and ends when the T wave is completed. Typically, duration usually ranges from 0.36–0.44 seconds, but this may vary depending on the heart rate. If the heat rate is rapid, the duration is shorter and vice versa. Certain medications can prolong the QT interval, in such cases monitoring this is critical. A prolonged QT interval puts the patient at risk for R-on-T phenomenon, which can result in dangerous arrhythmias.
- **ST segment**: This is an isoelectric period when the ventricles are in a plateau phase, completely depolarized and beginning recovery and repolarization. Deflection is usually isoelectric. If the ST segment is ≥0.5 mm below the baseline, it is considered depressed and may be an indication of myocardial ischemia. Depression may also indicate digitalis toxicity. If the ST segment is elevated ≥0.3 mm above baseline, this is an indication of myocardial injury.



## MAP

The MAP **(mean arterial pressure)** is most commonly used to evaluate perfusion as it shows pressure throughout the cardiac cycle. Systole is one-third and diastole two-thirds of the normal cardiac cycle. The MAP for a blood pressure of 120/60 is calculated as follows:

$$\text{MAP} = \frac{\text{Diastole} \times 2 + \text{Systole}}{3} \frac{60 \times 2 + 120}{3} = \frac{240}{3} = 80$$

Normal range for mean arterial pressure is 70–100 mmHg. A MAP of greater than 60 mmHg is required to perfuse vital organs, including the heart, brain, and kidneys.

### Oxygen Saturation as It Relates to Hemodynamic Status

Hemodynamic monitoring includes monitoring **oxygen saturation** levels, which must be maintained for proper cardiac function. The central venous catheter often has an oxygen sensor at the tip to monitor oxygen saturation in the right atrium.

- Increased oxygen saturation may result from left atrial to right atrial shunt, abnormal pulmonary venous return, increased delivery of oxygen or decrease in extraction of oxygen.
- Decreased oxygen saturation may be related to low cardiac output with an increase in oxygen extraction or decrease in arterial oxygen saturation with normal differences in the atrial and ventricular oxygen saturation.

## ELECTROCARDIOGRAM

The electrocardiogram records and shows a graphic display of the electrical activity of the heart through a number of different waveforms, complexes, and intervals:

- **P wave**: Start of electrical impulse in the sinus node and spreading through the atria, muscle depolarization
- **QRS complex**: Ventricular muscle depolarization and atrial repolarization
- **T wave**: Ventricular muscle repolarization (resting state) as cells regain negative charge
- **U wave**: Repolarization of the Purkinje fibers

A modified lead II ECG is often used to monitor basic heart rhythms and dysrhythmias. Typical placement of leads for 2-lead ECG is 3–5 cm inferior to the right clavicle and left lower ribcage. Typical placement for a 3-lead ECG is (RA) right arm near shoulder, (LA) $V_5$ position over 5th intercostal space, and (LL) left upper leg near groin.

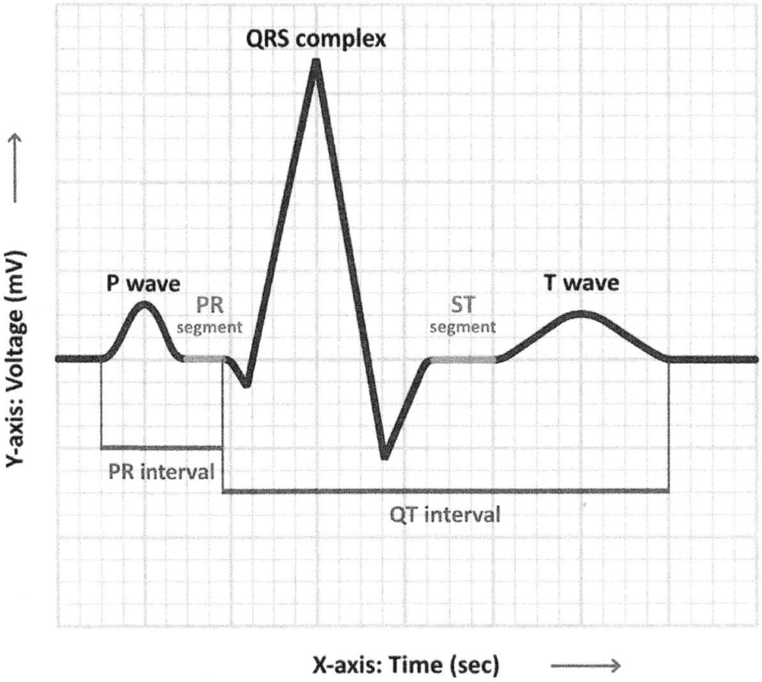


### ADMINISTRATION OF 12-LEAD ECG

The electrocardiogram provides a graphic representation of the electrical activity of the heart. It is indicated for chest pain, dyspnea, syncope, acute coronary syndrome, pulmonary embolism, and possible MI. The standard **12 lead ECG** gives a picture of electrical activity from 12 perspectives through placement of 10 body leads:

- 4 limb leads are placed distally on the wrists and ankles (but may be placed more proximally if necessary).
- Precordial leads:
  - V1: Right sternal border at 4th intercostal space
  - V2: Left sternal border at 4th intercostal space
  - V3: Midway between V2 and V4
  - V4: Left midclavicular line at 5th intercostal space
  - V5: Horizontal to V4 at left anterior axillary line
  - V6: Horizontal to V5 at left midaxillary line

In some cases, additional leads may be used:

- Right-sided leads are placed on the right in a mirror image of the left leads, usually to diagnose right ventricular infarction through ST elevation.

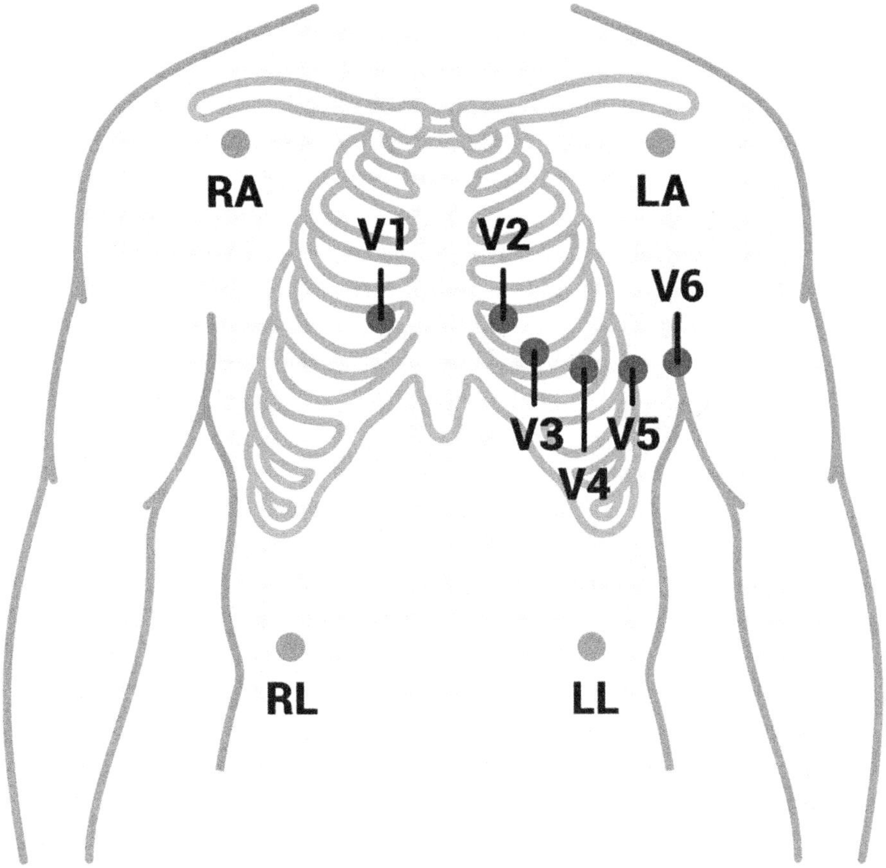




## Cardiac Output

Cardiac output (CO) is the amount of blood pumped through the ventricles during a specified period. Normal cardiac output is about 5 liters per minutes at rest for an adult. Under exercise or stress, this volume may multiply 3 or 4 times with concomitant changes in the heart rate (HR) and stroke volume (SV). The basic formulation for calculating cardiac output is the heart rate (HR) per minute multiplied by the stroke volume (SR), which is the amount of blood pumped through the ventricles with each contraction. The stroke volume is controlled by preload, afterload, and contractibility.

$$\mathrm{CO}\left(\frac{\mathrm{mL}}{\mathrm{min}}\right) = \mathrm{HR}\left(\frac{\mathrm{beats}}{\mathrm{min}}\right) \times \mathrm{SV}\ (\mathrm{mL})$$

The heart rate is controlled by the autonomic nervous system. Normally, if the heart rate decreases, stroke volume increases to compensate. The exception to this would be cardiomyopathies, so bradycardia results in a sharp decline in cardiac output.

## Cardiac Index

Cardiac index (CI) is the cardiac output (CO) divided by the body surface area (BSA). This is essentially a measure of cardiac output tailored to the individual, based on height and weight, measured in liters/min per square meter of BSA.

- Normal value: 2.2–4.0 L/min/$m^2$

## Stroke Volume

Stroke volume (SV) is the amount of blood pumped through the left ventricle with each contraction, minus any blood remaining inside the ventricle at the end of systole.

- Normal values: 60–100 mL
- Formula:

$$\text{SV (mL)} = \text{CO}\left(\frac{\text{mL}}{\text{min}}\right) \div \text{HR}\left(\frac{\text{beats}}{\text{min}}\right)$$

## Pulmonary Vascular Resistance and Ejection Fraction

**Pulmonary vascular resistance (PVR)** is the resistance in the pulmonary arteries and arterioles against which the right ventricle has to pump during contraction. It is the mean pressure in the pulmonary vascular bed divided by blood flow. If PVR increases, SV decreases.

- Normal value: 1.2–3.0 units or 100–250 dynes/sec/$cm^5$

**Ejection Fraction (EF)** is the percentage of the total blood volume of the heart that is pumped out with each beat. Dramatically decreased values indicate heart failure.

- Normal value: 60–70%

## Preload and Afterload

**Preload** refers to the amount of elasticity in the myocardium at the end of diastole when the ventricles are filled to their maximum volume and the stretch on the muscle fibers is the greatest. The preload value is based on the volume in the ventricles. The amount of preload (stretch) affects stroke volume because as stretch increases, the resultant contraction also increases (Frank-Starling Law). Preload may decrease because of dehydration, diuresis, or vasodilation. Preload may increase because of increased venous return, controlling fluid loss, transfusion, or intravenous fluids.

**Afterload** refers to the amount of systemic vascular resistance to left ventricular ejection of blood and pulmonary vascular resistance to right ventricular ejection of blood. Determinants of afterload include the size and elasticity of the great vessels and the functioning of the pulmonic and aortic valves. Afterload increases with hypertension, stenotic valves, and vasoconstriction.

## Assessing Jugular Venous Pressure

**Jugular venous pressure** (neck-vein) is used to assess the cardiac output and pressure in the right heart as the pulsations relate to changes in pressure in the right atrium. This procedure is usually not accurate if the pulse rate is >100. This is a non-invasive estimation of central venous pressure and waveform. Measurement should be done with the internal jugular if possible; if not, the external jugular may be used.

- **Elevate** the patient's head to 45° (and to 90° if necessary) with patient's head turned to the right.
- Position a **light** at an angle to illuminate veins and shadows.
- Measure the height of the **jugular vein pulsation** above the sternal joint, using a ruler.
    - Normal height is ≤4 cm above sternal angle.

Increased pressure (reflected in a height of >4 cm above the sternal angle) indicates increased pressure in the right atrium, and right heart failure. It may also indicate pericarditis or tricuspid stenosis. Laughing or coughing may trigger the Valsalva response and also cause an increase in pressure.

## Additional Cardiac Assessments

The **stress test**, also called an exercise tolerance test, is a commonly used assessment to screen for ischemic heart disease. In this test, the patient is put through exercise with increasing rigor, generally on a treadmill, while attached to an ECG to monitor their heart's rhythm. The patient is assessed for chest pain and dizziness as the rigor level is increased, which is a reflection of the heart's capacity to handle increasing workloads effectively. The stress test is not diagnostic on its own, but provides feedback on the direction of additional testing.

**Water-hammer pulse** is characterized by the alternation between a bounding heartbeat that is strong and forceful, and then collapse. This could be the result of a heightened stroke volume, decreased peripheral resistance, or these two factors together. To assess for this pulse, the patient is seated and one arm is raised vertically. Upon palpation of the radial pulse in the raised arm, the pulse resembles a tapping in the muscles of the forearm. This is often an indication of aortic regurgitation.

## Perfusion Pressure and Pulse Pressure

**Coronary perfusion pressure** directly affects coronary blood flow, and coronary perfusion occurs during diastole. Coronary artery perfusion pressure is equal to the diastolic blood pressure minus the pulmonary artery occlusion pressure. Normal values are 60–80 mmHg. Goal coronary perfusion when performing CPR to maintain enough perfusion necessary to achieve ROSC (return of spontaneous circulation) is thought to be 15 mmHg. During the cardiac cycle, *aortic pressure* causes the coronaries to be perfused, while *ventricular pressure* compresses the coronaries during systole, decreasing perfusion.

The **pulse pressure** is the difference between systolic and diastolic pressures, and this can be an important indicator. For example, with a decrease in cardiac output, vasoconstriction takes place in the body's attempt to maintain the blood pressure. In this case, the MAP may remain unchanged, but the pulse pressure narrows. Patients should be assessed for changes in pulse pressure that may be precipitated by medications, such as diuretics that alter fluid volume.



## Assessment of Lower Extremities

Assessment of lower extremities includes a number of different elements:

- **Appearance** includes comparing limbs for obvious differences or changes in skin or nails as well as evaluating for edema, color changes in skin, such as pallor or rubor. Legs that are thin, pale, shiny, and hairless indicate peripheral arterial disease.
- **Perfusion** should be assessed by checking venous filling time and capillary refill, skin temperature (noting changes in one limb or between limbs), bruits (indicating arterial narrowing), pulses (comparing both sides in a proximal to distal progression), ankle-brachial index and toe-brachial index.
- **Sensory function** includes the ability to feel pain, temperature, and touch.
- **Range of motion** of the ankle must be assessed to determine if the joint flexes past 90° because this is necessary for unimpaired walking and aids venous return in the calf.
- **Pain** is an important diagnostic feature of peripheral arterial disease, so the location, intensity, duration, and characteristics of pain are important.

### *Assessment of Pulse and Bruit*

Evaluation of the pulses of the **lower extremities** is an important part of assessment for peripheral arterial disease/trauma. Pulses should be first evaluated with the patient in supine position and then again with the legs dependent, checking bilaterally and proximal to distal to determine if intensity of pulse decreases distally. Pedal pulses should be examined at both the posterior tibialis and the dorsalis pedis. The pulse should be evaluated as to the rate, rhythm, and intensity, which is usually graded on a 0 to 4 scale:

0+= pulse absent
1+= weak, difficult to palpate
2+= normal as expected
3+= full
4+= strong and bounding

Pulses may be **palpable** or **absent** with peripheral arterial disease. Absence of pulse on both palpation and Doppler probe does indicate peripheral arterial disease.

**Bruits** may be noted by auscultating over major arteries, such as femoral, popliteal, peroneal, and dorsalis pedis, indicating peripheral arterial disease.

### *Assessing Perfusion of Lower Extremities*

Assessment of perfusion can indicate venous or arterial abnormalities:

- **Venous refill time**: Begin with the patient lying supine for a few moments and then have the patient sit with the feet dependent. Observe the veins on the dorsum of the foot and count the seconds before normal filling. Venous occlusion is indicated with times greater than 20 seconds.
- **Capillary refill**: Grasp the toenail bed between the thumb and index finger and apply pressure for several seconds to cause blanching. Release the nail and count the seconds until the nail regains normal color. Arterial occlusion is indicated with times of more than 2–3 seconds. Check both feet and more than one nail bed.
- **Skin temperature**: Using the palm of the hand and fingers, gently palpate the skin, moving distally to proximally and comparing both legs. Arterial disease is indicated by decreased temperature (coolness) or a marked change from proximal to distal. Venous disease is indicated by increased temperature about the ankle.

## *ABI*

#### Procedure

The ankle-brachial index **(ABI) examination** is done to evaluate peripheral arterial disease of the lower extremities.

1. Apply BP cuff to one arm, palpate brachial pulse, and place conductivity gel over the artery.
2. Place the tip of a Doppler device at a 45-degree angle into the gel at the brachial artery and listen for the pulse sound.
3. Inflate the cuff until the pulse sound ceases and then inflate 20 mmHg above that point.
4. Release air and listen for the return of the pulse sound. This reading is the brachial systolic pressure.
5. Repeat the procedure on the other arm and use the higher reading for calculations.
6. Repeat the same procedure on each ankle with the cuff applied above the malleoli and the gel over the posterior tibial pulse to obtain the ankle systolic pressure.
7. Divide the ankle systolic pressure by the brachial systolic pressure to obtain the ABI.

Sometimes, readings are taken both before and after 5 minutes of walking on a treadmill.

### Interpreting Results

Once the ABI examination is completed, the ankle systolic pressure must be divided by the brachial systolic pressure. Ideally, the BP at the ankle should be equal to that of the arm or slightly higher. With peripheral arterial disease the ankle pressure falls, affecting the ABI. Additionally, some conditions that cause calcification of arteries, such as diabetes, can cause a false elevation.

**Calculation** is simple:

$$\text{ABI} = \frac{\text{Ankle systolic}}{\text{Brachial systolic}}$$

The degree of disease relates to the **score**:

- >1.4: Abnormally high, may indicate calcification of vessel wall
- 1.0–1.4: Normal reading, asymptomatic
- 0.9–1.0: Low reading, but acceptable unless there are other indications of PAD
- 0.8–0.9: Likely some arterial disease is present
- 0.5–0.8: Moderate arterial disease
- < 0.5: Severe arterial disease

# Respiratory Assessment

## Assessment of the Respiratory System

If significant respiratory distress is present, one must stabilize the patient before doing a **respiratory history** or ask family if available:

- Question the patient about risk factors, such as smoking, exposure to smoke or other inhaled toxins, past lung problems, and allergies.
- Ask the patient about symptoms of respiratory problems, such as dyspnea, cough, sputum production, fatigue, ability to do ADLs and IADLs, and chest pain.
- Determine how long symptoms have been present, the length of periods of dyspnea, aggravating and alleviating factors, and the severity of symptoms.

When performing a **physical assessment**, one should assess vital signs, posture, pulse oximetry, check nails for clubbing, do a skin assessment, listen to lung sounds via auscultation and percussion, and look for accessory muscle use, signs of anxiety, and edema. Depending on condition, blood may be drawn for arterial blood gases, electrolytes, and CBC. Sputum cultures may be obtained.

**Review Video: Respiratory System**
Visit mometrix.com/academy and enter code: 783075

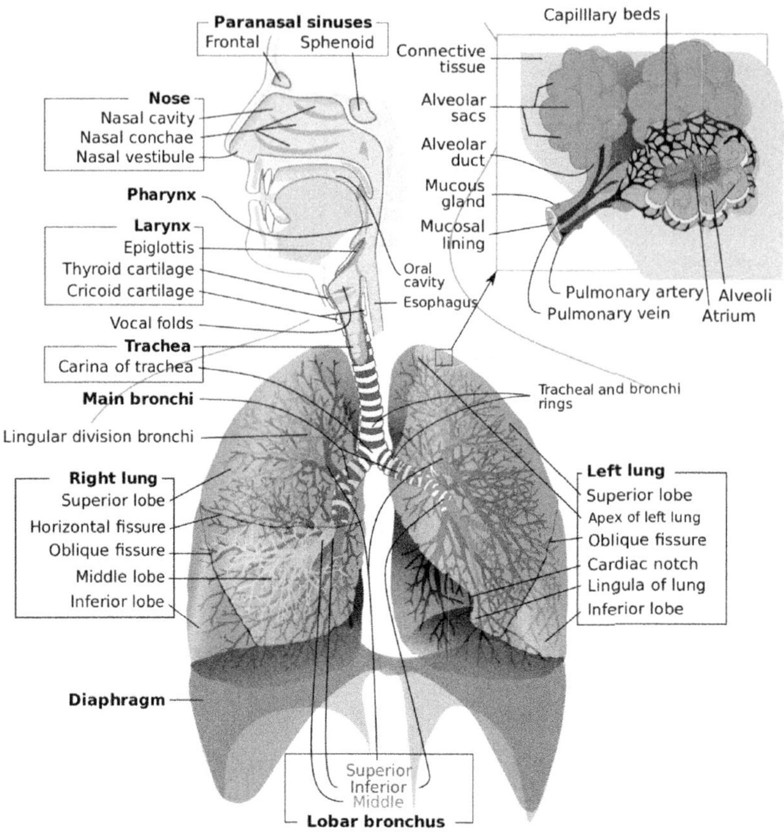


## PRIMARY AND SECONDARY MUSCLES USED FOR BREATHING

Muscles used for breathing are separated into primary and secondary muscle groups.

- The **primary muscle groups** are those that are used in normal, quiet breathing. When patients are in respiratory distress and breathing is more difficult, secondary muscle groups become activated. The muscles considered primary for breathing are the diaphragm and the external intercostal muscles. These muscles act by changing the pressure gradient, allowing the lungs to expand and air to flow in and out.
- The **secondary muscle groups** include the sternocleidomastoid, scaleni, internal intercostals, obliques, and abdominal muscles. These secondary muscle groups work when breathing is difficult, both in inspiration and expiration, in cases such as obstructions or bronchoconstriction. Use of these secondary muscle groups can often be seen on exam and may be described as see-saw or abdominal breathing (when the abdominal muscles are being used during exhalation) or retractions as the muscles activate and can be seen between rigid structures such as bone.

## NORMAL PHYSIOLOGICAL AIRWAY CLEARANCE

**Normal airway clearance** is caused by various aspects of the respiratory system. A thin layer of mucus lines the airways as a protective mechanism against debris and helps trap foreign objects before they enter the lower airways. Proper hydration keeps the mucosa adequately moist so it can trap foreign debris. As this debris lands in the mucus, the cilia in the respiratory tract act as an "elevator" to push the debris up to the larynx, where it can either be coughed up or swallowed and digested. An intact cough reflex is necessary for the debris to stimulate the cough, and normal muscle strength and nerve innervation of the diaphragm is required to produce a sufficiently forceful cough.

## Ventilation/Perfusion Ratio

In order to maintain homeostasis, the respiratory and cardiac systems need to maintain a careful balance. The **ventilation/perfusion ratio** indicates that ventilation of the lungs and perfusion to the lungs are within a normal balance. A normal ventilation/perfusion ratio is equal to 0.8. A ventilation/perfusion ratio higher than normal is indicative of ventilation that is too high, perfusion that is too low, or some combination of the two. This can occur because of hyperventilation (either physiological or caused by healthcare practitioners due to incorrect ventilator settings), pulmonary embolism, or hypotension. Essentially, a high ventilation/perfusion ratio means that there is more ventilation than perfusion. If the ventilation/perfusion ratio is lower than normal, then ventilation is too low, perfusion is too high, or some combination of the two. This can be caused by atelectasis, pneumonia, or lung disease. Whatever the cause, a low ventilation/perfusion ratio indicates that there is more perfusion than ventilation.

## Normal and Abnormal Breath Sound Terms

Normal breath sounds can be divided into three types. Vesicular breath sounds are low, soft sounds that can normally be heard over the peripheral lung space. Bronchovesicular breath sounds are moderate pitch breath sounds that are normally heard in the upper lung fields. Tracheal breath sounds are higher in pitch and heard over the trachea. Abnormal breath sounds are also known as adventitious lung sounds. Wheezes are high-pitched, expiratory sounds caused by air flowing through an obstructed airway. Stridor is also high-pitched, but is usually heard on inspiration in the upper airways. Coarse crackles are caused by an excessive amount of secretions in the airway and can be heard on inspiration and expiration. Fine crackles occur late in the expiratory phase and usually occur when the peripheral airways are being "popped" back open.

**Review Video: Lung Sounds**
Visit mometrix.com/academy and enter code: 765616

## Diagnostics and Tools Used During Pulmonary/Thoracic Trauma Assessment

The diagnostic procedures and tools used during assessment of **pulmonary and thoracic trauma/disease** will vary according to the type and degree of injury/disease, but may include:

- **Thorough physical examination** including cardiac and pulmonary status, assessing for any abnormalities.
- **Electrocardiogram** to assess for cardiac arrhythmias.
- **Chest x-ray** should be done for all those with injuries to check for fractures, pneumothorax, major injuries, and placement of intubation tubes. X-rays can be taken quickly and with portable equipment so they can be completed quickly during the initial assessment.
- **Computerized tomography** may be indicated after initial assessment, especially if there is a possibility of damage to the parenchyma of the lungs.
- **Oximetry and atrial blood gases** as indicated.
- **12-lead electrocardiogram** may be needed if there are arrhythmias for more careful observation.
- **Echocardiogram** should be done if there is apparent cardiac damage.

## Capnography with End-Tidal $CO_2$ Detector

**Capnometry** utilizes an **end-tidal $CO_2$ (ETCO) detector** that measures the concentration of $CO_2$ in expired air, usually through pH sensitive paper that changes color (commonly purple to yellow). Typically, the capnometer is attached to the ETT and a bag-valve-mask (BVM) ventilator. The capnogram provides data in the shape of a waveform that represents the partial pressure of exhaled gas. It is often used to confirm placement of endotracheal tubes as clinical assessment is not always sufficient, and it is a noninvasive mode of monitoring carbon dioxide in the respiratory cycle. Information provided by the capnogram includes:

- $PaCO_2$ level
- Type and degree of bronchial obstruction, such as COPD (waveform changes from rectangular to a fin-like)
- Air leaks in the ventilation system
- Rebreathing precipitated by need for new $CO_2$ absorber
- Cardiac arrest
- Hypothermia or reduced metabolism

The normal capnogram is a waveform that represents the varying $CO_2$ level throughout the breath cycle:

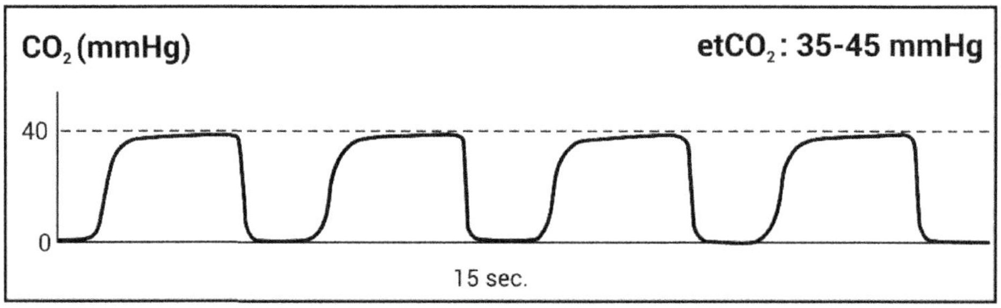


## Arterial Blood Gases

**Arterial blood gases** (ABGs) are monitored to assess effectiveness of oxygenation, ventilation, and acid-base status and to determine oxygen flow rates. Partial pressure of a gas is that exerted by each gas in a mixture of gases, proportional to its concentration, based on total atmospheric pressure of 760 mmHg at sea level. Normal values include:

- Acidity/alkalinity (pH): 7.35–7.45
- Partial pressure of carbon dioxide ($PaCO_2$): 35–45 mmHg
- Partial pressure of oxygen ($PaO_2$): ≥80 mmHg
- Bicarbonate concentration ($HCO_3^-$): 22–26 mEq/L
- Oxygen saturation ($SaO_2$): ≥95%

The relationship between these elements, particularly the $PaCO_2$ and the $PaO_2$ indicates respiratory status. For example, $PaCO_2$ >55 and the $PaO_2$ <60 in a patient previously in good health indicates respiratory failure. There are many issues to consider. Ventilator management may require a higher $PaCO_2$ to prevent barotrauma and a lower $PaO_2$ to reduce oxygen toxicity.

**Review Video: Blood Gases**
Visit mometrix.com/academy and enter code: 611909

# Endocrine, Immunologic, and Oncologic Assessment

## Assessing for Endocrine Disorders

The **endocrine system** comprises organs that produce hormones that are critical to growth, sexual development, and metabolism, so changes in these areas are suggestive of endocrine disorders. While symptoms may vary widely, there are often generalized symptoms that can be associated with most endocrine disorders. One should question the patient about fatigue and ability to perform ADLs, heat or cold intolerance, changes in sexual libido, sexual functioning, and secondary sexual characteristics, weight fluctuation, sleep problems, decreased concentration and memory, and mood changes. During the physical exam, one should assess the patient for edema, "moon" face or "buffalo hump," exophthalmos, hair loss, female facial hair, enlarged trunk with thin extremities, and enlarged hands and feet. Vital signs should be assessed for hypo or hypertension, and one should assess for changes in skin appearance and vision.

## Thyroid Imaging

Thyroid imaging plays a critical role in assessment of many thyroid diseases. This test may be used to determine the uptake characteristics of the thyroid gland in addition to the size and shape of the gland. In addition, **thyroid imaging** may determine how much iodine-131 is needed in order to safely ablate the gland when necessary. The radioactive iodine uptake scan (RAIU) is basically administration of iodine-123 with imaging performed 8 and 24 hours later:

Uptake of radioactive iodine is increased in disorders such as Graves' disease, "hot" nodules of various etiologies (including toxic multinodular goiter), TSH-secreting pituitary tumor, and iodine deficiency.

Uptake of radioactive iodine is decreased in the setting of thyroiditis and iodine excess.

**Ultrasound imaging** is used in thyroid disease to determine the size and structure of a thyroid nodule, such as to determine uniformity of shape, irregular contour, solid/cystic structure, and depth.



## Immunology

Immunology is the field of medicine that examines the body's ability to fight off infection. The body has a complicated system of cells and certain substances that react when an unknown agent attempts to cause an infectious process within the body. When a cell is altered to form a cancer cell, the body usually recognizes it as abnormal and attacks it. This prevents its replication and the development of more cancer cells. If immune cells are not functioning properly, the cancer cell could go on to reproduce more cells to eventually form a tumor that can potentially invade the surrounding tissues. Immunology also focuses on treatment research and ways in which the immune system can function more effectively in preventing cancer cell formation.

> **Review Video: Immune System**
> Visit mometrix.com/academy and enter code: 622899

## Cancer

Cancer is a potentially life-threatening disease that occurs due to irregular cell growth and reproduction. These cells can develop into a tumor that can occupy an area where normal body cells are usually found. **Cancer cells** also have the ability to metastasize, or extend, into other areas of the body. Cells within the body are constantly being replaced by normal cells. During this process, an abnormality in a cell's DNA can occur which causes it to become a malignant cancer cell. The body's immune system will usually attack and destroy this cell, but sometimes there can be a failure of the immune system to do this or the immune system is not able to destroy the cell. When this happens, the cancer cell can continue to reproduce itself until a tumor is formed. Some cancers can even attack normal, healthy cells within the body and alter their DNA so they will begin to reproduce as cancer cells.

## Stages of Cancer Development

There are three stages of the development of cancer:

- **Initiation** is the action of a cancer-causing substance entering the body, reacting with DNA, and causing DNA mutation. Examples include cigarette smoke, radiation exposure, etc. The effects of initiation are irreversible; it results in permanent genetic change. Any daughter cells produced from the division of the mutated cell will also carry the mutation.
- **Promotion** is the process in which the body is repeatedly exposed to the cancer-causing substance. This repeats the process mentioned above and increases the likelihood of cancer cells being reproduced.
- **Progression** occurs when the malignant cancer cells begin to outnumber the normal, healthy cells because of continued replication within the body. At this point, the body is no longer able to attempt to repair the damage done to DNA by the cancer-causing agents and the normal cells continue to replicate as cancer cells.

## Causes of Cancer

There are five main causes of cancer:

- **Radiation** can cause cancer by altering a cell's DNA. If the body is not able to repair the damages, the cell can reproduce as a cancer cell. Radiation exposure can be accidental or from diagnostic testing. UV light exposure is a form of radiation, also, and it causes skin cancer. Asbestos is considered a form of radiation, also, and causes mesothelioma tumors within the lungs.
- **Chemical carcinogens** can alter a cell's DNA to cause cancer. An example of this is cigarette smoke and exposure to tar within cigarettes.
- **Viruses** can cause cancer. Viruses that alter a cell's genetic material can stimulate the production of cancer cells.
- **The immune system** may be unsuccessful in repairing or destroying cells with altered DNA, which can lead to cancer. Certain cancer cells have the ability to alter the immune system so that it cannot recognize the formation of malignant cells within normal tissues.
- Cancer can also occur because of **inherited factors**. A person can inherit oncogenes responsible for causing certain types of cancer.

## Tumor Staging and Tumor Grading

Tumor staging and grading are two types of tumor severity assessment. They are assigned by the surgical pathologist. Tumor staging is a measurement of the size or extent of spread of a tumor. It is based on three parameters, known collectively as **TNM**. T stands for the size of the original local tumor, N specifies whether there is regional lymph node involvement, and M indicates whether there is distant metastatic spread. There is also a distinction between clinical staging prior to treatment and pathological staging after surgical resection. On the other hand, tumor grading is a histopathologic evaluation of the extent of differentiation of the tumor. Grading assesses the difference between the tumor and the surrounding tissues. Grade 1 tumors do not differ much in appearance from the normal tissue and are said to be well-differentiated. When the histopathological variation between normal and tumor tissues is large, graded as 3 or 4, the tumors are considered poorly differentiated (and more aggressive).

### IMPORTANT TERMS

- **Invasion** is the process in which cancer cells continue to reproduce and effectively take over an area of the body's normal, healthy tissue.
- **Angiogenesis** is the process in which a tumor causes the body to produce blood vessels that enable the tumor to survive and grow.
- **Metastasis** is the extension of cancer cells to other parts of the body. This occurs when the cancer cells continue to reproduce and spread into other tissues in the area where the original cancer started. It can also occur through the blood or lymph stream by carrying cancer cells to other tissues within the body. Certain cancers have a propensity for metastasizing to specific areas of the body. For example, prostate and breast cancers are more likely to metastasize to the spine.
- **Tumor heterogeneity** is the term used to describe the dissimilarities found between cancer cells within a tumor. The more heterogeneous a tumor is, the more difficult it can be to treat and the more types of treatments may be required to treat it.
- **Hyperplasia** is the process in which the quantity of cells within a certain tissue multiplies. This occurs in healthy tissue and in cancerous tissue.
- **Metaplasia** is when one type of cell is interchanged with another within a specific tissue. This occurs in response to chronic damage inflicted on a certain type of cell.
- **Dysplasia** is a change in normal cells. This can involve a change in any of the cell's characteristics.
- **Anaplasia** is used to explain cancer cells. It means that certain cells hold the characteristics that are seen with cancer cells.

## Neurological Assessment



### ASSESSMENT OF THE NEUROLOGICAL SYSTEM

Assessment of the neurological system includes:

- Assess the **health history** for any trauma, falls, alcoholism, drug abuse, medications taken, and family history of neurological problems.
- Ask about any presenting **neurological symptoms**, the circumstances in which they occur, whether they fluctuate, and any associated factors, such as seizures, pain, vertigo, weakness, abnormal sensations, visual problems, loss of consciousness, changes in cognition, and motor problems.

Assessment includes determining the level of consciousness and cognition. Posture and movements are assessed for abnormalities. Facial expression and movement are noted. Cranial nerve assessment is done. The patient is assessed for strength, coordination, and balance and the ability to perform ADLs. One should assess for clonus and test all reflexes, including Babinski, gag, blink, swallow, upper and lower abdominal, cremasteric in males, plantar, perianal, biceps, triceps, brachioradialis, patellar and ankle. Peripheral sensation is tested by touching the patient with cotton balls and the sharp and dull ends of a broken tongue blade.

**Review Video: What is the Function of the Nervous System**
Visit mometrix.com/academy and enter code: 708428

## ASSESSING FUNCTIONAL STATUS

**Functional abilities** include the acts needed to meet basic needs and perform *activities of daily living* (ADLs), such as eating and elimination, as well as those *activities that are essential to independent living* (IADLs), such as shopping. A thorough assessment of the patient's functional abilities will identify areas that should be concentrated upon during rehabilitation. One should observe the patient as he/she performs these functions and record the following:

- Degree of independence shown
- Ability to complete activity without rest
- Nerve function
- Muscle function and strength
- Motion
- Coordination
- Cardiac status
- Respiratory status
- Assistance required to complete activity

The facility usually provides one of the tools available to record a functional assessment. The most common tool used is the Functional Independence Measure (FIM). Other tools available include the Barthel Index, the PULSES Profile, and the Patient Evaluation Conference System.

## ASA CLASSIFICATION SYSTEM FOR THE EXTENT OF A BRAIN ATTACK INJURY

The American Stroke Association developed a **brain attack outcome classification system** to standardize descriptions of stroke injuries:

- **Number of impaired domains** (Potentially affected neurological domains: motor, sensory, vision, language, cognition, and affect): Level 0: no domains impaired; Level 1: one domain impaired; Level 2: two domains impaired; Level 3: greater than 2 domains impaired.
- **Severity of impairment**: A (minimal or no neurological deficit due to stroke); B (mild/moderate deficit); or C (severe deficit). Note: When more than one domain is affected, severity is measured by the domain with the most impairment.

Assessment of function determines the ability to **live independently**:

- **I**: Independent in basic activities of daily living (BADL), such as bathing, eating, toileting, and walking; and instrumental activities of daily living (IADL), such as telephoning, shopping, maintaining a household, socializing, and using transportation
- **II**: Independent in BADL but partially dependent in IADL
- **III**: Partially dependent in BADL (less than 3 areas) and IADL
- **IV**: Partially dependent in BADL (3 or more areas)
- **V**: Completely dependent in BADL (5 or more areas) and IADL

Level III requires much assistance and Levels IV and V cannot live independently.

## Administration of the NIHSS

The **National Institutes of Health Stroke Scale (NIHSS)** is administered with careful attention to directions. The examiner should record the answers and avoid coaching or repeating requests, although demonstration may be used with aphasic patients. The scale comprises 11 sections, with scores for each section ranging from 0 (normal) to 2, 3, or 4:

- **Level of consciousness**: Response to noxious stimulation (0–3), request for month and his/her age (0–2), request to open and close eyes, grip and release unaffected hand (0–2)
- **Best gaze**: Horizontal eye movement (0–2)
- **Visual**: Visual fields (0–3)
- **Facial palsy**: Symmetry when patient shows teeth, raises eyebrows, and closes eyes (0–3)
- **Motor, arm**: Drift while arm extended with palms down (0–4)
- **Motor, leg**: Leg drift at 30 degrees while patient supine (0–4)
- **Limb ataxia**: Finger-nose and heel-shin (0–2)
- **Sensory**: Grimace or withdrawal from pinprick (0–2)
- **Best language**: Describes action of pictures (0–3)
- **Dysarthria**: Reads or describes words on list (0–2)
- **Distinction and inattention**: Visual spatial neglect (0–2)

## Glasgow Coma Scale

The Glasgow coma scale (GCS) measures the depth and duration of coma or impaired level of consciousness and is used for post-operative assessment. The GCS measures three parameters: best eye response, best verbal response, and best motor response, with a total possible score that ranges from 3 to 15:

| | |
|---|---|
| **Eye opening** | 4: Spontaneous<br>3: To verbal stimuli<br>2: To pain (not of face)<br>1: No response |
| **Verbal** | 5: Oriented<br>4: Conversation confused, but can answer questions<br>3: Uses inappropriate words<br>2: Speech incomprehensible<br>1: No response |
| **Motor** | 6: Moves on command<br>5: Moves purposefully respond pain<br>4: Withdraws in response to pain<br>3: Decorticate posturing (flexion) in response to pain<br>2: Decerebrate posturing (extension) in response to pain<br>1: No response |

Injuries/conditions are classified according to the total score: 3–8 Coma; ≤8 Severe head injury likely requiring intubation; 9–12 Moderate head injury; 13–15 Mild head injury.

**Review Video: Glasgow Coma Scale**
Visit mometrix.com/academy and enter code: 133399

## Cranial Nerves

| | Name | Function | PE Test |
|---|---|---|---|
| I | Olfactory | Smell | Test olfaction |
| II | Optic | Visual acuity | Snellen eye chart; Accommodation |
| III | Oculomotor | Eye movement/pupil | Pupillary reflex; Eye/eyelid motion |
| IV | Trochlear | Eye movement | Eye moves down & out |
| V | Trigeminal | Facial motor/ sensory | Corneal reflex; Facial sensation; Mastication |
| VI | Abducens | Eye movement | Lateral eye motion |
| VII | Facial | Facial expression; Taste | Moves forehead, closes eyes, smile/frown, puffs cheeks; Taste |
| VIII | Vestibulo-cochlear (Acoustic) | Hearing; Balance | Hearing (Weber/Rinne tests); Nystagmus |
| IX | Glosso-pharyngeal | Pharynx motor/sensory | Gag reflex; Soft palate elevation |
| X | Vagus | Visceral sensory, motor | Gag, swallow, cough |
| XI | Accessory | Sternocleidomastoid and trapezius (motor) | Turns head & shrugs shoulders against resistance |
| XII | Hypoglossal | Tongue movement | Push out tongue; move tongue from side to side |

## ICP and Monroe-Kellie Hypothesis

Increasing **intracranial pressure (ICP)** is a frequent complication of brain injuries, tumors, or other disorders affecting the brain, so monitoring the ICP is very important. Increased ICP can indicate cerebral edema, hemorrhage, and/or obstruction of cerebrospinal fluid. The **Monroe-Kellie hypothesis** states that in order to maintain a normal ICP, a change in volume in one compartment must be compensated by a reciprocal change in volume in another compartment. There are 3 compartments in the brain: the brain tissue, cerebrospinal fluid (CSF), and blood. The CSF and blood can change more easily to accommodate changes in pressure than tissue, so medical intervention focuses on cerebral blood flow and drainage.

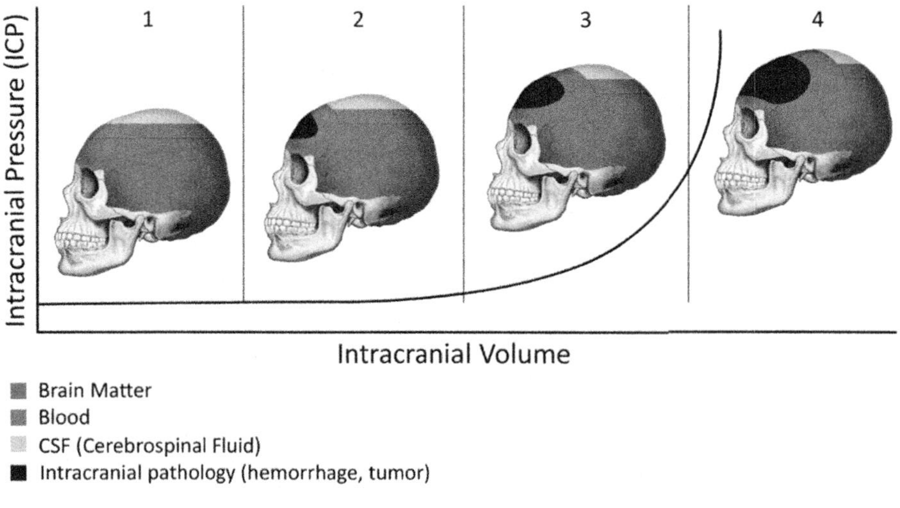

Normal ICP is 1–15 mmHg on transducer or 13.6–203.9 $mmH_2O$ on manometer. As intracranial pressure increases, **symptoms** include:

- Headache
- Alterations in level of consciousness
- Restlessness
- Slowly reacting or nonreacting dilated or pinpoint pupils
- Seizures
- Motor weakness
- Cushing's triad (late sign):
    - Increased systolic pressure with widened pulse pressure
    - Bradycardia in response to increased pressure
    - Decreased respirations

### *ICP Monitoring Devices*

The intracranial pressure (ICP) **monitoring device** may be placed during surgery or a ventriculostomy performed in which a burr hole is drilled into the frontal area of the scalp and an **intraventricular catheter** threaded into the lateral ventricle. The intraventricular catheter may be used to monitor ICP and to drain excess CSF. Other monitoring devices include:

- **Intracranial pressure monitor bolt** (subarachnoid bolt) is applied through a burr hole with the distal end of the monitor probe resting in the subarachnoid space.
- **Epidural monitors** are placed into the epidural space.
- **Fiberoptic monitors** may be placed inside the brain.

The intraventricular catheter is the most accurate. CSF may be drained continuously or intermittently and must be monitored hourly for amount, color, and character. For ICP measurement, the patient's head must be elevated to 30–45° and the transducer leveled to the tragus of the ear or outer canthus of the eye, depending on facility policy.



## Cerebral Blood Flow, MAP, and CPP

**Cerebral blood flow,** or the blood supply to the brain at any given moment, is influenced directly by one's **mean arterial pressure** (MAP). A MAP of greater than 60 mmHg is required to perfuse vital organs, including the brain. A MAP that falls below 60 mmHg risks ischemia and infarction. An excessively high MAP (greater than 100 mmHg) can also cause damage. A high MAP can result in increased oxygen demands by the heart, vascular injury, end organ damage, and stroke.

**Cerebral perfusion pressure** (CPP) is the pressure required to maintain adequate blood flow to the brain. CPP is based on mean arterial pressure (MAP) and intracranial pressure (ICP). Elevated ICP can be associated with a reduction in CPP.

$$CPP = MAP - ICP$$

- Normal CPP: 60–100 mmHg.
- <60 mmHg: Hypoperfusion occurs , resulting in focal or global ischemia.
- <30 mmHg: Hypoperfusion is marked and incompatible with life.
- >100 mmHg: Leads to hypertensive encephalopathy and cerebral edema (particularly if CPP >120 mmHg); Patients with chronic hypertension tolerate a higher level of CPP.

# Gastrointestinal Assessment

## Assessment of the Gastrointestinal System

Assessment of the gastrointestinal system includes:

- Ask about personal and family history of gastrointestinal problems and risk factors, such as alcoholism, smoking, drug and medicine use, and poor dietary habits.
- Ask about symptoms, such as GI discomfort, flatus, nausea, vomiting, diarrhea, and abdominal pain.
- Determine the defecation pattern and ask about weight fluctuations.

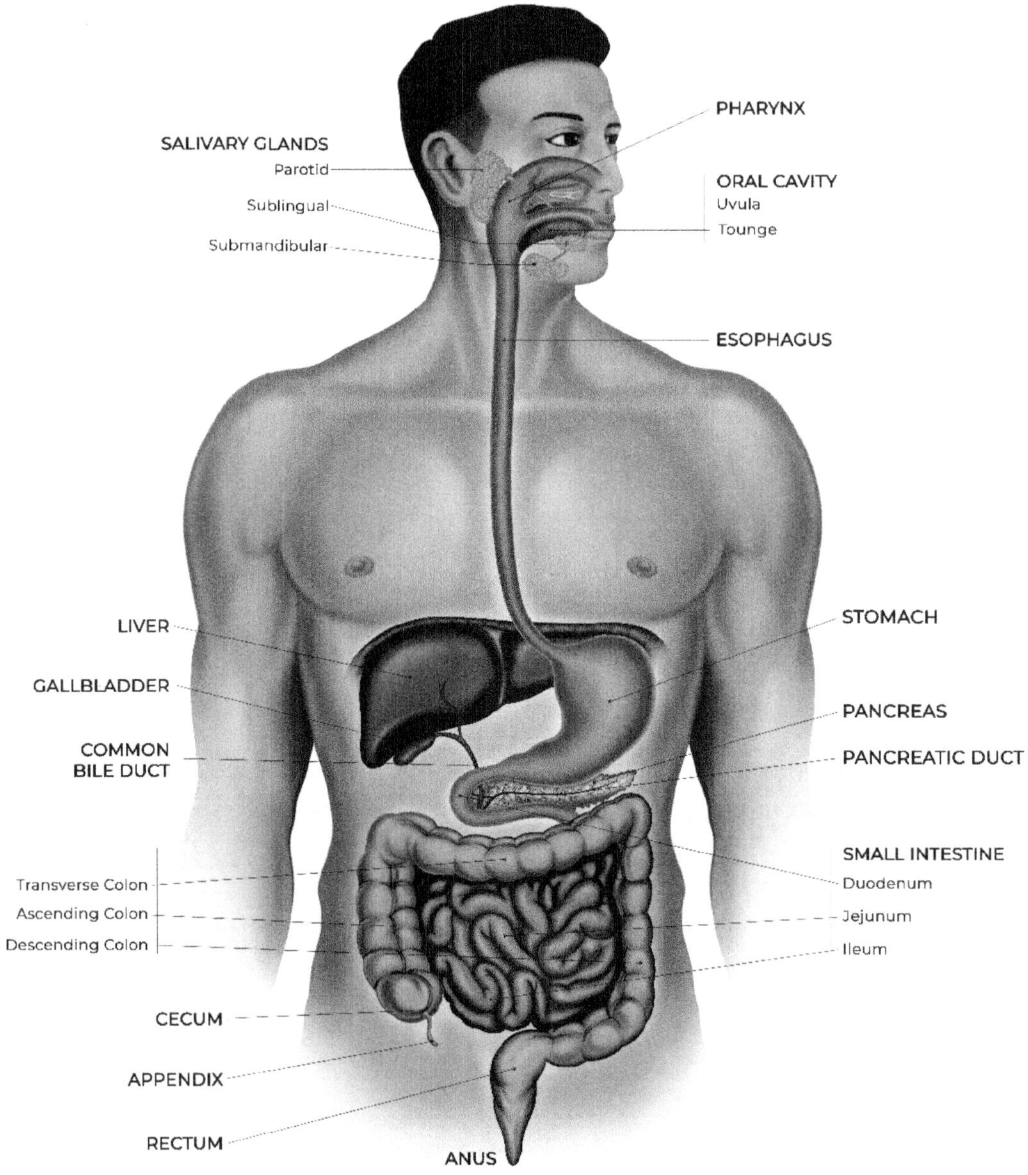

When performing a **physical assessment**, one must assess oral mucosa, tongue, teeth, pharynx, thyroid and parathyroid glands, skin color, moisture, turgor, nodules or lesions, bruises, scars, abdominal shape, and bowel sounds, assessing the abdomen in all 4 quadrants using the stethoscope diaphragm. The number of sounds heard determine if the intestines are functioning:

- **Absent**: no sounds in 3–5 minutes
- **Hypoactive**: only one sound in 2 minutes
- **Normal**: sounds heard every 5–20 seconds
- **Hyperactive**: 5–6 sounds in <30 seconds

One should examine the anal region for fissures, inflammation, tears, and dimples. Blood may be drawn for liver function studies, lipid profile, iron studies, CBC.

**Review Video: Gastrointestinal System**
Visit mometrix.com/academy and enter code: 378740

## ASSESSMENT FOR GALLBLADDER AND PANCREATIC DISEASE

Gallbladder and pancreatic assessments are prompted by the appearance of symptoms. Symptoms of gallbladder disease include epigastric discomfort following fatty food intake, abdominal distension, right upper quadrant pain, which may be colicky, nausea, and vomiting. Pain may occur intermittently.

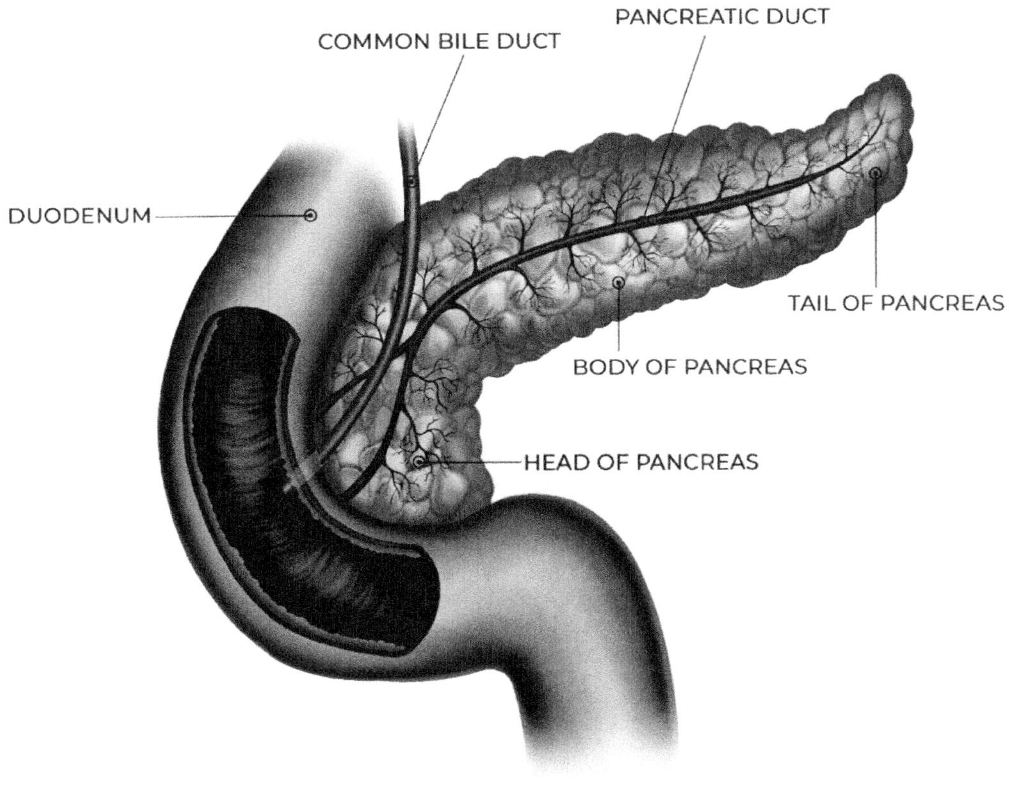

The patient with pancreatitis may have acute onset of severe abdominal pain, back pain, extensive vomiting, and dyspnea. Pancreatitis is most often related to gallstones or alcoholism, so history of alcohol use and examination for gallstones must be done:

- Assess for RUQ tenderness and mass, bowel sounds, and abdominal guarding.
- Assess the vital signs for hypotension, tachycardia, or fever and note any anxiety, agitation, or confusion.
- Note signs of hypoxia.
- Assess the skin for jaundice and bruising on the flanks and near the umbilicus.
- Blood is drawn to assess amylase and lipase, CBC, calcium, glucose, and bilirubin.

## Assessment for Liver Disease

The liver must be 70% damaged before lab tests show abnormalities. Assessment of risk factors and early symptoms are important to identify early disease. Risk factors for liver disease include alcoholism and drug abuse, risky sexual practices, exposure to infection or environmental toxins, and travel to countries with poor sanitation. One should question the patient about symptoms of liver disease, such as fatigue, itching, abdominal pain, anorexia, weight gain, fever, blood in stools or black stools, sleep problems, lack of menstruation, and lack of libido. Physical assessment includes checking vital signs and skin for scratches, pallor, jaundice, dryness, bruising, petechiae, abdominal veins and spider angiomas, and red palms:

- Assess for gynecomastia, abdominal distension, fluid waves, bowel sounds, liver margins, tenderness, consistency, and hardness and sharpness of the edge.
- Examine extremities for wasting, edema, and weakness.
- Assess neurological system for cognitive status, tremors, balance problems, slurred speech.
- Identify testicular atrophy.
- Blood should be drawn for serum enzymes and proteins, bilirubin, ammonia, clotting factors, and lipid profile.

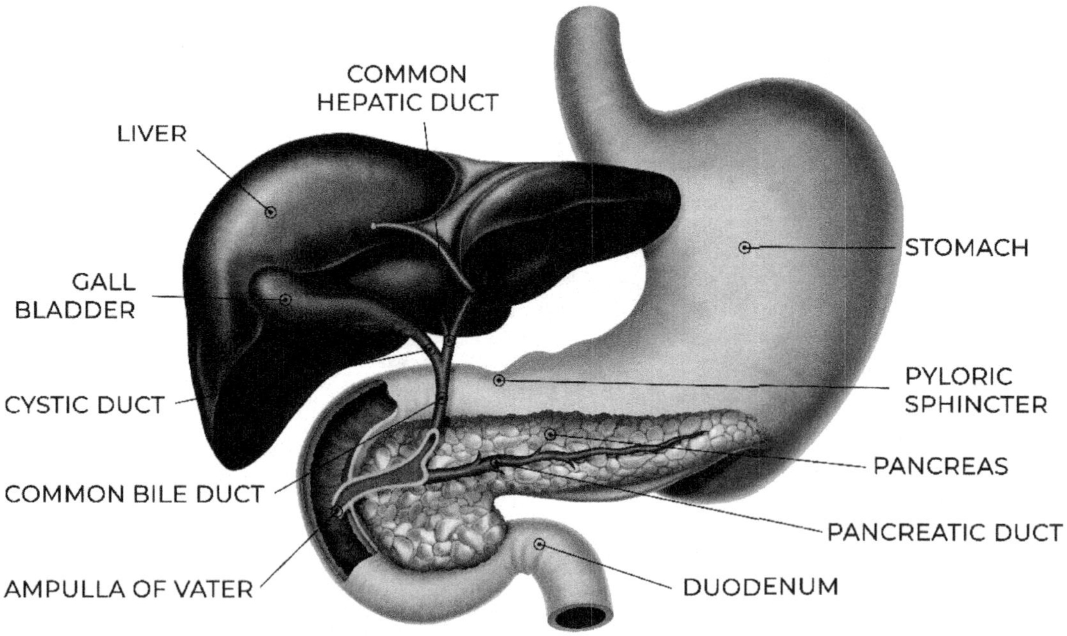

## ASSESSMENT OF NUTRITIONAL STATUS

Assessment of nutritional status begins with an assessment of the patient's intake. The patient is asked to report intake for the previous 24 hours. This may indicate the need for a **food diary** over a period of time:

- Compare the patient's nutritional intake with the requirements of the USDA's MyPlate.
- Measure height and weight and check against a BMI table to help determine nutritional status.
- Measure waist circumference.
- Assess the patient for physical signs of poor nutrition such as muscle wasting, obesity, hair breakage and loss, poor skin turgor, ulcers, bruising, and loss of subcutaneous tissue.
- Assess mucous membranes and condition of teeth, abdomen, extremities, and thyroid gland.

Nutritional status is connected to endocrine disease, infections, other acute and chronic diseases, digestion, absorption, excretion, and storage of nutrients, so these areas must also be assessed. Blood testing should include proteins, transferrin, electrolytes, vitamins A and C, carotene, and CBC. Test urine for creatinine, thiamine, riboflavin, niacin, albumin, and iodine.

### *ASSESSING NUTRITIONAL STATUS OF HOSPITALIZED PATIENTS*

Assessing the nutritional status of the hospital inpatient is an important part of forming a care plan. The two screening tools that are most commonly used are the **subjective global assessment (SGA)** and the **prognostic nutritional index (PNI)**. The SGA provides a nutritional assessment based on both the patient history and current symptoms. The patient is asked about any changes in weight and is also asked questions about his or her diet. The presence of symptoms that may lead to weight loss and poor nutritional status, such as diarrhea, nausea, and vomiting, as well as water retention (edema) and muscle wasting (cachexia), is also included in the SGA. The PNI is also used as an indicator of malnutrition and is especially helpful in predicting survival in cancer patients and determining how well a patient will recover from surgery. The PNI results from a calculation involving the measurement of serum albumin and absolute lymphocyte count.



# Genitourinary Assessment

## ASSESSMENT OF KIDNEYS AND URINARY TRACT

Assessment of kidneys and urinary tract includes:

- Assess the health history for family urinary system disease and risk factors, such as previous urinary disease, increased age, immobility, hypertension, diabetes, chemical exposure, chronic disease, radiation to the pelvis, STIs, alcohol or drug use, and complications of pregnancy and delivery.
- Determine daily fluid intake.
- Question symptoms such as flank or abdominal pain, hesitancy, urgency, difficulty or straining with voiding, difficulty emptying the bladder, urinary incontinence, fatigue, SOB, exercise intolerance from anemia, fever, chills, blood in the urine, and GI symptoms.

**Physical assessment** includes vital signs, kidney and bladder palpation, and percussion over the bladder after urination:

- Palpate for ascites and edema.
- Measure the DTRs and check gait and ability to walk heel-to-toe.
- Examine the genitalia and check the urethra and vagina for herniation, irritation, or tears.

Urine specimen is obtained via clean catch midstream technique for analysis and culture if indicated. Blood is taken for a CBC, and in males, prostate-specific antigen (PSA) levels will also be measured via blood specimen.

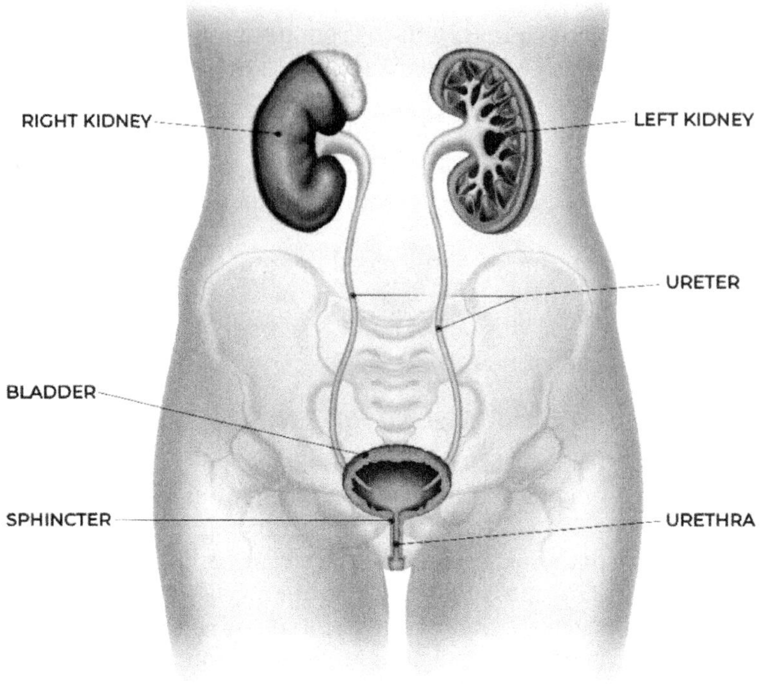


**Review Video: Urinary System**
Visit mometrix.com/academy and enter code: 601053

## Kidney Regulatory Functions Regarding Fluid Balance

Kidney regulatory functions include maintaining **fluid balance**. Fluid excretion balances intake with output, so increased intake results in a large output and vice versa:

- **Osmolality** (the number of electrolytes and other molecules per kg/urine) measures the concentration or dilution. With dehydration, osmolality increases; with fluid retention, osmolality decreases. With kidney disease, urine is dilute and the osmolality is fixed.
- **Specific gravity** compares the weight of urine (weight of particles) to distilled water (1.000). Normal urine is 1.010–1.025 with normal intake. High intake lowers the specific gravity, and low intake raises it. In kidney disease, it often does not vary.
- **Antidiuretic hormone** (ADH/vasopressin) regulates the excretion of water and urine concentration in the renal tubule by varying water reabsorption. When fluid intake decreases, blood osmolality rises, and this stimulates the release of ADH, which increases reabsorption of fluid to return osmolality to normal levels. ADH is suppressed with increased fluid intake, so less fluid is reabsorbed.

### ASSESSING SEXUAL HEALTH AND PREFERENCES

Bringing up the topic of sex gives a patient permission to ask questions and openly discuss **sexual concerns**:

- Ask for permission to ask questions about sexual health and preferences during the gynecological/urological portion of the health history.
- If the patient refuses, go on with the rest of the health history, otherwise continue.
- Ask first if the person has sex with men, women, or both.
- Be nonjudgmental and do not assume that those who are elderly or disabled do not have sex. Use layman terms according to the patient's age and education level.
- Ask if the person is having any problems with relationships or sexual intercourse.
- Ask if the person has ever been forced to have sex or if is afraid of anyone close to them.
- End by asking if there are any questions about expression of sexual feelings, contraception, safe sex practices, or risky behavior.
- Refer those with problems to their doctor, or a gynecologist, urologist, or sex therapist.

## Musculoskeletal Assessment

### ASSESSING RISK OF FALLING

Many factors must be examined and combined to determine the **fall risk** status of a patient. They include age, sensory deficits, mobility problems, neurological disorders, past history of falling, cognitive impairment, and depression. Some medications, such as those associated with postural hypotension and psychotropic medications, may increase the danger of falls. The presence of dizziness, acute or chronic illness, poor physical status, elimination requirements, medications, and environmental concerns contribute to the risk for falls.

Multiple factors increase risk, so careful history and physical exam are necessary as part of assessment. When the presence of risk factors shows a risk for falls, this information should be communicated to other caregivers by wristband, colored markers on doors, care plans, or other effective means. The factors are then modified as much as possible. The patient should be re-evaluated as their condition changes or after a fall to determine the cause.



### ASSESSING PATIENTS WITH DISABILITIES

A patient with **disabilities** may find it very difficult to obtain screening for health problems due to inaccessibility:

- Work with the patient to resolve barriers to obtain weight, mammography, bone density tests, and pap/pelvic exams on a regular basis.
- Ask how to best assist the patient during the assessment.
- Observe the patient carefully for nonverbal communication, such as grimacing.
- If sensation is affected, warn the patient before touching any part of the body.
- Always address all areas of the patient's history, including sexual history.
- Use an interpreter that is not a family member if needed.
- Give the patient extra time to respond to questions when there is aphasia or other communication problems.
- Address the impact of the disability on the ability to perform ADLs, health status in general, access to healthcare, financial status, emotional status, work, community roles, and family wellbeing.

# Integumentary Assessment

## General Skin Assessment

**Skin color** varies according to ethnicity. Color changes should be assessed to determine if they are local or extend over the entire body, and if they are permanent or transient. Pallor may indicate stress, impaired oxygenation, and vasoconstriction. Erythema may indicate vasodilation, local inflammation, and blushing. Cyanosis indicates impaired oxygenation, and jaundice indicates increased bilirubin.

**Temperature** is typically assessed by touching the skin with the back of the hand. Skin should be warm and equal bilaterally. Hypothermia may indicate impaired circulation, intravenous infusion, and immobilized limb (such as in a cast). Hyperthermia may indicate fever, infection, and excessive exercise.

**Review Video: Skin Assessment**
Visit mometrix.com/academy and enter code: 794925

## Effects of Age on Skin

**Age** is an important consideration when evaluating the skin because the characteristics of the skin change as people age.

- An **infant's** skin is thinner than an adult's because, while the epidermis is developed, the dermis layer is only about 60% of that of an adult and continues to develop after birth. The skin of premature infants is especially friable, allowing for transepidermal water loss and evaporative heat loss.
- During **adolescence**, the hair follicles activate, the thickness of the dermis decreases about 20%, and epidermal turnover time increases, so healing slows.
- As people **continue to age**, Langerhans' cells decrease in number, making the skin more prone to cancer, and the inflammatory reactions decrease. The sweat glands, vascularity, and subcutaneous fat all decrease, interfering with thermoregulation and contributing to dryness and irritation of the skin. The epidermal-dermal junction flattens, resulting in skin that is prone to tearing. The elastin in the skin degrades with age and solar exposure. The thinning of the hypodermis can lead to pressure injuries.

**Review Video: Integumentary System**
Visit mometrix.com/academy and enter code: 655980

### BRADEN SCALE

The Braden scale is a risk assessment tool that has been validated clinically as predictive of the risk of patient's developing pressure injuries. It was developed in 1988 by Barbara Braden and Nancy Bergstrom and is in wide use. The scale scores six different areas with five areas scored 1–4 points, and one area 1–3 points. The lower the score, the greater the risk.

| Area | Score of 1 | Score of 2 | Score of 3 | Score of 4 |
|---|---|---|---|---|
| Sensory perception | Completely limited | Very limited | Slightly limited | No impairment |
| Moisture | Constantly moist | Very moist | Occasionally moist | Rarely moist |
| Activity | Bed | Chair | Occasional walk | Frequent walk |
| Mobility | Immobile | Limited | Slightly limited | No limitations |
| Nutritional pattern | Very poor | Inadequate | Adequate | Excellent |
| Friction and shear | Problem | Potential problem | No apparent problem | |

## EENT Assessment

### EYE ASSESSMENT

Assessment of the eyes includes:

- **History**: Ask about blurring, blind spots, floaters, night blindness, halos, pain, photophobia, tearing, allergies, previous ocular problems, use of glasses or contact lenses, and changes in depth perception.
- **Extraocular muscles**: Ask patient to stare straight ahead and shine light from 12 inches. Reflection of light on the corneas should be identical on both eyes. Asymmetry indicates muscle weakness or paralysis.
- **External inspection**: Note symmetry. Use thumbs to pull lower lids down and ask patient to look upward and elevate upper lid at outer aspect and ask patient to look down to examine conjunctiva and sclera. Note redness, pallor, cyanosis, swelling, or excessive tearing. In darkened room, note pupillary response to light and size and symmetry. In lighted room, ask patient to look at a distance and then at an item 8 inches from eyes. Note pupillary constriction and convergence.
- **Ocular fundus (ophthalmoscope)**: Darken room, remove patient's eyeglasses, ask patient to stare at distant object, anchor upper eyelid, hold instrument 10 inches from patient at 15° lateral to patient's line of vision. Note the red reflex and move slowly toward patient, noting abnormalities, such as opaque areas (cataracts), and inspect the optic disc, retinal vessels, and macula.

## Vision Assessment

Assessment of vision includes:

- **Visual acuity**: Leave glasses or contact lenses in place and position the patient 20 feet from Snellen chart and shield one eye at a time, asking patient to read the chart down to the smallest line, and record that line as a numeric fraction to indicate errors.
- **Near vision**: Ask patient to read vision screener with text in different sizes. Hold screener approximately 14 inches from the eyes and test one eye at a time with the patient wearing usual glasses or contact lenses.
- **Visual fields**: Stand 2 feet in front of the patient at eye level and ask the patient to look straight ahead and cover one eye. Advance an item (finger, pencil) from the periphery toward the midline from multiple directions and ask the patient to note when the item is first seen. Estimate the angles. Normal findings: upward 50°, temporally 90°, downward 70°, and nasally 60°.

## Ear and Hearing Assessment

Assessment of the ears includes:

- **External ear**: Observe for symmetry, size, shape, erythema, crusting, scaling, and discoloration. Move the pinna and tragus to see if they are tender (otitis externa).
- **External ear canal**: Note size, evidence of edema, erythema, or discharge.
- **Internal ear canal and eardrum**: Use an otoscope. Pull the pinna up and back (adults) or down (infants, children under 3) and tilt the patient's head slightly to the opposite side to straighten the ear canal. Insert the otoscope and rotate it to view the entire eardrum. Note any discharge, foreign bodies, edema, or erythema. Note the amount and color of cerumen. Examine the eardrum for color, contour, and perforations.
- **Hearing acuity (estimate)**: Occlude one ear at a time (with a finger), obscure the patient's vision, whisper softly toward the unoccluded ear from 1–2 feet away, using numbers or simple words with equally accented syllables (e.g., "baseball"). Increase intensity of whispers as needed.

Tuning fork tests:

- **Weber test**: Place a vibrating tuning fork on top of the patient's head and ask where sound is heard (should be equal in both ears). An abnormal finding may indicate either conductive or sensorineural hearing loss.
- **Rinne test**: Place a vibrating tuning fork on the mastoid process and measure duration of sound. Then place a tuning fork at the external ear canal. Sound is normally heard twice as long through air as through bone.

## Nose and Sense of Smell Assessment

Assessment of the nose and smell includes:

- **History**: Ask about any nasal discharge, frequent URIs, sinusitis, PND, pain, history of trauma, nosebleeds, allergies, and changes in the sense of smell.
- **External inspection**
  - Anterior: Assess nose symmetry or deviation.
  - Lateral: Assess shape.
  - Inferior: Assess the nasal vestibule, applying gentle upward pressure on the tip of the nose to widen the nostrils, noting any difference in size or pain that may indicate local infection.
- **Internal inspection**: Maintaining gentle pressure on the tip, use a penlight to observe for signs of redness, polyps, deviation, or swelling. For further examination, use a nasal speculum or an otoscope, using care to rest the device against the alae nasi (outer aspect) rather than the septum.

- **Obstruction**: Compress one nostril at a time and ask patient to breathe in and note any impaired airflow. Place a flat metal tool beneath the nostrils and ask patient to breathe out and observe for equal misting.
- **Smell (olfactory nerve)**: Ask the patient to close their eyes, and hold one nostril at a time closed. Place an item with a familiar smell (vanilla, alcohol pad, coffee) beneath the nose at approximately 2 cm and ask the patient to identify.

### Mouth and Throat Assessment

Assessment of the mouth and throat includes:

- **Preparation**: Ask the patient to remove lipstick and any dentures.
- **Lips**: Note color, texture, moisture, symmetry, scaliness, cracks, and lesions.
- **Mucosa**: Use a tongue blade to improve visualization and note color, nodules, ulcerations, white patches, or other abnormalities.
- **Gums**: Note color and abnormalities such as a black line (lead poisoning), lesions, pallor, gingivitis.
- **Teeth**: Use a gloved thumb and index finger to check for absence of teeth, discoloration, misshapen teeth, or loose teeth.
- **Hard palate**: Note color and architecture. Note presence of *torus palatinus* (midline bony growth), including size and shape.
- **Tongue and floor of mouth**: Ask the patient to stick their tongue out and note symmetry, color, moisture, and texture. Note any ulcerations or nodules. Carefully inspect the sides by grasping the tongue tip with a gauze square and pulling tongue to the side, then palpate for any lesions. Examine the floor of the mouth.
- **Pharynx**: Ask the patient to open their mouth, relax their tongue, and say "ahhh." If visualization is inadequate, use a tongue blade at the midpoint of the tongue. Note that the soft palate rises (10th cranial nerve). Examine the soft palate, uvula, tonsils, and pharynx for signs of swelling, ulceration, pain, and asymmetry. Palpate any suspicious areas, if possible.



## Geriatric Assessment

### Age Categories of the Elderly

The elderly population can be divided into three groups. The age group ranging from 65-74 years are considered the **young-old**, from 75-84 are considered the **middle-old**, and 85 and older are considered **old-old**. There are many physical and psychological changes that occur as someone moves through these age groups. As this population increases in size, so does the number of those with physical and mental illnesses.

### Factors That Influence Presentation of Illness in Older Adults

There are three major factors that influence **how an illness will present in an older patient.** These factors, either alone or in combination with one another, have the potential to make an ordinarily standard clinical presentation confusing for the clinician.

- The first of these factors is **underreporting of illness or the symptoms associated** with illness. There are a number of reasons that illnesses are not reported: the patient may fear hospitalization, institutionalization, or loss of control, or the patient may be convinced that there really is no problem.
- Another factor is the **pattern of distribution of illness** amongst the elderly population. This affects presentation because there are a number of diseases and impairments that are prevalent among older adults, including congestive heart failure, arthritis, osteoporosis, and pneumonia; therefore, identifying and differentiating the primary diagnosis may be difficult.
- The last factor is an **altered response to illness**. This can make diagnosis and treatment very difficult because symptoms may be exaggerated by other problems, or they may be nonexistent.

## Age-Related Considerations When Evaluating Adult Patients

Because each individual patient is exposed to different environmental, psychological, and physical stressors that can affect the aging process, it is important to consider that some patients may experience adverse health impacts, while other patients of the same age may not be affected. As individuals age, the amount of wear on the body, as well as the likelihood of pathological changes, increases at different rates for every individual. Factors affecting the aging process include proper nutrition (or the lack thereof), level of physical activity, smoking, alcohol consumption, environmental or occupational exposures, and socioeconomic standing. Also, remember that as an individual ages, a disease or impairments with one organ or organ system will have a marked effect on other systems, because the body is not able to compensate as it once was. Symptoms may not be noticeable until other functions begin to decline. Most often, health issues manifest in the elderly as confusion, so close attention must be given to this symptom and investigated when present.

## Basic Patient Safety Assessments When Evaluating a Patient

There are four basic assessments that the nurse should make when **assessing a patient's safety** and identifying possible safety concerns:

- The first of these is the **mobility assessment**; different safety risks apply to patients who are mobile as opposed to those who are not. An immobile patient, for example, has a tendency to form pressure injuries, or bedsores.
- The next assessment is the evaluation of the patient's **level of awareness**; is the patient able to communicate to the nursing staff when something is wrong? If not, certain measures should be undertaken to ensure that the nursing staff is aware of a change in the patient's condition.
- An extension of this assessment is determining whether the patient is in **critical condition**; these patients must be monitored more closely for changes.
- An assessment of the patient's **mental status** is also important because the patient may not be able to make safe decisions on his or her own.

## Functional Evaluation of Elderly Patient

A functional evaluation of the elderly patient examines the patient's ability to carry out activities of daily living (ADL) that are critical in gauging the patient's ability to care for oneself without the need of assistance. Use the **Index of Independence in Activities of Daily Living Scale** to check foundational tasks such as taking a shower, getting dressed, eating, and going to the bathroom. Aged patients will be more likely to overstate what they are able to do and understate their limitations, while the patient's family will likely understate what the patient is able to handle. Assess mental ability with the following exams:

- Short Portable Mental Status Questionnaire (SPMSQ)
- Mini-Mental State Exam (MMSE)

The **Tinetti Balance and Gait Evaluation** exams are also important elements of the functional evaluation of an elderly patient. These tests, along with the simple **Up-and-Go test,** are used to assess the balance and gait issues that elderly patients have. The patient has to complete certain actions, such as sitting down and standing up from a chair, turning around, bending over, etc. The entire assessment takes approximately 15–20 minutes. The **Lawton and Brody: Instrumental Activities of Daily Learning** test is used to check whether the patient can do more complex activities important to daily living, second to the ADL's required for basic function. Examples of IADLs include the ability to go shopping, wash clothes, cook, etc. The **Index of Independence of Activities of Daily Living** is utilized to find what the patient is able do independently on a regular basis.

## Depression and Suicide in the Elderly

**Depression** commonly goes unidentified in an aging patient. Cognitive changes are often wrongly identified as dementia, confusion, or natural aging changes, rather than depression. It is important to be cognizant of the prevalence of this issue among the elderly, and treat appropriately.

**Suicide rates** for elderly patients are higher than any other age group. The compounding stress and emotional burden of losing loved ones, mobility, and independence often contribute to suicidal ideations. Other factors include seemingly unbearable psychological anguish, dissatisfaction, and unmet requirements. Suicide is more commonly seen in elderly males (seven times higher rate), Caucasians, unmarried individuals (divorced, separated, single), individuals who are poor and/or out of work, individuals with psychiatric or cognitive impairments, the very sick, individuals with substance additions, individuals that are grieving (particularly in the first year of loss or retirement), those without friends or community relationships, or those who have tried suicide before. Suicidal thoughts and attempts may be overt or covert.

As with patients of other age ranges, if an elderly patient hints at suicidal ideations or thoughts, this must be addressed directly by the nurse.

### Indications and Assessments for Delirium

**Delirium (acute confusion)** presents in a variety of indications. The patient may experience mental issues, including inattention or short attention span, difficulty remembering, trouble with perception, bafflement, and lack of decision-making. There may be changing moods, faulty ability to manage whims, stress, slight to moderate depression, visual or auditory hallucinations, confabulation, changing intellectual ability that worsens at night (sun-downing) and is more frequently seen in patients that have had prior dementia, psychomotor agitation including inability to sleep, tachycardia, enlarged pupils, and perspiration. The patient may appear restless, overcautious, not cautious enough, or appear lost/stunned. There may be tachycardia, high blood pressure, fever, rapid breathing, and there might be focal neurological indications.

Physical assessments include a complete history, physical examination, check of mind and neurological issues to determine what is causing the problem, foundation of lab work such as CBC, electrocardiogram, chest radiograph, urinalysis, urine toxicology, and other assessments that are deemed necessary, such as EED, CT, or blood work for drugs.



## Postpartum Assessment and Management

### Postpartum Assessment

The postpartum assessment includes the following elements:

- **Vital signs**
  - VS should be checked every 15 minutes and evaluated in relation to baseline VS and VS prior to delivery.
  - Normal BP varies from 90/60 to 140/90.
  - Falling BP and increased pulse may indicate uterine bleeding.
  - Pulse (60–90) is usually slightly decreased from that found during labor.
  - Respirations should be relaxed and not labored, usually 12–20/min.
- **Temperature**
  - Slight elevation immediately after delivery (≤100.4 °F), but this should return to normal within 24 hours.
- **Alertness**
  - The mother should be awake, alert, responsive, and able to hold the infant.
- **Fundus**
  - Fundus is palpated to determine if it is firm, midline, and in the expected position (at the umbilicus).
  - A boggy fundus may indicate uterine bleeding.
  - Bladder distention may cause the fundus to deviate from midline.

- **Lochia**
  - Lochia should be checked every 15 minutes for signs of excess bleeding, such as copious discharge or large clots.
  - Lochia must be observed while the fundus is massaged to determine if there is free flow of blood or expulsion of clots, which may indicate hemorrhage.
  - Lochia rubra should be present with moderate amount of discharge, not to exceed 1 saturated perineal pad/hr.
- **Perineum**
  - The perineal area should be examined and the amount of swelling and bruising noted, along with the condition of episiotomy (if present) and sutures.
  - Severe perineal/rectal pain requires further examination.
- **Bladder**
  - The bladder should be palpated to determine if it is distended.
  - The mother should be given the opportunity to urinate within the first hour after delivery before catheterization is considered.
  - The mother should spontaneously urinate >100 mL clear urine with no distention noted after urination.
- **Rectum**
  - Rectum should be examined for presence of tearing or hemorrhoids.
  - No severe rectal pain should be present.
  - If hemorrhoids are present, engorgement must be reported to physician, especially if they are larger than 2 cm in size.
- **Pain**
  - Mother should have only mild pain, <3 on a 1 to 10 scale.
  - Severe pain requires further examination to determine the cause.
  - Analgesia should be provided to control pain.
- **Legs/feet**
  - Feet and legs should be warm and pulses palpable.
  - Edema, which may have been present before delivery, should remain stable or decrease.
- **Anesthesia**
  - If the mother had an anesthetic, such as epidural or spinal, the level of anesthesia should be assessed every 15 minutes.

## The REEDA Episiotomy Perineal Assessment

The REEDA scale is used to assess the perineal area after an episiotomy. Score: 0 = healed, 1–5 = moderately healed, 6–10 = mildly healed, 11–15 = not healed

| | Redness | Edema | Ecchymosis | Approximation |
|---|---|---|---|---|
| **0** | None | None | None | Closed |
| **1** | <1 cm from incision | <0.25 cm bilaterally or 0.5 cm unilaterally of incision | Serous | Skin separation <3 mm |
| **2** | 1–2 cm from incision | <0.25 cm–1.0 cm bilaterally or 0.5–2.0 cm unilaterally of incision | Serosanguineous | Skin and subcutaneous fat separation |
| **3** | >2 cm from incision or affects vulvar area | >1 cm bilaterally or 2 cm unilaterally of incision | Bloody/ Purulent | Skin, subcutaneous fat, and fascial separation |

## Wound Care

Wound care of the postpartum mother is needed if the woman has had a Cesarean, episiotomy, or lacerations. In all cases, the patient should receive analgesia as needed. **Wound care**:

- **Cesarean**: Surgi-strips or staples may be in place and the wound covered with a sterile bandage. An ice pack may be applied 15 minutes at a time to help control pain and swelling in the first 24 hours. The initial sterile bandage is usually removed after 24 hours and then the wound left open to the air or covered with light sterile gauze. The woman is usually allowed to shower after 24 hours. The wound should be routinely checked to make sure it is intact and healing.
- **Episiotomy/Lacerations**: The suture line should be checked frequently for signs of infection, hematoma, or separation. Ice packs may be applied 15 minutes at a time for the first 24 hours to reduce swelling and pain. After 24 hours, warm Sitz baths for 20 minutes 2–4 times daily are usually advised, and the woman is cautioned to tighten buttocks muscles when sitting down to avoid stress on suture lines.

## Pain Assessment and Control

Assess the location, intensity, frequency, and type of pain present. **Uterine pain** occurs with assessment, cramping, and massage. Slow, deep breathing and relaxation can help the mother through this pain. Be sure your hands are warm during palpation and massage to decrease comfort. Administer analgesia as ordered and teach the mother the side effects and how to take the medicine when she goes home.

**Perineal pain** may be relieved by analgesics and anesthetic sprays used when pericare is performed following toileting. Ice packs are also helpful in the first 24–48 hours to decrease edema and inflammation. Apply moist heat via a sitz bath after the first 48 hours have passed.

The accumulation of intestinal gas also causes pain in the postpartum period. The use of rocking and ambulation will help. The mother should avoid gas-producing foods until the GI tract motility resumes normal functioning.



## Cesarean Section Management

### *Postoperative Assessment*

The initial assessments of the mother who has had a **Cesarean** and of the neonate are similar to those for vaginal birth, but the mother also must recover from a surgical procedure and anesthesia. These assessments constitute standard **postoperative care** during the first hour postpartum:

- **VS** are checked every 5 minutes until stable, then every 15 minutes for one hour, and finally every 30 minutes until the mother is released from the recovery area.
- **Abdominal dressing and perineal pad** are checked every 15 minutes for bleeding for the first hour; fundus gently palpated with a hand supporting the area of the incision.
- **IV oxytocin** is administered to promote contraction of the uterine muscles.
- If general anesthesia was administered, the patient should be positioned on her side and **turned** every 2 hours for 24 hours.
- If epidural or spinal anesthesia was administered, level of **anesthesia** should be checked every 15 minutes.
- **Intake and output** are monitored, and urine checked for signs of blood (indicating bladder trauma).
- **Analgesia** should be administered as needed to control pain.

### *Postoperative Care*

The mother who has had a **Cesarean** birth has both routine postpartum and surgical needs. The mother should deep-breathe and cough (while supporting the abdomen with a pillow) and use an **incentive spirometer** every 2–4 hours during the daytime for the first few days. The mother should sit on the side of the bed within 12 hours of surgery and ambulate within 24 hours. **Pain management** with PCA, oral, and parenteral medications and/or relaxation techniques helps the mother to ambulate and care for her infant. Epidural analgesia may continue for 24 hours after delivery and must be monitored carefully. Flatus and abdominal distention are common complaints, so the mother should avoid carbonated beverages and drinking through straws. Taking an antiflatulent (Mylicon), turning frequently, rocking, or lying on the left side may help to expel gas. The mother should be encouraged to breastfeed but may be more comfortable sitting with the baby supported by a pillow or lying on her side to prevent pressure on the incision.

### *Postoperative Guidelines by the Enhanced Recovery After Surgery (ERAS) Society*

The Enhanced Recovery After Surgery (ERAS) Society is focused on streamlining the surgical management of patients to minimize complication risks and encourage quicker recovery. They have specific guidelines for Cesarean sections, which include three focuses: preoperative, intraoperative, and postoperative care. Recommended postoperative care management of a Cesarean section include the following:

- Nausea and vomiting prevention: fluid reloading and administrative of antiemetic drugs
- Postoperative pain management: utilize NSAIDs and paracetamol in a multimodal approach to analgesia
- Perioperative nutritional care: encourage oral intake (drinking fluids and eating a regular diet) within 2 hours of delivery; chewing gum is considered effective if oral intake is delayed.
- VTE prophylaxis: compression stockings and early mobilization
- Removal of Foley catheter immediately after delivery (if placed)

## Chapter Quiz

Ready to see how well you retained what you just read? Scan the QR code to go directly to the chapter quiz interface for this study guide. If you're using a computer, simply visit the online resources page at **mometrix.com/resources719/nclexrn-31183** and click the Chapter Quizzes link.

# Psychosocial Integrity

## Psychological Assessment

### Elements of the Psychosocial Assessment

A psychosocial assessment should provide additional information to the physical assessment to guide the patient's plan of care and should include:

- Previous hospitalizations and experience with healthcare
- Psychiatric history: Suicidal ideation, psychiatric disorders, family psychiatric history, history of violence and/or self-mutilation
- Chief complaint: Patient's perception
- Complementary therapies: Acupuncture, visualization, and meditation
- Occupational and educational background: Employment, retirement, and special skills
- Social patterns: Family and friends, living situation, typical activities, support system
- Sexual patterns: Orientation, problems, and sex practices
- Interests/abilities: Hobbies and sports
- Current or past substance abuse: Type, frequency, drinking pattern, use of recreational drugs, and overuse of prescription drugs
- Ability to cope: Stress reduction techniques
- Physical, sexual, emotional, and financial abuse: Older adults are especially vulnerable to abuse and may be reluctant to disclose out of shame or fear
- Spiritual/cultural assessment: Religious/spiritual importance, practices, restrictions (such as blood products or foods), and impact on health/health decisions

### Cognitive Assessment

Individuals with evidence of dementia, delirium, or short-term memory loss should have cognition assessed. The **mini-mental state exam (MMSE)** or the **mini-cog test** are both commonly used. These tests require the individual to carry out specified tasks and are used as a baseline to determine change in mental status.

**MMSE:**

- Remembering and later repeating the names of 3 common objects
- Counting backward from 100 by 7s or spelling "world" backward
- Naming items as the examiner points to them
- Providing the location of the examiner's office, including city, state, and street address
- Repeating common phrases
- Copying a picture of interlocking shapes
- Following simple 3-part instructions, such as picking up a piece of paper, folding it in half, and placing it on the floor

*A score of ≥24/30 is considered a normal functioning level.*

**Mini-cog:**

- Remembering and later repeating the names of 3 common objects
- Drawing the face of a clock, including all 12 numbers and the hands, and indicating the time specified by the examiner

*A score of 3–5 (out of 5) indicates a lower chance of dementia but does not rule it out.*

## Confusion Assessment Method

The Confusion Assessment Method is an assessment tool intended to be used by those without psychiatric training in order to assess the progression of delirium in patients. The tool covers 9 factors, some factors have a range of possibilities, and others are rated only as to whether the characteristic is present, not present, uncertain, or not applicable. The tool also provides room to describe abnormal behavior. Factors indicative of delirium include:

- **Onset**: Acute change in mental status
- **Attention**: Inattentive, stable, or fluctuating
- **Thinking**: Disorganized, rambling conversation, switching topics, illogical
- **Level of consciousness**: Altered, ranging from alert to coma
- **Orientation**: Disoriented (person, place, and time)
- **Memory**: Impaired
- **Perceptual disturbances**: Hallucinations, illusions
- **Psychomotor abnormalities**: Agitation (tapping, picking, moving) or retardation (staring, not moving)
- **Sleep-wake cycle**: Awake at night and sleepy in the daytime

**The Confusion Assessment Method indicates delirium if there is an acute onset, fluctuating inattention, and disorganized thinking OR altered level of consciousness.*

## Hamilton Anxiety Scale

The Hamilton Anxiety Scale (HAS or HAMA) is utilized to evaluate the anxiety related symptomatology that may be present in adults as well as children. It provides an evaluation of overall **anxiety** and its degree of severity. This includes **somatic anxiety** (physical complaints) and **psychic anxiety** (mental agitation and distress). This scale consists of 14 items based on anxiety produced symptoms. Each item is ranked 0–4 with 0 indicating no symptoms present and 4 indicating severe symptoms present. This scale is frequently utilized in psychotropic drug evaluations. If performed before a particular medication has been started and then again at later visits, the HAS can be helpful in adjusting medication dosages based in part on the individual's score. It is often utilized as an outcome measure in clinical trials.

## Beck Depression Inventory

The Beck Depression Inventory (BDI) is a widely utilized, self-reported, multiple-choice questionnaire consisting of 21 items, which measures the **degree of depression**. This tool is designed for use in adults ages 17–80. It evaluates physical symptoms such as weight loss, loss of sleep, loss of interest in sex, fatigue, and attitudinal symptoms such as irritability, guilt, and hopelessness. The items rank in four possible answer choices based on an increasing severity of symptoms. The test is scored with the answers ranging in value from 0–3. The total score is utilized to determine the degree of depression. The usual ranges include: 0–9 no signs of depression, 10–18 mild depression, 19–29 moderate depression, and 30–63 severe depression.

## Evaluation for Suicidal or Homicidal Thoughts

During a risk assessment two of the most important areas to evaluate are the patient's **risk for self-harm or harm to others**. The staff member performing the assessment should very closely evaluate for any descriptions or thoughts the patient may have concerning these risks. Direct questioning on these subjects should be performed and documented. Close evaluation of any delusional thoughts the patient may be having should be carefully evaluated. Does the patient believe he or she is being instructed by others to perform either of these acts? Safety of the patient and others needs to be a top priority and carefully documented. If the patient indicates that they are having these thoughts or ideas, they must be placed in either suicidal or assault precautions with close monitoring per facility protocol.

## Suicide Risk Assessment

A suicide risk assessment should be completed and documented upon admission, with each shift change, at discharge, or any time suicidal ideations are suggested by the patient. This risk assessment should evaluate some of the following criteria:

- Would the patient sign a contract for safety?
- Is there a suicide plan? How lethal is the plan?
- What is the elopement risk?
- How often are the suicidal thoughts, and have they attempted suicide before?

Any associated symptoms of hopelessness, guilt, anger, helplessness, impulsive behaviors, nightmares, obsessions with death, or altered judgment should also be assessed and documented. The higher the score the higher the risk for suicide.

## Alcohol Use Assessment

The **Clinical Instrument for Withdrawal for Alcohol (CIWA)** is a tool used to assess the severity of alcohol withdraw. Each category is scored 0–7 points based on the severity of symptoms, except #10, which is scored 0–4. A score <5 indicates mild withdrawal without need for medications; for scores ranging 5–15, benzodiazepines are indicated to manage symptoms. A score >15 indicates severe withdrawal and the need for admission to the unit.

- Nausea/Vomiting
- Tremor
- Paroxysmal Sweats
- Anxiety
- Agitation
- Tactile Disturbances
- Auditory Disturbances
- Visual Disturbances
- Headache
- Disorientation or Clouding of Sensorium

The **CAGE** tool is used as a quick assessment to identify problem drinkers. Moderate drinking, (1–2 drinks daily or one drink a day for older adults) is usually not harmful to people in the absence of other medical conditions. However, drinking more can lead to serious psychosocial and physical problems. One drink is defined as 12 ounces of beer/wine cooler, 5 ounces of wine, or 1.5 ounces of liquor.

- **C** – *Cutting Down*: "Do you think about trying to cut down on drinking?"
- **A** – *Annoyed at Criticism*: "Are people starting to criticize your drinking?"
- **G** – *Guilty feeling*: "Do you feel guilty or try to hide your drinking?"
- **E** – *Eye opener*: "Do you increasingly need a drink earlier in the day?"

"Yes" on one question suggests the possibility of a drinking problem. "Yes" on ≥2 indicates a drinking problem

## Screening for Risk-Taking Behavior

The ability to assess outcomes and respond appropriately to risks are part of the decision-making process. Decision making can be impaired in patients with mental health disorders such as depression, anxiety, bipolar disorder, and personality disorders, as well as in patients who have experienced a brain injury or have a dependence on drugs or alcohol. Health care providers should screen patients for the presence of high-risk behaviors. This may be accomplished through a self-administered questionnaire or through a patient interview with a trained clinician. Examples of **high-risk behaviors** include substance use/abuse, high risk sexual behaviors, high risk driving behaviors such as drinking and driving, speeding or riding with a drunk driver, and violence related behaviors. Patients with an increased response to risk taking may exhibit signs of impulsivity and sensation seeking. Conversely, other patients may exhibit abnormally cautious behavior.

# Abuse and Neglect

## Indicators of Abuse That May Be Identified in the Patient History

The healthcare provider should always be aware of the presence of any **indicators** that may present a potential for or an actual situation that involves **abuse**. These indicators may present in the **patient's history**. Some examples of indicators concerning their primary complaint may include the following: vague description about the cause of the problem, inconsistencies between physical findings and explanations, minimizing injuries, long period of time between injury and treatment, and over-reactions or under-reactions of family members to injuries. Other important information may be revealed in the family genome, such as family history of violence, time spent in jail or prison, and family history of violent deaths or substance abuse. The patient's health history may include previous injuries, spontaneous abortions, or history of pervious inpatient psychiatric treatment or substance abuse.

During the collection of the patient history, the financial history, the patient's family values, and the patient's relationships with family members can also reveal actual or potential **abuse indicators**.

- The **financial history** may indicate that the patient has little or no money or that they are not given access to money by a controlling family member. They may also be unemployed or utilizing an elderly family member's income for their own personal expenses.
- **Family values** may indicate strong beliefs in physical punishment, dictatorship within the home, inability to allow different opinions within the home, or lack of trust for anyone outside the family.
- **Relationships** within the family may be dysfunctional. Problems such as lack of affection between family members, co-dependency, frequent arguments, extramarital affairs, or extremely rigid beliefs about roles within the family may be present.

During the collection of the patient history, the sexual, social, and psychological history of the patient should be evaluated for any signs of actual or potential abuse.

- The **sexual history** may reveal problems such as previous sexual abuse, forced sexual acts, sexually transmitted infections (STIs), sexual knowledge beyond normal age-appropriate knowledge, or promiscuity.
- The **social history** may reveal unplanned pregnancies, social isolation as evidenced by lack of friends available to help the patient, unreasonable jealousy of significant other, verbal aggression, belief in physical punishment, or problems in school.
- During the **psychological assessment** the patient may express feelings of helplessness and being trapped. The patient may be unable to describe their future, become tearful, perform self-mutilation, have low self-esteem, and have had previous suicide attempts.

## Observations That May Indicate Abuse

During the initial assessment, observations may also be made by the provider that can provide vital information about actual or potential abuse. **General observations** may include finding that the patient history is far different from what is objectively viewed by the provider or that there is a lack of proper clothing or lack of physical care provided. The home environment may include lack of heat, water, or food. It may also reveal inappropriate sleeping arrangements or lack of an environmentally safe housing situation. Observations concerning **family communications** may reveal that the abuser answers all the questions for the whole family or that others look to the controlling member for approval or seem fearful of others. Family members may frequently argue, interrupt each other, or act out negative nonverbal behaviors while others are speaking. They may avoid talking about certain subjects that they feel are secretive.

## Indicators of Abuse That May Be Evident During the Physical Assessment

During the **physical assessment** the provider should always be aware of any **indicators of abuse**. These indicators may include increased anxiety about being examined or in the presence of the abuser; poor hygiene; looks to abuser to answer questions for them; flinching; over or underweight; presence of bruises, welts, scars or cigarette burns; bald patches on scalp for pulling out of hair; intracranial bleeding; subconjunctival hemorrhages; black eye(s); hearing loss from untreated infection or injury; poor dental hygiene; abdominal injuries; fractures; developmental delays; hyperactive reflexes; genital lacerations or ecchymosis; and presence of STIs, rectal bruising, bleeding, edema, or poor sphincter tone.

## Domestic Violence

Men, women, elderly, children, and the disabled may all be victims of **domestic violence**. The violent person harms physically or sexually and uses threats and fear to maintain control of the victim. The violence does not improve unless the abuser gets intensive counseling. The abuser may promise not to do it again, but the violence usually gets more frequent and worsens over time. The provider should ask all patients in private about abuse, neglect, and fear of a caretaker. If abuse is suspected or there are signs present, the state may require **reporting**:

- Give victims information about community hotlines, shelters, and resources.
- Urge them to set up a plan for escape for themselves and any children, complete with supplies in a location away from the home.
- Assure victims that they are not at fault and do not deserve the abuse.
- Try to empower them by helping them to realize that they do not have to take abuse and can find support to change the situation.

**Review Video: Domestic Violence**
Visit mometrix.com/academy and enter code: 530581

## Assessment of Domestic Violence

According to the guidelines of the Family Violence Prevention Fund, **assessment** for domestic violence should be done for all adolescent and adult patients, regardless of background or signs of abuse. While females are the most common victims, there are increasing reports of male victims of domestic violence, both in heterosexual and homosexual relationships. The person doing the assessment should be informed about domestic violence and be aware of risk factors and danger signs. The interview should be conducted in private (special accommodations may need to be made for children <3 years old). The manager's office, bathrooms, and examining rooms should have information about domestic violence posted prominently. Brochures and information should be available to give to patients. Patients may present with a variety of physical complaints, such as headache, pain, palpitations, numbness, or pelvic pain. They are often depressed and may appear suicidal and may be isolated from friends and family. Victims of domestic violence often exhibit fear of spouse/partner, and may report injury inconsistent with symptoms.



## Steps to Identifying Victims of Domestic Violence

Identifying and assisting victims of domestic violence involves the following steps:

1. **Inquiry**: Non-judgmental questioning should begin with asking if the person has ever been abused—physically, sexually, or psychologically.
2. **Interview**: The person may exhibit signs of anxiety or fear and may blame himself or report that others believe he is abused. The person should be questioned if she is afraid for her life or for her children.

3. **Question**: If the person reports abuse, it's critical to ask if the person is in immediate danger or if the abuser is on the premises. The interviewer should ask if the person has been threatened. The history and pattern of abuse should be questioned, and if children are involved, whether the children are abused. Note: State laws vary, and in some states, it is mandatory to report if a child was present during an act of domestic violence as this is considered child abuse. The provider must be aware of state laws regarding domestic and child abuse, and all healthcare providers are mandatory reporters.
4. **Validate**: The interviewer should offer support and reassurance in a non-judgmental manner, telling the patient the abuse is not his or her fault.
5. **Give information**: While discussing facts about domestic violence and the tendency to escalate, the interviewer should provide brochures and information about safety planning. If the patient wants to file a complaint with the police, the interviewer should assist the person to place the call.
6. **Make referrals**: Information about state, local, and national organizations should be provided along with telephone numbers and contact numbers for domestic violence shelters.
7. **Document**: Record keeping should be legal, legible, and lengthy with a complete report and description of any traumatic injuries resulting from domestic violence. A body map may be used to indicate sites of injury, especially if there are multiple bruises or injuries.

## Injuries Consistent with Domestic Violence

There are a number of characteristic **injuries** that may indicate domestic violence, including ruptured eardrum; rectal/genital injury (burns, bites, or trauma); scrapes and bruises about the neck, face, head, trunk, arms; and cuts, bruises, and fractures of the face. The pattern of injuries associated with domestic violence is also often distinctive. The bathing-suit pattern involves injuries on parts of body that are usually covered with clothing as the perpetrator inflicts damage but hides evidence of abuse. Head and neck injuries (50%) are also common. Abusive injuries (rarely attributable to accidents) are common and include bites, bruises, rope and cigarette burns, and welts in the outline of weapons (belt marks). Bilateral injuries of arms/legs are often seen with domestic abuse. Defensive injuries are indicative of abuse.

Defensive injuries to the back of the body are often incurred as the victim crouches on the floor face down while being attacked. The soles of the feet may be injured from kicking at perpetrator. The ulnar aspect of hand or palm may be injured from blocking blows.

## Identifying and Reporting Neglect of the Basic Needs of Adults

**Neglect of the basic needs of adults is a common problem, especially among the elderly, adults with psychiatric or mental health problems, or those who live alone or with reluctant or incapable caregivers.** In some cases, **passive neglect** may occur because an elderly or impaired spouse or partner is trying to take care of a patient and is unable to provide the care needed, but in other cases, **active neglect** reflects a lack of caring which may be considered negligence or abuse. Cases of neglect should be reported to the appropriate governmental agency, such as adult protective services. Indications of neglect include the following:

- Lack of assistive devices, such as a cane or walker, needed for mobility
- Misplaced or missing glasses or hearing aids
- Poor dental hygiene and dental care or missing dentures
- Patient left unattended for extended periods of time, sometimes confined to a bed or chair
- Patient left in soiled or urine- and feces-stained clothing
- Inadequate food, fluid, or nutrition, resulting in weight loss
- Inappropriate and unkempt clothing, such as no sweater or coat during the winter and dirty or torn clothing
- A dirty, messy environment

# Family Dynamics

## FAMILY TYPES

A table of the different family types is provided below:

| Family Type | Description |
|---|---|
| **Nuclear** | This husband-wife-children model was once the most common family type but is no longer the norm. In this model, the husband is the provider, and the mother stays home to care for the children. This makes up only about 7% of current American families. |
| **Dual career/ dual earner** | This model, where both parents work, is the most common in American society, affecting about 66% of two-parent families. One parent may work more than another, or both may work fulltime. There may be disparities in income that affect family dynamics. |
| **Childless** | 10-15% of couples have no children because of infertility or choice. |
| **Extended** | These may include multigenerational families or shared households with friends, parents, or other relatives. Childcare responsibilities may be shared or primarily assumed by an extended family member, such as a grandparent. |
| **Extended kin network** | Two or more nuclear families live close together, share goods and services, and support each other, including sharing childcare. This model is common in the Hispanic community. |
| **Single-parent** | This is one of the fastest growing family models. Typically, the mother is the single parent, but in some cases, it is the father. The single parent may be widowed, divorced, or separated but more commonly has never married. In cases of divorce or abandonment, the child may have minimal or no contact with one parent, often the father. Single parents often face difficulties in trying to support and care for a child and may suffer economic hardship. |
| **Stepparent** | Because of the high rate of divorce, stepparent families are common. This can result in stress and conflict when a new child enters the picture. There may be jealousy and resentment on the part of siblings and estranged family members. In some cases, families can work together to achieve harmony and provide added support to children. |
| **Binuclear/co-parenting** | In this model, children share time between two primarily nuclear families because of joint custody agreements. While this may at times result in conflict, the child benefits from having a continued relationship with both parents. |
| **Cohabiting** | This model refers to unmarried heterosexual couples living together. The relationships within this model may vary, with some similar to the nuclear family. In some cases, people are in committed relationships and may avoid marriage because of economic or personal reasons. A planned child may strengthen the relationship, but an unplanned child may cause conflict. |
| **Same sex** | Whether those in same sex relationships marry or cohabit, they have the opportunity to create families using sperm donors, adoption, or surrogacy. |



## FAMILY THEORY

### *FAMILY DEVELOPMENTAL THEORY*

According to the family developmental theory, families move through different developmental stages, which are accompanied by certain tasks:

- **Marriage**: Get to know significant other, establish good relationships with new kin, and discuss parenthood.
- **Birth of first child**: Adjust to and bond with new baby, maintain spousal relationship.

- **Preschool children**: Provide for different children's needs while family grows, teach socialization skills, maintain healthy relationships between immediate family and extended family, cope with decreased energy and privacy.
- **School-age children**: Encourage academic achievement and good relationships with peers and teachers.
- **Teenagers**: Help teens balance freedom and responsibility, maintain good communication between parents and teens, renewed focus on career and marital relations.
- **Launching adult children**: Allow children to start their own life, jobs, etc., welcome new family members by marriage, help with aging parents' needs, and work on marital relationship.
- **Empty nest**: Maintain relationships with children and aging parents, establish stronger marital relationship.
- **Aging family**: Adjust to health issues, reduced income and loss of spouse/family members/friends.

*Limitation: The theory assumes a traditional, nuclear, middle-class family.*

### STRUCTURAL-FUNCTIONAL THEORY

According to the structural-functional theory, the family, a social system, serves society by performing functions needed for survival:

- **Affective**, or providing love and acceptance to each member
- **Socialization and social placement**, or teaching the children how to get along with others and fit into society as adults
- **Reproductive**, or producing of offspring to continue the family line
- **Economic**, or providing and distributing the necessary resources to the family members
- **Health care**, or providing basic necessities (food, clothing, shelter) and health care, as well as teaching basic hygiene to maintain good health

*Limitation: The theory assumes the traditional definition of family and doesn't address the changes that a family encounters.*

### FAMILY SYSTEMS THEORY

According to the family systems theory, the family is a system where members can only be understood in relationship to other family members. They are interdependent, so that as one member experiences a change, other family members will change to maintain equilibrium. Each member has specific roles, with certain rules governing them.

*Limitation: The theory is vague and therefore difficult to apply.*

### FAMILY STRESS THEORY

The stress theory has several different models. Most assume a stressor (sometimes more than one stressor can occur at the same time, termed **stressor pileup**), resources that are available to the family in coping with the stressor, and how the family perceives the stressor. These factors together will determine whether the family experiences stress or a crisis. Stress causes changes within the family, but it is usually short-lived. A crisis occurs when the family cannot recover from a stress using the resources at hand or the stress is too large for the family to handle.

### RESILIENCY MODEL

The resiliency model assumes that some families develop strength over time by facing changes common to all families. These strengths, as well as strong resources and relationships, help protect against crises when uncommon stressors are present. Families respond to stressful events in two phases. The **adjustment phase** occurs when the family makes minor changes to its roles and routines. When the family moves into the **adaptation phase**, it makes major changes to its structure and functions.

## FAMILY ASSESSMENT AND FACTORS THAT INFLUENCE RELATIONSHIPS AND PARENTING

Family assessment is the collection of data concerning the structure of the family and how family members relate to each other and society. It is an ongoing process, using assessment tools, such as a genogram (a map of a three generational family tree, including relationships and health histories), an ecomap (a chart depicting the relationships within and outside of the family and the support networks available to the family), interviews, questionnaires, and observations.

There are many factors that influence family relationships and parenting. These include: the type of family unit (nuclear, blended, single parent, gay, or lesbian), parental culture, parenting a foster child, adolescent parenting, parenting an adopted child, parenting by grandparents.

## FAMILY FUNCTIONING AND DYNAMICS

Cultural/lifestyle factors that affect family integration include the following:

- **Values**: Values based on attitudes, ideas, and beliefs often connect family members to common goals. However, these values may be influenced by many external factors, such as education, social norms, and attitudes of peers, extended family, and coworkers, so values may change, which may affect family integration.
- **Roles**: In some families, roles are clearly defined by gender and task (homemaker and breadwinner), but the roles blur or are shared in many families, and in some cases the father becomes the primary caregiver while the mother works. Other common roles include peacemaker, nurturer, and social planner. How these roles are perceived and actualized affects the manner in which a child is integrated into the family and cared for.
- **Decision making**: Family power structures vary widely, but in many families, power rests with one person who makes ultimate decisions and whose opinions affect other family members. In many traditional cultures (Hispanic, Asian, Middle Eastern) power lies with the father, grandfather, or other male family member. However, in American society, this may vary because of diversity. Power may be shared or rest with the mother or the father.
- **Socioeconomic**: Employment trends, marriage rates, and economic trends all affect family integration. Many people have become unemployed and are unable to support their families, resulting in severe stress, which may be exacerbated by the arrival of a new child or illness. The divorce rate is high, leaving many parents with inadequate funds to support a child. Even if both parents are employed, the cost of living continues to escalate, including the cost of caring for a child.

## IDENTIFYING PRIMARY CAREGIVER

Identifying the primary caregiver is especially important in the emergency care of infants and children, as their ability to report is limited and may not be reliable, depending on age. With the diversity of family models, one cannot assume that the mother, father, or person accompanying the child is the primary caregiver. In some cases, custodial arrangements designate one parent as custodial and the other as non-custodial, and they may or may not share legal rights over medical care for the child. Therefore, the nurse should ask who is the primary caregiver in order to glean information about the child and ask who has the legal right to make medical decisions to determine who should sign consent forms and make decisions.

## Impact and Complications When Patient Has Multiple Caregivers

Continuity of care is especially important for infants and young children, and the lack of stability in caregivers can lead to various problems. Even when children must have **multiple caregivers**, a primary care giver should be identified and should oversee care and ease the transitions whenever possible by introducing other caregivers and coordinating care activities. The greater the number of changes, the greater the impact on the child. The impacts/complications involved when a patient has multiple caregivers, either at the same time or sequentially, include:

- Inadequate communication of the patient's needs and condition
- Different approaches to caregiving, leading to confusion or discord
- Inability of the patient to adequately bond and form attachment with the caregivers
- Patient insecurity and impaired sociopsychological development
- Increased stress and anxiety
- Behavioral problems

Some children are able to adapt to multiple changes over time and can better handle the demands of change than others.

## Functional Coping Strategies of Families

Some families utilize a number of functional coping strategies to deal with stress. These families exhibit resilience in difficult situations. Strategies include:

- The family gathers information, increases organization, discusses issues, and tries to jointly solve problems.
- Family members draw together as a strengthened family unit to deal with stressful situations.
- The family attempts to carry on as normal a routine as possible while making accommodations as needed for a child who is ill. This provides the child with a sense of security.
- The family accepts those things that cannot be changed rather than wasting energy trying to deny or alter reality.
- The family communicates openly and directly, avoiding family secrets and including the child in discussions as appropriate to the child's age.
- The family uses humor to deflect stress.
- The family uses resources outside of the immediate family for support, such as extended family, spiritual advisors, and community agencies.

## Dysfunctional Coping Strategies of Families

Some families are not resilient when dealing with stressful situations and exhibit dysfunctional coping strategies, which include:

- Family members may resort to substance abuse, such as alcohol and/or drugs, rather than facing problems. This adds to the family dysfunction and negatively affects all members.
- The family may take out frustrations through domestic violence, aimed at the child or other family members. This can include physical, sexual, or mental abuse and can create an environment of fear within the family.
- The family denies problems and refuses to acknowledge that family dynamics have changed, attempting to carry on as usual.
- The family uses threats, aggression, and/or withholding of affection to retain control and maintain the family unit.
- The family may blame vulnerable members, such as the child, for the stressful situation, often scapegoating the member that they "blame" rather than dealing with the real problems.

## Methods to Get Parents More Involved in Their Child's Health at School

Most children spend a great deal of time at school, and children with health conditions are often monitored and supported by school health staff, such as the school nurse, health aide, psychologist, or counselor. Parents can be involved with their child's health at school by maintaining communication with these professionals to provide the most comprehensive care for their child. This may mean partnering with school officials to develop a care plan to use at school, signing documents approving medication administration at school, and attending meetings to discuss the effects of their child's health on the classroom experience. Parents provide the health care providers in the school system with much of the information needed for their child to have a sufficient school experience without health issues standing in the way. School nurses can reinforce this behavior by keeping in frequent contact with parents about their child's health, communicating when the child receives health services at school, and keeping records updated and accurate.

## Factors That Influence the Relationship Between the Child and Parents

Factors influencing parent-child relationships are cultural (some children consider themselves a part of the American culture, while their parents still hold true to the cultural practices of their home country), religious (some youth rebel against their religious upbringing, especially in the teen years), parenting style, and family structure (nuclear, extended, blended, gay/lesbian, single parent, adolescent parent, adoptive parenting, grandparents raising the children, and foster parenting).

## Appropriate Disciplinary Practices for Families to Use

Appropriate discipline practices should be discussed with parents. These include:

- Make rules clear and appropriate for the age of the child.
- Set the consequences before the rule has been broken, making sure they are appropriate for the broken rule and age of the child. The consequence should be administered directly after the rule has been broken, with a calm attitude.
- Use lots of praise when the child behaves appropriately.

## Temperament

Temperament is the way a person relates or responds to his environment and the people around him. Temperament is inborn, but it can be affected by how parents relate to the child/adolescent.

### *Attributes*

The nine attributes of temperament are:

- **Activity**: How active is the child is during normal activities?
- **Rhythmicity**: How regular are the child's normal physiological activities, such as bowel movements, sleep cycle, and eating patterns?
- **Approach-withdrawal**: How does the child respond to different stimuli, such as being drawn readily to a new stuffed animal or withdrawing from the noise of fireworks?
- **Adaptability**: How does the child adapt to new circumstances?
- **Intensity of reaction**: How forcefully does the child respond to new circumstances?
- **Threshold of responsiveness**: How much stimulus is needed before the child responds?
- **Mood**: How much positive vs. negative behavior is exhibited in different situations?
- **Distractibility**: How easily can the child be distracted and the behavior changed?
- **Attention span and persistence**: How long will the child continue an activity and how much distraction is needed to pull the child away from the activity (persistence)?

### *TYPES*

Types of temperament include:

- **Easy**: Easily adapts to new situations, gets along with others well, easy going behaviors
- **Difficult**: Responds negatively to new situations, behaviors are unpredictable, does well in highly structured environment
- **Slow-to-warm-up**: Moody, shy, slow to adapt to new situations, low activity level

## EFFECTS OF PARENTING STYLES ON TEMPERAMENT OF CHILDREN

Although children are born with their own temperament, the parenting style they grow up with can influence how this temperament manifests over time.

- **Authoritarian (autocratic)** parents desire obedience without question. They tend toward harsh punishments, using their power to make their children obey. They are emotionally withdrawn from their children and enforce strict rules without discussing why the rules exist. These children tend to have low self-esteem, be more dependent, and are introverted with poor social skills.
- **Authoritative (democratic)** parents provide boundaries and expect obedience, but use love when they discipline. They involve their children in deciding rules and consequences, discussing reasons for their decisions, but will enforce the rules consistently. They encourage independence and take each child's unique position seriously. These children tend to have higher self-esteem, good social skills, and confidence in themselves.
- **Indulgent (permissive)** parents stay involved with their children, but have few rules in place to give the children boundaries. These children have a difficult time setting their own limits and are not responsible. They disrespect others and have trouble with authority figures.
- **Indifferent (uninvolved)** parents spend as little time as possible with their children. They are self-involved, with no time or patience for taking care of their children's needs. Guidance and discipline are lacking and inconsistent. These children tend toward delinquency, with a lack of respect for others.

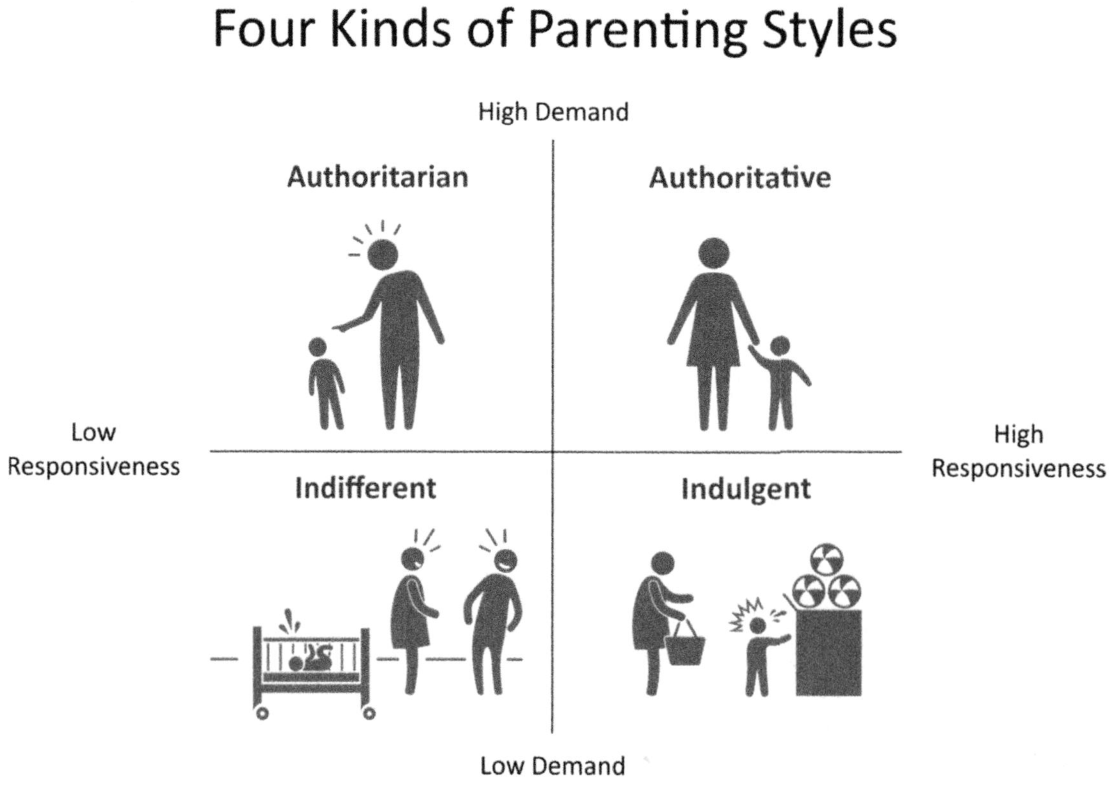

# Therapeutic Relationships

## THERAPEUTIC COMMUNICATION

### *FACILITATING COMMUNICATION*

Therapeutic communication begins with respect for the patient/family and the assumption that all communication, verbal and nonverbal, has meaning. Listening must be done empathetically. The following are some techniques that facilitate communication.

**Introduction**:

- Make a personal introduction and use the patient's name: "Mrs. Brown, I am Susan Williams, your nurse."

**Encouragement**:

- Use an open-ended opening statement: "Is there anything you'd like to discuss?"
- Acknowledge comments: "Yes," and "I understand."
- Allow silence and observe nonverbal behavior rather than trying to force conversation. Ask for clarification if statements are unclear.
- Reflect statements back (use sparingly): Patient: "I hate this hospital." Nurse: "You hate this hospital?"

**Empathy**:

- Make observations: "You are shaking," and "You seem worried."
- Recognize feelings:
  - Patient: "I want to go home."
  - Nurse: "It must be hard to be away from your home and family."
- Provide information as honestly and completely as possible about condition, treatment, and procedures and respond to the patient's questions and concerns.

**Exploration**:

- Verbally express implied messages:
  - Patient: "This treatment is too much trouble."
  - Nurse: "It seems like this treatment plan is a lot to handle. Can you explain what makes it 'too much trouble?'"
- Explore a topic but allow the patient to terminate the discussion without further probing: "I'd like to hear how you feel about that."

**Orientation**:

- Indicate reality:
  - Patient: "Someone is screaming."
  - Nurse: "That sound was an ambulance siren."
- Comment on distortions without directly agreeing or disagreeing:
  - Patient: "That nurse promised I didn't have to walk again."
  - Nurse: "I was not part of that conversation, but what I can see is that the doctor ordered physical therapy twice a day."

**Collaboration**:

- Work together to achieve better results: "Maybe if we talk about this, we can figure out a way to make the treatment easier for you."

**Validation**:

- Seek validation of the understanding of a patient's statement: "To make sure I understand, you are saying that when you take the medication, you feel that it is easier to breathe when you walk?"

### *Avoiding Non-therapeutic Communication*

While using therapeutic communication is important, it is equally important to avoid interjecting **non-therapeutic communication**, which can block effective communication. *Avoid the following:*

- Meaningless clichés: "Don't worry. Everything will be fine." "Isn't it a nice day?"
- Providing advice: "You should..." or "The best thing to do is...." It's better when patients ask for advice to provide facts and encourage the patient to reach a decision.
- Inappropriate approval that prevents the patient from expressing true feeling or concerns:
  - Patient: "I shouldn't cry about this."
  - Nurse: "That's right! You're an adult!"
- Asking for an explanation of behavior that is not directly related to patient care and requires analysis and explanation of feelings: "Why are you so upset?"
- Agreeing with rather than accepting and responding to patient's statements can make it difficult for the patient to change his or her statement or opinion later: "I agree with you," or "You are right."
- Making negative judgments: "You should stop arguing with the nurses."
- Devaluing the patient's feelings: "Everyone gets upset at times."
- Disagreeing directly: "That can't be true," or "I think you are wrong."
- Defending against criticism: "The doctor is not being rude; he's just very busy today."
- Changing the subject to avoid dealing with uncomfortable topics;
  - Patient: "I'm never going to get well."
  - Nurse: "Your family will be here in just a few minutes."
- Making inappropriate literal responses, even as a joke, especially if the patient is at all confused or having difficulty expressing ideas:
  - Patient: "There are bugs crawling under my skin."
  - Nurse: "I'll get some bug spray,"
- Challenging the patient to establish reality often just increases confusion and frustration:
  - "If you were dying, you wouldn't be able to yell and kick!"

## Communicating with Patients with Disabilities

Guidelines for communicating with individuals with disabilities:

- Do not assume that the person with disabilities also has impaired cognition.
- Always treat the person with respect and dignity.
- Use first names with the patient if asked to do so, but start out formally as with any patient.
- Offer to shake hands even when a prosthesis is present.
- Be patient if communication is impaired.
- Offer assistance, but allow the patient to tell you what is helpful; otherwise don't assist.

- When a wheelchair is used, sit down so the patient does not have to strain their neck to speak with you.
- If the patient requests directions, consider the obstacles that may be in the way and assist the person to find an appropriate way around them.

## Communication with Patients with Cognitive Disabilities

The person with cognitive disabilities may be easily distracted, so verbal communication should be attempted in a quiet area:

- Address people with dignity and respect.
- Be sensitive to understanding when describing abstract or complex ideas, frequently assessing understanding and using aids when helpful.
- Keep words and sentences very simple and try rephrasing when necessary. People may have difficulty in distinguishing your spoken words and deriving the meaning from them.
- Be very patient with people's attempts to speak to you since they may have difficulty in processing thoughts and changing them into spoken words.
- Use objects around you and gestures to illustrate your words since the patient may also use pointing and gesturing when unable to find the words to communicate with you. The person may prefer written communication, although some may be unable to read.
- The use of touch may be helpful to convey your regard during communication, but permission must first be granted.
- Give a few instructions at a time as to not overwhelm them.

## Communicating with Deaf or Hearing-Impaired Patients

Communicating with a person with deafness or hearing impairment:

- Try to communicate in a quiet environment if possible.
- Wave or touch the person to let him or her know you are trying to communicate.
- Determine the method the person uses to communicate: sign language, lip reading, hearing devices, or writing.
- Use signs only if proficient in doing so.
- Use a medical interpreter when communicating any critical information. Family/caregivers may be used only in emergency situations when an interpreter is not readily available.
- Address the person directly when you speak even though the person may be looking at an interpreter or your lips.
- Look at the person as the interpreter tells you what was said.
- Speak at a normal pace and cadence so the interpreter can keep up with you.
- If the person reads lips, face the person and speak clearly and normally, using normal volume.
- If writing a communication, do not speak while writing.
- Do not be afraid to check that the person understands you, and ask questions if you do not understand the person.



## Communication with People with Low Vision or Blindness

Communicating with a person with low vision or blindness:

- Greet the person with low vision or blindness, identifying yourself and others present.
- Ask the person about their preferences for levels of assistance, and implement with care as needed. Always gain permission before touching the patient.
- Always say goodbye when you are leaving.
- Alert the person to written communications, such as warning signs or printed notices.

- Face the person and touch briefly on the arm to let the person know you are speaking to him or her if you are in a group.
- Speak at normal loudness.
- Make any directions given specific in terms of the length of walk and obstacles, such as stairs.
- Use the position of hands on a clock face to advise on the location of items in relation to the individual (potatoes at 3 o'clock) as well as using *right* or *left*.
- Mention sounds that the person may hear in transit or on arrival at a destination.
- Do not be afraid to use the word *see*, as the person will probably use it as well.

## Communicating with a Patient on a Ventilator

When a patient on a ventilator is conscious, he or she may still be able to communicate by blinking, nodding, shaking the head, or pointing to a picture or word board:

- If the person is able to write, utilize white boards or paper and pen to communicate, being cognizant of IV lines that may be on the patient's dominant hand or arm.
- For patients with a tracheostomy, discuss the need for communication with the speech therapist and ask if a valve or an electric larynx can be used to permit speech.
- Remember the patient's glasses or hearing aids when attempting to communicate.
- Enlist the aid of a speech therapist if there is frustration on the part of the patient and family due to communication difficulty.

## Communicating with Persons with Speech Problems Due to a Stroke

Methods to communicate with stroke patients with speech problems:

- **Dysarthria**: Patients have problems forming the words to speak them aloud. Give them time to communicate, offer them a picture board or other means of communicating, and give encouragement to family members who are frustrated with the difficulty of trying to communicate.
- **Expressive aphasia**: The patients' efforts at speech are struggled, but single words may be clear. Encourage the patients to try to write and to practice the sounds of the alphabet. Resist the urge to finish sentences for the patients. Utilize yes/no questions when possible.
- **Receptive aphasia**: The patients have a problem comprehending the speech they hear. Communicate in simple terms and speak slowly. Test comprehension of the written word as an alternative method of communication.
- **Global aphasia**: The patient has both receptive and expressive aphasia. Use simple, clear, slow speech augmented by pictures and gestures.

## Communication Problems of Patients with Parkinson's Disease

Parkinson's disease causes problems with speaking in the majority (75–90%) of patients. The reason for this has been linked to dysfunction of the basal ganglia circuit. Speech is often reduced in pitch and loudness or is hoarse, given in a monotone and with a soft voice. Speech production may decrease because of the effort required to speak. **Speech therapy** can develop exercises for the patient that can assist them in remembering to speak slowly and carefully, as patients are not always aware that their **communication** is impaired:

- Allow time for the patient to communicate, asking for repetition if you do not understand the message.
- Help family by teaching ways to facilitate communication with the patient and encouraging them to assist the patient to do the exercises provided by the therapist.
- If speech volume is very low, suggest amplification devices that can be obtained through speech therapy. The patient can also be considered for intensive loudness-based therapy.

## Communication with Patients with Mental Health Conditions

Persons with mental health conditions appreciate being addressed with respect, dignity, and honesty:

- Speak simply and clearly, repeating as necessary.
- Encourage patients to discuss their concerns regarding treatment and medications to improve compliance.
- Use good eye contact and be attentive to your body language messages.
- Be alert to threats to safety; position oneself to have a direct exit if needed; maintain a calm manner, respectful language, and active listening.
- Don't try to avoid words or phrases pertaining to mental health problems, but if you do say something inappropriate, apologize honestly to the patient.
- Offer patients outlets for their thoughts and feelings.
- Learn more about their disorder and ways to use therapeutic communication to help them with their problem, such as re-orienting for those who are frequently disoriented.

## Cultural Competence and Cultural Sensitivity

Different cultures view health and illness from very different perspectives, and patients often come from a mix of many cultures, so the nurse must be not only accepting of cultural differences but must be sensitive and aware. There are a number of characteristics that are important for a nurse to have **cultural competence** and to thereby incopororate **cultural sensitivity** into practice:

- **Appreciating diversity**: This must be grounded in information about other cultures and understanding of their value systems.
- **Assessing own cultural perspectives**: Self-awareness is essential to understanding potential biases.
- **Assess the patient's individualized culture**: Utilize tools to assess how a patient's culture influences their interpretation of disease, medicine, health care providers, treatement approaches, and medical decision-making.
- **Understanding intercultural dynamics**: This must include understanding ways in which cultures cooperate, differ, communicate, and reach understanding.
- **Recognizing institutional culture**: Each institutional unit (hospital, clinic, office) has an inherent set of values that may be unwritten but is accepted by the staff.
- **Adapting patient service to diversity**: This is the application of cultural competence to practice.



## Cultural Characteristics

### *Hispanic Patients*

Many areas of the country have large populations of Hispanics and Hispanic Americans. As always, it's important to recognize that cultural generalizations don't always apply to individuals. Recent immigrants, especially, have cultural needs that the nurse must understand:

- Many Hispanics are Catholic and may like the nurse to make arrangements for a priest to visit.
- Large extended families may come to visit to support the patient and family, so patients should receive clear explanations about how many visitors are allowed, but some flexibility may be required.
- Language barriers may exist as some may have limited or no English skills, so translation services should be available around the clock.
- Hispanic culture encourages outward expressions of emotions, so family may react strongly to news about a patient's condition, and people who are ill may expect some degree of pampering, so extra attention to the patient/family members may alleviate some of their anxiety.

**Caring for Hispanic and Hispanic American patients** requires understanding of cultural differences:

- Some immigrant Hispanics have very little formal education, so medical information may seem very complex and confusing, and they may not understand the implications or need for follow-up care.
- Hispanic culture perceives time with more flexibility than American culture, so if parents need to be present at a particular time, the nurse should specify the exact time (1:30 PM) and explain the reason rather than saying something more vague, such as "after lunch."
- People may appear to be unassertive or unable to make decisions when they are simply showing respect to the nurse by being deferent.
- In traditional families, the males make decisions, so a woman waits for the father or other males in the family to make decisions about treatment or care.
- Families may choose to use folk medicines instead of Western medical care or may combine the two.
- Children and young women are often sheltered and are taught to be respectful to adults, so they may not express their needs openly.

### *Middle Eastern Patients*

There are considerable cultural differences among Middle Easterners, but religious beliefs about the segregation of males and females are common. It's important to remember that segregating the female is meant to protect her virtue. Female nurses have low status in many countries because they violate this segregation by touching male bodies, so parents may not trust or show respect for the nurse who is caring for their family member. Additionally, male patients may not want to be cared for by female nurses or doctors, and families may be very upset at a female being cared for by a male nurse or physician. When possible, these cultural traditions should be accommodated:

- In Middle Eastern countries, males make decisions, so issues for discussion or decision should be directed to males, such as the father or spouse, and males may be direct in stating what they want, sometimes appearing demanding.
- If a male nurse must care for a female patient, then the family should be advised that *personal care* (such as bathing) will be done by a female while the medical treatments will be done by the male nurse.

**Caring for Middle Eastern patients** requires understanding of cultural differences:

- Families may practice strict dietary restrictions, such as avoiding pork and requiring that animals be killed in a ritual manner, so vegetarian or kosher meals may be required.
- People may have language difficulties requiring a translator, and same-sex translators should be used if at all possible.
- Families may be accompanied by large extended families that want to be kept informed and whom patients consult before decisions are made.
- Most medical care is provided by female relatives, so educating the family about patient care should be directed at females (with female translators if necessary).
- Outward expressions of grief are considered as showing respect for the dead.
- Middle Eastern families often offer gifts to caregivers. Small gifts (candy) that can be shared should be accepted graciously, but for other gifts, the families should be advised graciously that accepting gifts is against hospital policy.
- Middle Easterners often require less personal space and may stand very close.

### *ASIAN PATIENTS*

There are considerable differences among different Asian populations, so cultural generalizations may not apply to all, but nurses caring for Asian patients should be aware of common cultural attitudes and behaviors:

- Nurses and doctors are viewed with respect, so traditional Asian families may expect the nurse to remain authoritative and to give directions and may not question, so the nurse should ensure that they understand by having them review material or give demonstrations and should provide explanations clearly, anticipating questions that the family might have but may not articulate.
- Disagreeing is considered impolite. "Yes" may only mean that the person is heard, not that they agree with the person. When asked if they understand, they may indicate that they do even when they clearly do not so as not to offend the nurse.
- Asians may avoid eye contact as an indication of respect. This is especially true of children in relation to adults and of younger adults in relation to elders.

**Caring for Asian patients** requires understanding of cultural differences:

- Patients/families may not show outward expressions of feelings/grief, sometimes appearing passive. They also avoid public displays of affection. This does not mean that they don't feel, just that they don't show their feelings.
- Families often hide illness and disabilities from others and may feel ashamed about illness.
- Terminal illness is often hidden from the patient, so families may not want patients to know they are dying or seriously ill.
- Families may use cupping, pinching, or applying pressure to injured areas, and this can leave bruises that may appear as abuse, so when bruises are found, the family should be questioned about alternative therapy before assumptions are made.
- Patients may be treated with traditional herbs.
- Families may need translators because of poor or no English skills.
- In traditional Asian families, males are authoritative and make the decisions.

## Grief and Loss

### GRIEF

Grief is an emotional response to a **loss** that begins at the time a loss is anticipated and continues on an individual timetable. While there are identifiable stages or tasks, it is not an orderly and predictable process. It involves overcoming anger, disbelief, guilt, and a myriad of related emotions. The grieving individual may move back and forth between stages or experience several emotions at any given time. Each person's grief response is unique to their own coping patterns, stress levels, age, gender, belief system, and previous experiences with loss.

### KUBLER-ROSS'S FIVE STAGES OF GRIEF

**Kubler-Ross** taught the medical community that the dying patient and family welcomes open, honest discussion of the dying process and felt that there were certain **stages** that patients and family go through. The stages may not occur in order, but may vary or some may be skipped. Stages include:

- **Denial**: The person denies the diagnosis and tries to pretend it isn't true. During this time, the person may seek a second opinion or alternative therapies. They may use denial until they are better able to emotionally cope with the reality of the disease or changes that need to be made. Patients may also wish to save family and friends from pain and worry. Both patients and family may use denial as a coping mechanism when they feel overwhelmed by the reality of the disease and threatened losses.
- **Anger**: The person is angry about the situation and may focus that rage on anyone.

- **Bargaining**: The person attempts to make deals with a higher power to secure a better outcome to their situation.
- **Depression**: The person anticipates the loss and the changes it will bring with a sense of sadness and grief.
- **Acceptance**: The person accepts the impending death and is ready to face it as it approaches. The patient may begin to withdraw from interests and family.

| **Review Video: The Five Stages of Grief** |
| --- |
| Visit mometrix.com/academy and enter code: 648794 |

## Anticipatory Grief

Anticipatory grief is the mental, social, and somatic reactions of an individual as they prepare themselves for a **perceived future loss**. The individual experiences a process of intellectual, emotional, and behavioral responses in order to modify their self-concept, based on their perception of what the potential loss will mean in their life. This process often takes place ahead of the actual loss, from the time the loss is first perceived until it is resolved as a reality for the individual. This process can also blend with past loss experiences. It is associated with the individual's perception of how life will be affected by the particular diagnosis as well as the impending death. Acknowledging this anticipatory grief allows family members to begin looking toward a changed future. Suppressing this anticipatory process may inhibit relationships with the ill individual and contribute to a more difficult grieving process at a later time. However, appropriate anticipatory grieving does not take the place of grief during the actual time of death.

## Disenfranchised Grief

Disenfranchised grief occurs when the loss being experienced cannot be openly acknowledged, publicly mourned, or socially supported. Society and culture are partly responsible for an individual's response to a loss. There is a **social context** to grief; if a person incurring the loss will be putting himself or herself at risk if grief is expressed, disenfranchised grief occurs. The risk for disenfranchised grief is greatest among those whose relationship with the individual they lost was not known or regarded as significant. This is also the situation found among bereaved persons who are not recognized by society as capable of grief, such as young children, or needing to mourn, such as an ex-spouse or secret lover.

## Grief vs. Depression

Normal grief is preoccupied with self-limiting to the loss itself. Emotional responses will vary and may include open expressions of anger. The individual may experience difficulty sleeping or vivid dreams, a lack of energy, and weight loss. Crying is evident and provides some relief of extreme emotions. The individual remains socially responsive and seeks reassurance from others.

By contrast, **depression** is marked by extensive periods of sadness and preoccupation often extending beyond two weeks. It is not limited to the single event. There is an absence of pleasure or anger and isolation from previous social support systems. The individual can experience extreme lethargy, weight loss, insomnia, or hypersomnia. Crying is absent or persistent and provides no relief of emotions. Professional intervention is often required to relieve depression.

## Loss

Loss is the blanket term used to denote the absence of a valued object, position, ability, attribute, or individual. The aspect of **loss** as it is associated with the death of an animal or person is a relatively new definition. Loss is an individualized and subjective experience depending on the **perceived attachment** between the individual and the missing aspect. This can range from little or no value of attachment to significant value. Loss also can be represented by the **withdrawal of a valued relationship** one had or would have had in the future.

Depending on the unique and individual responses to the perception of loss and its significance, reactions to the loss will vary. Robinson and McKenna summarize the aspects of loss in three main attributes:

- Something has been removed.
- The item removed had value to that person.
- The response is individualized.

## MOURNING

Mourning is a public grief response for the death of a loved one. The various aspects of the mourning process are partially determined by **personal and cultural belief systems**. Kagawa-Singer defines mourning as "the social customs and cultural practices that follow a death." Durkheim expands this to include the following: "mourning is not a natural movement of private feelings wounded by a cruel loss; it is a duty imposed by the group." Mourning involves participation in religious and culturally appropriate customs and rituals designed to publicly acknowledge the loss. These rituals signify they are adjusting to the change in their relationships created by the loss, as well as mark the beginning of the reorganization and forward movement of their lives.

## BEREAVEMENT

Bereavement is the emotional and mental state associated with having suffered a **personal loss**. It is the reactions of grief and sadness initiated by the loss of a loved one. Bereavement is a normal process of feeling deprived of something of value. The word bereave comes from the root "reave" meaning to plunder, spoil, or rob. It is recognized that the lost individual had value and a defining role in the surviving individual's life. Bereavement encompasses all the acts and emotions surrounding the feeling of loss for the individual. During this grieving period, there is an increased mortality risk. A **positive bereavement experience** means being able to recognize the significance of the loss while still recognizing the resilience and value of life.

### *RISK FACTORS COMPLICATING BEREAVEMENT*

The caregiver should assess for multiple **life crises** that take energy away from the grieving process. An important factor is the grieving individual's history with past grieving experiences. Assess for other recent, unresolved, or difficult losses that may need to be addressed before the individual can move toward resolution of the current loss. Age, mental health, substance abuse, extreme anger, anxiety, or dependence on the individual facing the end of life can add additional stressors and handicap natural coping mechanisms. Income strains, community support, outside and personal responsibilities, the absence of cultural and religious beliefs, the difficulty of the disease process, and age of the loved one lost can also present additional risk factors.

## INTERVENTIONS FOR PATIENTS AND FAMILY EXPERIENCING LOSS AND GRIEF

Loss is painful and frightening. Loss can occur through death or loss of health, self-esteem, or relationships. Loss can also occur from threats, such as fire, flood, theft, or severe weather. The severity of the loss, preparation for it, and the maturity, stability, and coping mechanisms of the person all affect the grieving process. Multiple losses and substance abuse can complicate grief and recovery. Previous life experience and cultural and religious beliefs can help in resolution of grief. Many emotions are triggered, and if the loss is not acknowledged, the person may become depressed or develop health problems. **Interventions** for those experiencing grief and loss include:

- Teach patients to recognize symptoms, such as SOB, empty feelings in the chest or abdomen, deep sighing, lethargy, and weakness as signs of grief.
- Assist the patient and family to heal themselves by accepting the loss, recognizing the pain from it, making changes to adapt to and assimilate the loss, and moving toward new relationships and activity.
- Refer to groups or counseling for more intense support if needed.

## Supporting Families and Patients as They Receive Bad News

It is often best if the patient can **receive bad news** while being **supported** by family, friends, physicians, nurses, support staff, social workers, and clergy if they so desire. However, the patient may not want family members or others to be present, and this too should be respected.

- Provide privacy and ensure that there will be no interruptions.
- Provide seating for all participants.
- Do not provide too much information at once, as the opening statement may be all that the patient can comprehend at one time.
- Allow time for reactions before providing more information.
- Wait for the patient to signal the need for more information and then provide an honest answer in layman's terms. Information may not be absorbed and may need to be repeated as the patient and family are ready for it later after the initial conference.
- Use techniques of therapeutic communication. People may need others to sit and listen and provide comforting empathy many times before having a conversation about problem solving.

## Spirituality

Spirituality provides a connection of the self to a higher power and a way of finding meaning in life experiences. It provides guidance for behavior and can help to clarify one's purpose in life. It can offer hope to those who are ill or facing loss and grief and can give comfort, support, and guidance. **Spirituality** is not always connected to a religion and is highly individualized. A person may lose faith and confidence in his/her spiritual beliefs during trying times:

- Ask patients about their spiritual beliefs.
- Listen attentively and do not offer opinions about their beliefs or share your own unless invited.
- Show respect for their views and offer to obtain spiritual support by calling a spiritual leader or setting up a spiritual ritual that has meaning for them.

This support can help them to regain their beliefs and endure illness by helping them to rise above their suffering and find meaning in this experience.

## Palliative and Hospice Care

**Palliative care** attempts to make the rest of the patient's life as comfortable as possible by treating distressing symptoms to keep them controlled. It does not attempt to cure but only to control discomfort caused by the disease. Palliative care does not require terminal illness/prognosis and can be implemented for any patient with chronic disease and suffering.

**Hospice care** uses palliative care as it supports the patient and family through the dying process. Hospice teams support the daily needs of the patient and family and provide needed equipment, medical expertise, and medications to control symptoms. They offer spiritual, psychological, and social support to the patient and family as needed and desired. Assistance with end-of-life planning is given to help the patient and family accomplish goals important to them. Bereavement support is also given. The team consists of the attending physician, hospice physician advisor, nurses, social worker, clergy, hospice aides, and volunteers. Hospice care is given in the home when the patient has family who are willing to assume care with the assistance of the hospice team. Hospice care also occurs in hospice facilities, hospitals, and extended care facilities. To qualify for Hospice care, the patient must be deemed terminal and given a 6-month or less life expectancy by two separate physicians. Should the patient survive 6 months in hospice, they can be extended for two 90-day periods, and then an unlimited number of 60-day periods per physician order.

# Psychosocial Pathophysiology

## Developmental Delays and Intellectual Disability

Developmental delays occur when a patient does not progress mentally at the same rate as the general population. Intellectual disability is a condition in which individuals may have difficulty adapting to changing environments, need guidance in decision-making, and have self-care or communication deficits. Behaviors range from shy and passive to hyperactive and aggressive. Intellectual disability may be inherited (Tay-Sachs), toxin-related (maternal alcohol consumption), perinatal (hypoxia), environmental (lack of stimulation/neglect), or acquired (encephalitis, brain injury). **Diagnosis** involves performance results from standardized tests with behavior analysis. Intellectual disability classifications are based on IQ:

- **55–69 (mild, 85% of cases):** Educable to about 6$^{th}$ grade level. May not be diagnosed until adolescence. Usually able to learn skills and be self-supporting but may need assistance and supervision.
- **40–54 (moderate, 10% of cases):** Trainable and may be able to work and live in sheltered environments or with supervision.
- **25–39 (severe, 3–4% of cases):** Language usually delayed and can learn only basic academic skills and perform simple tasks.
- **≤25 (profound, 1–2% of cases):** Usually associated with neurological disorder with sensorimotor dysfunction. Require constant care and supervision.

**Nursing considerations:** Always treat patients according to their developmental level, not their physical age. This is especially important when considering education and consent. People with developmental delays are at increased risk for injury and abuse.

## Personality Disorder

A personality disorder is a fixed and enduring set pattern or traits of behavior that **deviate from expected behaviors within a culture**. These disorders inhibit the individual's ability to have meaningful interpersonal relationships, to be fulfilled, or to enjoy life. Onset usually occurs during adolescence or early adulthood. A personality disorder is an attitude directed toward the whole world including one's own self. This attitude is expressed through thoughts, feelings, and behaviors. Many times, the behaviors will become less extreme as the person gets older.

### *DSM Classification Groupings*

The DSM-5-TR lists 10 personality disorders grouped into three clusters: A, B, and C.

- **Cluster A** includes disorders that are characterized by odd or eccentric behaviors and a tendency for social awkwardness and withdrawal.
- **Cluster B** includes disorders that are characterized by erratic, highly emotional, dramatic, or impulsive behaviors.
- **Cluster C** includes disorders that are characterized predominantly by fearful or anxious symptoms.

### Specific Diagnoses Included in Cluster A for Personality Disorders

**Cluster A:** The classification of Cluster A for personality disorders includes the diagnoses of paranoid, schizoid, and schizotypal personality disorders.

- The **paranoid** individual is very distrustful and suspicious of others. They believe that other people are up to no good, are keeping secrets, and may intend to harm them. There is usually no basis or evidence to support this belief.
- The **schizoid** individual exhibits a consistent social detachment. Many of their behaviors indicate a restricted emotional response and can include appearing cold and indifferent, having no desire for close personal relationships, having no desire for intimacy, choosing solidarity over socializing, and usually having no close friends or relatives.
- Like the schizoid individual, the **schizotypal** individual tends to lack intimate relationships, but this is due to social ineptitude and fear rather than a lack of interest in relationship. They also experience cognitive and perceptual distortions, seeing or hearing things that are not there, and hold odd or superstitious beliefs.

### Specific Diagnoses Included in Cluster B for Personality Disorders

**Cluster B:** The classification of Cluster B for personality disorders includes the diagnoses of antisocial, borderline, histrionic, and narcissistic personality disorders.

- The **antisocial** individual exhibits a blatant disregard for other people. They frequently lie, manipulate, exploit, and commit illegal acts.
- The **borderline** individual has a markedly unstable self-image. They are very impulsive, self-destructive, have unstable and intense interpersonal relationships, mood instability, inappropriate and intense anger, and may have recurrent suicidal or self-mutilating behaviors.
- The **histrionic** individual is extremely emotional and desires to be the center of attention. They often perform attention-seeking behaviors and have frequent, intense, and short-lived relationships.
- The **narcissistic** individual has a great sense of self-importance and is often arrogant. They lack empathy for others and can be exploitative and manipulative, and they tend to react violently if they perceive disrespect or opposition.

### Specific Diagnoses Included in Cluster C for Personality Disorders

**Cluster C***:* The classification of Cluster C for personality disorders includes the diagnoses of avoidant, dependent, and obsessive-compulsive personality disorders.

- The **avoidant** individual is socially inhibited and consequently avoids interaction with others. They are very sensitive to criticism or rejection and often have feelings of inadequacy.
- The **dependent** individual has very low self-esteem and will be submissive and dependent in behaviors and relationships, making them susceptible to being taken advantage of. If they lose their primary supportive relationship, they will quickly seek to establish another one.
- The **obsessive-compulsive** individual will have an extreme preoccupation with minute details, and will possess an inflexible perfectionism and desire for control. They also exhibit cold, unfeeling, and superior attitudes towards others.

## Bipolar Disorder

Bipolar disorder causes severe mood swings between hyperactive states and depression, accompanied by impaired judgment because of distorted thoughts. The hypomanic stage may allow for creativity and good functioning in some people, but it can develop into more severe mania, which may be associated with psychosis and hallucinations with rapid speech and bizarre behavior, and then into periods of profound depression. While most cases are diagnosed in late adolescence, there is increasing evidence that some children present with symptoms earlier; especially at risk are children with a bipolar parent. Bipolar disorder is associated with high rates of suicide, so early diagnosis and treatment is critical.

**Symptoms** may be relatively mild or involve severe rapid cycling between mania and depression.

**Treatment** includes both medications (usually given continually) to prevent cycling and control depression and psychosocial therapy, such as cognitive therapy, to help control disordered thought patterns and behavior. Psychiatric referral should be made.

## Obsessive-Compulsive Disorder

Anxiety disorders also include the diagnosis of obsessive-compulsive disorder (OCD). OCD involves either **obsessions** or **compulsions** that are persistent impulses or thoughts that are uncontrollable by the person. These thoughts lead to an **abnormally elevated anxiety response**. Some examples of obsessions can include fear of dirt, germs, robbery, contracting a medical disease, unintentional discarding of important information, having images of a sexual nature, or things not being symmetrical or completed. Compulsions are when the individual is driven to perform certain repetitive behaviors in ritualistic order with the outcome being resolution of the anxiety caused by the obsession.

Some examples of **compulsive repetitive behaviors** can include hand washing, checking locks, counting objects found routinely within their normal day, hoarding, ordering or arranging items, or saying words silently.

**Review Video: Obsessive-Compulsive Disorder (OCD)**
Visit mometrix.com/academy and enter code: 499790

### *Comorbidities*

When an individual has two or more disorders occurring at the same time, these disorders are considered to share **comorbidity**. Obsessive-compulsive disorder (OCD) is often found sharing comorbidity with other psychological disorders. Many times, individuals with OCD also have Tourette's syndrome, depression, panic attacks, mood disorders, social and specific phobias, eating disorders, or personality disorders. It has been found that Tourette's syndrome and OCD actually cause similar brain dysfunctions. Depression is commonly seen in patient's suffering from OCD due to the isolating effects it can have upon their lifestyle. It is also common for these individuals to have substance abuse problems due to trying to self-medicate to solve their struggles with OCD.

## Depression

Depression is a mood disorder characterized by profound feelings of sadness and withdrawal. It may be acute (such as after a death) or chronic with recurring episodes over a lifetime. The cause appears to be a combination of genetic, biological, and environmental factors. A major depressive episode is a depressed mood, profound and constant sense of hopelessness and despair, or loss of interest in all or almost all activities for a period of at least two weeks. Some drugs may precipitate depression: diuretics, Parkinson's drugs, estrogen, corticosteroids, cimetidine, hydralazine, propranolol, digitalis, and indomethacin. Depression is associated with neurotransmitter dysregulation, especially serotonin and norepinephrine. Major depression can be mild, moderate, or severe.

**Symptoms** include changes in mood, sadness, loss of interest in usual activities, increased fatigue, changes in appetite and fluctuations in weight, anxiety, and sleep disturbance.

**Treatment** includes tricyclic antidepressants (TCAS) and SSRIs, but SSRIs have fewer side effects and are less likely to cause death with an overdose. Counseling, undergoing cognitive behavioral therapy, treating underlying cause, and instituting an exercise program may help reduce depression.

**Review Video: Major Depression**
Visit mometrix.com/academy and enter code: 632694

### *Anxiety and Depression Due to Intensive Care Stays*

Anxiety and depression affect over half of patients who are treated in intensive care not only during the stay but also after discharge, especially if care is long-term or if their needs for moderate or high care continue. Additionally, studies have shown that those who suffer depression during and after ICU stays have increased risk of mortality over the next two years. Patients with anxiety may appear restless (thrashing about the bed), have difficulty concentrating, exhibit tachycardia and tachypnea, experience insomnia and feelings of dread, and complain of various ailments, such as stomach ache and headache. Symptoms of depression may overlap (and patients may have both anxiety and depression) and may also include fatigue, insomnia, withdrawal, appetite change, irritability, pessimistic outlooks, feelings of worthlessness, sadness, and suicidal ideation. Brief screening tools for anxiety and depression should be used with all ICU patients and interventions per psychological referral made as needed.

## Anxiety Disorders

Anxiety is a human emotion and experience that everyone has at some point during their life. Feelings of uncertainty, helplessness, isolation, alienation, and insecurity can all be experienced during an **anxiety response**. Many times, anxiety occurs without a specific known object or source. It can occur because of the unknown. Anxiety occurs throughout the life cycle, and therefore anxiety disorders can affect people of all ages. Populations that are most commonly affected include women, smokers, people under the age of 45, individuals that are separated or divorced, victims of abuse, and people in the lower socioeconomic groups. An individual can have one single anxiety disorder, experience more than one anxiety disorder, or have other mental health disorders all occurring at the same time.

**Review Video: Different Types of Anxiety Disorders**
Visit mometrix.com/academy and enter code: 366760

### *Generalized Anxiety Disorder*

Generalized anxiety disorder can be very insidious and occurs when an individual consistently experiences **excessive anxiety and worry**. This anxiety and worry will be present almost every day and lasts for a period of at least six months. The worry and anxiety will be uncontrollable, intrusive, and not related to any medical disease process. It will pertain to real-life events, situations, or circumstances and may occur along with mild depression symptoms. The individual will also experience three or more of the following symptoms: fatigue, inability to concentrate, irritability, insomnia, restlessness, loosing thought processes or going blank, and muscle tension. The continued anxiety and worry will eventually affect daily functioning and cause social and occupational disturbances.

#### Comorbidities

Individuals with generalized anxiety disorder (GAD) will often have **other mental health disorders**. When a person has more than one psychological disorder occurring at the same time, these disorders are considered to be **comorbid**. Most patients suffering from GAD will have at least one more psychiatric diagnosis. The most common comorbid disorders can include major depressive disorder, social or specific phobias, panic disorder, and dysthymic disorder. It is also common for these individuals to have substance abuse problems, and they may look to alcohol or barbiturates to help control their symptoms of anxiety.

### LEVELS OF ANXIETY

There are four main levels of anxiety that were named by Peplau. They are as follows:

- **Mild anxiety** is associated with normal tensions of everyday life. It can increase awareness and motivate learning and creativity.
- **Moderate anxiety** occurs when the individual narrows their field of perception and focuses on the immediate problem. This level decreases the perceptual field; however, the person can tend to other tasks if directed.
- **Severe anxiety** leads to a markedly reduced field of perception and the person focuses only on the details of the problem. All energy is directed at relieving the anxiety and the person can only perform other tasks under significant persuasion.
- **Panic** is the most extreme level of anxiety and associated with feelings of dread and terror. The individual is unable to perform any other tasks no matter how strongly they are persuaded to do so. This level can be life-threatening with complete disorganization of thought occurring.

### PHYSICAL SYMPTOMS

Anxiety produces a very physical response and effects the largest body systems, such as cardiovascular, respiratory, GI, neuromuscular, urinary tract, and skin. Symptoms vary and can increase upon a continuum depending upon the level of anxiety the person is experiencing.

- **Cardiovascular symptoms** can include palpitation, tachycardia, hypertension, feeling faint or actually fainting, hypotension, or bradycardia.
- **Respiratory symptoms** can include tachypnea, shortness of breath, chest pressure, shallow respirations, or choking sensation.
- **GI symptoms** can include revulsion toward food, nausea, diarrhea, and abdominal pain or discomfort.

Even though anxiety occurs psychologically, it can produce extreme **physical responses** from the neuromuscular system, urinary tract, and skin. These symptoms can range from mild to severe depending upon the degree of anxiety the person is experiencing.

- **Neuromuscular symptoms** can include hyperreflexia, being easily startled, eyelid twitching, inability to sleep, shaking, fidgeting, pacing, wobbly legs, or clumsy movements.
- **Urinary tract symptoms** can include increased frequency and sensation of need to urinate.
- **Skin symptoms** can include flushed face, sweaty palms, itching, sensations of being hot and/or cold, pale facial coloring, or diaphoresis.

### BEHAVIORAL AND AFFECTIVE RESPONSES

Behavioral and affective symptoms along with a multitude of physical symptoms are observable in anxious patients. The effects of these responses can affect the person experiencing the anxiety along with their relationships with others.

- Some **behavioral responses** can include restlessness and physical tension, hypervigilance, rapid speech, social or relationship withdrawal, decreased coordination, avoidance, or flight.
- **Affective responses** are the patient's emotional reactions and can be described subjectively by the individual. Patients may describe symptoms such as edginess, impatience, tension, nervousness, fear, frustration, jitteriness, or helplessness.

### *Cognitive Responses*

Anxiety not only produces physical and emotional symptoms, but it can also greatly affect the individual's intellectual abilities. **Cognitive responses** to anxiety occur in three main categories. These include sensory-perceptual, thought difficulties, and conceptualization. Responses that affect the patient's **sensory-perceptual fields** can include feeling that their mind is unclear or clouded, seeing objects indistinctly, perceiving a surreal environment, increased self-consciousness, or hypervigilance. **Thinking difficulties** can include the inability to remember important information, confusion, inability to focus thoughts or attention, easily distracted, blocking thoughts, difficulty with reasoning, tunnel vision, or loss of objectivity. **Conceptual difficulties** can include the fear of loss of control, inability to cope, potential physical injury, developing a mental disorder, or receiving a negative evaluation. The patient may have cognitive distortion, protruding scary visual images, or uncontrollable repetition of fearful thoughts.

**Review Video: Different Types of Anxiety Disorders**
Visit mometrix.com/academy and enter code: 366760

## Panic Attacks

Panic attacks are short episodes (peaking in 5-10 minutes) of intense anxiety that can result in a wide variety of **symptoms** that include:

- Dyspnea
- Palpitations
- Hyperventilation
- Nausea and vomiting
- Intense fear or anxiety
- Pain and pressure in the chest
- Dizziness and fainting
- Tremors

Panic attacks may be associated with agoraphobia, depression, or intimate partner violence and abuse (IPVA), so a careful history is important. Typically, patients believe they are dying or having a heart attack and require reassurance and treatment, such as diazepam or lorazepam, in the ED for the acute episode. In severe cases, ASA may be given and EKG done to rule out cardiac abnormalities. Patients should be referred for psychiatric evaluation for ongoing medications such as SSRIs (sertraline, paroxetine, fluoxetine) to prevent recurrence. Panic attacks become chronic panic disorders if they are recurrent, with each attack each followed by at least a month of fear of another attack.

## PTSD

Patients that experience a traumatic event may re-experience the trauma through distressing thoughts and recollections of the event. In addition, psychological effects of the trauma may include difficulty sleeping, emotional lability and problems with memory and concentration. Patients may also wish to avoid places or activities that remind them of their trauma. These are all characteristics of **post-traumatic stress disorder (PTSD)** and may cause patients extreme distress and significantly impact their quality of life.

**Signs and symptoms**: Nightmares, flashbacks, insomnia, symptoms of hyperarousal including irritability and anxiety, avoidance, and negative thoughts and feelings about oneself and others.

**Diagnosis**: PTSD is diagnosed through psychological assessment and criteria defined in the Diagnostic and Statistical Manual of Mental Disorders, Fifth Edition (DSM-5-TR).

**Treatment**: Pharmacologic therapy may be utilized to help control the symptoms of PTSD. Non-pharmacologic therapy options include group and individual/family therapy, cognitive behavioral therapy, and anxiety management/relaxation techniques. Hypnosis may also be utilized.

## Stress

### Relationship Between Stress and Disease

Stress causes a number of physical and psychological changes within the body:

- Cortisol levels increase
- Digestion is hindered and the colon stimulated
- Heart rate increases
- Perspiration increases
- Anxiety and depression occur and can result in insomnia, anorexia or weight gain, and suicide
- Immune response decreases, making the person more vulnerable to infections
- Autoimmune reaction may increase, leading to autoimmune diseases

The body's **compensatory mechanisms** try to restore homeostasis. When these mechanisms are overwhelmed, pathophysiological injury to the cells of the body result. When this injury begins to interfere with the function of the organs or systems in the body, symptoms of dysfunction will occur. If the conditions are not corrected, the body changes the structure or function of the affected organs or systems.

### Adaptation of Cells to Stress

The most common stressors to cells include the lack of oxygen, presence of toxins or chemicals, and infection. **Cells react to stress** by making the following changes:

- **Hypertrophy**: Cells swell, leading to an overall increase in the size of the affected organ.
- **Atrophy**: Cells shrivel and the overall organ size decreases in size.
- **Hyperplasia**: The cells divide and overgrowth and thickening of the tissue results.
- **Dysplasia**: The cells are changed in appearance as a result of irritation over an extended period of time, sometimes leading to malignancy.
- **Metaplasia**: Cells change type as a result of stress.

If the stress that caused the cells to change continues, the cells become injured and die. When enough cells die, organ and systemic failure occur.

### Psychological Response to Stress

When stress is encountered, a person **responds** according to the threat perceived to compensate. The threat is evaluated as to the amount of harm or loss that has occurred or is possible. If the stress is benign (such as with marriage), then a challenge is present that demands change. Once the threat or challenge is defined, the person can gather information, resources, and support to make the changes needed to resolve the stress to the greatest degree possible. Immediate psychological response to stress may include shock, anger, fear, or excitement. Over time, people may develop chronic anxiety, depression, flashbacks, thought disturbances, and sleep disturbances. Changes may occur in emotions and thinking, in behavior, or in the person's environment. People may be more able to adapt to stress if they have many varied experiences, a good self-esteem, and a support network to help as needed. A healthy lifestyle and philosophical beliefs, including religion, may give a person more reserve to cope with stress.



### Impact of Different Kinds of Stress

Everyone encounters **stress** in life and it **impacts** each person differently. There are the small daily "hassles," major traumatic events, and the periodic stressful events of marriage, birth, divorce, and death. Compounded stress experienced on a daily basis can impact health status over time. Stressors that occur suddenly are the hardest to overcome and result in the greatest tension. The length of time that a stressor is present affects the impact with long-term, relentless stress, such as that generated by poverty or disability, resulting in disease more often. If there is **ineffective coping**, a person will suffer greater changes resulting in even more stress. The nurse can help patients to recognize those things that induce stress in their lives, find ways to reduce stress when possible, and teach effective coping skills and problem-management.

## Violence and Aggression

Violence and aggression are sometimes seen in critical care settings. The nurse must be aware of signs of impending violence or aggression in order to intervene and prevent injury to self or staff.

- **Violence** is a physical act perpetrated against an inanimate object, animal, or other person with the intent to cause harm. Violence often results from anger, frustration, or fear. It often occurs because the perpetrator believes that he is threatened in some way. Violence may occur suddenly without warning or following an escalating pattern of aggressive behavior.
- **Aggression** is the communication of a threat or intended act of violence that often occurs before the act of violence is carried out. This communication can occur verbally or nonverbally. Gestures, shouting, increasing volume of speech, invasion of personal space, and prolonged eye contact are all examples of aggression. The nurse should promptly recognize all forms of aggression and redirect or remove the patient from the situation to avoid an act of violence.

### *Management of Patients with Violent Behavior*

Patients may exhibit **violent behavior** for a number of reasons, including metabolic disorders (hypoglycemia), neurological disorders (brain tumor), psychiatric disorders (schizophrenia), or substance abuse (drugs and alcohol). Patients who make threats or have a history of violent behavior should be approached with caution.

**Diagnosis** includes history, physical exam, CBC and chemistry panel, toxicology screening, ECG, and, in some cases, CT scans or lumbar punctures. Violent behavior tends to escalate from anxiety to defensiveness to aggression, so identifying these signs and providing support through information, setting limits, using restraints, and seclusion can avoid injuries. Handcuffs should not be removed in the ED, and patients who are so violent they must be restrained should not be allowed to leave the ED against medical advice.

**Pharmacologic treatment** includes:

- **Antipsychotic drugs**: Haloperidol 5 mg IM (1–2 mg for elderly patients)
- **Benzodiazepines**: Lorazepam 2–4 mg IM/IV (often in conjunction with antipsychotic drugs)
- **Hypnotics**: Droperidol 2.5 mg IM/IV

## Homicidal Ideation

Homicidal ideation, the intention to kill another person, can occur for a variety of reasons:

- **Sociopathy/psychopathy**: These patients usually appear quite normal and may even seem charming, but they can be very dangerous because they lack empathy for others. Some are involved in gangs in which violent behavior is expected and valued.
- **Psychosis**: Uncontrolled schizophrenia and paranoia may result in a patient behaving in a homicidal manner. In some cases, these changes may be brought about by pathology, such as TBI or brain tumor.
- **Medications**: Medications such as antidepressants, SSRIs, and antipsychotics as well as interferon have been associated with homicidal ideation in some patients. Patients on multiple medications may experience an involuntary intoxication that results in rage reactions and sometimes even the death of others.

Indications of homicidal ideation may include verbal threats, use of weapons, and violent behavior. Patients who express homicidal ideation or have attempted homicide require immediate psychiatric referral and may require restraint. The nurse should conduct a complete review of medications and notify security personnel if the patient poses a danger.

## Psychosis

Psychosis is a severe reaction to stressors (psychological, physical) that results in alterations in affect and impaired psychomotor and behavioral functions, including the onset of hallucinations and/or delusions. Psychosis is not a diagnosis but is a symptom that may be caused by a mental disorder (such as schizophrenia or bipolar disease) or a physical disorder (such as a brain tumor or Alzheimer's disease). Psychosis may also be induced by some prescription drugs (muscle relaxants, antihistamines, anticonvulsants, corticosteroids, antiparkinson drugs), illicit drugs (cocaine, PCP, amphetamines, cannabis, LSD), and alcohol. Treatment depends on identifying the underlying cause of the psychosis and initiating treatment. For example, if caused by schizophrenia, then antipsychotic drugs and hospitalization in a mental health facility may be indicated. In most cases of drug-induced psychosis, stopping the drug alleviates the symptoms although some may benefit from the addition of a benzodiazepine or antipsychotic drug until symptoms subside.

## Suicidal Ideation

Patients may attempt suicide for many reasons, including severe depression, social isolation, situational crisis, bereavement, or psychotic disorder.

**Suicidal indications** are as follows:

- Depression or dysphoria
- Hostility to others
- Problems with peer relationships, and lack of close friends
- Post-crisis stress (divorce, death in family, graduation, college)
- Withdrawn personality; quiet or lonely appearance or behavior
- Change in behavior (dropping grades, unkempt appearance, change in sleeping patterns)
- A sudden increase in positive mood may indicate patient has a plan
- Co-morbid psychiatric problems (bipolar, schizophrenia)
- Substance abuse

The following are indicators of **high risk for repeated suicide attempt**:

- Violent suicide attempt (knives, gunshots)
- Suicide attempt with low chance of rescue
- Ongoing psychosis or disordered thinking
- Ongoing severe depression and feeling of helplessness
- History of previous suicide attempts
- Lack of social support system

**Nursing considerations:** Take all suicidal ideations seriously; do not minimize them. Suicidal patients should be watched continuously, given plastic utensils, break-away wall rails/shower heads, no cords/sharp instruments.

## Substance Abuse

Substance abuse is the abuse of drugs, medicines, or alcohol that causes mental and physical problems for the abuser and family. Abusers use substances out of boredom, to hide negative self-esteem, to dampen emotional pain, and to cope with daily stress. As the abuse continues, abusers become unable to take care of daily needs and duties. They lack effective coping mechanisms and the ability to make healthy choices. They can't identify and prioritize stress or choose positive behavior to resolve the stress in a healthy way. Some family members may act as codependents because of their desire to feel needed by the abuser, to control the person, and to stay with him or her. The nurse can help the family to confront an individual with their concerns about the person and their proposals for treatment. Family members can enforce consequences if treatment is not sought. Family members may also need counseling to learn new behaviors to stop enabling the abuser to continue substance abuse.

### *Pathophysiology of Addiction*

Genetic, social, and personality factors may all play a role in the development of **addictive tendencies**. However, the main factor of the development of substance addiction is the pharmacological activation of the **reward system** located in the central nervous system (CNS). This reward systems pathway involves **dopaminergic neurons**. Dopamine is found in the CNS and is one of many neurotransmitters that play a role in an individual's mood. The mesolimbic pathway seems to play a primary role in the reward and motivational process involved with addiction. This pathway begins in the ventral tegmental area of the brain (VTA) and then moves forward into the nucleus accumbens located in the middle forebrain bundle (MFB). Some drugs enhance mesolimbic dopamine activity, therefore producing very potent effects on mood and behavior.

### *Indicators of Substance Abuse*

Many people with substance abuse (alcohol or drugs) are reluctant to disclose this information, but there are a number of **indicators** that are suggestive of substance abuse:

**Physical signs** include:

- Burns on fingers or lips
- Pupils abnormally dilated or constricted, eyes watery
- Slurring of speech, slow speech
- Lack of coordination, instability of gait, tremors
- Sniffing repeatedly, nasal irritation, persistent cough
- Weight loss
- Dysrhythmias
- Pallor, puffiness of face
- Needle tracks on arms or legs
- Odor of alcohol/marijuana on clothing or breath

**Behavioral signs** include:

- Labile emotions, including mood swings, agitation, and anger
- Inappropriate, impulsive, or risky behavior
- Lying
- Missing appointments
- Difficulty concentrating, short term memory loss, blackouts
- Insomnia or excessive sleeping; disoriented, confused
- Lack of personal hygiene

### *Alcohol Withdrawal*

Chronic abuse of ethanol (alcoholism) can lead to physical dependency. Sudden cessation of drinking, which often happens in the inpatient setting, is associated with **alcohol withdrawal syndrome.** It may be precipitated by trauma or infection and has a high mortality rate, 5–15% with treatment and 35% without treatment.

**Signs/symptoms:** Anxiety, tachycardia, headache, diaphoresis, progressing to severe agitation, hallucinations, auditory/tactile disturbances, and psychotic behavior (delirium tremens).

**Diagnosis:** Physical assessment, blood alcohol levels (on admission).

**Treatment** includes:

- Medication: IV benzodiazepines to manage symptoms; electrolyte and nutritional replacement, especially magnesium and thiamine.
- Use the CIWA scale to measure symptoms of withdrawal; treat as indicated.
- Provide an environment with minimal sensory stimulus (lower lights, close blinds) & implement fall and seizure precautions.
- Prevention: Screen all patients for alcohol/substance abuse, using CAGE or other assessment tool. Remember to express support and comfort to patient; wait until withdrawal symptoms are subsiding to educate about alcohol use and moderation.

## EATING DISORDERS

### *ANOREXIA NERVOSA*

Eating disorders are a profound health risk and can lead to death, especially for adolescent girls, although boys also have eating disorders, often presenting as excessive exercise. Anorexia nervosa is characterized by profound fear of weight gain and severe restriction of food intake, often accompanied by abuse of diuretics and laxatives, which can cause electrolyte imbalances, kidney and bowel disorders, and delay or cessation of menses.

- **Symptoms** include growth retardation, amenorrhea (missing 3 consecutive periods), unexplained and sometimes precipitous weight loss (at least 15% below normal weight), dehydration, loss of appetite, hypoglycemia, hypercholesterolemia, or carotenemia with yellowing of skin, emaciated appearance, osteoporosis, bradycardia, and food obsessions and rituals.
- **Diagnosis** includes complete history, physical, and psychological exam with CBC and chemical panels to rule out other disorders.
- **Treatment** includes volume and electrolyte replacement initially with referral to psychiatric care for long-term management of the disorder and nutritional plans.

### *BULIMIA NERVOSA*

Bulimia nervosa includes binge eating followed by vomiting (at least 2 times monthly for at least 3 months), often along with diuretics, enemas, and laxatives. Some may engage in periods of fasting or excessive exercise rather than vomiting to offset the effects of binging. Gastric acids from purging can damage the throat and teeth. While bulimics may maintain a normal weight, they are at risk for severe electrolyte imbalances that can be life-threatening. Binge eating affects 2–5% of females and includes grossly overeating, often resulting in obesity, depression, and shame. Symptoms include hypokalemia, metabolic acidosis, fluctuations of weight, dental caries and loss of enamel, knuckle scars (from contact with teeth while inducing vomiting), parotid and submandibular gland enlargement, and insulin-dependent diabetes. Diagnosis includes complete history, physical, and psychological exam with CBC and chemical panels to rule out other disorders. Treatment includes volume and electrolyte replacement initially with referral to psychiatric care for long-term management of the disorder and nutritional plans, as well as SSRIs, naltrexone, and ondansetron.

# Psychosocial Interventions

## Behavior Modification

Behavior modification is a type of systematic therapy that works toward the goal of replacing **maladaptive behaviors** with **positive behaviors**. This type of therapy can be utilized with individuals, groups, or entire communities. The hope of this approach is to get rid of the unwanted behaviors by utilizing positive reinforcement directed toward the desired behaviors. After experiencing **positive reinforcement**, the participant will want to repeat the good behaviors to gain the reward. These new behaviors will then become habits over time and will replace the old behaviors. This type of therapy can be very effective with eating disorders, smoking cessation, or addictions.

## Cognitive-Behavioral Therapy

Cognitive-Behavioral Therapy (CBT) focuses on the impact that thoughts have on behavior and feelings, encouraging the individual to use the power of rational thought to alter perceptions. CBT centers on the concept of unlearning previous behaviors and learning new ones, questioning behaviors, and doing homework. This approach to counseling is usually short-term, about 12–20 sessions. The first sessions obtain a history, middle sessions focus on the problems, and the last sessions review and reinforce newly learned habits and thought patterns. Individuals are assigned homework during the sessions to practice new ways of thinking and to develop new coping strategies. The therapist helps the individual identify goals and then find ways to achieve those goals. CBT acknowledges that all problems cannot be resolved, but one can deal differently with problems. The therapist asks questions to determine the individual's areas of concern and encourages the individual to question his or her own motivations and needs. CBT is goal-centered, so each counseling session is structured toward a particular goal, such as coping techniques.

## Aaron Beck's Cognitive Therapy

Aaron Beck discovered that during psychotherapy patients often had a second set of thoughts while undergoing free association. Beck called these **automatic thoughts**, which were labeled and interpreted, according to a personal set of rules. Beck called dysfunctional automatic thoughts **cognitive disorders**. Beck identified a triad of negative thoughts regarding the self, environment, and world. The key concepts in **Aaron Beck's cognitive therapy** include the following:

- **Therapist/patient relationship**: Therapy is a collaborative partnership. The goal of therapy is determined together. The therapist encourages the patient to disagree when appropriate.
- **Process of therapy**: The therapist explains the following: one's perception of reality is not reality. The interpretation of sensory input depends on cognitive processes. The patient is taught to recognize maladaptive ideation, identifying the following: observable behavior, underlying motivation, his or her thoughts and beliefs. The patient practices distancing the maladaptive thoughts, explores his or her conclusions, and tests them against reality.
- **Conclusions**: The patient makes the rules less extreme and absolute, drops false rules, and substitutes adaptive rules.

## Recovery Model

The Recovery Model approach to mental health shifts control of treatment options to the patient rather than the physician deciding the plan of care. This has been effective in those patients who have the capacity to make decisions to allow them to be more independent and take a more active role in the decision-making regarding their treatment plan. The goal of this model is to allow the patient to be more **autonomous** so that they may achieve the ultimate goals of gaining employment, finding housing, and living independently. The more independent the patient can become, the more they progress to making independent decisions about the treatment of their mental health issues. This model is not appropriate for those patients who are so incapacitated by their illness that they do not understand they are ill. The amount of independence and decision-making that is turned over to the patient should increase as they become more stable.

## ACCEPTANCE AND COMMITMENT THERAPY

Acceptance and commitment therapy (ACT) is a "third wave" of CBT that emphasizes contextual and experiential learning through psychological flexibility. Rather than avoiding or changing dysfunctional thoughts, clients are taught to observe them without judgment or resistance. ACT uses six core processes to help clients develop psychological flexibility:

- **Cognitive defusion:** This involves detaching from thoughts their personally ascribed meanings and undesirable functions.
- **Acceptance:** This process allows thoughts, emotions, and sensations to exist without attempting to change their content or frequency.
- **Self as context:** This involves fostering an understanding that the client's thoughts do not define them.
- **Contact with the present moment:** This involves fully experiencing sensations, thoughts, and feelings while adopting an objective, nonjudgmental perspective of the here and now.
- **Values:** Therapists help clients understand that values are ongoing, dynamic, and constantly evolving principles that guide them toward living a purposeful and meaningful life.
- **Committed action:** This process involves taking proactive steps toward leading a value-driven life by integrating all five core processes into sustained behavioral change.

## SINGLE-SESSION THERAPY

Single-session therapy is the **most frequent form of counseling** because individuals often attend only one session for various reasons even if more are advised. Individuals may not have insurance or believe that one session is sufficient. Sessions typically last 1 hour. The goal is to identify a problem and reach a solution in one session. The therapist serves as a facilitator to motivate the individual to view the problem as part of a pattern that can be changed and to identify a solution. The therapist may use a wide range of techniques that culminates in a **plan for the individual** (e.g., homework exercises) so the individual can begin to make changes.

## SOLUTION-FOCUSED THERAPY

Solution-focused therapy aims to **differentiate methods** that are effective from those that are not, and to identify areas of strengths so they can be used in problem solving. The premise of solution-focused therapy is that change is possible but that the individual must identify problems and deal with them in the real world. This therapy is based on questioning to help the individual establish goals and find solutions to problems:

- **Pre-session**: The patient is asked about any differences he or she noted after making the appointment and coming to the first session.
- **Miracle**: The patient is asked if any miracles occurred or if any problems were solved, including what, if anything, was different and how this difference affected relationships.
- **Exception**: The patient is asked if any small changes were noted and if there were any problems that no longer seemed problematic and how that manifested.
- **Scaling**: The patient is asked to evaluate the problem on a 1–10 scale and then to determine how to increase the rating.
- **Coping**: The patient is asked about how he or she is managing.

## TRAUMA-INFORMED CARE

Trauma-informed care acts on the premise that many individuals have experienced some sort of trauma, and therefore every patient should be approached with sensitivity and care. Traumatic events are deeply individualized, and what may have been traumatic to one individual, may not be to the next. Withholding judgment of what qualifies as trauma is imperative for the psychiatric-mental health nurse.

The five elements of **trauma-informed care** include the following:

- **Safety**: Ensuring that the patient feels emotionally and physically safe must be the first priority in order to create a conducive environment for treatment.
- **Choice**: Treatment cannot be forced and must honor the individual's right to choose.
- **Collaboration**: The patient and the nurse must work collaboratively through shared decision-making.
- **Trustworthiness**: The patient must trust the nurse in order for treatment to be effective. Trustworthiness can be established by communicating what is happening and what will happen next to the patient.
- **Empowerment**: Empower the patient with tools to cope on their own so that their recovery extends outside the walls of treatment.

## PSYCHIATRIC AND MENTAL HEALTH PROGRAMS

A variety of psychiatric and mental health programs are available and should be evaluated, according to the needs of the individual patient.

- **Inpatient programs** provide a secure environment and comprehensive care, often with psychologists, psychiatrists, occupational therapists, social workers, and other allied health personnel. Programs may be tailored to one specific type of patient (e.g., criminally insane, substance abusers) or to a general population. They may offer short-term or long-term care.
- **Outpatient programs** provide assessment and treatment, such as group therapy, cognitive-behavioral therapy, and family therapy. Programs may be community-based, targeting specific groups of people, such as alcoholics or the homeless.
- **Partial/day hospitalization programs** provide daily inpatient care during prescribed hours (e.g., 8 a.m. to 3 p.m.) as well as outpatient services. The stay is usually short-term (1–2 weeks) and may serve as a transition from inpatient to outpatient care.

## NONVIOLENT CRISIS INTERVENTION AND DE-ESCALATION TECHNIQUES

Nonviolent crisis intervention and de-escalation techniques begin with self-awareness because the normal response to aggression is a stress response (freezing, fight/flight, fear). The nurse must control these responses in order to deal with the situation. The nurse should recognize signs of impending conflict (clenched fists, and sudden change in tone of voice or body stance, and change in eye contact). Steps include:

- Maintain social distance (≥12 feet) if possible and stay at the same level as the person (sitting or standing).
- Speak in a quiet calm tone of voice, limiting eye contact and avoiding changes in voice tone, facial expression, and gestures (especially avoid pointing or waving a finger at the person).
- Ask the person's name (if necessary) and use the name when addressing the person.
- Validate the person by acknowledging their issue: "I can see that you are angry about the changes in your treatment."
- Show empathy without being judgmental: "I'm sorry you are upset."
- Ignore questions that are challenging and avoid arguing.
- Practice active listening by paraphrasing and clarifying.
- Assist the person to explore options and the results of those options: "What is it that you would like to do?"

## Physical Restraints

Restraints are used to restrict movement and activity when other methods of controlling patient behavior have failed and there is a risk of harm to the patient or others. There are two primary types of **physical restraints**: violent (behavioral) and non-violent (clinical). Violent restraints are more commonly used in the psychiatric unit or when individuals exhibit aggressive behavior. More commonly, non-violent restraints are used to ensure that the individual does not interfere with safe care. Non-violent restraints are commonly used in the confused elderly or intubated patient to prevent pulling out lines/removing equipment. The federal government and the Joint Commission have issued strict **guidelines** for temporary restraints or those not part of standard care (such as post-surgical restraint):

- Each facility must have a written policy and restraints are only used when ordered by a physician (usually require written/signed order every 24hrs and within 4 hours of restraint initiation).
- An assessment must be completed frequently, including circulation, toileting, and nutritional needs (generally every 1–2 hours).
- All alternative methods should be tried before applying a restraint and the least restrictive effective restraint should be used.
- A nurse must remove the restraint, assess, and document findings at least every 2 hours, every hour for violent restraints.

*Key: Least restrictive option for the least amount of time.*

## Chemical Restraints

Chemical restraints involve the use of pharmacological sedatives to manage an individual's behavior problems. This type of restraint is indicated only when severe agitation/violence puts the patient at risk for injury to themselves or others. **Chemical restraints** inhibit the individuals' physical movements, making their behavior more manageable. It is important to realize that medication used on an ongoing basis as part of treatment is not legally considered a chemical restraint, even though the medications may be the same. There is little consensus about the use of chemical restraints, although benzodiazepines and antipsychotics are frequently used to control severe agitation (haloperidol, lorazepam, etc.). Oral medications should be tried first before injections, as oral medication is less coercive. It is important for the nurse to realize that chemical restraints are used as a last resort when other measures (such as de-escalation and environmental modification) have failed and there is an immediate risk of harm to the patient or others.

# Chapter Quiz

Ready to see how well you retained what you just read? Scan the QR code to go directly to the chapter quiz interface for this study guide. If you're using a computer, simply visit the online resources page at **mometrix.com/resources719/nclexrn-31183** and click the Chapter Quizzes link.

# Basic Care and Comfort

## Functional Status and Rehabilitation

### ADLs

**Activities of daily living** (ADLs) are a group of activities that are used to evaluate a patient's return to normal function; these are activities that the patient had performed on a daily basis before hospitalization, and will be expected to perform once he or she has completed rehabilitation. The **rate** at which the patient accomplishes these activities, in addition to the **level of independence** maintained by the patient when performing the activities, can help caregivers determine the amount of rehabilitation required, and can also be used to monitor the progress of the patient during the rehabilitation process. ADLs are grouped into 3 different areas: **personal or physical**, **instrumental**, and **occupational**.

#### *Grouping ADLs*

The first group of ADLs, the **physical or personal group**, contains those daily activities that relate to the patient's ability to take care of him or herself. Included in this group are activities related to health management, nutritional needs, elimination of bladder and bowel contents, exercise, self-esteem, coping/stress management, cognitive abilities, communication, sexual health and ability, and relationship roles. The second group of ADLs, the **instrumental group**, contains activities such as shopping, answering the phone, and other activities that involve leaving home. The third group, **occupational activities**, includes activities that are required of being a parent, husband, or wife, as well as those required on the job.

### Rehabilitation

Rehabilitation is an area of health care that is dedicated to helping patients improve and/or restore functions and abilities after a disease or injury. Although rehabilitation is usually thought of in relation to **physical therapy** (which is one of the many areas of rehabilitation), it also encompasses **drug and alcohol rehabilitation**, as well as **occupational therapy** for physically and mentally ill patients. The general goals of all types of rehabilitation include an improvement in overall function; the promotion of independence, satisfaction, and well-being; and the preservation of the individual's self-esteem in the face of illness or debilitating disease or injury.

### Assessing Potential for Rehabilitation

There are various factors that are considered when assessing a patient to determine whether he or she will benefit from **rehabilitation**. A patient with the inability to perform any of the ADLs will automatically be considered for rehabilitation. At this point, however, other factors must be considered. First and foremost is whether or not the patient has a **desire to improve his or her functions** through rehabilitation; if the patient is not interested in improvement, the rehabilitation potential is poor. If the patient wants to improve function and increase independence, the potential for rehabilitation is greater. Another factor is whether or not the patient has **support at home**; even if the patient improves greatly during his or her rehabilitation stay, he or she will still most likely need some support at home. If the patient has no support at home, rehabilitation may eventually fail.

### Diseases and Illnesses That Commonly Require Rehabilitation

There are some diseases, illnesses, and injuries that almost always require rehabilitation at some point during their course; in these cases, rehabilitation may be initiated before the patient even leaves the hospital to be transferred to a rehabilitation facility. It is important to know which diseases usually require rehabilitation, because the sooner evaluation and rehabilitation are initiated, the better the patient's chance of recovery. The following are diseases, illnesses, and injuries that **commonly require rehabilitation**: AIDS, amyotrophic lateral sclerosis (ALS), limb amputation, traumatic or ischemic brain injury, spinal cord injury, burns, Guillain-Barré syndrome, hip or knee replacement, multiple sclerosis (MS), and most types of cancer.

## REHABILITATION SETTINGS

There are various kinds of rehabilitation settings, depending on the needs of the patient. Once the need for rehabilitation has been determined and the patient has been evaluated regarding specific rehabilitation needs, he or she can be placed in an appropriate rehabilitation setting. A **long-term acute care hospital** is a rehabilitation facility that is best for patients who are physically and psychologically stable but are receiving medical treatment such as dialysis or ventilation and thus require medical support. A **subacute care unit** is appropriate for patients who require more limited treatment, such as cancer patients. A **comprehensive inpatient rehabilitation facility** is just what the name suggests; it addresses the needs of a broad range of different patients, from burn victims to amputees. The comprehensive rehabilitation center has a "team" of medical specialists that includes a rehabilitation medicine physician, nurses trained in rehabilitation, occupational therapists, physical therapists, social workers, and speech-language pathologists. **Outpatient rehab** is designed for the high-functioning patient who can return home after rehab sessions.

## INTERVENTIONS TO CONSIDER WHEN BEGINNING REHABILITATION PROCESS

When a patient is to be considered for rehabilitation, he or she must undergo a rather extensive **evaluation** in order to increase the likelihood that he or she will succeed during rehabilitation. This process of evaluation, which includes various interventions, should take place in the early stages of illness, when the patient is still in the hospital. The goal is to forestall any **secondary complications** that may inhibit the rehabilitation process. These **interventions** include health management, in which the patient and family are educated about his or her disease(s); nutritional status assessment and support; initiation of bowel and bladder management in order to prevent infection; exercises; assessment of cognitive function; and education involving self-esteem, relationship roles, sexual activity, and coping mechanisms.

## OCCUPATIONAL THERAPY

Occupational therapy is defined as the use of creative activities in the treatment of individuals with disabilities, whether physical or mental. The purpose of occupational therapy is to provide those individuals with the skills that are necessary to live life as fully and independently as possible; after completion of occupational therapy, the individual should be able to perform at his or her **maximum potential**. The occupational therapist will typically provide the patient with **interventions** tailored to his or her disability. The OT will also visit the patient's home and/or place of employment in order to assess potential problems and provide **adaptive solutions**. As part of occupational therapy, the patient will receive regular **assessments** of his or her skills, as well as specific training. The occupational therapist is also responsible for educating the patient's family, caretakers, friends, and coworkers.

The philosophy of occupational therapy is based on the idea that **occupation** (meaning, loosely, either an activity or activities in which an individual engages) is a **basic human need**, one that is important to an individual's health and overall well-being in that it is in and of itself therapeutic in nature. The basic assumptions of occupational therapy are based on the idea of occupational therapy as stated by its creator, **William Rush Dunton**. Dunton states that occupational therapy is a human need because an individual's occupation has an effect on his or her health and general well-being. It creates **structure** in the individual's life and allows for him or her to manage and organize time. Another assumption is that individuals have different sets of values and, therefore, will value different occupations; for each person, however, the occupation that he or she chooses is meaningful to him or her.

### *AREAS IN WHICH OCCUPATIONAL THERAPY MAY BE INSTITUTED AND PRACTICED*

Although occupational therapy is an important part of the overall rehabilitation process for hospitalized individuals, it is also beneficial in other areas because occupational therapy deals not only with physical disabilities but with **emotional and cognitive disabilities** as well. Occupational therapy as related to **physical disabilities** may be practiced in outpatient clinics, pediatric hospitals or units, acute care rehabilitation facilities, and long-term, or comprehensive, inpatient rehabilitation centers. Occupational therapy as related to **mental disabilities** may be practiced in mental health clinics, acute and long-term psychiatric hospitals, prisons, and gateway or halfway houses. Occupational therapists may also work at schools, childcare facilities, workplaces, or shelters, or they may even work with individuals in their own homes.

### Assistive Devices

**Crutches** should be properly fitted before client attempts ambulation. Correct height is one hand-width below axillae. The handgrips should be adjusted so the client supports the body weight comfortably with elbows slightly flexed rather than locked in place. The client should be cautioned not to bear weight under the axillae as this can cause nerve damage but to hold the crutches tight against the side of the chest wall. The type of gait used depends on the type of injury.

A **cane** should be held in the opposite hand of the side of injury. When holding the cane in neutral position, the elbow should be bent at about a 15-degree angle and if holding the cane straight down to the side of the body, the top of the cane should be in line with the crease of the wrist.

The same is true of a **walker**, the elbow should be bent at 15 degrees when standing up straight and grasping the handles, and the handle grasps should be in line with to the crease of the wrists. The client should be able to move the walker forward without leaning over.

## Bowel and Bladder Training

### Bladder Training

Bladder training usually requires the person to keep a toileting diary for at least three days so patterns can be assessed. There are a number of different approaches:

- **Scheduled toileting** is toileting on a regular schedule, usually every 2-4 hours during the daytime.
- **Habit training** involves an attempt to match the scheduled toileting to a person's individual voiding habits, based on the toileting diary. This is useful for people who have a natural and fairly consistent voiding pattern. Toileting is done every 2-4 hours.
- **Prompted voiding** is often used in nursing homes and attempts to teach people to assess their own incontinence status and prompts them to ask for toileting.
- **Bladder retraining** is a behavioral modification program that teaches people to inhibit the urge to urinate and to urinate according to an established schedule, restoring normal bladder function as much as possible. Bladder training can improve incontinence in 80% of cases.

#### *Prompted Voiding*

Prompted voiding is a communication protocol for people with mild to moderate **cognitive impairment**. It uses positive reinforcement for recognizing being wet or dry, staying dry, urinating, and drinking liquids.

- Ask patient **every two hours** (8 a.m. to 4-8 p.m.) whether they are wet or dry.
- Verify if they are correct and give **feedback**, "You are right, Mrs. Brown, you are dry."
- **Prompt** patient, whether wet or dry, to use the toilet or urinal. If yes, assist them, record results, and give positive reinforcement by praising and visiting for a short time. If no, repeat the request again once or twice. If they are wet, and decline toileting, change and tell them you will return in two hours and ask them to try to wait to urinate until then.
- Offer **liquids** and record amount.
- **Record** results of each attempt to urinate or wet check.

### *Bladder Retraining*

Bladder retraining teaches people to control the urge to urinate. It usually takes about three months to rehabilitate a bladder muscle weakened from frequent urination, causing a decreased urinary capacity. A short urination interval is gradually lengthened to every 2-4 hours during the daytime as the person suppresses bladder urges and stays dry.

- The patient keeps a **urination diary** for a week.
- An individual program is established with **scheduled voiding times and goals**. For example, if a patient is urinating every hour, the goal might be every 80 minutes with increased output.
- The patient is taught **techniques** to withhold urination, such as sitting on a hard seat or on a tightly rolled towel to put pressure on pelvic floor muscles, doing five squeezes of pelvic floor muscles, deep breathing, and counting backward from 50.
- When the patient consistently meets the goal, a **new goal** is established.

### *The Knack to Control Urinary Incontinence*

The **knack** is the use of precisely timed muscle contractions to prevent **stress incontinence**. It is "the knack" of squeezing up before bearing down. The knack is a preventive use of **Kegel exercises**. Women are taught to contract the pelvic floor muscles right before and during events that usually cause stress incontinence. For example, if a woman feels a cough or sneeze coming, she immediately contracts the pelvic floor muscles and holds until the stress event is over. This contraction augments support of the proximal urethra, reducing the amount of displacement that usually takes place with compromised muscle support, thereby preventing incontinence. It is particularly useful if used before and during stress events, such as coughing, sneezing, lifting, standing, swinging a golf club, or laughing. Studies have shown that women who are taught this technique for mild to moderate urinary incontinence and use it consistently are able to decrease incontinence by 73-98%.

## Bowel Training

Bowel training for defecation includes keeping a bowel diary to chart progress:

- **Scheduled defecation** is usually daily, but for some people 3-4 times weekly, depending on individual bowel habits. Defecation should be at the same time, so work hours and activities must be considered. Defecation is scheduled for 20-30 minutes after a meal when there is increased motility.
- **Stimulation** is necessary. Drinking a cup of hot liquid may work, but initially many require rectal stimulation, inserting a gloved, lubricated finger into the anus and running it around the rim of the sphincters. Some people require rectal suppositories, such as glycerine. Stimulus suppositories, such as Dulcolax (bisacodyl), or even Fleet enemas are sometimes used, but the goal is to reduce use of medical or chemical stimulants.
- **Position** should be sitting upright with knees elevated slightly if possible and leaning forward during defecation.
- **Straining** includes attempting to tighten abdominal muscles and relax sphincters while defecating.
- **Exercise** increases the motility of the bowel by stimulating muscle contractions. **Walking** is one of the best exercises for this purpose, and the person should try to walk 1 or 2 miles a day. If the person is unable to walk, then other activities, such as chair exercises that involve the arms and legs and bending can be very effective. Those who are bed bound need to turn from side to side frequently and change position.
- **Kegel exercises** increase strength of the pelvic floor muscles. Kegel exercises for urinary incontinence and fecal incontinence are essentially the same, but the person tries to pull in the muscles around the anus, as though trying to prevent the release of stool or flatus. The person should feel the muscles tightening while holding for 2 seconds and then relaxing for 2 seconds, gradually building the holding time to 10 seconds or more. Exercises should be done 4 times a day.

### *Management Strategies for Constipation and Fecal Impaction*

Management strategies for constipation and impaction include:

- **Enemas** and **manual removal of impaction** may be necessary initially.
- Add **fiber** with bran, fresh/dried fruits, and whole grains, to 20-35 grams per day.
- Increase **fluids** to 64 ounces each day.
- **Exercise** program should include walking if possible, and exercises on a daily basis.
- Change in **medications** causing constipation can relieve constipation. Additionally, the use of stool softeners, such as Colace (docusate), or bulk formers, such as Metamucil (psyllium), may decrease fluid absorption and move stool through the colon more quickly. Overuse of laxatives can cause constipation.
- Careful **monitoring** of diet, fluids, and medical treatment, especially for irritable bowel syndrome.
- **Pregnancy-related constipation** may be controlled through dietary and fluid modifications and regular exercise.
- **Delayed toileting** should be avoided and bowel training regimen done to promote evacuation at the same time each day. During travel, stool softeners, increased fluid, and exercise may alleviate constipation.

### *Purpose of Fiber in the Diet*

Most constipation is caused by insufficient **fiber** in the diet, especially if people eat a lot of processed foods. An adequate amount of fiber is 20-30 grams daily. There are both soluble and insoluble forms of fiber, and both add bulk to the stool and are not absorbed into the body. Some foods have both types:

- **Soluble fiber** dissolves in liquids to form a gel-like substance, which is why liquids are so important in conjunction with fiber in the diet. Soluble fiber slows the movement of stool through the gastrointestinal system. Food sources include bananas, potatoes, dried beans, nuts, apples, oranges, and oatmeal.
- **Insoluble fiber** changes little with the digestive process and increases the speed of stool through the colon, so too much can result in diarrhea. Food sources of insoluble fiber include wheat bran, whole grains, seeds, skins of fruits, vegetables, and nuts.

# Wound and Skin Assessment

## Assessing Etiologic Factors

Wounds should be evaluated for **etiology** (the origin of the wound) during the initial assessment to ensure proper treatment. Wounds can arise from a number of different etiologies:

- **Pressure**: Wounds that occur over bony prominences, such as the heels and coccyx, may be related to pressure, shear, or friction. The skin should be carefully examined for discolorations or changes in texture that might indicate compromise.
- **Arterial**: Arterial insufficiency is associated with a decrease in pedal pulses, and cool atrophic (shiny, dry) skin. It may result in small punctate-type ulcers, frequently on the dorsum of foot.
- **Venous stasis**: A decrease in venous circulation often results in hemoglobin leaking into the tissues of the lower leg, causing a brown discoloration. Tissue is often edematous, and ulcers are most common near the medial malleolus.
- **Diabetic neuropathy/ischemia**: Neuropathy can result in a lack of sensation to pain so that injuries to the feet may go unnoticed. Diabetes may also cause damage to small vessels, resulting in ischemia that can lead to ulcerations.
- **Trauma**: Injuries resulting from accidents or other types of trauma may vary considerably with some resulting in extensive damage to bones, tissues, organs, and circulation. Additionally, the wounds may be contaminated. Each wound must be assessed individually for multiple factors.

- **Burns**: Burn wounds may be chemical, thermal, or electric and should be assessed according to the area, the percentage of the body burned, and the depth of the burn.
- **Infection**: An infected surgical or wound site can result in pain, edema, cellulitis, drainage, erosion of the sutures and ulceration of the tissue. Surgical sites must be assessed carefully and laboratory findings reviewed.

## Assessing Oxygenation

Assessment of oxygenation includes:

- **Color**: Impaired oxygenation may cause a change in the color of the skin, including pallor and cyanosis, especially in the extremities and about the mouth and nose. Individuals with darker skin may take on a gray, ashy appearance.
- **Respiratory rate**: As oxygenation falls, air hunger may occur with the patient becoming increasingly dyspneic.
- **Oxygen saturation**: While normal oxygen saturation is greater than 95%, as oxygenation is impaired, the level may fall below 92%. Oxygen saturation loses accuracy if the level falls below 80%, so blood gas analysis should be done in those cases.
- **Blood gas analysis**: $PO_2$ should be greater than 80 mmHg but may fall below 60 mmHg (indicating hypoxemia).
- **Altered mental status**: As oxygen levels fall, the patient may exhibit confusion.
- **Blood lactate level**: Results higher than 2 mEq/L indicate impaired tissue oxygenation.

## Neurological/Neurovascular Assessment

Neurological/neurovascular assessment includes:

- **Cranial nerve assessment**: Assess cranial nerves I through VII.
- **Inspection of muscles**: Determine if they are of normal size, strength, and tone and equal bilaterally. Note any involuntary movements (twitches, tremors).
- **Balance assessment**: Assess gait, Romberg test (feet together, eyes closed for 20 seconds), rapid alternating movements, finger-to-finger or finger-to-nose, and heel-to-shin test.
- **Sensory assessment**: Assess spinothalamic tracts for perception of pain, temperature, and light touch. Assess posterior column tract with vibration, position, fine touch, stereognosis, graphesthesia, two-point discrimination, extinction, and point location testing.
- **Reflexes**: Assess deep tendon reflexes (biceps reflex, triceps reflex, brachioradialis reflex, quadriceps reflex, Achilles reflex, and clonus) and superficial cutaneous reflexes (abdominal reflexes, cremasteric reflex, and plantar reflex).
- **Developmental status**: An age-appropriate assessment should determine if the patient's development is within normal parameters. Older adults may exhibit slower response times than younger adults and may exhibit tremors and unsteady gait related to age changes.

## Elements of Wound Assessment

### *Location and Size*

**Wound location** should be described in terms of anatomic position using landmarks (such as sternal notch, umbilicus, lateral malleolus), correct medical terminology, and directional terms:

- Anterior (in front)
- Posterior (behind)
- Superior (above)
- Inferior (below)

**Wound size** should be carefully described through actual measurement rather than association (the size of a dime). Measurements should be done with a disposable ruler in millimeters or centimeters. The current standard for measurement:

$$\text{length} \times \text{width} \times \text{depth} = \text{dimension}$$

However, a clear description requires more detail. The measurement should be done at the greatest width and greatest length. More than two measurements may be needed if the wound is very irregularly shaped. The depth of the wound should be measured by inserting a sterile applicator and grasping or marking the applicator at skin level and then measuring the length below. Ideally, the wound should be photographed as well, following protocols for photography.

### *Wound Bed Tissue*

Wound bed tissue should be described as completely as possible, including color and general appearance:

- **Granulation tissue** is slightly granular in appearance and deep pink to bright red and moist, bleeding easily if disturbed.
- **Clean non-granular tissue** is smooth and deep pink or red and is not healing.
- **Hypergranulation** is excessive, soft, flaccid granulating tissue that is raised above the level of the periwound tissue, preventing proper epithelization, and may reflect excess moisture in the wound.
- **Epithelization** should appear at wound edges first and then eventually cover the wound. It is dry and light pink or violet in color.
- **Slough** is necrotic tissue that is viscous, soft, and yellow-gray in appearance and adheres to the wound.
- **Eschar** is hard dark brown or black leathery necrotic tissue that accumulates with death of the tissue.

### *Wound Margins*

Wound margins and the tissue surrounding the wound should be described carefully and with correct terminology:

- **Color** should be described using color descriptions and such terms as blanched, erythematous (red), or ecchymosed (purple, green, yellow).
- **Skin texture** may be normal, indurated (hardened), or edematous (swollen). Note if there is cellulitis or maceration evident.
- **Wound edges** may be diffuse (without clear margins), well defined, or rolled. A healing ridge may be evident if granulation has begun. Note if the wound is closed (as with a surgical incision) or open (as with dehiscence or ulcerations). Note if wound edges are attached or unattached (indicating undermining or tunneling).
- **Tunneling or undermining** should be assessed by probing the wound margins with a moist sterile cotton applicator, using clock face locators (toward the head is 12 o'clock, for example). Tunneling may be described as extending from 3 o'clock to 4 o'clock. A large area is usually described as undermining. The size should be measured or estimated as closely as possible.

### *Distribution, Drainage, and Odor*

**Distribution** of lesions should be clearly delineated if there is more than one lesion over an area. The arrangement of the lesions can be helpful for diagnosis and treatments.

- Linear (in a line)
- Satellites (small lesions around a larger one)
- Diffuse (scattered freely over an area)

**Drainage** may vary considerably from nothing at all to copious outpourings of discharge.

- Serous drainage is usually clear to slightly yellow.
- Serosanguineous drainage is a combination of serous drainage and blood.
- Sanguineous drainage is bloody.
- Purulent discharge may be thick and milky, yellow, brownish, or green, depending upon the infective agent.

**Odor** requires more subjective assessment, but the odor and type of discharge together can provide useful information. Some infective agents, such as *Pseudomonas*, produce distinctive odors, which may be described in various ways: musty, foul, sweet.

### *Wound Exudate*

Wound exudate is fluid found in the wound, consisting of blood serum, debris from cells, bacteria, and white blood cells (leukocytes). **Wound exudate** can occur in small to large amounts and, depending on the presence of an organism, may be colored clear or pale yellow (serous), pink or blood tinged (serosanguineous), red (sanguineous), or white/yellow (purulent pus). Consistency can range from thin to milky to thick, and odor may occur. When fluid covers less than one-third of the dressing, it is termed small in amount. Fluid covering one-third to two-thirds of the dressing is considered moderate, and fluid covering over two-thirds of the surface of the dressing is considered large. The presence of exudate can occur when the wound is left untreated or when venous insufficiency, congestive heart failure, malnutrition, kidney or liver disease, or infection is present. One must remember that some odors may be caused by the reaction of the wound fluid on the dressing. Odor can also be caused when the dressing is not changed often enough.

### *Wound Measurement*

Wound measurement determines the progress of healing and must be done accurately and consistently each time. When the wound is a surgical one, it is sufficient to measure length and width, but depth is important for pressure injuries:

- One should use millimeters or centimeters, not inches, in measurement.
- Linear measurement utilizes a plastic or paper ruler marked in centimeters, measuring the greatest length and the greatest width or making the measurements perpendicular to each other. This is the most common method, but it doesn't take into account the shape of the wound and can overestimate the surface area involved when the measurement is multiplied length by width.
- The outline of the wound may also be traced onto an acetate sheet marked in centimeters and the surface area determined by counting the squares.
- Depth is then determined by inserting a sterile moist cotton applicator into the deepest part of the wound.
- Undermining and tunneling tracts are measured in the same manner.

**Measuring Wounds**

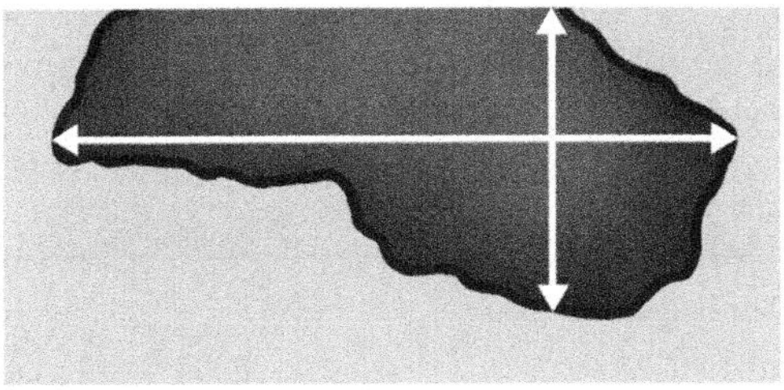

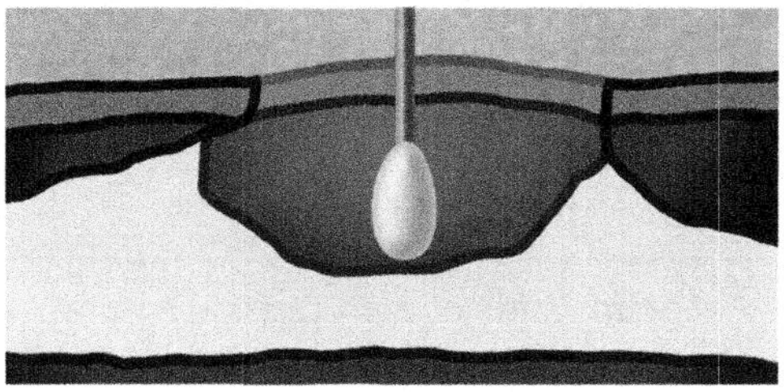

Basic Care and Comfort

### Digital Methods of Wound Measurement

A number of different tools are available for measuring and monitoring wounds using digital equipment. These tools are often more accurate than manual measurements and maintain a historical record that can be easily accessed to track changes. Most tools are software applications that can be loaded onto a smartphone (camera-enabled) or iPad, requiring only that the healthcare provider position the device and take photos. Some programs, such as WoundDesk (Digital MedLab) are primarily management software to improve documentation, but others, such as Scout (WoundVision) provide visual and infrared imaging and both physical and physiological (blood flow, metabolic activity) monitoring. Another program, WoundZoom, contains a 3D sensor and can provide an image of the wound that includes the length, depth, and breadth. Swift Skin and Wound, a widely-used program, offers a wound management system (Swift App for measurement, Swift HealX to calibrate size, color, lighting, and Swift dashboard to display data) that includes wound measurement, imaging, and tracking.

### *Assessment of Periwound Environment*

The periwound environment includes the area around the wound and is an important part of wound assessment:

- Note signs of inflammation such as warmth, erythema, and edema.
- Palpate the skin for firmness and fluctuation that may indicate a subcutaneous abscess.
- Look for signs of breakdown from tape.
- Observe for signs of pale, moist, soft skin that may be maceration caused by exudate from the wound.
- Check the skin for flakiness or evidence of dryness, as the surrounding skin may be too dry if the dressing wicks the moisture out of the skin.
- Examine the skin for signs of circulatory impairment, such as abnormal hair distribution, rubor, or pallor.
- Note evidence of undermining or tunneling that extends under the tissue.

### *Documentation of the Wound Assessment*

The care provider can use the acronym **ASSESSMENT** to help document the thorough assessment of a wound:

- **A**natomically locate the wound on the body and include the age of the wound
- **S**ize of the wound in centimeters: length, width, and depth, including shape and stage of the wound
- **S**inus tracts, tunneling, fistulas, and undermining at the edges
- **E**xudate color, amount, and consistency
- **S**epsis present in the wound or systemically
- **S**urrounding skin color, edema, status
- **M**argins of the wound, attachment to the wound bed, rolling, presence of maceration
- **E**rythema, presence of epithelialization or eschar
- **N**ecrotic tissue presence, odor of wound, visible blood vessels
- **T**issue of wound bed, amount of granulation present, wound tenderness, tension, and temperature

## Assessment Characteristics of Arterial, Neuropathic, and Venous Ulcers

The assessment process is important in delineating between the arterial, neuropathic, or venous origin of the ulcer. Characteristics of each must be known and closely examined:

**Location**

- **Arterial**: Ends of toes, pressure points, traumatic nonhealing wounds
- **Neuropathic**: Plantar surface, metatarsal heads, toes, and sides of feet
- **Venous**: Between knees and ankles, medial malleolus

**Wound Bed**

- **Arterial**: Pale, necrotic
- **Neuropathic**: Red (or ischemic)
- **Venous**: Dark red, fibrinous slough

**Exudate**

- **Arterial**: Slight amount, infection common
- **Neuropathic**: Moderate to large amounts, infection common
- **Venous**: Moderate to large amounts

**Wound Perimeter**

- **Arterial**: Circular, well-defined
- **Neuropathic**: Circular, well-defined, often with callous formation
- **Venous**: Irregular, poorly-defined

**Pain**

- **Arterial**: Very painful
- **Neuropathic**: Pain often absent because of reduced sensation
- **Venous**: Pain varies

**Skin**

- **Arterial**: Pale, friable, shiny, and hairless, with dependent rubor and elevational pallor
- **Neuropathic**: Ischemic signs (as in arterial) may be evident with co-morbidity
- **Venous**: Brownish discoloration of ankles and shin, edema common

**Pulses**

- **Arterial**: Weak or absent
- **Neuropathic**: Present and palpable, diminished in neuroischemic ulcers
- **Venous**: Present and palpable

## Assessing for Wound Complications

### *Chronic Inflammation*

Chronic inflammation of a wound can last for months, delaying wound healing. The immune system may fail to adequately phagocytose debris and dead tissue in the wound and fight infection, and wound care may be inadequate, such as failure to debride the wound or clear infection. Chronic inflammation is caused by debris, necrotic tissue, repeated injury to the wound, and continued effects of histamine release from mast cells. The blood vessels stay dilated, causing warmth, redness, and swelling. The wound-encircling erythema is a ring of redness in light skin or a ring of darkness in dark skin. Pain may be absent or intense if there is infection or arterial vascular disease present. Necrotic tissue may extend over all or part of the wound bed and may be light or dark in color and hard, soft, or stringy. Exudate may be thick, yellow, brown, or green with an odor. The exudate should be cleansed from the wound so that the odor of the wound bed itself can be determined.

### *UNDERMINING*

Undermining occurs at the edges of a wound and may result from shear injuries. The tissues pull away from the base of the wound and a cavity occurs under the intact skin of the wound periphery. The opening of the wound is thus smaller than the area of tissue damage beneath the surface of the skin surrounding the wound. The degree of undermining should be documented by using the face of the clock to describe the location of the undermining in relation to the opening and by recording the depth of the undermining into surrounding tissues by gently probing with a moist sterile cotton applicator. There are two basic **types of undermining**:

- **Initial**: This is related to discharge of liquefied necrotic tissue, leaving undermining that circles the wound. The wound usually lacks signs of epithelialization.
- **Late**: This is related to external pressure (after discharge undermining), and leaves more localized undermining, often in the direction of a bony prominence. The wound shows signs of epithelialization in non-undermined areas.

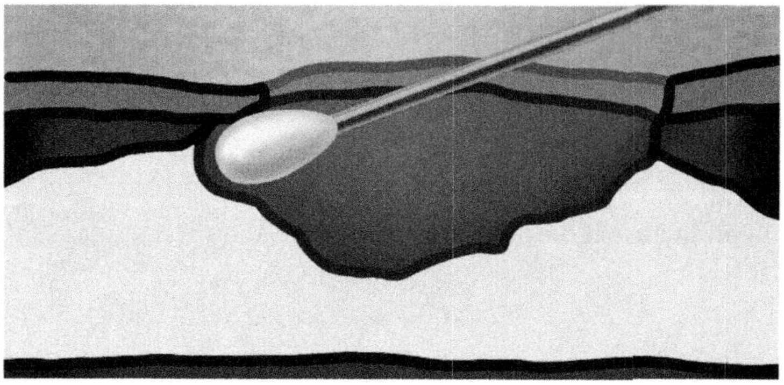

### *WOUND TUNNELING*

Wound tunneling is a form of undermining that creates a tract that leads away from the wound through subcutaneous tissues between muscles. Tunneling occurs when the fascia that holds muscles together in bundles is cut. Tunneling must be measured with a sterile moist cotton applicator and documented as to depth and width, using the clock face to describe location (3 to 4 o'clock) and then packed loosely to stimulate the healing process. If tunneling ends in a dead space, infection of the wound can progress through the tunnel to cause development of abscess. Tunneling may be caused by infection, pressure that causes tissue necrosis (over bony prominences), or foreign bodies, such as a suture or dressing material left in the wound. It is important for tunnels to heal prior to wound closure to prevent abscess formation, necessitating surgical drainage later. Tunnels are common in surgical wounds in which dehiscence occurs, and the tunnels can join together to form sinus tracts.

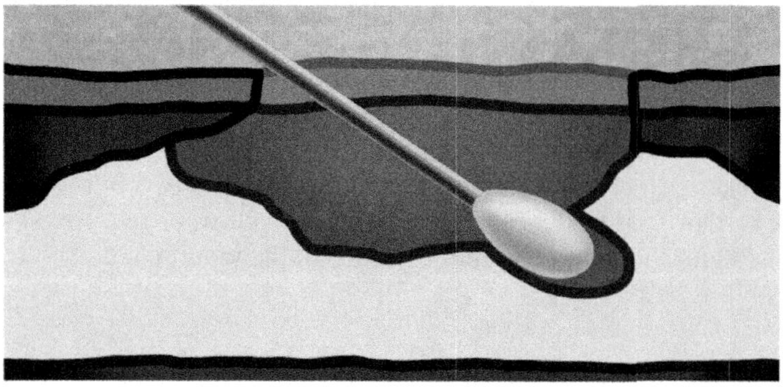

# Wound Classification Systems

## Classification of Wounds by Cause

Wounds can be classified in various ways. The most common classification of wounds is that according to cause:

- **Vascular wounds:** Vascular changes can result in wounds that occur most commonly in the lower extremities, such as those that result from arterial insufficiency and ischemia, those that relate to changes in the lymphatic system, and those related to venous insufficiency.
- **Neuropathic wounds:** Neuropathic changes that occur with chronic diseases, such as diabetes, and chronic alcoholism can decrease sensation and circulation, resulting in ulcerations.
- **Pressure injuries:** Shear friction and pressure, especially over bony prominences such as the sacral area and heels, causes erosion of the tissue.
- **Traumatic wounds:** Trauma often results in contaminated wounds.
- **Surgical wounds:** Surgery can result in wounds that are originally contaminated or originally clean, depending upon the type of surgery and the reason.
- **Infected wounds:** Inflammation and infection may result in deteriorating wounds or fistulas.
- **Self-inflicted wounds:** Vary widely, from minor cuts to traumatic gunshot wounds.
- **Dysfunctional healing wounds:** Hypergranulation/keloid formation can change the character of a wound and prevent adequate healing.

## Modified Wagner Ulcer Classification System for Foot Ulcers

The modified Wagner Ulcer Classification System divides foot ulcers into six grades, based on lesion depth, osteomyelitis or gangrene, infection, ischemia, and neuropathy:

- **Grade 0**: At risk but no open ulcers
- **Grade 1**: Superficial ulcer, extending into subcutaneous tissue; superficial infection with or without cellulitis
- **Grade 2**: Full-thickness ulcer to tendon or joint with no abscess or osteomyelitis
- **Grade 3**: Full-thickness ulcer that may extend to bone with abscess, osteomyelitis, or sepsis of joint and may include deep plantar infections, abscesses, fasciitis, or infections of tendon sheath
- **Grade 4**: Gangrene in one area of foot, but the foot is salvageable
- **Grade 5**: Gangrene of entire foot, requiring amputation

While this classification system is useful in predicting outcomes, it does not contain information about the size of the ulcer or the type of infection, so it should be only one part of an assessment, as more detailed information is needed to fully evaluate an ulcer.

## University of Texas Diabetic Foot Wound Classification System

The University of Texas created a wound classification system to account for the shortcomings of the Wagner classification system. Although the Wagner system is still used today, it has limitations at predicting outcome after grade 3 and lacks certain aspects of the wound assessment, making it less comprehensive in nature. The University of Texas wound classification system considers the wound's depth and infection status, as well as the presence of peripheral arterial occlusive disease, and evaluates the wound by both grade (0 through 3) and Stage (A, B, C, or D), which are defined as follows:

| Stage | Grade 0 | Grade 1 | Grade 2 | Grade 3 |
|---|---|---|---|---|
| A | Lesion (pre- or post-ulcerative) is completely epithelialized | Ulcer is superficial and does not involve tendon or bone | Ulcer penetrates to the tendon | Ulcer penetrates to the bone/joint space |
| B | Infection present | Infection present | Infection present | Infection present |
| C | Ischemia present | Ischemia present | Ischemia present | Ischemia present |
| D | Both infection and ischemia present | Both infection and ischemia present | Both infection and ischemia present | Both infection and ischemia present |

## S(AD) SAD Classification System

S(AD) SAD stands for Size (Area and Depth), Sepsis, Arteriopathy, and Denervation. The S(AD) SAD classification system for lower-extremity neuropathic disease is one of many that builds upon the original or modified Wagner classification system and assigns a 0-3 grade based on 5 categories: area, depth, sepsis, arteriopathy, and denervation.

- **Grade 0**: No pathology is evident.
- **Grade 1**: Ulcer is <10 $mm^2$, involving subcutaneous tissue with superficial slough or exudate, diminution or absence of pulses, and reduced sensation.
- **Grade 2**: Ulcer is 10-30 $mm^2$, extending to tendon, joint, capsule, or periosteum with cellulitis, absence of pulses except for neuropathy dominant ulcers that have palpable pedal pulses.
- **Grade 3**: Ulcer is >30 $mm^2$, extending to bones and/or joints; seen with osteomyelitis, gangrene, and Charcot's foot.

This grading system is useful, but as with most other classification systems, it doesn't provide a simple way to distinguish those wounds that follow an atypical pattern or may be consistent with the grade in some areas and inconsistent in others.

## CEAP Classification for Chronic Venous Disorders

### Clinical (C0-C6)

- 0: No apparent venous disease
- 1: Telangiectasia/reticular veins
- 2: Varicose veins
- 3: Edema
- 4: Skin changes
- 5: Healed ulcer
- 6: Active ulcer

**Etiologic**

- $E_C$: Congenital
- $E_P$: Primary
- $E_S$: Secondary
- $E_N$: No cause identified

**Anatomic distribution**

- $A_S$: Superficial veins
- $A_D$: Deep veins
- $A_P$: Perforating veins
- $A_N$: No location identified

**Pathophysiological classification**

- $P_R$: Reflux
- $P_O$: Obstruction
- $P_{R,O}$: Reflux and obstruction
- $P_N$: No pathophysiology identified

## Staging System for Pressure Injuries

Pressure-related injuries result from pressure with or without shear and/or friction over bony prominences. The National Pressure Injury Advisory Panel developed a staging system to ensure that definitions for pressure injuries were standardized:

- **Suspected deep tissue injury**: Skin discolored, intact or blood blister
- **Stage I**: Intact skin with non-blanching reddened area
- **Stage II**: Abrasion or blistered area without slough but with partial-thickness skin loss
- **Stage III**: Deep tissue injury with exposed subcutaneous tissue; tunneling or undermining may be evident with or without slough or epibole (rolling inward of wound edge)
- **Stage IV**: Deep tissue injury, full thickness, with necrosis into muscle, bone, tendons, and/or joints
- **Unstageable**: Eschar and/or slough prevents staging prior to debridement

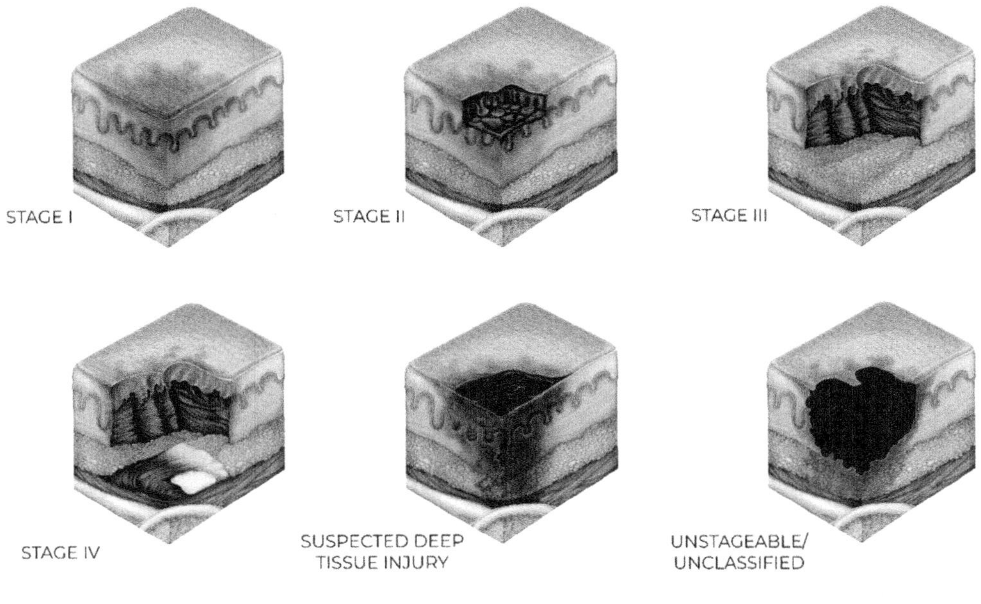

# Pressure Injuries

## Assessment of Pressure Injuries

When assessing a tissue injury, it is necessary to determine whether it is a pressure injury or non-pressure injury because the treatment protocol may vary depending upon whether the injury is caused by pressure, venous or arterial insufficiency, or neuropathic disorders. The clinical basis for this determination should be clearly outlined.

- The pressure injury should be classified according to the stage and the characteristics, including size (length, width, and depth).
- Pain associated with the pressure injury should be described.
- Photographs should be taken if a protocol is in place.
- Pressure injuries should be monitored daily and any changes carefully documented.
- The injury should be evaluated for signs of infection.

It is important to differentiate between colonization, which is very common, and infection, which usually presents with symptoms such as periwound erythema, induration, and increased pain as well as delayed healing of the wound. Wound culture and blood tests should be done if there are indications of infection. Treatment should be determined according to the characteristics of the wound.

## Causes of Pressure Injuries

### *Pressure Intensity, Pressure Duration, and Tissue Tolerance*

**Pressure injuries** are caused primarily by pressure, but there are numerous additional considerations:

- **Pressure intensity***:* Capillary closing pressure (10–32 mmHg) is the minimal pressure needed to collapse capillaries, reducing tissue perfusion. This pressure can be easily exceeded in the sitting or supine position if weight is not shifted.
- **Duration of pressure**: Low pressure for long periods and high pressure for short periods can both result in pressure injuries.
- **Tissue tolerance***:* The tissue tolerance is the ability of the skin to tolerate and redistribute pressure, preventing anoxia. Both extrinsic and intrinsic factors can affect tissue tolerance. Extrinsic factors include shear (the skin stays in place but the underlying tissue slides), friction (moving the skin against bedding or other objects), and moisture. Intrinsic factors include poor nutrition, advanced age, low blood pressure, stress, smoking, and low body temperature.

### *Shear and Friction*

**Shear** occurs when the skin stays in place and the underlying tissue in the deep fascia over the bony prominences stretches and slides, damaging vessels and tissue and often resulting in undermining. Shear is one of the most common causes of pressure injuries, which are often described as pressure ulcers but are technically somewhat different, although the effects of shearing are often combined with pressure. The most common cause of shear is elevation of the head of the bed over 30°. Friction against the sheets holds the skin in place while the body slides down the bed, resulting in pressure and damage in the sacrococcygeal area. The underlying vessels are damaged and thrombosed, leading to undermining and deep ulceration.

**Friction** is a significant cause of pressure injuries because it acts with gravity to cause shear. Friction by itself results only in damage to the epidermis and dermis, such as abrasions or denudement referred to as "sheet burn." Friction and pressure can combine, however, to form tissue injury.

### *Measures to Control Shear and Friction*

Because **shear** and **friction** are primary factors in the development of pressure injuries, measures to reduce them are essential:

- The head of the bed should never be elevated more than 30°; however, bed-bound patients may not be able to feed themselves at this angle. If the bed is elevated higher, the patient should be carefully positioned, using a pull sheet or overhead trapeze to make sure the patient is at the right position. The bed should be lowered as soon as possible.

*Note*: Elevating the foot of the bed to prevent sliding and shear simply increases pressure to the sacrococcygeal area, solving one problem by creating another.

- Making sure that the skin is dry; using fine cornstarch-based powders may help prevent the skin from "sticking" to the sheets.
- Pull sheets or mechanical lifting devices should be used to lift, move, or transfer the patient.
- Medical treatments may reduce restlessness.
- Heel and elbow protectors provide protection.

## Management of Pressure Injuries

### *Measures to Promote Mobility*

**Mobility** is a problem for many patients with pressure injuries because their restricted mobility is often the cause of the injury in the first place. However, promoting mobility to the extent possible improves circulation, aids healing, and decreases risk of developing further pressure injury:

- Bed-bound patients must be repositioned on a scheduled basis and should receive passive ROM exercises and active bed exercises if tolerated daily. The patient's head should be elevated only to 30° for short periods of time.
- Patients with limited mobility should be evaluated by physical and occupational therapists in order to develop an individualized plan for activities. Patients may need assistive devices, such as walkers, canes, or wheelchairs. Because the wound must be protected without compromise to circulation, the amount and type of mobility or exercises must be designed with respect to the area and stage of the pressure injury as well as underlying pathology or co-morbid conditions.

### *Measures to Control Fecal Incontinence*

**Control of fecal incontinence** is necessary to prevent deterioration of tissue that can increase the risk of pressure injuries and to prevent contamination of existing pressure injuries:

- Assess incontinence to determine cause and whether it is temporary, related to health problems, or chronic.
- Determine the type of incontinence:
  - Passive, in which the person is unaware.
  - Urge, which is the inability to retain stool.
  - Seepage, after a bowel movement or around a blockage.
- Use medications as indicated to control diarrhea or constipation.
- Place on a bowel-training regimen with scheduled bowel movements, using suppositories, stool softeners, and bulk formers as indicated, according to cause of incontinence. Use skin moisture barriers and absorbent pads or adult briefs as needed.
- Modify diet as needed with foods to control diarrhea or constipation.
- Ensure adequate fluid intake.
- Consider fecal pouches or fecal containment devices if incontinence cannot be otherwise controlled.

### *MEASURES TO CONTROL URINARY INCONTINENCE*

**Control of urinary incontinence** is necessary to prevent deterioration of the tissue that can increase the risk of pressure injuries:

- Assess incontinence to determine cause and whether it is temporary, related to health problems, or chronic.
- A temporary Foley catheter may be used in some cases while tissue heals, but long-term use is contraindicated because of the danger of infections.
- Medications may be indicated to treat urinary infections or frequency. Scheduled toileting with reinforcement may help to decrease incidence.
- Use absorbent pads or adult briefs that wick liquid away from the body, and establish a regular schedule for changing.
- Cleanse soiled skin with no-rinse wipes, as they are less drying to skin than soap and water.
- Use skin moisture barrier ointments to protect skin from urine.
- Use protective and support devices as needed.
- Avoid positioning on existing pressure injuries.

## Pressure Redistribution

### TISSUE INTERFACE PRESSURES

Tissue interface pressure is the amount of pressure exerted on the body by a surface that the body is lying or sitting on. Small sensors are placed between the patient and the surface to measure pressures in localized areas. The measurement is important to assess whether the pressure is great enough to occlude the capillaries in the area, increasing the risk of tissue ischemia and injury formation. The force that closes capillaries is 12-32 mmHg. This range is used as a comparison along with patient condition, skin condition, nutrition, and other factors to decide whether a support surface relieves enough pressure in a specific location on that particular patient. However, research has not demonstrated that there is a specific threshold at which pressure will cause harm, so the tissue interface pressure should only be used as a guide and not a substitute for observation.

### PRESSURE INJURY PREVENTION

Every patient should be assessed for **risk factors** for pressure injuries. These include immobility, inactivity, moisture and incontinence, poor nutritional state and intake, friction and shear, decreased sensation, mental status changes, fragile skin condition, and certain medications. Tools are available for assessing patient risk for pressure injuries, including the Gosnell Scale and the Braden Scale. Use of these scales provides consistency in assessment from patient to patient and can be used to assess changes in risk level as a result of interventions. Once the risk factors are defined, prevention can concentrate on alleviating these factors. Interventions are designed, and patient and family teaching is performed. Interventions are specific for each patient, disease status, and individual situation. Several solutions for risk factors are possible, and solutions must be individualized for the patient.

### *Turning and Repositioning to Reduce Pressure*

Measures to reduce pressure include turning and repositioning.

- Goals for repositioning and a turning schedule of at least every 2 hours should be established for each individual, with documentation required.
- Devices, such as pillows or foam, should be used to correctly position patients so that bony prominences are protected and not in direct contact with each other.
- Re-position patients carefully to avoid friction or shear.
- Assistive devices should be used if necessary to move patients.
- Use chairs of correct size and height and use pressure relieving devices for the seats.
- Limit chair time for those who are acutely ill to no more than 2 hours.
- Patients should be taught or reminded to redistribute weight every 15 minutes. A timer may be used to remind patients.
- Use the 30° lateral position rather than the 90° side-lying position.

#### Positioning Strategies in the Bed and Chair

Passive repositioning should be performed on the patient in both the bed and the chair:

- **Bed**: When positioned on his or her side, the patient should be turned to a 30° laterally-inclined position rather than a 90° side-lying position, which puts pressure on the trochanter. Two people should use a turn sheet, draw sheet, and pillows to pull up in bed, turn, and position the patient. Pillows should be placed under the head, under the legs to keep heels off the bed, behind the back, and between the ankles and knees.
- **Chair**: Patients in chairs need repositioning hourly as well. The patient should be assisted to stand and sit down again. Small changes in seated patients include changing leg position from dependent to elevated. The body should be in proper alignment, using pillows or cushions if needed. Patients who are cognizant and able to shift position should be instructed to do so every 15 minutes while seated.

### *Use of Support Surfaces to Prevent Pressure Injuries*

A support surface redistributes pressure to prevent pressure injuries and reduce shear and friction. There are various types of support surfaces for beds, examining tables, operating tables, and chairs. General use guidelines include:

- Pressure redistribution support surfaces should be used in beds, operating tables, and examining tables for at-risk individuals.
- Patients with multiple injuries or with stage II to stage IV injuries require support surfaces.
- Chairs should have gel or air support surfaces to redistribute pressure for chair bound patients, critically ill patients, and those who cannot move independently.
- Support surface material should provide at least an inch of support under areas to be protected when in use to prevent bottoming out. (Check by placing hand palm-up under overlay below the pressure point.)
- Static support surfaces are appropriate for patients who can change position without increasing pressure to an injury.
- Dynamic support surfaces are needed for those who need assistance to move or when static pressure devices provide less than an inch of support.

### CATEGORIES OF SUPPORT SURFACES

There are five elements that are used to categorize support surfaces:

- **Pressure redistribution** may be preventive (≤32 mmHg, but not consistently) or therapeutic (≤32 mmHg, consistently). Preventive devices are used for those at risk or with stage I or II injuries. Therapeutic devices are used for those with stage III and IV pressure injuries.
- **Device forms** are varied and may supplement or replace existing equipment. Devices include chair cushions, mattress overlays, pressure-reducing mattresses, and specialty bed systems used in place of traditional hospital beds.
- **Active support surfaces** are powered, requiring attachment to an electrical motor for utilization, (dynamic) or non-powered (static).
- **Medium** may be different types of foam, water, gels, or air.
- **Medicare reimbursement group**:
    - Group 1: Used as a preventive measure and includes overlays and mattresses.
    - Group 2: Used as a therapeutic measure and includes non-powered and powered overlays and mattresses.
    - Group 3: Used as a therapeutic measure and includes air-fluidized beds.

### FUNCTIONS OF SUPPORT SURFACES

Support surfaces are designed for a number of functions:

- **Pressure redistribution** occurs through *immersion* (spreading the pressure out) and *envelopment* (conforming to shape without increasing pressure). The aim is to reduce pressure on the skin to less than the capillary closing pressure (<32 mmHg), but lower pressures may be necessary for elderly patients. *Interface pressure measurement* is measurement of the pressure exerted between the body and the support surface. This measurement is currently used to evaluate the pressure redistribution efficiency of devices although it has not been demonstrated through research that this measurement can predict clinical performance. Thin, flexible sensors are placed under the support surface and the patient and computerized readings indicate if the support surface is adequate. A number of new measurement devices are now marketed that show colored-coded computerized pictures demonstrating different levels of pressure.
- **Temperature control** is important because temperature increases can lead to skin breakdown. Skin temperature relates to the specific heat of the material in the support surface. Specific heat (the ability to conduct heat) varies considerably from one type of material to another. Air has a low specific heat, and water has a high specific heat. Material with high specific heat may conduct heat away from the body, decreasing skin temperature.
- **Moisture control** prevents moisture damage to skin, but there are wide ranges of materials in use in support surfaces. Some materials, such as rubber or plastic, may increase perspiration and moisture, while some porous materials, such as some foams, may reduce perspiration.
- **Friction/shear control** is more difficult to achieve although some surface coverings, such as those with Gortex, are purposely slick to decrease friction. However, proper positioning, lifting, and repositioning still must be done.

# Alternative, Complementary, and Non-Pharmacologic Interventions

## Complementary Therapy

Complementary therapies are often used, either alone or in conjunction with conventional medical treatment. These methods should be included if this is what the patient/family chooses, empowering the family to take control of their plan of care. Complementary therapies vary widely and most can easily be incorporated. The **National Center for Complementary and Alternative Medicine** recognizes the following:

- **Whole medical systems**: Chinese medicine (acupressure, acupuncture), naturopathic and homeopathic medicines, and Ayurveda
- **Mind-body medicine**: Prayer, artistic creation, music and dance therapy, biofeedback, focused relaxation, and visualization
- **Biological medicine**: Aromatherapy, herbs, plants, trees, vitamins and minerals, and dietary supplements
- **Manipulation**: Massage and spinal manipulation
- **Energy medicines**: Magnets, electric current, pulsed fields, Reiki, qi gong, and laying-on of the hands

### *Precautions*

The use of alternative and complementary therapies should be thoroughly discussed by patients and their physician. Patients should be encouraged to use therapies that are shown to have a beneficial, complementary effect on conventional medical treatment. These therapies include the use of massage, superficial stimulation, relaxation, distraction, hypnosis, and guided imagery.

- Encourage patients to practice the techniques until they are proficient in their use to give them a chance to prove their value.
- Teach the patient how the therapies work to encourage the patient to believe in them to contribute to the placebo effect.
- Caution the patient against abandoning current medical treatment.
- Inform the patient of the high cost of alternate therapies that can divert needed funds and result in little or no benefit.
- Provide the patient with resources in the form of books, pamphlets, and informative websites that prove the results of scientific research so that they can evaluate alternative therapies for themselves.

## Whole Medical Systems

Whole medical systems are different philosophies and methods of explaining and treating health and illness. Some systems include:

- **Homeopathic medicine**: This European system uses small amounts of diluted herbs and supplements to help the body to recover from disease by stimulating an immune response.
- **Naturopathic medicine**: This is a European system that uses various natural means (herbs, massage, acupuncture) to support the natural healing forces of the body.
- **Chinese medicine**: Centers on restoring the proper flow of life forces within the body to cure disease by using herbs, acupressure and acupuncture, and meditation.
- **Ayurveda**: This is an Indian system that tries to bring the spirit into harmony with the mind and body to treat disease via yoga, herbs, and massage.

## Essential Oils

Essential oils (concentrated oils from plants) are either inhaled (aromatherapy) or diluted and applied to the skin. Essential oils are believed to reduce stress, aid sleep, improve dermatitis, and aid digestion. Commonly used essential oils include eucalyptus, lavender, lemon, peppermint, rosemary, rose, and tea tree. Oils may cause skin irritation when applied to the skin.

## Cupping

Cupping is an ancient practice still used in Southeast Asia and the Middle East to reduce pain, promote healing, and improve circulation. With dry cupping, cups are heated by placing something flammable (such as paper or herbs) inside the cup and setting it on fire to heat the cup, which is then immediately placed on the back along the meridians (generally on both sides of the spine) to form a vacuum that draws blood to the skin and causes circular bruises believed to heal that part of the body. Wet cupping includes leaving the heated cup in place for three minutes, removing it, making small cuts in the skin, and then applying suction cups again to withdraw blood. Cupping should be avoided in children under 4 and limited to short periods in older children.

## Acupuncture

Alternative systems of medical practice include acupuncture, homeopathy, and naturopathy. **Acupuncture**, an ancient Oriental practice, uses stainless steel or copper needles inserted into superficial skin layers at points where energy or life force called *qi* is believed to occur. The needles are supposed to restore balance and the flow of *qi*. The NIH has recognized the effectiveness of acupuncture for certain side effects of other cancer treatments, such as nausea, vomiting, and pain. However, there is limited scientific evidence to support the principles expounded. Acupuncturists are certified through either formal coursework or apprenticeships, and there is also board certification in this area for physicians. The needles used are classified as class II, which means they have manufacturing and labeling requirements.

## Herbal Remedies and Regulations

In the United States, most **herbal preparations** are classified as dietary supplements. That means that they are not subject to the same rigorous manufacturing, safety, efficacy, and control practices as pharmaceutical drugs. Herbal supplements are only governed by the Dietary Supplement and Health Education Act (DSHEA). As long as no specific disease treatment or curative claims are made, the supplement can be marketed without limitation and safety concerns must be pursued by the FDA after the fact. Nevertheless, some herbal remedies have been undergoing clinical trials in the U.S. to substantiate their health-enhancing or traditional/historical or international use claims. However, the focal point of these studies is still only on the effectiveness of the specific supplement. In Europe, there has been some movement toward greater regulation and licensing of herbal products, but not to the extent of formal drug regulations.

### *Toxicities Associated with Herbal Remedies*

Use of herbal preparations has been associated with a variety of **toxicities**, primarily in categories such as cardiovascular problems, hypersensitivity reactions, disorientation, gastrointestinal problems, and liver malfunction. Because quality control measures are relatively lax for these remedies, contamination from infectious agents and toxic metals can potentially cause other side effects. Many of these herbal medicines **interact with conventional drugs**, thus altering their pharmacodynamics. For example, St. John's wort, which is primarily used for depressive disorders or as a sedative, interacts with a wide range of traditional pharmacologic agents and suppresses their levels in the bloodstream. Kava kava, made from dried roots of a type of pepper bush, is used as a sedative, but it also has been associated with hepatic failure and via interactions with several other drugs can actually induce a comatose state. Ginseng is an Asian remedy touted for its curative properties in a number of diseases. However, it can react with steroidal drugs and induce shaking and manic episodes. These are just a few examples of potential dangers.

## Non-Pharmaceutical Pain Relief

Non-pharmaceutical methods to relieve pain that can be used exclusively or combined with medications include massage, heat, cold, electrical stimulation, distraction, relaxation, imagery, visualization, and music. Other **alternatives or adjuncts to pain medication** include hypnosis, magnets, acupuncture, acupressure, and therapeutic touch. Herbs, aromatherapy, reflexology, homeopathic medicine, and prayer may also be accepted by the patient. Any method that the patient feels may help that isn't harmful should be used to help get relief.

## MIND-BODY MEDICINE FOR PAIN AND DISEASE

Mind-body medicine (prayer, artistic creation, music and dance, biofeedback, relaxation, and visualization) can help distract people from pain or other symptoms if they are able to concentrate on the method. This can result in the inhibition of pain stimuli by stimulating the **descending control system**. These methods work if the patient can use them to create alternate sensations in the brain, but will not work if the patient is unable to concentrate due to intense pain.

Relaxation that occurs as a result of using these methods helps to reduce muscular tension that can make pain worse and reduces fatigue caused by chronic pain. Relaxation has been proven to be the most helpful after surgery. Postoperative patients report a greater feeling of control over their pain and tend to request fewer opioids to control pain. Biofeedback can help patients to recognize the feelings of both tension and relaxation and provide a way to indicate their success in managing muscle tension.

## USE OF VISUALIZATION

There are a number of methods used for **visualization** to reduce anxiety and promote healing. Some include audiotapes with guided imagery, such as self-hypnosis tapes, but the patient can be taught basic **techniques** that include:

- Sit or lie comfortably in a **quiet place** away from distractions.
- Concentrate on **breathing** while taking long slow breaths.
- **Close the eyes** to shut out distractions and create an image in the mind of the place or situation desired.
- Concentrate on that **image**, engaging as many senses as possible and imaging details.
- If the mind wanders, breathe deeply and **bring consciousness back** to the image or concentrate on breathing for a few moments and then return to the imagery.
- End with positive imagery.

Sometimes, patients are resistive at first or have a hard time maintaining focus, so **guiding** them through visualization for the first few times can be helpful.

## STIMULATION OF THE SKIN TO REDUCE PAIN

Skin, muscles, fascia, tendons, and the cornea contain **nociceptors** that are nerve endings that respond to painful stimuli. Massage, transcutaneous electrical nerve stimulation (TENS), heat and cold provide stimulation to other nerves that transfer only sensation, not pain. These signals block some of the transfer of the nociceptor impulses:

- **Massage** not only sends alternate sensation to the brain, but also results in relaxation that decreases the muscular tension that contributes to pain.
- **TENS** works well on incisional and neuromuscular pain by providing a gentle electrical stimulation that overrides the painful impulses from the area and may stimulate endorphins.
- **Heat therapy** increases blood flow and oxygen to promote healing and stimulates neural receptors, decreasing pain. Heat also helps loosen tense muscles that may be contributing to pain.
- **Cold therapy** decreases circulation and reduces production of chemicals related to inflammation, thereby reducing pain.

## Temperature-Controlled Therapies

### *Methods of Heating and Cooling*

There are a number of different ways to **heat** (thermotherapy) or **cool** (cryotherapy) for **healing**:

- **Conduction**: Conveyance of heat, cold, or electricity through direct contact with the skin, such as with hot baths, ice packs, and electrical stimulation.
- **Convection**: Indirect transmission of heat in a liquid or gas by circulation of heated particles, such as with whirlpools and paraffin soaks.
- **Conversion**: Heating that results from converting a form of energy into heat, such as with diathermy and ultrasound.
- **Evaporation**: Cooling caused by liquids that evaporate into gases on the skin with a resultant cooling effect, such as with perspiration or vapo-coolant sprays.
- **Radiation**: Heating that results from transfer of heat through light waves or rays, such as with infrared or ultraviolet light.

### *Superficial Heat*

Superficial heat with externally applied heat sources penetrates only the superficial layers of the skin (1–2 cm after about 30 minutes), but it is believed to relax deeper muscles by reflex, decrease pain, and increase metabolisms (2–3 times for every 10 °C increase in skin temperature). Therapeutic temperature range is 40–45 °C. **Superficial heat modalities** include:

- **Moist heat packs** placed on the skin and secured by several layers of towels to provide insulation, applied for 15–30 minutes.
- **Paraffin baths** (52–54 °C) with the hand, foot, or elbow dipped 7 times, cooling between dippings, and then wrapping with plastic and towels for 20 minutes.
- **Fluidotherapy** uses hot-air warmed (38.8–47.8 °C) cellulose particles into which a hand or foot is submerged for 20–30 minutes.

**Passive and active range of motion exercises** are done after superficial heat treatment. Contraindications include cardiac disease, peripheral vascular disease, malignant tumor, bleeding, and acute inflammation.

**Deep heat** differs from superficial heat in that the heat is generated internally using ultrasound, short wave, and microwave diathermy rather than applied to the surface of the skin. Deep heating has penetrance to 3–5 cm.

### *Shortwave Diathermy*

Shortwave diathermy uses electromagnetic waves (usually 27.12 MHz) to **increase the temperature in subcutaneous tissue** and is used along with passive and active range of motion exercises to **improve range** in painful conditions such as inflammation of the muscles, tendons, and bursae. The radio waves (eddy currents) are transmitted through a capacitor or inductor in a continuous or pulse waveform. Temperatures increase about 15 °C in fatty tissue and 4–6 °C in muscular tissue. Shortwave diathermy should not be used over any organs containing fluid, including the eyes, heart, head, or over pacemakers as the diathermy may disrupt the settings. Because this treatment may increase cardiac demand, it should be avoided in those with preexisting cardiac conditions and should not be used over malignancies. Additionally, it is contraindicated in areas of inflammation because heating the tissue increases inflammation. It cannot be used over prostheses as the metal may heat and damage tissue. Shortwave diathermy should avoid the epiphyses in children, as it may stimulate abnormal growth.

### *Microwave Diathermy*

Microwave diathermy is used similarly to shortwave diathermy but has a lower rate of heat increase and penetrance so it is used for muscles and joints near the surface rather than deep muscles, such as the hip. Heat is created by electromagnetic waves (usually 2.45 GHz or 915 MHz) and raises temperature in fatty tissues by about 10–12 °C and in muscular tissue by 3–4 °C. **Treatment** is usually given for 15–30 minutes per session and is followed by range of motion exercises (passive and active) to increase flexibility. Contraindications are similar to those of shortwave diathermy in that this treatment should not be used where increase in temperature may be detrimental, such as over organs containing fluid, areas of inflammation, and epiphyses of children. Additionally, it should not be used over prostheses or pacemakers and should be avoided in those with cardiac disease.

### *Cryotherapy*

Cryotherapy uses therapeutic cold treatment to cool the surface of the skin and underlying subcutaneous tissues in order to decrease blood flow, pain, and metabolism. Initially response to cold therapy causes **vasoconstriction** to occur within the first 15 minutes but if the tissues are cooled to -10 °C, then the body responds with **vasodilation**. Cryotherapy affects sensory response so the person will at first feel cold, which progresses to burning, aching, and finally to numbness and tingling. Treatment is usually given for 15–30 minutes. **Treatment modalities** include:

- **Ice packs** such as refrigerated gel packs (-5 °C) or plastic bags filled with water and ice chips are applied directly to the skin for 10–15 minutes for superficial cooling and 15–20 minutes for greater penetrance.
- A **towel dipped in ice and water slurry** is wrapped around limb to provide cold therapy, but this is best used only for emergency situations when ice packs are unavailable, as the towel must be changed frequently as the skin warms the towel rapidly.
- **Ice massage** is applied directly to the affected area for 5–10 minutes, usually rubbing the ice in circular motions on the skin surface. An ice massager is easily made by filled a paper cup with water and freezing it with a tongue depressor or Popsicle stick (to use as a handle) inserted into the center as the water starts to freeze. Then, the paper can be torn away from the bottom and sides when the ice is solid. Ice massage is often followed by friction massage.
- **Ice baths** (13–18 °C) are used for limbs, such as the lower leg, foot, or hand. The body part is immersed for 20 minutes.

Cryotherapy is usually followed by **active and passive exercises**. Contraindications include impaired circulation or sensation, cardiac disease, Raynaud's disease, and nerve trauma.

### *Whirlpool Baths*

Whirlpool baths are used to increase **circulation** and promote **healing**. They are tubs with a turbine that mixes air with water, which is pressurized and flows into the tub water to create turbulence. Tubs are usually large enough to accommodate the full body although smaller limb-sized whirlpool tubs are available. Water temperature is 95–104 °F (adjusted for the individual) and should be deep enough to completely submerge the affected part. The body part should be cleaned with soap and water before immersion or a shower taken. If the full body is treated, then the patient should wear a swimming suit. During the whirlpool treatment, the muscles relax from the heat and **range of motion exercises** can be done while in the water. Typically, treatments last about 20 minutes, but the patient should be monitored, especially for the first 5 minutes, as some people become lightheaded and can lose consciousness.

### *Contrast Baths*

Contrast baths (alternating hot and cold) are used in the sub-acute phase of healing (after edema begins to subside) for **strains and sprains**. It is believed that contrast baths increase the circulation and help to further decrease edema by a pumping action as the **vasoconstriction and vasodilation** alternate. Two containers are filled with water, one with hot and the other with cold. The hot water should be maintained at about 100–110 °F and the cold at 55–65 °F. The cycle begins and ends with immersion in cold water. Cold water immersions usually last about 1 minute and hot water immersions 4 minutes. Typically, the affected limb is immersed in the cold water for 1 minute, removed, and immediately immersed in hot water for 4 minutes. This cycle is repeated about 3–4 times.

### Therapeutic Ultrasound

Ultrasound treats soft-tissue injuries (such as myositis, bursitis, and tendinitis) with sound waves (frequency 0.8–3.0 MHz). Ultrasound utilizes a **piezoelectric crystal** that vibrates, producing sound waveforms, which are transmitted from the transducer through a gel substance into the tissue. The sound waves bounce off of the bone in an irregular pattern that causes an increase in temperature in the connective tissue, such as collagen fibers. Temperatures of the tissue may increase up to 43.5 °C, increasing metabolism in the area, neural conduction, as well as blood flow. Ultrasound is used to **decrease both contractures and scarring**. During treatment, the transducer passes in a circular motion about the skin surface, staying in contact with the gel medium. If a distal limb is submerged in water, the treatment is given with the head of the transducer 0.5–1.0 in from the skin surface. Treatment is followed by range of motion exercises, passive and active. Contraindications are similar to other heat-producing modalities and include peripheral vascular disease, but ultrasound may be used over metal prostheses.

### TENS

Transcutaneous electrical nerve stimulation (TENS) uses electrical stimulation to stimulate **peripheral sensory nerve fibers** to reduce acute or recurrent pain. TENS machines may be 2-lead or 4-lead and have adjustments for both frequency (1–20 Hz) and pulse width (50–300 μs, 10–50 mA). Stimulation can be intermittent or continuous. TENS units are small and battery-powered with wires and adhesive electrodes attached so that they can be worn while the person goes about usual activities. The positioning of the electrodes and the settings depend upon the site and type of injury, following guidelines provided by the manufacturer. The TENS machine can be used for a number of hours, but if used for days at a time, it will be less effective. TENS treatment is contraindicated with demand pacemakers and should not be used on the head or neck or over irritated skin.

## Postmortem Care and Services

### Postmortem Decomposition

The process of postmortem decomposition begins almost immediately after death. **Livor mortis** occurs as the blood vessels become more permeable and red blood cells begin to break down, resulting in the pooling of blood and staining of tissue that occurs in dependent parts of the body (**lividity**). The skin may appear splotchy within 4-5 hours, but lividity with bluish-purplish-red discoloration is very evident by 5-6 hours. The discoloration remains after compression by about 12 hours and, as red cells break down, a marbling discoloration occurs, and Tardieu spots (tiny dark spots) result from capillary rupture. When lividity occurs, the rest of the body takes on a grey hue. The color of the lividity may vary depending on the cause of death, and the face is often deep reddish-purple in those with cardiac-related death. While liver mortis is occurring, the body also goes through rigor mortis, muscle contracture and stiffening, and algor mortis, cooling of the body to ambient temperature.

### Rigor Mortis

Immediately after death, the body tends to be flaccid. However, changes occur within a few hours. **Rigor mortis** is an exaggerated contraction of muscles that occurs 2-6 hours after death when stores of **adenosine phosphate (ATP)**, which is necessary for muscle relaxation, are depleted. Rigor mortis is progressive, beginning with the internal organs and progressing to small muscles in the head and neck (such as the eyelids) and on to larger muscles in the trunk and extremities. Rigor mortis may be more pronounced in those with large muscles while those who are thin and frail may have less rigor mortis. Ambient temperatures may affect the onset and duration of rigor mortis with high temperatures speeding and low temperatures slowing the changes. Chemical activity usually peaks around 12 hours after death and persists for around 18 hours following this peak, but it may persist for another 48 hours or more before the muscles relax.

## Algor Mortis

Normal body temperature is about 37 °C, but when body functions cease at death, **algor mortis** (cold death), a gradual decrease in body temperature, begins within approximately one hour, and the body starts to cool by about 1 °C every hour until it reaches **ambient temperature**. The exterior surface temperature cools more rapidly than the internal temperature, and the overall rate of cooling may vary depending on the patient's internal temperature at the time of death, the ambient temperature of the environment, the patient's size (muscle mass, fat), and the presence and thickness of clothing or blankets. High temperatures (internal or external) slow the cooling process. As the body cools, the skin loses elasticity and takes on a waxy appearance. This stage of the process of death ends when the temperature begins to rise again as part of **decomposition**, generally within 24 hours.

## Death Vigil

A death vigil entails staying with a dying person and ensuring that the person is never left alone. In some cases, the death vigil may be over within hours, but other patients may die slowly over a number of days, and family members can become exhausted, so they should be encouraged to take turns sitting vigil or to take periodic rest periods. In some cultures, a death vigil means a large number of people are present, but in other cases only one or two close family members. In either case, the nurse and nursing assistant can support this practice by helping to make the room comfortable with adequate seating and encouraging friends/family to maintain a quiet and peaceful environment (low lights, soft music, limited conversation, and distractions). The provider should assist with any cultural traditions that the family desires and ask the family if they want a visit from a spiritual leader/advisor (such as a priest or shaman) and help with arrangements.

## Postmortem Care

The body should be prepared in order to provide a clean, peaceful impression for those family members who desire an opportunity to say good-bye before transport to a funeral home. Kindly caring for the body shows respect to the family, the continued value of the deceased, as well as modeling grief-facilitating behaviors for others present. Religious or other rituals the family may find comforting should be encouraged, as should participation in the preparation of the body. Explain the process and what to expect as care is given. Unless otherwise indicated by protocol or the need for autopsy, any tubes, drains, and other medical devices should be removed. Bandages should be applied, as fluids may still be expressed. A waterproof pad or incontinence brief underneath the body is helpful for containing fluids. Packing of the vagina or rectum is unnecessary. Wash the body and comb the hair. Consider dressing the body in something normalizing. It should be noted that the body may "sigh" as it is rolled and the lungs are compressed. If the area is kept cool, the decomposition process will be slowed, allowing the family time to grieve.

## Providing Support When Notifying Family and Coworkers at Time-of-Death

The provider should prepare to notify family and coworkers near and at the time of death by asking family members **before death is imminent** who should be notified in the event the patient's condition worsens and how that notification should be carried out (telephone, text) and should post this information prominently in the patient's **chart**. Because of HIPAA regulations regarding privacy and confidentiality, only those coworkers and friends that the patient and/or family have indicated should be notified can be contacted. (Health information remains protected under HIPAA for 50 years after a patient's death). If calling to notify a person of a death, the nurse should prepare the person first: "I'm sorry to say that I have some bad news." Then, the provider should briefly explain that the patient has died, avoiding euphemisms, which may be misunderstood and should answer any questions the person may have. The provider should express sympathy, "I'm so sorry for your loss," but avoid clichés such as, "He is in a better place."

### Death Pronouncement

The death pronouncement itself is fairly straightforward, but it can be complicated by the presence of family members or friends, so the provider must remain sensitive to their needs and emotions. Protocols for **death pronouncement** may vary somewhat but generally include:

- Gather information from medical health record and staff members if not present at the time of death
- Identify the patient, verifying patient's ID number
- Description of the body's appearance and location
- Verbal and tactile stimulation utilized and lack of response
- Check of pupillary reflex and finding of fixed and dilated pupils
- Assessment of respiratory status and lack of breathing/lung sounds
- Assessment of cardiac status and lack of pulse noted on palpation and auscultation of apical pulse for at least 60 seconds
- Note and record the official time of death
- Note family and physician notifications
- File report to the CDC for those conditions that require notification if part of responsibility
- Describe notification of appropriate authorities for suspicious death or when regulations require notification of the medical examiner

### Documentation Needed at the Time of Death

Documentation needed at the time of death includes:

- Deceased name, birthdate, address, and unique patient number
- Date and time of documentation
- Reason for attending to the deceased
- List of those present at time of death
- Description of circumstances, including location and complications or disease processes that may have contributed to death
- Outline of death confirmation according to established protocol
- Outcome of assessment and time of death
- Interactions with others present, including staff members and family members
- Specific notifications, such as of spouse, children, or physician
- Description of any special requests or concerns, such as cultural practices
- Discussion regarding organ donation and plans
- Plans for disposition of body (funeral home, autopsy, body/organ donation)
- Notification of medical examiner if required by circumstances/regulations
- Signature, including full name, role, any professional ID number, and contact information

## Chapter Quiz

Ready to see how well you retained what you just read? Scan the QR code to go directly to the chapter quiz interface for this study guide. If you're using a computer, simply visit the online resources page at **mometrix.com/resources719/nclexrn-31183** and click the Chapter Quizzes link.

# Pharmacological and Parenteral Therapies

## Principles of Pharmacology

### Principles of Pharmacokinetics

**Pharmacokinetics** relates to the route of administration, the absorption, the dosage, the frequency of administration, the distribution, and the serum levels achieved over time.

- The **drug's rate of clearance (elimination)** and **doses needed** to ensure therapeutic benefit are considered. Most drugs are cleared through the kidneys, with water-soluble compounds excreted more readily than protein-soluble compounds.
- **Volume of distribution** (IV drug dose divided by plasma concentration) determines the rate at which the drug passes into tissue. Drug distribution depends on the degree of protein binding and ion trapping that takes place.
- **Elimination half-life** is the time needed for the concentration of a particular drug to decrease to half of its starting dose in the body. Approximately five half-lives are needed to achieve steady-state plasma concentrations if giving doses intermittently.
- **Context-sensitive half-life** is the time needed to reach 50% concentration after withdrawal of a continuously-administered drug.
- **Recovery time** is the length of time it takes for plasma levels to decrease to the point that the effect is eliminated. This is affected by plasma concentration.
- **Effect-site equilibrium** is the time between administration of a drug and clinical effect (the point at which the drug reaches the appropriate receptors) and must be considered when determining dose, time, and frequency of medications.
- The **bioavailability** of drugs may vary, depending upon the degree of metabolism that takes place before the drug reaches its site of action.

### Principles of Pharmacodynamics

**Pharmacodynamics** relates to biological effects (therapeutic or adverse) of drug administration over time. Drug transport, absorption, means of elimination, and half-life must all be considered when determining effects. Responses may include continuous responses, such as blood pressure variations, or dichotomous responses in which an event either occurs or does not (such as death). Information from pharmacodynamics provides feedback to modify medication dosage (pharmacokinetics). Drugs provide biological effects primarily by interacting with receptor sites (specific protein molecules) in the cell membrane. Receptors include voltage-sensitive ion channels (sodium, chloride, potassium, and calcium channels), ligand-gated ion channels, and transmembrane receptors. Agonist drugs exert effects after binding with a receptor, while antagonist drugs bind with a receptor but have no effects, so they can block agonists from binding. The total number of receptors may vary, upregulating or downregulating in response to stimuli (such as drug administration). Dose-response curves show the relationship between the amount of drug given and the resultant plasma concentration and biological effects.

### First Pass Metabolism and Drug Clearance

**First pass metabolism** is the phenomenon that occurs to ingested drugs that are absorbed through the gastrointestinal tract and enter the hepatic portal system. Drugs metabolized on the first pass travel to the liver, where they are broken down, some to the extent that only a small fraction of the active drug circulates to the rest of the body. This first pass through the liver greatly reduces the bioavailability of some drugs. Routes of administration that avoid first pass metabolism include intravenous, intramuscular, and sublingual.

**Drug clearance** refers to the ability to remove a drug from the body. The two main organs responsible for clearance are the liver and the kidneys. The liver eliminates drugs by metabolizing, or biotransforming, the substance or excreting the drug in the bile. The kidneys eliminate drugs by filtration or active excretion in the urine. Drugs use either renal or hepatic methods of clearance. Kidney and liver dysfunction inhibit the clearance of drugs that rely on that organ for removal. Toxicity results from poor clearance.

## Enterohepatic Recirculation of Drugs and Renally Excreted Drugs

**Enterohepatic recirculation** refers to the process whereby a drug is effectively removed from circulation and then reabsorbed. The drug is secreted in bile, which is collected in the gall bladder and emptied into the small intestine, from which part of it is reabsorbed and part excreted in the feces. This reabsorption reduces the clearance of these drugs and increases their duration of action. Generally, drugs susceptible to enterohepatic recirculation are generally those with a molecular weight greater than 500 g/mol and those that are amphipathic (have both a lipophilic portion and a polar portion).

**Renally excreted** drugs are metabolized (biotransformed) by the liver to a form that can be excreted by the kidneys. Others are excreted by the kidneys unchanged. Infants with decreased renal function demonstrate decreased urine output or elevated levels of BUN and creatinine. The nurse should avoid using drugs that depend on the kidneys for clearance if the infant has renal impairment, as overdose may result.

## Absorption in Relation to Routes of Medication Administration

The absorption rate of a drug depends on its transfer from its site of administration to the circulatory system. Different **routes of administration** have different absorption characteristics:

- **Oral**: Ingested medications pass from the gastrointestinal tract into the bloodstream. Most absorption occurs in the small intestine and is affected by gastric motility and emptying rate, drug solubility in gastrointestinal fluids, and food presence. Orally administered drugs are susceptible to first pass metabolism by the liver.
- **Intravenous**: Medications directly administered to the bloodstream have 100% absorption. Peak serum levels are rapidly achieved. Some drugs are not tolerated intravenously, due to vein irritation or toxicity, and others must be given as an infusion.
- **Intramuscular**: Medications injected into a muscle are absorbed fairly rapidly because muscle tissue is highly vascularized. Drugs in lipid vehicles absorb more slowly than those in aqueous vehicles.
- **Subcutaneous**: Medications injected beneath the skin absorb more slowly because the dermis is less vascularized than muscle. Hypoperfusion and edema decrease absorption further.

## Blood Drug Levels

Plasma drug levels are used for **therapeutic drug monitoring** because, although plasma is often not the site of action, plasma levels correlate well with therapeutic (effective) and toxic (dose-related adverse effects) responses to most drugs. The therapeutic range of a drug is that between the minimum effective concentration (level at which there is no therapeutic benefit) and the toxic concentration (level at which toxic effects occur). To achieve drug plateau (steady state), the drug half-life (time needed to decrease drug concentration by 50%) must be considered. Most drugs reach plateau with administration equal to four half-lives and completely eliminate a drug in 5 half-lives. Because drug levels fluctuate, peak (highest drug concentration) and trough (lowest drug concentration) levels may be monitored. Samples for trough levels are taken immediately prior to administration of another dose, while peak samples are taken at various times, depending on the average peak time of the specific drug, which may vary from 30 minutes to 2 hours or so after administration.

## Side Effects of Medications

All drugs can have side effects, and some are toxic at certain levels or in combination with other drugs. Some side effects will be minor and may go away after a week or two. Others can be severe or life-threatening, such as anaphylaxis. Common side effects include nausea, vomiting, diarrhea, and rashes. Side effects may vary with individuals according to age, gender, and condition and may be related to non-compliance with treatment, incorrect dosage, polypharmacy, or drug interactions. Drug compendiums will list all possible side effects according to system or incidence. Pharmacologically similar medications usually have some common side effects among the drugs in that class. Nursing actions include:

- Always question the patient about allergies or previous drug reactions before administering medication.
- Educate the patient about possible side effects of all medications.
- Watch out for drug-drug and food-drug combinations that are dangerous.

## Drug Interactions

Drug interactions occur when one drug interferes with the activity of another in either the pharmacodynamics or pharmacokinetics:

- With **pharmacodynamic interaction,** both drugs may interact at receptor sites causing a change that results in an adverse effect or that interferes with a positive effect.
- With **pharmacokinetic interaction**, the ability of the drug to be absorbed and cleared is altered, so there may be delayed effects, changes in effects, or toxicity. Interactions may include problems in a number of areas:
  - **Absorption** may be increased or (more commonly) decreased, usually related to the effects within the gastrointestinal system.
  - **Distribution** of drugs may be affected, often because of changes in protein binding.
  - **Metabolism** may be altered, often causing changes in drug concentration.
  - **Biotransformation** of the drug must take place, usually in the liver and gastrointestinal system, but drug interactions can impair this process.
  - **Clearance interactions** may interfere with the body's ability to eliminate a drug, usually resulting in increased concentration of the drug.

### *Specific Interactions*

Some drugs will either increase or inhibit the actions of other drugs. They may interfere with receptor-site binding or the way in which the drug is metabolized or excreted. Certain drugs may cause drowsiness when taken together or with alcohol. Some foods will inhibit drug action, such as the inhibition of warfarin by vitamin-K-containing foods. Other foods may cause toxic levels of a drug to accumulate. Grapefruit juice, for example, is metabolized by the same enzyme that metabolizes about 50 drugs, including digoxin and statins, and this can prevent the liver from breaking down drugs and lead to severe reactions. The nurse should always obtain a complete medication list from the patient, including prescription and over-the-counter medications, herbals, vitamins, minerals, and dietary supplements that are taken regularly and occasionally. All medications taken should be checked for **potential interactions with drugs or foods**.

# Principles of Adult Medication Administration

## Drug Classification

The following are different ways to classify drugs:

- **Therapeutic classification**: The common uses for the drug will place it in a certain therapeutic classification.
- **Pharmacological classification**: The action of the drug determines which pharmacological category a drug will be in.

All drugs have a **chemical name** and a **generic name,** which is simpler. A company making the drug can give it a **trade or brand name**. The generic form of a drug is generally cheaper but may differ in efficacy from a brand name drug due to a difference in the amount of drug that is absorbed for use in the body. The Controlled Substances Act restricts usage of certain drugs and classifies them according to schedules that include:

- **Schedule I**: Ecstasy, LSD, marijuana, peyote, mescaline, psilocybin, heroin, and others
- **Schedule II**: Amphetamine, cocaine, codeine, fentanyl, Dilaudid, Demerol, Ritalin, morphine, opium, and others
- **Schedule III**: Anabolic steroids, barbiturates, codeine, Vicodin, and pentothal
- **Schedule IV**: Xanax, Librium, Klonopin, Valium, Ativan, Versed, phenobarbital, Restoril, Ambien
- **Schedule V**: Lomotil and others

## 5 Rights of Medication Administration

The 5 rights of medication administration are used to prevent/reduce medication errors in the hospital setting. Often these 5 rights are integrated into the scanning requirements of electronic documentation. The **5 rights of medication administration** must also be incorporated into the prescriber's order:

- **Right Patient**: Confirm the patient's identity using two identifiers, often being their full name and date of birth. Scanning will also confirm the patient's identity with their bar code and electronic health record.
- **Right Drug**: Check the name of the drug with the prescriber's order. By scanning the medication, the drug name will also be checked against the order.
- **Right Dose**: Check the dose of the drug with the prescriber's order. Some medications require a second nurse confirm any dosage calculations utilized before administration. Ensure the dosage is appropriate and contact the prescriber if there are any concerns.
- **Right route**: Routes include oral (PO), subcutaneous, intradermal, IV, or IM, amongst others. The route must also be confirmed with the prescriber's order.
- **Right time/frequency**: The drug may be administered as a one-time dose, PRN (as needed), or recurring administration (twice daily, every 8 hours, etc.).

## Clinical Situations That Have Implications for Medication Administration

It is quite important to recognize clinical situations involving patients that may have **implications for the administration of medications**. For example, many patients have co-morbid conditions that will impact decisions about their medication administration. A patient with non-insulin-dependent diabetes and coronary artery disease who is being treated for a hip fracture would require oral hypoglycemic medications, cardiovascular medications, pain medication, and anti-coagulants. Another example would be an insulin-dependent diabetic patient with concomitant hypertension and renal failure. This patient would require insulin, anti-hypertensive medications, and dosing adjustments of medications secondary to renal failure. The nurse who is responsible for the patient must ensure that the correct dosages of each prescribed medication are administered on time. Potential negative side effects and drug-drug interactions should be avoided, and the patient should be monitored for adverse reactions to newly prescribed drugs.

## Routes of Drug Administration

The route of administration is the manner by which a drug is introduced into the body. The most **common routes of administration** are:

- Enteral (oral, rectal, or by feeding tube)
- Topical (on the skin, in the eyes or nose, vaginal, or inhaled)
- Parenteral (IV, subcutaneous, intramuscular, intracardiac, intraosseous, intradermal, intrathecal, intraperitoneal, transdermal, transmucosal, intravitreal, and epidural)

There are many variations on these three basic routes of administration. The FDA acknowledges 111 different routes of administration. When deciding on the route of administration, the doctor and pharmacist consider:

- How fast the patient requires the drug
- How effective it will be by a given route
- The likelihood of toxicity
- The discomfort it will cause
- How likely the patient is to comply with the route
- How likely the route is to play into the patient's addictive habits

### *Injections*

The three most common types of injections and the preferred injection sites are as follows:

- **Subcutaneous Injection**: Deliver the drug under the skin with a ½ inch, 24- or 25-gauge needle held at a 45° angle to reach the fat. Choose the upper arm, abdomen, thigh, or lower back as the site. The maximum amount of subcutaneous medication is 0.5 mL. An example is insulin for a patient with diabetes.
- **Intramuscular Injection**: Deliver the drug into the muscle at a 90° angle to reach the deep tissue. Standard needle length is 1 to 1.5 inches depending on the weight of the individual. CDC guidelines recommend the use of a 22- to 25-gauge needle for adult intramuscular injections. Recommended sites for injection on the adult include deltoid (most recommended), vastus lateralis (thigh), ventrogluteal (hip), or dorsogluteal (buttocks). The maximum recommended amount of IM medication is 3 mL. An example is Vitamin B12 for a patient with pernicious anemia.
- **Intravenous Injection**: Deliver the drug into a vein of the arm, hand, leg, foot, scalp, or neck with an Angiocath, butterfly, or Insyte Autoguard needle. Use a size from 14 gauge to 26 gauge, depending on the fluid and the patient. The nurse sets the drip rate per minute by adjusting the clamp and monitoring the drip chamber. An example of a drug requiring intravenous injection is Zoledronate, which is given yearly to prevent bone fractures for individuals with osteoporosis.

Two less frequently used forms of injection are: Intradermal (into the skin) for Mantoux TB test, and intraosseous access (IO) into the bone, which is used in emergency situations when other access sites are not available.

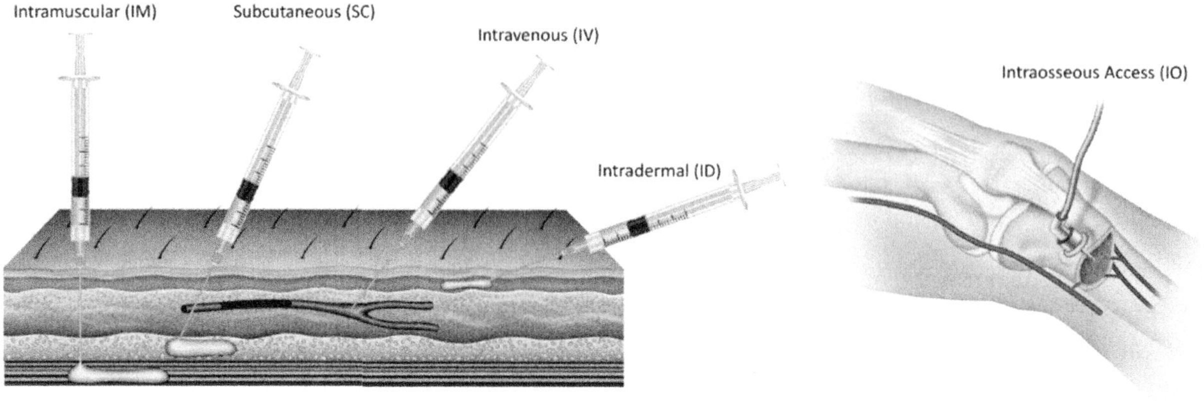


## HERBAL-DRUG CONTRAINDICATIONS

Patients on certain medications should not take some herbals. Some **contraindications for common herbals** include:

- **Echinacea**: Anti-anxiety meds, antifungals, heart medications, HIV medications, anabolic steroids, methotrexate, NSAIDs
- **Gingko Biloba**: Anticoagulants, NSAIDs, aspirin, acetaminophen
- **Garlic**: Anticoagulants, oral hypoglycemics, NSAIDs
- **Licorice**: Diuretics, digoxin, antihypertensives
- **St. John's Wort**: Antidepressants, anticoagulants, Tamoxifen, oral contraceptives, HIV medications, anesthetics. Action is similar to MAO inhibitor
- **Valerian**: Sedatives, anti-seizure meds, anesthetics, alcohol, opioids
- **Feverfew**: Anticoagulants, migraine meds, NSAIDs
- **Ginger**: Anticoagulants, NSAIDs
- **Ginseng**: Anticoagulants, antihypertensives, NSAIDs, opioids. Do not take when pregnant or lactating
- **Goldenseal**: Antihypertensives, diabetic medications, meds for kidney diseases. Do not take when pregnant or lactating
- **Kava-kava**: Alcohol, anti-seizure meds, antidepressants, sedatives, anesthetics, antipsychotics, NSAIDS, opioids
- **Saw Palmetto**: Hormone therapy
- **Hawthorn**: Digoxin

# Medication Dosage Calculations

## Abbreviations for Different Units of Measure

| Abbreviation | Meaning |
|---|---|
| ss | One half, 1/2 |
| L | Liter |
| mL | Milliliter |
| tsp | Teaspoon (5 mL) |
| tbsp | Tablespoon (15 mL) |
| Fl oz | Fluid ounce (30 mL) |
| gr | Grain |
| qs, qs ad | Dispense a sufficient quantity or add a sufficient quantity to make |
| aq | Water |
| ad | Up to |
| aa | Of each |
| gtt | Drop |
| G, g, gm | Gram |
| kg | Kilogram |
| mg | Milligram |
| mcg | Microgram |
| mEq | Milliequivalent |
| ds | Days' supply |
| lb | Pound |
| c | Cup |

## Roman Numerals

| | |
|---|---|
| I | 1 |
| II | 2 |
| III | 3 |
| IV | 4 |
| V | 5 |

| | |
|---|---|
| VI | 6 |
| VII | 7 |
| VIII | 8 |
| IX | 9 |
| X | 10 |

| | |
|---|---|
| L | 50 |
| C | 100 |
| D | 500 |
| M | 1000 |

## Conversion Factors

Conversion factors are used to change from one unit of measure to another. For instance, if a drug is prescribed in milliliters and the patient wants to know their dose in teaspoons, you will have to use a conversion factor.

| Conversion Factors | |
|---|---|
| 1 kg | 2.2 lb |
| 1 tsp | 5 mL |
| 1 tbsp | 3 tsp (15 mL) |
| 1 fl oz | 29.57 mL (often rounded to 30 mL) |
| 1 cup | 8 oz |
| 1 L | 33.8 oz |
| 1 gr | 64.8 mg |

### *Converting Between Grams, Kilograms, Milligrams, and Micrograms*

A gram (g) is the basic metric unit of mass or weight. All other metric units of mass are centered around the gram. Metric units of measure can be easily converted from one form to another by moving the decimal place. A kilogram (kg) is $10^3$ or 1000 times larger than a gram. Therefore, to convert grams to kilograms, the decimal place must be moved to the left three places. Milligrams (mg) and micrograms (mcg) are smaller than a gram. A milligram is $10^{-3}$ or 1000 times smaller than a gram, whereas a microgram is $10^{-6}$ or 1,000,000 times smaller than a gram. To convert grams to milligrams, the decimal place must be moved to the right three places. To convert grams to micrograms, the decimal place must be moved to the right six places.

| Unit of Measure | Kilogram | Gram | Milligram | Microgram |
|---|---|---|---|---|
| Conversion factor | $10^3$ | 1 | $10^{-3}$ | $10^{-6}$ |
| Sample conversion | 0.008 | 8 | 8000 | 8,000,000 |

**Review Video: Measurement Conversions**
Visit mometrix.com/academy and enter code: 316703

## Adding and Subtracting Fractions

In order to **add or subtract fractions**, you must first convert the fractions to an equivalent fraction so that both fractions have the same denominator (the number on the bottom of the fraction). An easy way of doing this is to multiply the two denominators together and multiply the numerators (the top number of the fraction) by the original denominator of the opposite fraction (cross-multiplication):

$$\frac{1}{4}+\frac{1}{6}=$$

Cross-multiply the numerators by the opposite denominator, and multiply the denominators to get a common denominator:

$$\frac{6}{24}+\frac{4}{24}=$$

Once the fractions are converted to have the same common denominator, the numerators (the numbers on the top of the fraction) can simply be added:

$$\frac{6}{24}+\frac{4}{24}=\frac{10}{24}$$

Reduce the fraction by converting it to its smallest possible form. Divide each part of the final fraction by a common whole number until the numbers cannot be divided any further:

$$\frac{10}{24}\div\frac{2}{2}=\frac{5}{12}$$

**Review Video: Adding and Subtracting Fractions**
Visit mometrix.com/academy and enter code: 378080

## Multiplying and Dividing Fractions

In order to **multiply fractions**, simply multiply the numerators (top numbers) and denominators (bottom numbers) separately. Then, reduce the final fraction to the smallest possible form by dividing the numerator and denominator by a common whole number until the numbers cannot be divided further.

Example:

$$\frac{1}{4}\times\frac{6}{8}=\frac{6}{32}$$

Reduce the fraction:

$$\frac{6}{32} \div \frac{2}{2} = \frac{3}{16}$$

In order to **divide fractions**, use the same process as multiplying fractions except flip the second fraction upside down. The mathematical term for a fraction that is flipped upside down is called the reciprocal. Then, reduce the fraction to its smallest possible form.

Example:

$$\frac{1}{4} \div \frac{6}{8} =$$

Flip the second fraction:

$$\frac{1}{4} \times \frac{8}{6} = \frac{8}{24}$$

Reduce the fraction:

$$\frac{8}{24} \div \frac{8}{8} = \frac{1}{3}$$

**Review Video: Multiplying and Dividing Fractions**
Visit mometrix.com/academy and enter code: 473632

## Dimensional Analysis

A useful method for solving problems involving unit conversions is **dimensional analysis**. In this method conversion factors (example: $\left(\frac{1\text{ g}}{1{,}000\text{ mg}}\right)$) or their reciprocals (example: $\left(\frac{1{,}000\text{ mg}}{1\text{ g}}\right)$) may be used to obtain the required unit. Consider this drip rate example:

$$\text{Drip rate} = \frac{25\text{ mL}}{1\text{ hour}} \times \frac{10\text{ gtt}}{1\text{ mL}} \times \frac{1\text{ hour}}{60\text{ min}} = \frac{250\text{ gtt}}{60\text{ min}} = 4.2\,\frac{\text{gtt}}{\text{min}}$$

In this example, the flow rate (25 mL/hour) was given, as was the conversion factor of 10 gtt (drops) per mL. Those values plus the conversion of 1 hour = 60 minutes can be used to solve the problem.

One way to check that the problem was set up and solved correctly is to make sure the units cancel out across the problem to give the desired dimensions. This problem asked for drip rate, which is measured in drops (gtt) per unit of time (minutes in this problem). Below, the mL and hour in the numerator cancel out the mL and hour in the denominator because 1 hour ÷ 1 hour = 1 and 1 mL ÷ 1 mL = 1, so the resulting units match the units required for the answer.

$$\text{Drip rate} = \frac{25\,\cancel{\text{mL}}}{1\,\cancel{\text{hour}}} \times \frac{10\text{ gtt}}{1\,\cancel{\text{mL}}} \times \frac{1\,\cancel{\text{hour}}}{60\text{ min}} = \frac{250\text{ gtt}}{60\text{ min}} = 4.2\,\frac{\text{gtt}}{\text{min}}$$

## Decimals

To **multiply decimals**, first multiply the numbers as if there were no decimals present. Then, place a decimal point at the end of the number (to the right) and move the decimal place to the left the number of spaces equal to the total number of decimal places in the original numbers.

Example: 5.68 × 1.25

The total number of decimal places = 2 + 2 = 4

At first, multiply the numbers ignoring the decimal places: 568 × 125 = 71,000

Place a decimal place at the end of this number: 71,000

Move the decimal place to the left a total number of spaces equal to the total number of decimal places in the original numbers (in this case, four spaces): 7.1

To **convert a decimal to a percent**, move the decimal two places to the *right* and add a % sign.

Example: 0.30 = 30%

To **convert a percent to a decimal**, move the decimal point two places to the *left* and remove the % sign.

Example: 65% = 0.65

**Review Video: Decimals**
Visit mometrix.com/academy and enter code: 837268

**Review Video: How to Multiply Decimals**
Visit mometrix.com/academy and enter code: 731574

**Review Video: Converting Percentages to Decimals and Fractions**
Visit mometrix.com/academy and enter code: 287297

## Sample Ratio and Proportion Calculation Problem

*You are to prepare an IV for a patient that contains potassium chloride 10 mEq in 500 mL. All you have in stock is potassium chloride 40 mEq/10 mL. How much of the stock solution should be added to the 500 mL IV bag in order to prepare the 10 mEq solution?*

In order to solve this type of proportion problem, it is easiest to use cross multiplication. In cross multiplication, you summarize the information into two fractions where three values are known, and one value is unknown. Then, you cross-multiply to solve for the unknown value.

We know that the stock solution we have contains 40 mEq/10 mL, so this is our first fraction or proportion. We also know that we need to end with 10 mEq, but we don't know how much volume equates to 10 mEq. Therefore, our second fraction will be 10 mEq over an unknown volume:

$$\begin{aligned} \frac{10\text{ mEq}}{?\text{ mL}} &= \frac{40\text{ mEq}}{10\text{ mL}} \\ 10\text{ mEq} \times 10\text{ mL} &= 40\text{ mEq} \times ?\text{ mL} \\ ?\text{ mL} &= \frac{(10 \times 10)}{40}\text{mL} \\ &= 2.5\text{ mL} \end{aligned}$$

The correct answer is 2.5 mL. This means that 2.5 mL of the 40 mEq/10 mL stock solution must be added to the 500 mL IV bag in order to prepare a 10 mEq/500 mL solution (although in reality the exact concentration would become 10 mEq/502.5 mL because nothing would be removed from the 500 mL IV bag when the 2.5 mL is added).

It's always a good idea to review your answer to ensure that it is reasonable. If the stock solution is 40 mEq/10 mL and we need 10mEq, that means that our answer will be one-fourth of 10 mL because 10 mEq is one-fourth of 40 mEq. Because 2.5 mL is one-fourth of 10 mEq, our answer is correct.

## Sample IV Flow Rate/Drip Rate Problem

*An IV antibiotic was prescribed for a patient to be administered at a rate of 25 mL/hour. What volume (in mL) of IV solution would be needed to last 8 hours? What is the drip rate if the IV is running through at a rate of 10 gtt/mL?*

Flow rates can be expressed in mL/hour or mL/min depending upon what type of pump is being used to administer the IV:

$$\textbf{Flow rate} = \frac{\text{mL of IV solution}}{\text{hours or minutes}}$$

In this problem, the IV flow rate is given, and it is asking how many mL of solution are needed to run over an 8-hour time frame. In order to figure this out, the flow rate must be multiplied by the time period:

Flow rate (mL/hour) × hours = total mL administered

25 mL/hour × 8 hours = **200 mL** administered over 8 hours

The drip rate is the number of drops of IV solution that are administered per minute.

$$\textbf{Drip rate} = \frac{\text{gtt of IV solution}}{\text{minute}}$$

In order to calculate the drip rate from the flow rate, the mL of solution must be converted into drops (gtt). A conversion factor will be given for this. In this problem, the rate is 10 gtt/mL. If the flow rate is given in hours, then the time must be converted into minutes to calculate the drip rate.

$$\text{Drip rate} = \frac{25\text{ mL}}{1\text{ hour}} \times \frac{10\text{ gtt}}{1\text{ mL}} \times \frac{1\text{ hour}}{60\text{ min}} = \frac{250\text{ gtt}}{60\text{ min}} = 4.2\frac{\text{gtt}}{\text{min}}$$

**Review Video: Calculating IV Drip Rates**
Visit mometrix.com/academy and enter code: 396112

## Sample Amount of Glucose in Solution Problem

*How many grams of glucose are there in a 500 mL bag of glucose 5% solution? How many grams are contained in a 500 mL bag of glucose 0.5% solution?*

A concentration is the amount of substance in a volume of solution. Concentrations can be expressed as weight to volume (g/100 mL), volume to volume (mL/100 mL) or weight to weight (g/100 g).

A percentage is the quantity of substance in 100. Because concentrations are also expressed as an amount per 100, no conversion or decimal place movement is required to convert the percentage into a concentration. To solve this problem, multiply the concentration of the solution by the volume of the bag to find the total amount of glucose contained within the bag:

$$\text{Glucose } 5\% = \frac{5\text{ g}}{100\text{ mL}} \times \frac{500\text{ mL}}{\text{bag}} = \frac{(5 \times 500)}{100} = 25\text{ g}$$

$$\text{Glucose } 0.5\% = \frac{0.5\text{ g}}{100\text{ mL}} \times \frac{500\text{ mL}}{\text{bag}} = \frac{(0.5 \times 500)}{100} = 2.5\text{ g}$$

Ensure that these answers are reasonable and make sense. If there is 5% glucose in a solution (5 g/100 mL), then a 500 mL bag will have five times as much as a 100 mL bag. Because 5 × 5 = 25, our answer of 25 g makes sense. For the 0.5% solution, move the decimal place to the left one place to find the answer in comparison to the answer for a 5% solution. Therefore, 2.5 g is a reasonable answer.

## Child Dosage Calculation

In most cases, the manufacturer's instructions will provide children's (pediatric) dosing for a medication. However, there are some instances in which pediatric dosing is not provided and must be calculated. Formulas for estimating a pediatric dose will typically use age, weight, or body surface area.

**Young's Rule (Age, >2 yr)**

$$\text{child dose} = \frac{\text{age of child (yr)}}{\text{age of child (yr)} + 12} \times \text{adult dose}$$

**Fried's Rule (Age, <2 yr)**

$$\text{child dose} = \frac{\text{age of child (mo)}}{150 \text{ mo}} \times \text{adult dose}$$

**Clark's Rule (Weight)**

$$\text{child dose} = \frac{\text{weight of child (lb)}}{150 \text{ lb}} \times \text{adult dose}$$

**Mosteller Formula (BSA)**

All BSA calculations are based on the general formula below:

$$\text{child dose} = \frac{\text{child BSA}}{\text{average adult BSA}} \times \text{adult dose}$$

The Mosteller formula is specifically a way to estimate a child's BSA based on height and weight. Plugging the Mosteller formula into the general equation gives the following formula:

$$\text{child dose} = \frac{\sqrt{\text{height (in)} \times \text{weight (lb)}}}{96.8} \times \text{adult dose}$$

BSA-based calculations tend to provide the most reasonable estimates, followed by weight-based. Age-based calculations are rarely used. BSA-based calculations are sometimes used in dosage calculations for chemotherapy regimens.

## Geriatric Dosage Calculation

Children are not the only patients who require dosing adjustments. Elderly (geriatric) patients also have a reduced ability to metabolize medications and may require dosage decreases. Geriatric dosage adjustments are usually listed in the manufacturer's instructions but can also be found in the *Geriatric Dosage Handbook*. Patient who are very frail or who have gastrointestinal diseases (e.g., Crohn's disease, ulcerative colitis) may also absorb and metabolize medications differently and may require dosage adjustments.

# Pharmacologic Pain Management

## WHO Pain Ladder

The WHO pain ladder was developed as an algorithm for treating pain through medications with progressively increasing potency. The approach can be used effectively with both adult and pediatric patients. Beginning with the least potent medication option, each step adds a stronger analgesic until optimum pain relief is reached.

The **WHO pain ladder** has three steps.

- **Step 1**: The patient is given a non-opioid medication which may be used alone or in conjunction with other adjuvant therapies.
- **Step 2**: If the patient reports no change in the pain level, mild- to moderate-level pain-relieving opioids are introduced along with adjuvants if they have not been previously introduced.
- **Step 3**: Uncontrolled pain is then treated with opioids for moderate to severe pain. Adjuvants may also be continued.

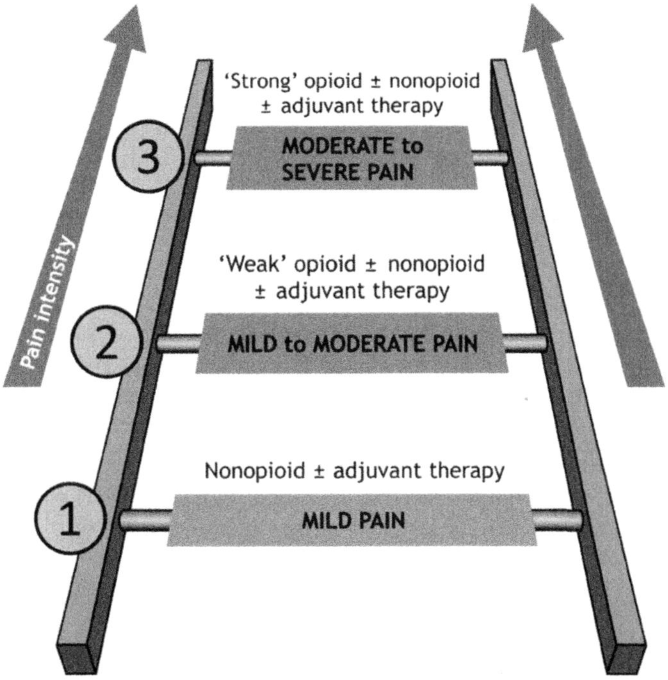


**Review Video: Adjuvants**
Visit mometrix.com/academy and enter code: 178200

## Scheduling of Pain Medications

For mild to moderate pain, patients may take **acetaminophen** alternating with an **NSAID** such as ibuprofen on a regularly scheduled basis or as needed (PRN) at the onset of pain or when pain is anticipated (such as before a dressing change). However, for severe chronic pain, long-acting **opioid pain medications**, such as time-released morphine, fentanyl, and oxycodone, should be given regularly around the clock, because these medications help not only control but also prevent pain. The patient should not skip a dose when free of pain, because this makes control more difficult when the pain recurs. In addition to **time-scheduled medications**, the patient may need **short-acting supplementary medications**, such as Percocet, to take on a PRN basis. When taking short-acting medications, the patient should take the medication at the onset of pain, before anticipated pain, or at the onset of increased pain, rather than waiting until the pain is severe, because the goal should always be to keep the pain under control.

## ACETAMINOPHEN

Acetaminophen remains one of the safest analgesics for **long-term use**. It can be used to treat mild pain or as an adjuvant with other analgesics for more severe pain. Nonspecific musculoskeletal pain and osteoarthritis are particularly responsive to acetaminophen therapy. Acetaminophen also has a limited **anti-inflammatory nature**.

Acetaminophen should, however, be used cautiously in persons with altered liver or kidney function, as well as those with a history of significant alcohol use, regardless of liver function compromise. It should be dosed separately from any opioid analgesic, which should be given separately as well. This allows for individual titration of each drug to assess the individual needs and side effects separately.

## NSAIDs

NSAIDs act by inhibiting the cyclooxygenase (COX) enzyme, which controls prostaglandin formation. COX-1 affects platelet clumping, gastric blood flow, and mucosal integrity. COX-2 affects pain, inflammation, and fever. COX-1 and 2 inhibitors include aspirin and ibuprofen. Ibuprofen has a lower occurrence of side effects, such as gastric bleeding, than aspirin does. A COX-2 inhibitor, such as Celebrex, must be used with caution due to increased cardiovascular risks when used for over 18 months. NSAIDs are useful for both arthritis and bone cancer pain and work well with opioids for relief of postoperative and other severe pain. NSAIDs may increase the effects of antiseizure drugs and warfarin. Smaller doses are needed if kidney function is impaired.

**Review Video: NSAID Side Effects**
Visit mometrix.com/academy and enter code: 569064

## LOCAL ANESTHETIC PAIN RELIEF

Local anesthetics block neural conduction of pain through the application of the anesthetic directly to the nerve endings in the area of pain. It can be injected prior to minor surgery or suturing. It can be injected intercostally for thoracic or high abdominal surgeries. The addition of a vasoconstrictor prolongs effectiveness of the anesthetic. A cream containing local anesthetics (EMLA) can be rubbed on the skin to decrease pain from IV starts or lumbar punctures. It should be applied 60–90 minutes prior to the procedure. A lidocaine 5% patch is approved to relieve pain from postherpetic neuralgia. The patient applies up to 3 patches for 12 hours at a time. Local anesthetics can be applied via the use of an epidural catheter to provide pain control for surgery, childbirth, or postoperative pain control. Opioids can be infused along with the anesthetic agent. Patients using an epidural catheter for postoperative pain tend to ambulate sooner, suffer fewer complications as a result, and go home more quickly.

## OPIOIDS

### *GUIDELINES FOR OPIOID USE*

**Opioid analgesic therapy** is a widely used method of chronic pain control. By adhering to clinical guidelines, pain control can be safely optimized. **Intramuscular administration** should be used as a last resort except in the presence of a "pain emergency" when no other treatment is readily available. Such cases are rare since subcutaneous delivery is almost always an alternative. Noninvasive routes such as **transdermal** and **transmucosal**, which bypass the enteral route, are optimal for continuous pain control and are often effective in eliminating breakthrough pain as well. Changing from one opioid to another, or altering the delivery method, may become necessary under the assumption that incomplete cross-tolerance among opioids occurs. Changing analgesics or method of delivery may result in a decreased drug requirement. When altering opioid delivery regimens, use **morphine equivalents** as the common factor for all dose conversions. This method will help reduce medication errors. Side effects such as sedation, constipation, nausea, and myoclonus should be anticipated in every care plan, and require both prevention and treatment methods.

### *Side Effects of Opioid Analgesics*

Examples of **opioid analgesics** are numerous and include morphine, hydromorphone, oxymorphone, methadone, meperidine, fentanyl, sufentanil, levorphanol, codeine, oxycodone, hydrocodone, nalbuphine, and buprenorphine. Opioid analgesics have multiple effects on most of the organ systems of the body. Central nervous system (CNS) effects include respiratory depression, analgesia, euphoria, sedation, miosis, cough suppression, truncal rigidity, nausea, and vomiting. Cardiovascular effects are usually slight and include bradycardia, hypotension, reduced blood volume, and increased cerebral blood flow. Gastrointestinal effects can include constipation, decreased gastric motility, and decreased hydrochloric acid. Genitourinary effects are urinary retention and decreased renal function. Other effects are sweating, flushing, and histamine release with itching.

### *Opioid Use During Last Few Hours of Life*

Assessment of pain continues in the **last hours of life**, and medication is adjusted according to assessment. Pain does not necessarily increase as death approaches. It can be assumed that if pain was present prior to loss of consciousness it will continue in the patient's unconscious state. It should be assessed for and treated accordingly. Research has confirmed that administering opioids at the end of life does not hasten nor prolong the dying process. The patient's **prior medication regimen** should be continued. However, adjustments may be made in consideration of reduced renal or hepatic clearance. The **route of administration** should also be assessed for appropriateness and adjusted as needed (e.g., loss of consciousness, inability to swallow).

### *Oral Transmucosal Fentanyl Citrate*

Oral transmucosal fentanyl citrate consists of **fentanyl** on an oral applicator. The patient applies the dosage (starting at 200 mcg) to the **buccal mucosa** between the cheek and gum for rapid absorption and subsequent pain relief. This makes transmucosal fentanyl particularly useful for managing **breakthrough pain**. Pain relief generally begins within 5 minutes, but the patient should be instructed to wait 15 minutes after the previous dose has been completed before taking another dose. Swallowing even part of the dose rather than having it completely absorbed through the oral mucosa can affect the timing of pain relief onset. **Peak effect** occurs in 20–40 minutes with the total pain relief duration lasting 2–3 hours. Side effects can include somnolence, nausea, and dizziness. Consuming drinks such as coffee, tea, and juices that alter the oral secretion pH can also alter the absorption rate of transmucosal fentanyl.

### *Methadone*

Methadone is useful for treating **severe or chronic pain** and may be particularly helpful in the presence of **neuropathic pain**. It has a long-acting pain relief factor for a lower cost than many comparable medications. However, the exact dosing ratios with morphine remain unclear within the available research. Metabolism of methadone can also be swayed (either increased or decreased) by many other medications normally taken by patients with chronic conditions. Methadone can also be used to treat opioid addiction. US law for the prescription of methadone for addiction in detoxification or maintenance programs requires a special license and patient enrollment. The words "for pain" need to be clearly stated in the prescription. Methadone can cause drowsiness, weakness, headache, nausea, vomiting, constipation, sweating, and flushing, as well as sedation, decreased respirations, or an irregular heart rate.

### *Oxycodone*

Oxycodone, a synthetic formulation, is a long-acting opioid for **moderate to severe pain relief**. Side effects are similar to those of morphine. It has a similar pain relief ratio, with the possibility of less nausea and vomiting. Because of its extended-release nature, the medication cannot be cut or crushed for administration. Oxycodone does not carry any greater addiction risk than other types of opioids; however, public sensationalism related to this formulation may create hesitation for use among patients. Pharmacies may also limit the amount of this medication they will make available to an individual. Oxycodone should be used cautiously in patients with a history of hypothyroidism, Addison disease, urethral stricture, prostatic hypertrophy, or lung or liver disease.

### Hydromorphone

Hydromorphone is available as tablets, liquid, suppository, and parenteral formulations. It offers the advantage of being synthetic, allowing for its use in the presence of a true **morphine allergy**. It is also helpful when significant side effects have occurred in the past or pain has been inadequately controlled with other medications. It may also be useful for controlling cough. However, neurotoxicity may occur, particularly myoclonus, hyperalgesia, and seizures. It should also be used cautiously in the presence of kidney, liver, heart, and thyroid disease, seizure disorders, respiratory disease, prostatic hypertrophy, or urinary problems. Common *side effects* include dizziness, lightheadedness, drowsiness, upset stomach if taken without food, vomiting, and constipation.

### Titration of Morphine for Pain Control

Morphine titration protocols vary according to the type of morphine used, the severity of pain, and the patient's tolerance:

| Type | Peak | Duration (hours) |
|---|---|---|
| **Short-acting** | 60 minutes | 4–5 |
| **Long-acting** | 3-4 hours | 8–24 |
| **IM** | 30–60 minutes | 4–5 |
| **SQ** | 50–90 minutes | 4–5 |
| **IV** | 20 minutes | 4–5 |
| **Rectal** | 20–60 minutes | 3–7 |

For example, **optimal dosage** is usually calculated by starting with short-acting oral morphine at 30 mg every 3–4 hours with doses increased by 25–50% for moderate pain or 50–100% for severe pain each time until the patient has at least 50% reduction in pain on a scale of 1–10 or a behavior scale. The dose may need to be reduced if excessive sedation occurs. Once the patient's pain is controlled on short-acting morphine and 24-hour dosage needs are calculated, the patient could be switched to extended-release. **Breakthrough pain** is usually treated with dosages that are 10% of the 24-hour dose. Dosages may be repeated or increased if there is inadequate relief of pain at the peak time. Increasing the dose prior to peak time will result in increased drowsiness.

### Morphine Use for Chronic Cancer Pain

One advantage of morphine for chronic cancer pain is that it has no **ceiling dose**. As tolerance to the medication increases or the disease progresses in severity, the dose can be gradually increased to an infinite level. It is also available in many different forms for administration, including intravenous, intramuscular, immediate release, sustained release, long-acting, liquid oral preparations, and suppositories. Morphine is often used as the **equivalency standard** for other opioid analgesics. Common *side effects* of morphine include sedation, respiratory depression, itching, nausea, chronic spasms or twitching of muscle groups, and constipation. Constipation is experienced by all patients receiving opioids. This inevitability should be planned for and treated aggressively. Hallucinations are common when morphine is initiated. After the first few days, most patients will overcome the respiratory depression, nausea, itching, and extreme sedation as tolerance for the medication is developed.

### Dosages for Morphine, Codeine, Hydromorphone, and Levorphanol

The dosages for both the enteral and parenteral routes of morphine, codeine, hydromorphone, and levorphanol are as follows:

- **Morphine**: Enteral dosage is 30 mg (available as continuous and sustained-release formulations to last 12–24 hours); parenteral dosage is 10 mg.
- **Codeine**: Enteral dosage is 200 mg (not generally recommended); parenteral dosage is 130 mg.
- **Hydromorphone**: Enteral dosage is 7.5 mg (available as a continuous-release formula lasting 24 hours); parenteral dosage is 1.5 mg.
- **Levorphanol**: In acute pain episodes, enteral dosage is 4 mg; parenteral dosage is 2 mg. For chronic pain, dosage is equivalent for both enteral and parenteral at 1 mg. Levorphanol has a long half-life, increasing the chances of dosage accumulation over time.

Adhering to the statement "If the gut works, use it," as much as 90 percent of all patients will at least start out able to use oral medications instead of other routes.

### Calculation for Converting Medication Regimen Between Two Opioids

Calculate the current 24-hour drug dose, or the total amount given in a 24-hour period. Multiply the current 24-hour dose times the ratio of the 24-hour equivalent dose for the new drug over the 24-hour equivalent of the old drug. This calculation provides the **equivalent 24-hour dose** for the new drug. Divide the new dose amount by the number of doses to be provided during the day. This amount equals the new **target dosage**.

$$\text{current 24 hr dose} \times \frac{\text{new drug 24 hr equiv dose}}{\text{current drug 24 hr equiv dose}} = \text{new 24 hr dose}$$

$$\frac{\text{new 24 hr dose}}{\text{doses per day}} = \text{new target dosage}$$

## Ketamine

Ketamine is a dissociative anesthetic that can provide pain relief as an alternate or complement to an opioid. The dissociative quality is an effective way to help the patient separate from the sensation of pain. Ketamine treatment begins with an initial bolus of 0.1 mg/kg IV. If there is no improvement, a second bolus with double the dosage is provided in 5 minutes. This can be repeated as needed. Boluses should be followed by a decrease in the patient's current opioid dose by 50% and an infusion of ketamine. **Infusion dosing** for ketamine is 0.015 mg/kg/min, or about 1 mg/min for a 70 kg person. If IV access cannot be attained, subcutaneous infusion is a possibility with dosing of 0.3–0.5 mg/kg. Consider concurrent treatment with a **benzodiazepine** to prevent hallucinations or frightful dreams and observe for increased secretions, as these are all possible side effects of ketamine. The secretions may be treated with glycopyrrolate, scopolamine, or atropine as needed.

## Treating Breakthrough Pain

The three basic types of breakthrough pain, and their treatment measures are as follows:

- **Incident pain**: Pain that can be specifically tied to an activity or event, such as a dressing change or physical therapy. These events can be anticipated and treated with a rapid-onset, short-acting analgesic just prior to the painful event.
- **Spontaneous pain**: This type of pain is unpredictable and cannot be pinpointed to a relationship with any certain time or event. There is no way to anticipate spontaneous pain. In the presence of neuropathic pain, adjuvant therapy may be useful. Otherwise, a rapid-onset, short-acting analgesic is used.
- **End-of-dose failure**: Pain that specifically occurs at the end of a routine analgesic dosing cycle when medication blood levels begin to taper off. Careful evaluation of end-of-dose failure can help prevent it sooner. It may indicate an increased dose tolerance and the need for medication dose alterations.

## Treating Neuropathic Pain

Treatment options for neuropathic pain are often different from the methods used to treat other types of pain. The three drug classes most commonly used and proven effective for treating neuropathic pain are **anticonvulsants**, **anesthetics**, and **antidepressants**. Some are given on an as-needed basis, but most require consistent dosing with **24-hour symptom control**. Examples of the most common medications include amitriptyline, nortriptyline, duloxetine, gabapentin, topical lidocaine, opioids, and pregabalin. Medication choice is dependent on factors such as the type and progression of the disorder and the associated physical and emotional problems, such as nerve injury, muscle weakness or spasms, anxiety, depression, or sleep disturbances.

**Review Video: Neuropathic Pain**
Visit mometrix.com/academy and enter code: 780523

## Treating Bone Pain

Treatment options for bone pain may depend on the causative agent related to the pain, such as the primary cancer site, severely weakened bones, or fractures. **Systemic treatment choices** include chemotherapy, radiation, and hormone therapy. **Hormone therapy** is used in the presence of estrogen and androgen receptors within the cancer cells. **Bisphosphonates**, such as ibandronate, zoledronate, and alendronate, may help strengthen the bones, slow damage, and prevent fractures; they can also help reduce pain. However, side effects can include fatigue, fever, nausea, vomiting, and anemia. **Surgery** may also be considered to remove cancerous cells or reinforce weakened areas of bone. **Opioids** and **NSAIDs/COX-2 inhibitors** are most often used for pain relief and need to be provided on a consistent basis.

Morphine combined with ibuprofen provides the benefit of a centrally acting opioid with a peripherally acting NSAID. Ibuprofen also acts as an effective adjuvant analgesic agent to enhance the relief provided by the opioid without increasing opioid side effects.

## Measures Taken During Pain Crisis

During a pain crisis, assess for a change in the mechanism or location of the pain and attempt to differentiate between **terminal anxiety** or agitation and the **physical causes** of pain. Begin with a rapid increase in **opioid treatment**. If the pain is unresponsive to opioid titration, switching to **benzodiazepines**, such as diazepam and lorazepam, may produce a more effective response. If terminal symptoms remain unresponsive, assess for **drug absorption**. While invasive routes of medication delivery are generally avoided unless necessary, the only guaranteed route of drug delivery is the IV route. If there is any question about absorption, it is appropriate to establish parenteral access. IM delivery should be considered as a last resort. When all accessible resources have been exhausted, seek a pain management consultation as quickly as possible. Alternative methods of terminal pain control include radiotherapy, anesthetic, or neuroablative procedures.

## Concerns Surrounding Use of Pain Medications with End-of-Life Patients

Common concerns surrounding the use of pain medications with end-of-life patients include:

- **Adequacy**: Patients are often concerned that medication may not be adequate to control pain and that chronic or breakthrough pain will occur. Patients may be concerned that if they take adequate pain medication, it will be less effective later when pain may be worse.
- **Sedation/addiction**: Some patients and family members are concerned about the risks of addiction, and others may be concerned about the effects of the medication on the patient's cognition, as some patients may become confused, disoriented, or sedated, depending on the medication or dosage.
- **Adverse effects**: Nausea and vomiting may be almost as debilitating to a patient as the pain it is intended to alleviate. Constipation, a common adverse effect, may be very uncomfortable for a patient. Some medications may result in itching and others may cause myoclonus, both of which are uncomfortable for the patient.

## ADDICTION CHALLENGES

In the presence of **addiction challenges**, it becomes important to choose a **long-acting opioid** that can facilitate around-the-clock dosing and minimize the need for short-term medications used for breakthrough doses. **Short-term medication** use should be very limited or eliminated entirely if possible. Whenever possible, **nondrug adjuvants** such as relaxation techniques, distraction, biofeedback, TNS, and therapeutic communication should be used in place of short-term medications. When short-term medication therapy is needed, a **nonopioid** is best. Limit the amount of medication available to the patient at any given time and monitor for compliance with pill counts and urine toxicology screens as necessary. In some instances, a referral to an addictions specialist is recommended.

## TOLERANCE AND PSEUDOTOLERANCE

**Tolerance** is the adaptation of the body to continued exposure to a drug or chemical. The effects of the drug at the same level of exposure are minimized over time. Additional dosing is required to maintain the same outcomes.

**Pseudotolerance** is the misguided perception of the health care provider that a patient's need for increasing doses of a drug is due to the development of tolerance, when the reality is that disease progression or other factors are responsible for the increase in dosing needs.

## ADDICTION AND PSEUDOADDICTION

**Addiction** is a primary and constant neurobiologic disease with genetic, psychosocial, and environmental factors that create an obsessive and irrational need or preoccupation with a substance. Addictive behaviors include unrestricted, continued cravings, as well as compulsive and persistent use of a drug despite harmful experiences and side effects.

**Pseudoaddiction** is an assumption that the patient is addicted to a substance when in actuality the patient is not experiencing relief from the medication. It is prolonged, unrelieved pain that may be the result of undertreatment. This situation may lead the patient to become more aggressive in seeking medicated relief, thus resulting in the inappropriate "drug seeker" label.

**Review Video: Addiction**
Visit mometrix.com/academy and enter code: 460412

## PHYSICAL DEPENDENCE

Physical dependence occurs when the body adapts to a drug, requiring increasing dosages over time to gain the same effect, and withdrawal of that drug then will result in an **abstinence syndrome** (withdrawal). Physical dependence can be described as a form of **addiction**. While physical dependence was commonly thought of as being related to narcotic drugs (such as morphine, methadone, fentanyl), many different types of drugs may cause some degree of physical dependence. For example, abruptly stopping a beta-blocker may result in cardiac arrhythmias or cardiac arrest. Abruptly stopping SSRIs may result in severe depression and anxiety. Thus, when considering stopping a patient's drugs near the end of life, physical dependence must be considered as many drugs should be **tapered** to avoid withdrawal effects. Drugs that affect the **central nervous system**, such as ethanol, barbiturates, and benzodiazepines, pose considerable risk of dependence and may result in severe withdrawal symptoms.

# Cardiovascular Pharmacology

## Anti-Hypertensive Medications

The classes of anti-hypertensive medications are as follows: Diuretics, sympatholytics, vasodilators, calcium channel blockers, and angiotensin-converting enzyme inhibitors (ACE inhibitors).

- Diuretics include hydrochlorothiazide, chlorthalidone, chlorothiazide, indapamide, metolazone, amiloride, spironolactone, triamterene, furosemide, bumetanide, ethacrynic acid, and torsemide.
- Sympatholytics are clonidine, methyldopa, guanabenz, guanadrel, guanethidine, reserpine, labetalol, prazosin, and terazosin.
- Vasodilators include diazoxide, hydralazine, minoxidil, and nitroprusside sodium.
- Calcium channel blockers include amlodipine, nimodipine, isradipine, nicardipine, nifedipine, bepridil, diltiazem, and verapamil.
- ACE inhibitors include benazepril, captopril, enalapril, fosinopril, lisinopril, moexipril, quinapril, ramipril, and losartan.

**Review Video: Side Effects of ACE Inhibitors and ARBs**
Visit mometrix.com/academy and enter code: 525864

## Diuretics

Diuretics increase **renal perfusion and filtration**, thereby reducing preload and decreasing peripheral and pulmonary edema, hypertension, CHF, diabetes insipidus, and osteoporosis. There are different types of diuretics: loop, thiazide, and potassium sparing.

### *Loop Diuretics*

Loop diuretics inhibit the reabsorption of sodium and chloride (primarily) in the ascending loop of Henle. They also cause increased secretion of other electrolytes, such as calcium, magnesium, and potassium, and this can result in imbalances that cause dysrhythmias. Other side effects include frequent urination, postural hypotension, and increased blood sugar and uric acid levels. They are short-acting so are less effective than other diuretics for control of hypertension.

- **Bumetanide** (Bumex) is given intravenously after surgery to reduce preload or orally to treat heart failure.
- **Ethacrynic acid** (Edecrin) is given intravenously after surgery to reduce preload.
- **Furosemide** (Lasix) is used for the control of congestive heart failure as well as renal insufficiency. It is used after surgery to decrease preload and to reduce the inflammatory response caused by cardiopulmonary bypass (post-perfusion syndrome).

**Review Video: Diuretics**
Visit mometrix.com/academy and enter code: 373276

### *Thiazide Diuretics*

Thiazide diuretics inhibit the **reabsorption of sodium and chloride** primarily in the early distal tubules, forcing more sodium and water to be excreted. Thiazide diuretics increase secretion of potassium and bicarbonate, so they are often given with supplementary potassium or in combination with potassium-sparing diuretics. Thiazide diuretics are the first line of drugs for treatment of **hypertension**. They have a long duration of action (12–72 hours, depending on the drug) so they are able to maintain control of hypertension better than short-acting drugs. They may be given daily or 3–5 days per week. There are numerous thiazide diuretics, including:

- Chlorothiazide
- Chlorthalidone
- Hydrochlorothiazide

Side effects include, dizziness, lightheadedness, postural hypotension, headache, blurred vision, and itching, especially during initial treatment. Thiazide diuretics cause sensitivity to sun exposure, so people should be counseled to use sunscreen.

### *Potassium-Sparing Diuretics*

Potassium-sparing diuretics inhibit the **reabsorption of sodium** in the late distal tubule and collecting duct. They are weaker than thiazide or loop diuretics, but do not cause a reduction in potassium level; however, if used alone, they may cause an increase in potassium, which can cause weakness, irregular pulse, and cardiac arrest. Because potassium-sparing diuretics are less effective alone, they are often given in a combined form with a thiazide diuretic (usually chlorothiazide), which mitigates the potassium imbalance. Typical side effects include dehydration, blurred vision, nausea, insomnia, and nasal congestion, especially in the first few days of treatment.

- **Spironolactone** (Aldactone) is a synthetic steroid diuretic that increases the secretion of both water and sodium and is used to treat congestive heart failure. It may be given orally or intravenously.
- **Eplerenone** is an antimineralocorticoid similar to spironolactone but with fewer side effects.

## Antidysrhythmic Drugs

Antidysrhythmic drugs include a number of drugs that act on the conduction system, the ventricles and/or the atria to control dysrhythmias. There are four classes of drugs that are used as well as some that are unclassified:

- **Class I:** 3 subtypes of sodium channel blockers (quinidine, lidocaine, procainamide)
- **Class II:** β-receptor blockers (esmolol, propranolol)
- **Class III:** Slows repolarization (amiodarone, ibutilide)
- **Class IV**: Calcium channel blockers (diltiazem, verapamil)
- **Unclassified:** Miscellaneous drugs with proven efficacy in controlling arrhythmias (adenosine, electrolyte supplements)

## Smooth Muscle Relaxants

Smooth muscle relaxants decrease peripheral vascular resistance, but may cause hypotension and headaches.

- Sodium nitroprusside (Nipride) dilates both arteries and veins; rapid-acting and used for reduction of hypertension and afterload reduction for heart failure.
- Nitroglycerin (Tridil) primarily dilates veins and is used sublingual or IV to reduce preload for acute heart failure, unstable angina, and acute MI. Nitroglycerin may also be used prophylactically after PCIs to prevent vasospasm.
- Hydralazine (Apresoline) dilates arteries and is given intermittently to reduce hypertension.

**Review Video: Muscle Relaxants**
Visit mometrix.com/academy and enter code: 862193

## Calcium Channel Blockers

Calcium channel blockers are primarily arterial vasodilators that may affect the peripheral and/or coronary arteries.

- Side effects: Lethargy, flushing, edema, ascites, and indigestion.
- Nifedipine (Procardia) and nicardipine (Cardene) are primarily arterial vasodilators, used to treat acute hypertension. Diltiazem (Cardizem) and Verapamil (Calan, Isoptin) dilate primarily coronary arteries and slow the heart rate, thus are used for angina, atrial fibrillation, and SVT. *Note:* Nifedipine (Procardia) should be avoided in older adults due to increased risk of hypotension and myocardial ischemia.

**Review Video: Calcium Channel Blockers and Antiarrhythmics**
Visit mometrix.com/academy and enter code: 942825

## Additional Vasodilators

**B-type natriuretic peptide (BNP)** (Nesiritide [Natrecor]) is type of vasodilator (non-inotropic), which is a recombinant form of a peptide of the human brain. It decreases filling pressure, vascular resistance, and increases U/O.

- May cause hypotension, headache, bradycardia, and nausea. It is used short term for worsening decompensated CHF; contraindicated in SBP<90, cardiogenic shock, contrictive pericarditis, or valve stenosis.

**Alpha-adrenergic blockers** block alpha receptors in arteries and veins, causing vasodilation.

- May cause orthostatic hypotension and edema from fluid retention.
- Labetalol (Normodyne) is a combination peripheral alpha-blocker and cardiac β-blocker that is used to treat acute hypertension, acute stroke, and acute aortic dissection.
- Phentolamine (Regitine) is a peripheral arterial dilator that reduces afterload. It is used for HTN crisis in patients with pheochromocytoma, as well as a subcutaneous injection for extravasation of vessicants.

**Selective specific dopamine DA-1-receptor agonists:**

- Fenoldopam (Corlopam) is a peripheral dilator affecting renal and mesenteric arteries and can be used for patients with renal dysfunction or those at risk of renal insufficiency.

## Inotropic Agents

Inotropic agents are drugs used to increase cardiac output and improve contractibility. IV inotropic agents may increase the risk of death, but may be used when other drugs fail. Oral forms of these drugs are less effective than intravenous. Inotropic agents include:

- **β-Adrenergic agonists**:
  - **Dobutamine** improves cardiac output, treats cardiac decompensation, and increases blood pressure. It helps the body to utilize norepinephrine. Side effects include increased or labile blood pressure, increased heart rate, PVCs, N/V, and bronchospasm.
  - **Dopamine** improves cardiac output, blood pressure, and blood flow to the renal and mesenteric arteries. Side effects include tachycardia or bradycardia, palpitations, BP changes, dyspnea, nausea and vomiting, headache, and gangrene of extremities.

- **Phosphodiesterase III inhibitors**:
  - **Milrinone** (Primacor) increases strength of contractions and cause vasodilation. Side effects include ventricular arrhythmias, hypotension, and headaches.
- **Digoxin (Lanoxin)** increases contractibility and cardiac output and prevents arrhythmias.

**Review Video: Antiadrenergics—Alpha- and Beta-Blockers**
Visit mometrix.com/academy and enter code: 947779

## Medications for Heart Failure

A patient with heart failure may be prescribed with one or multiple of the drugs below:

- **ACE inhibitors:** Captopril (Capoten), enalapril (Vasotec), and lisinopril (Prinivil). Decrease afterload/preload and reverse ventricular remodeling; they also prevent neuropathy in DM. Contraindicated with renal insufficiency, renal artery stenosis, and pregnancy.
  - Side effects include cough (#1), hyperkalemia, hypotension, angioedema, dizziness, and weakness.
- **Angiotensin receptor blockers (ARBs):** Losartan (Cozaar) and valsartan (Diovan). Decrease afterload/preload and reverse ventricular remodeling, causing vasodilation and reducing blood pressure. They are used for those who cannot tolerate ACE inhibitors.
  - Side effects include cough (less common than with ACE inhibitors), hyperkalemia, hypotension, headache, dizziness, metallic taste, and rash.
- **β-Blockers:** Metoprolol (Lopressor), carvedilol (Coreg) and esmolol (Brevibloc). Slow the heart rate, reduce hypertension, prevent dysrhythmias, and reverse ventricular remodeling. Contraindicated in bradyarrythmias, decompensated HF, uncontrolled hypoglycemia/diabetes mellitus, and airway disease.
  - Side effects: bradycardia, hypotension, bronchospasm, may mask signs of hypoglycemia.
- **Aldosterone agonist:** Spironolactone (Aldactone). Decreases preload and myocardial hypertrophy and reduces edema and sodium retention but may increase serum potassium.
- **Furosemide (Lasix)** is used for the control of congestive heart failure as well as renal insufficiency. It is used after surgery to decrease preload and to reduce the inflammatory response caused by cardiopulmonary bypass (post-perfusion syndrome).

**Review Video: Antihypertensives: ACE inhibitors and ARBs**
Visit mometrix.com/academy and enter code: 525864

## Digoxin

Digitalis drugs, most commonly administered in the form of digoxin (Lanoxin), are derived from the foxglove plant and are used to increase myocardial contractility, left ventricular output, and slow conduction through the AV node, decreasing rapid heart rates and promoting diuresis. Digoxin does not affect mortality, but increases tolerance to activity and reduces hospitalizations for heart failure. Therapeutic levels (0.5-2.0 ng/mL) should be maintained to avoid digitalis toxicity, which can occur even if digoxin levels are within therapeutic range, so observation of symptoms is critical. Because patients with heart failure are often on diuretics which decrease potassium levels, they are at increased risk for toxicity.

**Symptoms of toxicity** are as follows:

- Early signs: Increasing fatigue, lethargy, depression, and nausea and vomiting; progress to severe diarrhea, blurred vision/yellow or green halos around lights, fatigue/weakness
- Arrythmias: SA or AV block, VT/VF, PVCs, and bradycardia

**Treatment** consists of the following:

- Monitor serum levels and symptoms.
- Digoxin immune FAB (Digibind) may be used to bind to digoxin and inactivate it if necessary.

## Glycoprotein IIB/IIIA Inhibitors

Glycoprotein IIB/IIIA Inhibitors are drugs that are used to inhibit platelet binding and prevent clots prior to and following invasive cardiac procedures, such as angioplasty and stent placement. These medications are used in combination with anticoagulant drugs, such as heparin and aspirin for the following:

- Acute coronary syndromes (ACS), such as unstable angina or myocardial infarctions
- Percutaneous coronary intervention (PCI), such as angioplasty and stent placement

These medications are contraindicated in those with a low platelet count or active bleeding:

- **Eptifibatide (Integrilin)**: Used with both heparin and aspirin for ACS and PCI and affects platelet binding for 6-8 hours after administration. Should not be used in patients with renal problems.
- **Tirofiban (Aggrastat)**: Used with heparin for PCI patients with reduced dosage for those with renal problems and affects platelet binding for only 4-8 hours after administration.

## Pharmacologic Measures to Maximize Perfusion

The primary focus of pharmacologic measures to **maximize perfusion** is to reduce the risk of **thromboses**:

- **Antiplatelet agents**, such as aspirin, Ticlid, and Plavix, which interfere with the function of the plasma membrane, interfering with clotting. These agents are ineffective to treat clots but prevent clot formation.
- **Vasodilators** may divert blood from ischemic areas, but some may be indicated, such as Pletal, which dilates arteries and decreases clotting, and is used for control of intermittent claudication.
- **Antilipemic**, such as Zocor and Questran, slow progression of atherosclerosis.
- **Hemorheologic agents**, such as Trental, reduce fibrinogen, reducing blood viscosity and rigidity of erythrocytes; however, clinical studies show limited benefit. It may be used for intermittent claudication.
- **Analgesics** may be necessary to improve quality of life. Opioids may be needed in some cases.
- **Thrombolytics** may be injected into a blocked artery under angiography to dissolve clots.
- **Anticoagulants**, such as Coumadin and Lovenox, prevent blood clots from forming.

### *Administration of Fibrinolytic (Thrombolytic) Infusions for MI*

Fibrinolytic infusion is indicated for acute myocardial infarction under these conditions:

- Symptoms of MI, <6-12 hours since onset of symptoms
- ≥1 mm elevation of ST in ≥2 contiguous leads
- No contraindications and no cardiogenic shock

**Fibrinolytic agents** should be administered as soon as possible, within 30 minutes is best. All agents convert plasminogen to plasmin, which breaks down fibrin, dissolving clots:

- Streptokinase and anistreplase (1st generation)
- Alteplase or tissue plasminogen activator (tPA) (2nd generation)
- Reteplase and tenecteplase (3rd generation)

**Contraindications**

- Present or recent bleeding or history of severe bleeding
- History of intracranial hemorrhage
- History of stroke (<3 months unless within 3 hours)
- Aortic dissection or pericarditis
- Intracranial/intraspinal surgery or trauma within 3 months or neoplasm, aneurysm, or AVM

**Relative contraindications**

- Active peptic ulcer
- >10 minutes of CPR
- Advanced renal or hepatic disease
- Pregnancy
- Anticoagulation therapy
- Acute uncontrolled hypertension or chronic poorly controlled hypertension
- Recent (2–4 weeks) internal bleeding
- Non-compressible vascular punctures

# Respiratory Pharmacology

## Pharmacological Agents Used for Asthma

Numerous pharmacological agents are used for control of asthma, some that are long-acting to prevent attacks and others that are short-acting to provide relief for acute episodes. Listed with each are the standard med and dosage used for urgent care:

- **β-Adrenergic agonists** include both long-acting and short-acting preparations used for relaxation of smooth muscles and bronchodilation, reducing edema, and aiding clearance of mucus. Medications include salmeterol, sustained-release albuterol and short-acting albuterol, and levalbuterol. Albuterol 2.5–5.0 mg every 20 minutes, 3 doses by nebulizer.
- **Anticholinergics** aid in preventing bronchial constriction and potentiate the bronchodilating action of β-Adrenergic agonists. The most commonly used medication is ipratropium bromide 500 mcg every 20 minutes, 3 doses by nebulizer.
- **Corticosteroids** provide anti-inflammatory action by inhibiting immune responses and decreasing edema, mucus, and hyper-responsiveness. Because of numerous side effects, glucocorticosteroids are usually administered orally or parenterally for ≤5 days (prednisone, prednisolone, methylprednisolone) and then switched to inhaled steroids. If a person receives glucocorticoids for more than 5 days, then dosages are tapered. Methylprednisolone 60–125 mg IV is the standard dose for respiratory failure. The Global Initiative for Asthma (GINA) recommends daily inhaled corticosteroids for all individuals with severe asthma to reduce the risk of exacerbations.
- **Methylxanthines** are used to improve pulmonary function and decrease the need for mechanical ventilation. Medications include aminophylline and theophylline.
- **Magnesium sulfate** is used to relax smooth muscles and decrease inflammation. If administered intravenously, it must be given slowly to prevent hypotension and bradycardia. When inhaled, it potentiates the action of albuterol. Standard dosage: 2 g (8 mmol), 1 dose by IV over 20 minutes.
- **Heliox** (helium-oxygen) is administered to decrease airway resistance with airway obstruction, thereby decreasing respiratory effort. Heliox improves oxygenation of those on mechanical ventilation.
- **Leukotriene inhibitors** are used to inhibit inflammation and bronchospasm for long-term management. Medications include montelukast.

### Additional Pulmonary Pharmacology

There is a wide range of agents used for pulmonary pharmacology, depending upon the type and degree of pulmonary disease. Agents include:

- **Opioid analgesics**: Used to provide both pain relief and sedation for those on mechanical ventilation to reduce sympathetic response. Medications may include fentanyl or morphine sulfate.
- **Neuromuscular blockers**: Used for induced paralysis of those who have not responded adequately to sedation, especially for intubation and mechanical ventilation. Medications may include pancuronium and vecuronium. However, there is controversy about the use of such blockers, as induced paralysis has been linked to increased mortality rates, sensory hearing loss (pancuronium), atelectasis, and ventilation-perfusion mismatch.
- **Human B-type natriuretic peptides**: Used to reduce pulmonary capillary wedge pressure. Medications include nesiritide.
- **Surfactants**: Reduces surface tension to prevent the collapse of alveoli. Beractant (Survanta) is derived from bovine lung tissue and calfactant from calf lung tissue. They are administered as inhalants.
- **Alkalinizers**: Used to treat metabolic acidosis and reduce pulmonary vascular resistance by achieving an alkaline pH. Medications include sodium bicarbonate and tromethamine (THAM).
- **Pulmonary vasodilator (inhaled nitric oxide)**: Used to relax the vascular muscles and produce pulmonary vasodilation. Some studies show it reduces the need for extracorporeal membrane oxygenation (ECMO).
- **Methylxanthines**: Used to stimulate muscle contractions of the chest and stimulate respirations. Medications include aminophylline, caffeine citrate, and doxapram.
- **Diuretics**: Used to reduce pulmonary edema. Medications include loop diuretics such as furosemide and metolazone.
- **Nitrates**: Used for vasodilation to reduce preload and afterload, which in turn reduces myocardial need for oxygen. Medications include nitroglycerin and nitroprusside sodium.
- **Antibiotics**: Used for treatment of respiratory infections, including pneumonia. Medications are used according to the pathogenic agent and may include macrolides such as azithromycin (Zithromax) and erythromycin.
- **Antimycobacterials**: Used for treatment of TB and other mycobacterial diseases. Medications include isoniazid, ethambutol, rifampin, streptomycin sulfate, and pyrazinamide.
- **Antivirals**: Used to inhibit replication of a virus early in a viral infection. Effectiveness decreases as time passes because the replication process has already begun. Medications include ribavirin and zanamivir.

## Endocrine Pharmacology

### Oral Hypoglycemic Agents

Oral hypoglycemic agents are **anti-diabetic treatments** generally used in the treatment of Type II Diabetes. There are five classic categories of oral hypoglycemic agents: sulfonylureas, biguanides, meglitinides, competitive inhibitors of alpha-glucosidases (located in the intestinal brush border), and thiazolidinediones. More recently, two additional novel classes of oral hypoglycemics, DPP-4 inhibitors and SGLT2 inhibitors, were introduced with proven effectiveness when used in conjunction with changes in diet and exercise. Some examples of sulfonylurea oral hypoglycemic agents include the first-generation agents tolbutamide, tolazamide, chlorpropamide, and acetohexamide; and second-generation agents glyburide, glimepiride, and glipizide. The biguanide oral hypoglycemic agent is metformin. Metformin has the distinct advantage of not causing weight gain or hypoglycemic reactions. The meglitinide agent is repaglinide. Examples of alpha-glucosidase inhibitors are acarbose and miglitol. Alpha-glucosidase inhibitors bind tightly to intestinal alpha-glucosidases and decrease the postprandial rise in glucose levels. The only available thiazolidinedione oral hypoglycemic agent is currently pioglitazone; troglitazone was removed from US market in 2000, and rosiglitazone was removed from US market in 2011. Examples of DPP-4 inhibitors include linagliptin, vildagliptin, sitagliptin, and saxagliptin. Examples of SGLT2 inhibitors include canagliflozin, dapagliflozin, and empagliflozin.

### Insulin Used to Treat Glycemic Disorders

There are a number of different types of **insulin** with varying action times. Insulin is used to metabolize **glucose** for those whose pancreas does not produce insulin (type 1 diabetes) or does not produce sufficient insulin (type 2 diabetes). People may need to take a combination of insulins (short- and long-acting) to maintain glucose control. Duration of action may vary according to the individual's metabolism, intake, and level of activity:

- **Humalog** (Lispro H) is a rapid-acting insulin with onset in 5–15 minutes, peaking at 45–90 minutes and lasting 3–4 hours.
- **Regular** (R) is a relatively fast-acting insulin with onset in 30 minutes, peaks in 2–5 hours, and lasts 5–8 hours.
- **NPH** (N) insulin is intermediate-acting with onset in 1–3 hours, peaking at 6–12 hours, and lasting for 16–24 hours.
- **Insulin Glargine** (Lantus) is a long-acting insulin with onset in 3–6 hours, no peak, and lasting for 24 hours.
- **Combined NPH/Regular** (70/30 or 50/50) has an onset of 30 minutes, peaks at 7–12 hours, and lasts 16–24 hours.

## Immunologic Pharmacology

### Immunosuppressant Drugs

| Drugs | Actions | Side effects |
|---|---|---|
| **Corticosteroids** | Depress cell-mediated immune response, humoral immune response, and inflammation, reducing proliferation of T cells and B cells. Used with transplantations and to prevent GVHD disease. | Weight gain, edema, Cushing syndrome, hyperglycemia, bruising, and osteoporosis. Abruptly stopping drugs may trigger Addisonian crisis. |
| **Ciclosporin (cyclosporine)** | Inhibit activation of T cells. Used to prevent transplantation rejection and to treat autoimmune diseases and nephrotic syndrome. | Tremor, excessive facial hair, gingivitis, bone marrow suppression with increased risk of infection and cancer, especially skin cancer. |
| **Intravenous immuno-globulin G (IVIG)** | Used to combat immunosuppression by increasing antibodies to prevent infection or treat acute infection, such as Guillain-Barre. Used off-label for many different disorders and infections. | Dermatitis, headache, renal failure, and venous thrombosis. Infections can occur because IVIG is extracted from pooled plasma. |

**Review Video: Immunomodulators and Immunosuppressors**
Visit mometrix.com/academy and enter code: 666131

### Chemotherapy

Chemotherapy may be offered during palliative care to enhance patient comfort, wellbeing, and symptom control for **enhanced quality of life**. It is understood that the treatment is not expected to provide a cure and should not be given as a means to maintain a sense of false hope within the patient or family. It should be clear that the expectation of treatment is **prolonged survival** and **control of cancer-related symptoms**. Not all patients will benefit from palliative chemotherapy. The decision to provide chemotherapy is based on the clinical indicators and the patient's wishes. The benefit and cost ratios of treatment need to be considered. Tumor response to treatment, metastasis, and other disease specific factors will help define chemotherapy's usefulness for an individual patient. Patients also need to be aware that chemotherapy involves a commitment to repeated travel, hospitalizations, invasive procedures, and assessments in order to make an informed decision.

### Chemotherapeutic Agents

The major chemotherapy agents are alkylating agents, antimetabolites, plant alkaloids, antitumor antibiotics, and steroid hormones.

- **Alkylating agents** work directly by attacking the DNA of cancers such as chronic leukemias, Hodgkin's disease, lymphomas, and lung, breast, prostate, and ovary cancers.
- **Nitrosoureas** inhibit repair in damaged DNA. They are able to cross the blood-brain barrier and are frequently used to treat brain tumors, lymphomas, multiple myeloma, and malignant melanoma.
- **Antimetabolites** block cell growth. This class of chemotherapeutic drugs is used to treat leukemias, choriocarcinoma, and gastrointestinal, breast, and ovary cancers.
- **Antitumor antibiotics** are a broad category of agents that bind to DNA and prevent RNA synthesis and are used with a wide variety of cancers.
- **Plant (vinca) alkaloids** are extracted from plants and block cell division. These are used to treat acute lymphoblastic leukemia, Hodgkin and non-Hodgkin lymphomas, neuroblastomas, Wilms tumor, and lung, breast, and testes cancers.
- **Steroid hormones** have an unclear action but may be useful in treating hormone-dependent cancers such as ovary and breast cancer.

### Routes of Delivery

Chemotherapy treatments may be provided orally, intramuscularly, intravenously, intra-arterially, intralesionally (directly into the tumor), intraperitoneally, intrathecally, or topically. **Oral chemotherapy** is the easiest and often used in the home. **Intravenous delivery** is the most common chemotherapy route but **intramuscular delivery** may have more lasting effects. The goal of **intra-arterial chemotherapy** is to introduce the agent directly into the blood supply feeding the tumor or affected organ. Ovarian cancer with tumors greater than 2 cm in diameter may be treated with **intraperitoneal therapy**. Acute lymphocytic leukemia is primarily treated with **intrathecal administration**. **Intralesional treatments** are used for melanoma and Kaposi sarcoma. **Topical treatment** is most common with skin cancers.

### Side Effects

Not every patient will experience every symptom, or in the same degree. **Side effects** can vary greatly; some can be easily controlled with additional medications. Many side effects are due to the effects of the chemotherapy on **cells**, such as bone marrow, hair, and gastrointestinal cells, which have a rapid mitotic rate and rapid turnover. Common side effects can include bone marrow suppression, hair loss (alopecia), mouth ulcers, sore throat and gums, heartburn, nausea, vomiting, loss of appetite, weight loss, anorexia and cachexia, anemia, nerve and muscle problems, dry or discolored skin, kidney and bladder irritation, fatigue, and increased bruising, bleeding, and infection. The patient's sexual function can also be affected, including possible infertility.

### Risks

**Infection** is a common concern of chemotherapy because of the decreased number of **neutrophils** in the patient's system. **Neutropenia** is silent but dangerous, leaving no neutrophils to fight the threat of infections. Neutropenia can cause a septic situation, which can be life-threatening. Severe **anemia** may result in the need for blood transfusions. **Neurological damage** may include mild alterations in taste or smell, peripheral neuropathy, mental status changes, or seizures. Some anticancer drugs can cause **heart damage** if not monitored closely. Many anticancer drugs cause **kidney damage**, as well as increasing the risk of drug toxicity from decreased renal function. Anticancer drugs can also cause **cataracts** and **retina damage**.

### PALLIATIVE SEDATION

Palliative sedation is a treatment method focused on controlling and easing symptoms that have proven otherwise refractory or unendurable in nature. This process was originally named **terminal sedation**. It was changed to palliative sedation to emphasize the differences between symptom management and euthanasia. The purpose of palliative sedation is **symptom control**; it does not hasten or cause death. Through the monitored use of medications such as midazolam or propofol, relief can be provided through varying levels of unconsciousness. Among terminally ill patients, palliative sedation is most often used to calm persistent agitation and restlessness. The second most frequent need is for pain control, followed by confusion, shortness of breath, muscle twitching or seizures, and anguish.

## Hematologic Pharmacology

### ANTICOAGULANTS

Common anticoagulants used at home and in the hospital setting are discussed below, including possible complications and the antidotes for each:

- **Antithrombin activators**: Heparin (unfractionated) and derivatives, LWM (Dalteparin, Enoxaparin, tinzaparin), and Fondaparinux.
    - Possible complications: Thrombocytopenia, bleeding/hemorrhage, osteopenia, hypersensitivity.
    - Antidote: Protamine sulfate 1% solution—dosage varies according to drug and drug's dosage. (1 mg protamine neutralizes 100 units of heparin or 1 mg of enoxaparin.)
- **Direct thrombin inhibitors**: Hirudin analogs (bivalirudin, desirudin, lepirudin). Others: Apixaban, Argatroban, and dabigatran.
    - Possible complications: Bleeding/hemorrhage, GI upset, backpain, hypertension, headache.
    - No antidote is available.
- **Direct Xa inhibitor**: Rivaroxaban
    - Possible complications: Bleeding/hemorrhage.
    - No antidote is available.
- **Antithrombin (AT)**: Recombinant human AT, Plasma-derived AT
    - Possible complications: Bleeding/hemorrhage, hypersensitivity.
    - No antidote is available.
- **Warfarin**
    - Possible complications: Bleeding/hemorrhage. Drug interactions may cause thrombosis or increased risk of bleeding.
    - Antidote: Vitamin $K_1$ usually at 2.5 mg PO or 0.5–1.0 mg IV. If ineffective, FFP or fresh whole blood may be administered.

#### *HEPARIN*

##### PHARMACOLOGY

Heparin is an **anticoagulant** derived from the intestinal mucosa of the pig and the lung of the pig. The mechanism of action of heparin is to bind to the surface of the endothelial cell membrane. The activity of heparin depends upon plasma protease inhibitor antithrombin III. Antithrombin III inhibits thrombin and other anti-clotting proteases. In addition, heparin binding causes a change in antithrombin III inhibitor form, resulting in increased antithrombin-protease complex formation activity. After antithrombin-protease complex formation, heparin is subsequently released and is available to bind to more antithrombin molecules.

### Risk Factors

The major risk factor of heparin use is hemorrhage. Predisposing factors for hemorrhage include advanced age and renal failure. Prolonged use of heparin can result in osteoporosis and fractures. Other risk factors of heparin use include transient thrombocytopenia, severe thrombocytopenia, paradoxical thromboembolism, and heparin-induced aggregation of platelets. These risks can be reduced by careful selection of patients who receive heparin therapy, careful control of the dosage of heparin, and meticulous monitoring of the partial thromboplastin time, or PTT. It is important to remember that thrombocytopenia or the development of a thrombus may be due to heparin itself.

### Contraindications

There are numerous contraindications to the use of heparin, including: hypersensitivity to heparin; diseases of the hematologic system (hemophilia, purpura, or thrombocytopenia); uncontrolled hypertension; intracranial bleed; infectious endocarditis; active tuberculosis; gastrointestinal ulcers; cancer of the gastrointestinal visceral organs; severe liver dysfunction; severe kidney dysfunction; and threatened miscarriage or abortion. Heparin is contraindicated in the following medical procedures: following brain surgery; following spinal cord surgery; following eye surgery; after a lumbar puncture; and after regional anesthesia blocks. The effects of heparin may be reversed by stopping heparin or by the use of a specific antagonist (protamine sulfate).

**Review Video: Heparin - An Injectable Anti-Coagulant**
Visit mometrix.com/academy and enter code: 127426

## *Warfarin*

### Pharmacology

Warfarin causes a deficiency in prothrombin in the plasma and is used as an **anti-thrombotic agent** and to decrease the risk of embolism in humans. This agent causes the liver to manufacture less of the proteins necessary for blood coagulation. Since it is 99% bound to albumin in the plasma, warfarin has a high bio-availability. The mechanism of action of warfarin involves prothrombin, factor VII, factor IX, factor X, and protein C. Warfarin inhibits the g-carboxylation of the glutamate residues in the aforementioned factors. The mechanism of action of warfarin also involves vitamin K. Warfarin has a slow onset of action, usually 24 hours, and a typical duration of 2–5 days. Using increased dosages of warfarin as loading dosages will serve to speed up the onset of anti-coagulation. Patients on warfarin must discontinue this medication five days before planned surgery due to its longer duration.

### Drug-Drug Interactions

Warfarin has many drug-drug interactions, the most serious of which increases the risk of bleeding. Sulfinpyrazone and phenylbutazone interact with warfarin to cause enhanced decrease in prothrombin, increased inhibition of platelets, and increased risk of peptic ulcer. The following drugs can have adverse effects when co-administered with warfarin: antibiotics such as metronidazole, azithromycin, clarithromycin, dirithromycin, erythromycin, roxithromycin, and telithromycin; broad-spectrum antibiotics such as amoxicillin, imipenem, levofloxacin; antifungal agents such as fluconazole, miconazole, and ketoconazole; barbiturates; and trimethoprim-sulfamethoxazole, amiodarone, cimetidine, and disulfiram. Aspirin inhibits metabolism of the warfarin and nonsteroidal anti-inflammatory drugs (NSAIDs) inhibit the clotting of platelets. The third-generation cephalosporins increase the risk of bleeding with warfarin because these drugs destroy the intestinal bacteria that produce vitamin K. Always check on possible drug-drug interactions when administering warfarin and monitor patients who might be at risk.

**Review Video: Warfarin - Uses and Side Effects**
Visit mometrix.com/academy and enter code: 844117

## THROMBOLYTICS

Thrombolytics are drugs used to dissolve clots in myocardial infarction, ischemic stroke, DVT, and pulmonary embolism. **Thrombolytics** may be given in combination with heparin or low-weight heparin to increase anticoagulation effect. Thrombolytics should be administered within 90 minutes but may be given up to 6 hours after an event. They may increase the danger of hemorrhage and are contraindicated with hemorrhagic strokes, recent surgery, or bleeding. Thrombolytics include:

- **Alteplase tissue-type plasminogen activator** (t-PA) (Activase) is an enzyme that converts plasminogen to plasmin, which is a fibrinolytic enzyme. t-PA is used for ischemic stroke, MI, and pulmonary embolism and must be given IV within 3–4.5 hours or by catheter directly to the site of occlusion within 6 hours.
- **Reteplase** (Retavase) is a plasminogen activator used after MI to prevent CHF (contraindicated for ischemic strokes). It is given in 2 doses, a 10-unit bolus over 2 minutes and then repeated in 30 minutes.
- **Tenecteplase** (TNKase) is used to treat acute MI with large ST elevation. It is administered in a one-time bolus over 5 seconds and should be administered within 30 minutes of the event.

**Contraindications** to thrombolytic therapy include:

- Evidence of cerebral or subarachnoid hemorrhage or other internal bleeding or history of intracranial hemorrhage, recent stroke, head trauma, or surgery (ruled out by CT scan before administration for ischemic stroke)
- Uncontrolled hypertension, seizures
- Intracranial AVM, neoplasm, or aneurysm
- Current anticoagulation therapy
- Low platelet count (<100,000 $mm^3$)

**Review Video: Antiplatelets and Thrombolytics**
Visit mometrix.com/academy and enter code: 711284

**Review Video: Thrombolytics**
Visit mometrix.com/academy and enter code: 832357

# Neurological Pharmacology

## ANTICONVULSANTS

### Carbamazepine (Tegretol)

*Use*: Partial, tonic-clonic, and absence seizures; analgesia for trigeminal neuralgia

*Side effects*: Dizziness, drowsiness, nausea, and vomiting. Toxic reactions include severe skin rash, agranulocytosis, aplastic anemia, and hepatitis

### Clonazepam (Klonopin)

*Use*: Akinetic, absence, and myoclonic seizures; Lennox-Gastaut syndrome

*Side effects*: Behavioral changes, hirsutism or alopecia, headaches, and drowsiness. Toxic reactions include hepatotoxicity, thrombocytopenia, ataxia, and bone marrow failure.

**Ethosuximide (Zarontin)**

*Use*: Absence seizures

*Side effects*: Headaches and gastrointestinal disorders. Toxic reactions include skin rash, blood dyscrasias (sometimes fatal), hepatitis, and lupus erythematosus.

**Felbamate (Felbatol)**

*Use*: Lennox-Gastaut syndrome

*Side effects*: Headache, fatigue, insomnia, and cognitive impairment. Toxic reactions include aplastic anemia and hepatic failure. It is recommended only if other medications have failed.

**Fosphenytoin (Cerebyx)**

*Use*: Status epilepticus prevention and treatment during neurosurgery

*Side effects*: CNS depression, hypotension, cardiovascular collapse, dizziness, nystagmus, and pruritus.

**Gabapentin (Neurontin)**

*Use*: Partial seizures; post-herpetic neuralgia

*Side effects*: Dizziness, somnolence, drowsiness, ataxia, weight gain, and nausea. Toxic reactions include hepatotoxicity and leukopenia.

**Lamotrigine (Lamictal)**

*Use*: Partial and primary generalized tonic-clonic seizures; Lennox-Gastaut syndrome

*Side effects*: Tremor, ataxia, weight gain, dizziness, headache, and drowsiness. Toxic reactions include severe rash, which may require hospitalization.

**Levetiracetam (Keppra)**

*Use*: Partial onset, myoclonic, and generalized tonic-clonic seizures

*Side effects*: Idiopathic generalized epilepsy, dizziness, somnolence, irritability, alopecia, double vision, sore throat, and fatigue. Toxic reactions include bone marrow suppression and liver failure.

**Oxcarbazepine (Trileptal)**

*Use*: Partial seizures

*Side effects*: Double or abnormal vision, tremor, abnormal gait, GI disorders, dizziness, and fatigue. A toxic reaction is hepatotoxicity.

**Phenobarbital (Sezaby)**

*Use*: Tonic-clonic and cortical local seizures; acute convulsive episodes; insomnia

*Side effects*: Sedation, double vision, agitation, and ataxia. Toxic reactions include anemia and skin rash.

**Phenytoin (Dilantin)**

*Use*: Tonic-clonic and complex partial seizures

*Side effects*: Nystagmus, vision disorders, gingival hyperplasia, hirsutism, dysrhythmias, and dysarthria. Toxic reactions include collapse of cardiovascular system and CNS depression.

**Primidone (Mysoline)**

*Use*: Grand mal, psychomotor, and focal seizures

*Side effects*: Double vision, ataxia, impotence, lethargy, and irritability. Toxic reactions include skin rash.

**Tiagabine**

*Use*: Partial seizures

*Side effects*: Concentration problems, weak knees, dysarthria, abdominal pain, tremor, dizziness, fatigue, and agitation.

**Topiramate (Topamax)**

*Use*: Partial and tonic-clonic seizures; migraines

*Side effects*: Anorexia, weight loss, somnolence, confusion, ataxia, and confusion. Toxic reactions include kidney stones.

**Valproate/Valproic acid (Depakote, Depakene)**

*Use*: Complex partial, simple, and complex absence seizures; bipolar disorder

*Side effects*: Weight gain, alopecia, tremor, menstrual disorders, nausea, and vomiting. Toxic reactions include hepatotoxicity, severe pancreatitis, rash, blood dyscrasias, and nephritis.

**Zonisamide (Zonegran)**

*Use*: Partial seizures

*Side effects*: Anorexia, nausea, agitation, rash, headache, dizziness, and somnolence. Toxic reactions include leukopenia and hepatotoxicity.

## Hypertonic Saline Solution

Hypertonic saline solution (HSS) has a sodium concentration higher than 0.9% (NS) and is used to reduce intracranial pressure/cerebral edema and treat traumatic brain injury. Concentrations usually range from 2.0–23.4%. The hypertonic solution draws fluid from the tissue through osmosis. As edema decreases, circulation improves. HSS also expands plasma, increasing CPP, and counteracts hyponatremia that occurs in the brain after injury.

**Administration**:

- Peripheral lines: HSS <3% only
- Central lines: HSS ≥3%

HSS can be administered continuously at rates varying from 30–150 mL/hr. Rate must be carefully controlled. Fluid status must be monitored to prevent hypovolemia, which increases risk of renal failure. Boluses (typically 30 mL of 23.4%) may be administered over 15 minutes for acute increased ICP or transtentorial herniation.

**Laboratory monitoring** includes:

- Sodium (every 6 hours): Maintain at 145–155 mmol/L. Higher levels can cause heart/respiratory/renal failure.
- Serum osmolality (every 12 hours): Maintain at 320 mOsm/L. Higher levels can cause renal failure.

### MANNITOL

Mannitol is an osmotic diuretic that increases excretion of both sodium and water and reduces intracranial pressure and brain mass, especially after traumatic brain injury. Mannitol may also be used to shrink the cells of the blood-brain barrier in order to help other medications breach this barrier. Mannitol is administered per intravenous infusion:

- 0.5–2.0 g/kg in a 15–25% solution over 30–60 minutes
- A repeated dose of 0.25–1.0 g/kg every 4–6 hours based on patient response

Cerebral spinal fluid pressure should show decrease within 15 minutes. Fluid and electrolyte balances must be carefully monitored as well as intake and output and body weight. Concentrations of 20–25% require a filter. Crystals may form if the mannitol solution is too cold and the mannitol container may require heating (in 80 °C water) and shaking to dissolve crystals, but the solution should be cooled to below body temperature prior to administration. Mannitol cannot be administered in polyvinylchloride bags as precipitates form. Side effects include fluid and electrolyte imbalance, nausea, vomiting, hypotension, tachycardia, fever, and urticaria.

## Gastrointestinal Pharmacology

### HISTAMINE RECEPTOR ANTAGONISTS

Histamine (H) receptor antagonists (actually reverse agonists) are used to treat conditions in which excessive stomach acid causes heartburn and GERD. They block histamine 2 ($H_2$) (parietal) cell receptors in the stomach, thereby decreasing acid production. These drugs are used less commonly now than proton-pump inhibitors. **Common $H_2$ antagonists** include:

- **Cimetidine**: The first $H_2$ antagonist, it is used less frequently than others because of inhibition of enzymes that results in drug interactions, especially with contraceptive agents and estrogen.
- **Famotidine (Pepcid)**: This may be combined with an antacid to increase the speed of effects as it has a slow onset. It may be used pre-surgically to reduce post-operative nausea.
- **Nizatidine**: The last $H_2$ antagonist developed, it is used to treat ulcers and GERD. It is about equal in potency and action to ranitidine, which was discontinued due to the presence of NDMA, a cancer-causing contaminant, when stored in high temperatures.

### ANTACIDS

Antacids are medications used to reduce stomach acids by raising the pH and neutralizing the acids present. They are commonly used to treat heartburn or indigestion. Adverse reactions are relatively rare unless taken to excess or with renal impairment. Drugs include:

- **Aluminum hydroxide** may cause constipation and with renal impairment, hypophosphatemia and osteomalacia.
- **Magnesium hydroxide** (Milk of Magnesia) may cause diarrhea and with renal impairment can cause hypermagnesemia.
- **Aluminum hydroxide with magnesium hydroxide** may cause nausea, vomiting and diarrhea, yeast infection (thrush), or hypophosphatemia.

- **Calcium carbonate** (TUMS, Titralac) may cause gastric distention. Excess calcium intake may cause toxic reactions, including kidney stones and renal failure, so excess intake should be avoided.
- **Alka-Seltzer** combines sodium bicarbonate with aspirin and citric acid so this compound may cause gastric irritation, nausea and vomiting, and tarry stools.
- **Bismuth subsalicylate** (Pepto-Bismol). Pepto-Bismol may react with sulfur in the body to create a black tongue and black stools, but this is temporary. Pepto-Bismol has been associated with Reye's syndrome in children with influenza or chickenpox.

## Proton Pump Inhibitors

Proton pump inhibitors (PPIs) are now used more frequently than histamine receptor antagonists. PPIs interfere with an acid-producing enzyme in the stomach wall, reducing stomach acid. PPIs are used to treat GERD, stomach ulcers, and *H. pylori* (with antibiotics). PPIs are similar in action and include:

- Esomeprazole (Nexium)
- Lansoprazole (Prevacid)
- Omeprazole (Prilosec)
- Pantoprazole (Protonix)
- Rabeprazole (Aciphex)
- Omeprazole/sodium bicarbonate (Long-acting form of omeprazole)

Common side effects include gastrointestinal upset (nausea, diarrhea, and constipation), headache, and rash. In rare instances, PPIs may cause severe muscle pain; however, they are usually well-tolerated with few adverse effects. PPIs may interfere with the absorption of some drugs, such as those that are affected by stomach acid. Absorption of ketoconazole is impaired, and absorption of digoxin is increased, sometimes leading to toxicity. Omeprazole impacts the hepatic breakdown of drugs more than other PPIs and may cause increased levels of diazepam, phenytoin, and warfarin.

## Anti-Lipids

Anti-lipid medications are frequently used to **lower cholesterol levels** if dietary modifications are unsuccessful in order to decrease coronary artery disease. There are several **types** of medications aimed at lowering cholesterol levels, with the most common being :

- **Statins** (3-hydroxy-3-methylglutaryl coenzyme A reductase inhibitors), such as atorvastatin (Lipitor), rosuvastatin (Crestor), fluvastatin (Lescol), lovastatin (Altoprev), pravastatin, and simvastatin (Zocor), inhibit the liver enzyme that produces cholesterol, but different statins vary in the ability to reduce cholesterol and in drug/other interactions (protease inhibitors, erythromycin, grapefruit juice, niacin, and fibric acids). Adverse effects include rhabdomyolysis (which causes severe muscle pain and weakness), headache, rash, weakness, and gastrointestinal disorders.
- **Nicotinic acid** (Niacor) decreases synthesis of lipoprotein, lowers low-density lipoprotein (LDL) and triglycerides, and increases high-density lipoprotein (HDL). It is used for low elevations of cholesterol and may be combined with statins. Adverse effects include flushing, hyperglycemia, gout, upper gastrointestinal disorders, and hepatotoxicity. Liver function must be monitored.
- **Bile acid sequestrants,** such as cholestyramine (Questran, Prevalite), colesevelam (WelChol), and colestipol HCL (Colestid), decrease LDL, increase HDL, and do not affect triglyceride levels. They bind to bile acids in the intestines so that more are excreted in the stool rather than returned to the liver, so the liver has to produce bile acids by converting cholesterol. Adverse effects include gastrointestinal disorders and decrease in absorption of other drugs.

Additional anti-lipid drugs include cholesterol absorption inhibitors (ezetimibe), fibric acid derivatives, and omega-3-acid ethyl esters.

## Serotonin Antagonists

Serotonin antagonists block 5-$HT_2$ receptors of serotonin in the central and peripheral nervous systems and gastrointestinal system. An open channel can result in agitation, nausea, and vomiting, but antagonists close the channel and reduce these symptoms. Serotonin antagonists are frequently used to prevent and treat nausea associated with chemotherapy and anesthesia. Medications include:

- **Metoclopramide** (Reglan) is used to reduce nausea and vomiting from a wide range of causes. It is also a prokinetic drug that increases gastrointestinal contractions and promotes faster gastric emptying, so it is used for heartburn, GERD, and diabetic gastroparesis.
- **Ondansetron** (Zofran) reduces vagal stimulation of the medulla oblongata (vomiting center) and is used for nausea related to chemotherapy.
- **Granisetron** (Sancuso) is used to reduce nausea related to chemotherapy, surgery, and radiation.

Serotonin antagonists have fewer side effects than other antiemetics, but they may cause muscle cramping, agitation, diarrhea/constipation, dizziness, and headache.

## Laxatives

The following are different types of laxatives:

- **Bulk formers** have high fiber content and both soften stool and create more formed stools. These include products such as Metamucil, Citrucel, and FiberCon, which are usually added to liquids because without adequate fluids, they can increase constipation.
- **Lubricants** include both oral mineral oil and glycerin suppositories. They coat the stool, preventing fluid absorption and keeping the stool soft. Mineral oil absorbs fat soluble vitamins and should be used only temporarily
- **Saline**, such as Milk of Magnesia and Epsom Salt, contain ions, such as magnesium phosphate, magnesium hydroxide, and citrate, which are not absorbed through the intestines and draw more fluid into the stool. The magnesium in the preparations also stimulates the bowel. People with impairment of kidney function should avoid magnesium products, and saline laxatives should be used infrequently to avoid dependence. Epsom Salt often has a purging effect and is rarely used.
- **Stool softeners** (emollients, such as Colace) use wetting agents, such as docusate sodium, to increase liquid in the stool, thereby softening it. They should not be used with mineral oil because of increased absorption of the oil through the intestines.
- **Hyperosmotics** (available by prescription) contain materials that are not digestible and serve to retain fluid in the stool. Products, such as Kristalose and MiraLAX soften the stool but may result in increased abdominal distension and flatus, especially initially. There are three types of hyperosmolar laxatives: lactulose, polymer, and saline. Lactulose types use a form of sugar and work similarly to saline laxatives, but more slowly, and may be used for long-term treatment. The salines empty the bowels quickly and are used short-term. The polymers contain polyethylene glycol, which retains fluid in the stool and is used short-term.
- **Combinations** use two or more types, such as stool softener with stimulant, and should be used only short-term.

## Stimulants

Stimulants increase intestinal motility, moving the stool through the bowel faster and reducing the absorption of fluids so that the stool remains softer. Common ingredients include cascara in Castor oil and senna in Senokot. Stimulants work quickly and are effective but can result in electrolyte imbalance, Abdominal distension, and cramping. Chronic use may cause a cycle of constipation and diarrhea. Stimulant suppositories, such as Dulcolax, are also available.

**Review Video: Gastrointestinal Drugs**
Visit mometrix.com/academy and enter code: 455152

# Integumentary Pharmacology

## Pharmacologic Treatment of Wound Pain

### *Topical Anesthetics*

There are numerous different types of pain medications that may be used to control pain from wounds, including **topical anesthetics**:

- **Lidocaine 2–4%** is frequently used during debridement or dressing changes. Lidocaine is useful only superficially and may take 15–30 minutes before it is effective.
- **Eutectic Mixture of Local Anesthetics (EMLA Cream)** provides good pain control. The wound is first cleansed and then the cream is applied thickly (1/4 inch) extending about 1/2 inch past the wound to the periwound tissue. The wound is then covered with plastic wrap, which is secured and left in place for about 20 minutes. The wrapped time may be extended to 45–60 minutes if necessary, to completely numb the tissue. The tissue should remain numb for about 1 hour after the plastic wrap is removed, allowing time for the wound to be cleansed, debrided, and/or redressed.

**Review Video: Dermatology Drugs List**
Visit mometrix.com/academy and enter code: 886820

### *Regional Anesthesia*

Regional anesthesia (injectable subcutaneous and perineural medications) is administered locally about the wound or as nerve blocks. Medications include lidocaine, bupivacaine, and tetracaine in solution. Epinephrine is sometimes added to increase vasoconstriction and reduce bleeding, although it is avoided in distal areas of the limbs (hands and feet) to prevent ischemia.

- **Field blockade** involves injecting the anesthetic into the periwound tissue or into the wound margins. The effect may be decreased by inflammation. The effects last for limited periods of time.
- **Regional nerve blocks** may involve single injections, the effects of which are limited in duration but can provide pain relief for treatments. Techniques that use continuous catheter infusions are longer lasting and can be controlled more precisely. Blocks may involve nerves proximal to affected areas, such as peripheral nerve blocks, or large nerve blocks near the spinal cord, such as percutaneous lumbar sympathetic blocks (LSB). Long-term blocks may use alcohol-based medications to permanently inactivate the nerves.

# Psychosocial Pharmacology

## Antipsychotic Medications

### *First-Generation*

There are a variety of first-generation antipsychotics available, though their use is becoming less prominent now that atypical antipsychotic agents are available. Some **first-generation antipsychotics** include:

- Chlorpromazine
- Thioridazine hydrochloride
- Haloperidol
- Pimozide
- Fluphenazine hydrochloride
- Molindone hydrochloride
- Trifluoperazine hydrochloride

**Possible side effects** include photosensitivity, sexual dysfunction, dry mouth, dry eyes, nasal congestion, blurred vision, constipation, urinary retention, exacerbation of narrow-angle glaucoma, various cardiac effects, extrapyramidal effects, dyskinesia, sedation, cognitive dulling, amenorrhea, menstrual irregularities, hyperglycemia or hypoglycemia, increased appetite, and weight gain. The most common extrapyramidal symptom caused by antipsychotic agents is tardive dyskinesia, in which clients are unable to control their movements, such as tics, lip-smacking, and eye blinking. The extrapyramidal system is a group of neural connections outside of the medulla that control movement. **Extrapyramidal effects** are the result of drug influence on the extrapyramidal system and include:

- Akinesia (inability to start movement)
- Akathisia (inability to stop movement)
- Dystonia (extreme and uncontrolled muscle contraction, torticollis, flexing, and twisting)

### *Second-Generation*

Second-generation antipsychotics (SGAs), also called atypical antipsychotics, are used for bipolar disorders, schizophrenia, and psychosis, and include aripiprazole (Abilify), clozapine (Clozaril), olanzapine (Zyprexa), quetiapine (Seroquel), risperidone (Risperdal), and ziprasidone (Geodon). Females report more side effects than males, but the recommended doses for males and females are identical. Women were underrepresented when SGAs were clinically tested, because researchers feared teratogenic effects on fetuses:

- Side effects include constipation, increased appetite, weight gain, urinary retention, various sexual side effects, increased prolactin, menstrual irregularities, increased risk of diabetes mellitus, decreased blood pressure, dizziness, agranulocytosis, and leucopenia.
- Atypical antipsychotics may interact with fluvoxamine, phenytoin, carbamazepine, barbiturates, nicotine, ketoconazole, phenytoin, rifampin, and glucocorticoids.
- The use of atypical antipsychotic agents correlates with significant weight gain. Overweight and obese clients are likely to develop insulin resistance and glucose intolerance, which may lead to diabetes mellitus. Data show clozapine and olanzapine as the greatest offenders. Ziprasidone seems to present the lowest risk.

**Review Video: Antipsychotic Drugs**
Visit mometrix.com/academy and enter code: 369601

## Antidepressants

### *Indications for Treatment with Antidepressant*

The main **indicator** for use of an antidepressant is simply **depression**. This can be further expanded to include major depression, atypical depression, and anxiety disorders. Depression-type symptoms commonly include loss of interest in usual or pleasurable activities, decreased levels of energy, having a depressed mood, decreased ability to concentrate, loss of appetite, or suicidal thoughts. Antidepressants are also commonly used to treat **anxiety disorders** that include panic attacks, obsessive-compulsive disorder (OCD), social phobias, and post-traumatic stress disorder. They may also be beneficial in treating chronic pain syndromes, premenstrual syndrome, insomnia, attention deficit hyperactivity disorder, or bed-wetting.

### *SSRIs*

Selective serotonin reuptake inhibitors (SSRIs) prevent the reuptake of serotonin at the presynaptic membrane. This increases the amount of serotonin in the synapse for neurotransmission. This class of antidepressants has been shown to reduce depression and anxiety symptoms. Common side effects are usually short in duration and include headache, GI upset, and sexual dysfunction. They do not cause significant anticholinergic, cardiovascular, or significant patient sedation side effects. Examples of SSRIs include citalopram (Celexa), escitalopram (Lexapro), fluoxetine (Prozac), fluvoxamine (Luvox), paroxetine (Paxil), and sertraline (Zoloft). These drugs are not highly lethal in overdose.

### Monitoring

SSRI monitoring includes the following:

- Monitor for increased depression and suicidal ideation, especially in adolescents.
- Inform patients of the following:
  - Smoking decreases effectiveness.
  - Fatal reactions may occur with monoamine oxidase inhibitors.
  - Taking SSRIs with benzodiazepines or alcohol has an additive effect.
  - Some drugs, such as citalopram, may increase the effects of β-blockers and warfarin.
- Avoid cimetidine, which is prescribed for ulcers and gastroesophageal reflux disease, and St. John's wort.
- Inform patients of possible decreased libido and sexual functioning.
- Monitor for insomnia and gastrointestinal upset.

## *Tricyclic Antidepressants*

Tricyclic antidepressants not only block the reuptake of serotonin and norepinephrine, they also act to block muscarinic cholinergic receptors, histamine H1 receptors, and alpha1 noradrenergic receptors. These receptors do not affect depression symptoms, but their blockade is implicated in some of the side effects associated with tricyclics. The blockade of the muscarinic receptors produces anticholinergic side effects such as dry mouth, blurred vision, constipation, urinary retention, and tachycardia. The blockade of the histamine receptors is associated with drowsiness, low blood pressure, and weight gain. The alpha1 noradrenergic receptor blocking action produces the side effects associated with orthostatic hypotension, vertigo, and some memory disturbances.

### Mechanism of Action and Necessary Evaluations

Most of the tricyclic antidepressants have very similar mechanisms of action and side effects. Although their exact **mechanism of action** is unknown, they are believed to act to inhibit the reuptake of both serotonin and norepinephrine. These drugs have a high **first-pass rate of metabolism** and are excreted by the kidneys. A complete **physical and history** should be obtained before starting a patient on tricyclic drugs. Because this class of antidepressants can cause death with an overdose, an initial **suicide risk assessment** must be obtained, and continued assessments for this risk are necessary. This class of drug can cause a prolongation in the electrical conduction of the heart. Therefore, a **baseline ECG** should be performed in children, young teenagers, anyone with cardiac electrical conduction problems, and adults over age 40.

### Monitoring

Tricyclics monitoring includes the following:

- Observe for toxicity.
- Inform patients not to take with monoamine oxidase inhibitors.
- Observe for decreased therapeutic response to hypertensives (e.g., clonidine, guanethidine).
- Monitor other medications; the patient should avoid other central nervous system depressants, including alcohol. Some medications potentiate the effects of tricyclics, including bupropion, cimetidine, haloperidol, selective serotonin reuptake inhibitors, and valproic acid.
- Inform the patient to avoid prolonged exposure to sunlight or sunlamps.
- Administer major dosage of the drug at bedtime if the patient experiences drowsiness.
- Monitor for sedation, cardiac arrhythmias, insomnia, gastrointestinal upset, and weight gain.

## *MAOIs*

The **mechanism of action** for monoamine oxidase inhibitors (MAOIs) is exactly what their name indicates. These drugs act to inhibit the enzyme **monoamine oxidase (MAO)**. There are actually two of these enzymes, **MAO-A** and **MAO-B**, and this class of medication inhibits both. These enzymes act to metabolize serotonin and norepinephrine. By inhibiting the production of these enzymes, there are increased levels of **serotonin** and **norepinephrine** available for neurotransmission. Medications that selectively inhibit MAO-B have no antidepressant effects and can be used to treat disease processes such as Parkinson's.

#### Side Effects

Side effects associated with the use of monoamine oxidase inhibitors (MAOIs) are similar to antipsychotic medications. They can include symptoms such as GI upset, vertigo, headaches, sleep disturbances, sexual dysfunction, dry mouth, visual disturbances, constipation, peripheral edema, urinary hesitancy, weakness, increased weight, or orthostatic hypotension. The elderly population is at greatest risk for problems with **orthostatic hypotension** and should have lying, sitting, and standing blood pressure checks to monitor for this side effect. Orthostatic hypotension can lead to injuries related to falls, such as fractures. The most dangerous side effect can be an extreme **elevation in blood pressure** or **hypertensive crisis**. Hypertension can develop due to the presence of increased levels of **tyramine**. These levels increase because **monoamine oxidase**, which normally metabolizes tyramine, is inhibited. Increased levels of tyramine produce a vasoconstrictive response by the body that leads to increased blood pressure. Symptoms associated with hypertensive crisis can include severe occipital headache, palpitations, chest pain, diaphoresis, nausea and vomiting, flushed face, or dilated pupils. Complications associated with hypertensive crisis include hemorrhagic stroke, severe headache, or death. It is vital that patients receive in-depth education about the symptoms of hypertension, the need for close monitoring of blood pressure, and methods for sustaining a low-tyramine diet.

#### Diet Restrictions

Monoamine oxidase inhibitors can lead to increased levels of **tyramine** in the nerve cell. These increased levels can lead to a dangerous and possibly fatal increase in **blood pressure**. Certain **foods that contain tyramine** should be avoided to help prevent hypertensive episodes. Foods high in tyramine include strong or aged cheeses, cured meats, smoked or processed meats, pickled or fermented foods, sauces, such as soy or teriyaki sauce, soybeans, snow peas or broad beans, dried or overripe fruits, meat tenderizers, products containing monosodium glutamate, yeast-extract spreads, alcoholic beverages, and improperly stored foods or spoiled foods.

## Anti-Anxiety Medications

### *Benzodiazepines*

Benzodiazepines are the most commonly prescribed medications for **anxiety**. Some of the more commonly prescribed include chlordiazepoxide, lorazepam, diazepam, flurazepam, and triazolam. Benzodiazepines act to enhance the neurotransmitter **GABA**. This neurotransmitter inhibits the firing rate of neurons and therefore leads to a decline in anxiety symptoms. Indications for their use can include anxiety, insomnia disorders, alcohol withdrawal, seizure control, skeletal muscle spasticity, or agitation. They can also be utilized to reduce the anxiety symptoms preoperatively or before any other type of medical procedure such as cardiac catheterization or colonoscopy. This class of drug is also the treatment of choice for alcohol withdrawal.

#### Side Effects

There are several common side effects associated with the use of benzodiazepines. One of the most common is the effect of **drowsiness**. Patients should be advised to use caution when operating motor vehicles or machinery. Activity will help decrease this effect. Other side effects include feelings of detachment, irritability, emotional lability, GI upset, dependency, or development of tolerance. The elderly population is at high risk for the development of **dizziness** or **cognitive impairment**, which places them at high risk for falls with associated injuries. When discontinuing a benzodiazepine after long-term use, the drug should be weaned off to prevent withdrawal side effects.

#### Treatment of Insomnia

Benzodiazepines are used to treat **insomnia** because of their **sedative-hypnotic effects**. There are three different types of insomnia, which include the inability to fall asleep, inability to stay asleep, or the combination of both. Many times, insomnia can be helped by a change in habits or talking about worries or stress the patient may be experiencing. When using a sedative-hypnotic to treat sleep disturbances, the medication should have rapid onset and allow the patient to wake up feeling refreshed instead of tired and groggy. When administered at bedtime, most benzodiazepines will produce a sleep-inducing effect and should be used on a short-term basis.

> **Review Video: Sedatives, Hypnotics, and Insomnia Management**
> Visit mometrix.com/academy and enter code: 666132
>
> **Review Video: Chronic Insomnia**
> Visit mometrix.com/academy and enter code: 293232

### *Use of Buspirone for Treatment of Anxiety*

Due to the addictive potential of benzodiazepines, the use of **nonbenzodiazepines** to treat anxiety has increased. One of the most commonly used nonbenzodiazepine medications is the drug **buspirone**. This medication is highly effective in treating anxiety and its associated symptoms such as insomnia, poor concentration, tension, restlessness, irritability, and fatigue. Buspirone has no addiction potential, is not useful in alcohol withdrawal and seizures, and is not known to interact with other CNS depressants. Because it may take several weeks of continual use for the effects of this drug to be realized by the patient, it cannot be used on an as-needed basis. Buspirone does not increase depression symptoms and therefore is useful in treating anxiety associated with depression. Side effects associated with medication can include GI upset, dizziness, sleepiness, excitement, or headache.

# Geriatric Pharmacology

## Medication Considerations for Elderly Patients

An elderly patient has an increased chance of adverse effects from medications. Approximately 1/3 of hospitalizations that are related to side effects of drugs and 1/2 of drug-associated fatalities happen in patients that are at least 60 years of age. In the United States, expenses for prescriptions for elderly patients make up 30% of every prescription filled and 40–50% of non-prescription drugs. Elderly patients spend more than $3 billion annually on these medications. Most elderly individuals have at least one ongoing health condition, including arthritis, high blood pressure, heart problems, diabetes, or other conditions, often requiring more than one drug for treatment. There are more adverse drug reactions (ADR) amongst elderly patients, 10% of whom require hospitalization for treatment for the side effects. Frequently seen adverse reactions include edema, queasiness, vomiting, anorexia, vertigo, loose stools, infrequent and difficult stools, bewilderment, and urinary retention. Be careful not to misidentify these as another condition or symptom of aging.

## Pharmacokinetics of Older Adults

Pharmacokinetics involves four steps: Absorption, distribution, metabolism, and elimination. All of these steps are affected by the age of the patient as the organs involved degenerate from wear and tear:

1. **Absorption** of most drugs occurs in the small intestine. Drug absorption in older adults may be delayed or decreased due to decreased blood flow to the small intestine. This could change the blood levels of drugs achieved in the geriatric patient.
2. **Distribution** of the drug is altered due to a change in body composition. Elderly patients have decreased total body water and lean muscle mass. This relative increase in total body fat may increase the duration of action of lipid-soluble drugs.
3. Most drugs are **metabolized** by either the liver or the kidneys. Decreased function of these organs leads to delayed metabolism and elimination of certain medications.
4. **Renal function** and **elimination effectiveness** diminish with age, often decreasing the kidney's ability to remove toxins and medications from the body. For this reason, drugs may remain in the body longer, therefore requiring smaller doses among the elderly.

## Beers Criteria

The Beers Criteria, also called the Beers List, identifies inappropriate medication use among older adults. The list is used to determine which medications are beneficial compared to those that impose risks for older adults. Because older adults are at risk of polypharmacy and inappropriate medication use, the Beers Criteria helps healthcare providers identify which medications are truly necessary and are in the patient's best interests to use. All medications that the patient takes are identified, and indications are given as to whether the medications should be avoided among those older than age 65. The recommendations are then rated for strength, and the quality of the research supporting the recommendations is identified.

## Difficulties the Elderly Population May Encounter with Medication Use

Common difficulties with medication use amongst the elderly include:

- Overuse of prescription medications
- Medication adherence and compliance issues (e.g., providing incorrect or incomplete past medical history to the professional, or using medicine that is out of date, changing dose without practitioner's orders to do so)
- Misunderstanding of how the medicine is supposed to be used due to problems with comprehension, hearing, or proper education style
- Not remembering the reason, amount, or how often the drug should be used (may result in repeating the medicine when it has already been taken)
- Difficulty affording the medication
- Vision issues resulting in misreading the label and taking the wrong dosage
- Problems getting the bottle open, dealing with small pills, cutting pills in half, and using inhalers
- More than one medical worker or more than one pharmacy can lead to inadvertent redundancy of the same medication, as can using the generic and brand name of the same thing at the same time

## Common Adverse Outcomes of Frequently Used Prescription Medications

Certain physical and psychological states may be an adverse outcome resulting from a prescribed medication:

- **Bewilderment:** Digoxin, cimetidine, dopamine agent, antihistamine, hypnotic, sedative, anticholinergic, anticonvulsant
- **Anorexia**: Digoxin
- **Low energy or weakness:** Diuretic, antidepressant, antihypertensive
- **Absentmindedness**: Barbiturate
- **Difficult bowel movements**: Anticholinergic
- **Loose stool:** Oral antacid
- **GI upset:** Iron, NSAID, salicylate, corticosteroid, estrogen, alcohol
- **Ringing in the ears (tinnitus)**: Analgesic
- **Urinary retention:** Anticholinergic, alpha-agonist
- **Orthostatic low blood pressure:** Antihypertensive, sedative, diuretic, antidepressant
- **Depression:** Benzodiazepine
- **Vertigo:** Sedative, antihypertensive, anticonvulsant, diuretic

## Adverse Outcomes of Histamine Blockers, Ibuprofen, and Beta-Blockers

**Histamine blockers** in the elderly can cause paradoxical central nervous system provocation that has an outcome of ataxia in this population. Antihistamines may cause problems with vision and walking, leading to falls, which may cause unforeseen hospital visits or require a nursing home. Antihistamines can also interfere with the effectiveness of other medications or enhance other medications' negative side effects.

Some elderly patients are already dealing with decreased renal functioning. **Ibuprofen** has the ability to worsen these issues leading to nephrosis, cirrhosis, and congestive heart failure.

If the patient is older, a **beta-blocker** is not a good option for treating hypertension due to their decreased beta-adrenergic receptor sensitivity for the elderly patient. Elderly patients need smaller amounts of calcium entry antagonists, ACE inhibitors, or diuretics. Too high a dose (in the elderly) will cause moodiness, impotence, weariness, and lessened ability to think clearly. Elderly patients are particularly prone to congestive heart failure and peripheral vascular insufficiency due to beta-adrenergic toxins.

## Polypharmacy

Polypharmacy is a term used to describe inappropriate use of multiple medications at one time. It occurs when medications are taken that are not indicated, medications that have adverse interactions with one another are taken together, and patients take contraindicated medications. Polypharmacy is a common problem in the geriatric population. Most office visits result in new prescriptions being written and patients may accumulate many different medications in their home. Polypharmacy greatly increases the patient's risk of having an adverse drug reaction.

To manage polypharmacy and prevent complications, obtain a detailed drug history at each visit. This should include nonprescription medications and herbal remedies. Educating patients about the problem of polypharmacy is very important. This can occur in the clinician's office or with a community education program. Assist elderly patients with medication identification, recommending pill boxes to help the patient divide medications and minimize risks for medication misuse.

## MASTER Rules for Rational Drug Therapy

Although drugs are often very useful and effective in treating illnesses, there is a point when it becomes dangerous to the patient. Drug resistance, drug interactions, and drug intolerances are all common problems, especially among elderly patients, because an iatrogenic illness can develop. For these reasons, it is important to limit drugs to only those that are absolutely necessary. To help the practitioner decide whether a drug should be used or not, they must remember the **MASTER rules**.

- **M** is for **minimizing** the number of drugs a patient is taking.
- **A** is for considering **alternate** treatments that may be as or more effective than using a drug.
- **S** is for **start** low and increase slowly. Only give the patient the minimum amount, and be careful when increasing doses.
- **T** is for **titration** of drugs; tailor the amount given over time to the individual patient.
- **E** is for **education** of the patient about the drugs he or she is taking.
- **R** is for **regular** reviewing of drugs and doses.

# Chapter Quiz

Ready to see how well you retained what you just read? Scan the QR code to go directly to the chapter quiz interface for this study guide. If you're using a computer, simply visit the online resources page at **mometrix.com/resources719/nclexrn-31183** and click the Chapter Quizzes link.

# Reduction of Risk Potential

## Cardiovascular Diagnostics

### Cardiac Enzymes

While creatine kinase (CK) and CK-MB levels used to be the mainstay for diagnosing acute myocardial infarction, they are no longer commonly used in the United States. CK is a reflection of muscular infarction, but is not specific to the heart muscle. CK-MB adds slightly more specificity to the heart but not as much as the gold standard, which is **troponin**. Troponin, which is found in cardiac and skeletal muscle, is a type of protein. Both troponin I and T (isolates of troponin) are found in the myocardium, but troponin T is also found in skeletal muscle, so it is less specific than troponin I. Troponin I, therefore, may be used to detect a myocardial infarction after non-cardiac surgery and to detect acute coronary syndrome. Troponin is released into the bloodstream when injury to the tissue (such as the myocardium) occurs and causes damage to the cell membranes, as occurs with myocardial injury.

- **Troponin I** (<0.05 ng/mL): Appears in 2–6 hours, peaks at 15–20 hours and returns to normal in 5–7 days. Exhibits a second but lower peak at 60–80 hours (biphasic).
- **Troponin T** (<0.2 ng/mL): Increases 2–6 hours after MI and stays elevated. Returns to normal in 7 days. (Less specific than troponin I)

### Echocardiography

Echocardiography is a non-invasive ultrasound technology that is very useful for assessing and diagnosing anatomic heart abnormalities, blood flow, and valvular lesions:

- The **standard "2D Echo"** is used best for basic structural imaging, such as valvular lesions and assessment of pericardial disorders.
- The **transesophageal (TEE)** probe is an improved version of echocardiography, which allows better visualization of the left atrium and more precise evaluation of the valvular structure. TEE is also the best modality for evaluation of the thoracic aorta in the setting of suspected aortic dissection or aneurysm.
- **Doppler imaging** is used to measure blood flow, often in the context of velocity across a valve and a pressure gradient.
- **Bubble study** (which is done by injecting saline contrast that has been agitated to include bubbles) is an addition to echocardiography allowing the study to determine if there is right to left blood flow through a patent foramen ovale or a more distal intrapulmonary shunt of blood.

### Stress Echocardiography

Basic **cardiac stress testing** consists of exercise EKG testing (EET) and exercise imaging testing. The exercise imaging testing may be broken down into exercise, or "stress" echocardiography, and exercise myocardial perfusion imaging.

**Exercise imaging testing** is usually performed with echocardiography. Stress echocardiography is performed similarly to **exercise EKG testing** and also requires that the patient meet at least 85% maximum heart rate in order to attain optimum sensitivity and specificity. (The maximum heart rate formula is 220 minus the person's age.) Of note, chemicals may substitute for exercise during the "stress" portion of the test. This may be performed with dobutamine (beta-1-agonist: cannot be used after beta-blocker administration) or adenosine (causes diffuse coronary dilatation, leading to decreased perfusion pressure and unmasking of defects, and cannot be used with asthma). Stress imaging allows the study to determine the actual area of ischemia and whether or not this is a reversible defect. Additional information obtained during echocardiography is cardiac output and measurement of viability.

# Endocrine Diagnostics

## Glucose Laboratory Test

Glucose is manufactured by the liver from ingested carbohydrates and is stored as glycogen for use by the cells. If intake is inadequate, glucose can be produced from muscle and fat tissue, leading to increased wasting. High levels of glucose are indicative of diabetes mellitus, which predisposes people to skin injuries, slow healing, and infection. **Fasting blood glucose levels** are used to diagnose and monitor this condition:

- Normal values: 70–99 mg/dL
- Impaired: 100–125 mg/dL
- Diabetes: ≥126 mg/dL

There are a number of different conditions that can increase glucose levels, including stress, renal failure, Cushing syndrome, hyperthyroidism, and pancreatic disorders. Medications, such as steroids, estrogens, lithium, phenytoin, diuretics, tricyclic antidepressants, may increase glucose levels. Other conditions, such as adrenal insufficiency, liver disease, hypothyroidism, and starvation can decrease glucose levels.

### *Collecting a Point-of-Care Glucose Test*

Conducting a point-of-care blood glucose test includes:

- **Precautions**: Ask if the patient is taking medications that might interfere with readings (Sodium-glucose inhibitors, fluoroquinolones, hormones, cholesterol-lowering drugs). Use the device for only one patient or follow manufacturer's guidelines for cleaning and disinfection between patients. Use standard precautions. Check the expiration dates on test-strip vials.
- **Components**: Devices may vary by manufacturer, but generally include the testing device, test strips, and a control solution to check the accuracy of the readings. The control solution should be used to check test strips before initial use of the system, when opening a new container of test strips, and when results seem abnormally high or low.
- **Procedure**: Use the lancet on the side of the fingertip or the forearm (depending on the device). Note that a sample from the fingertip may be more accurate. The first drop is typically discarded and the second drop applied to the test strip. If obtaining a venous blood sample for testing, only test tubes containing sodium heparin should be used. The test strip is inserted into the device for the recommended time until the reading is displayed. Then, the strip is removed and discarded as biohazardous waste.

## Hemoglobin A1c Laboratory Test

Hemoglobin A1c comprises hemoglobin A with a glucose molecule because hemoglobin holds onto excess blood glucose, so it shows the average blood glucose levels over a 3-month period and is used primarily to monitor long-term diabetic therapy:

- Normal value: <6%

## Basic Thyroid Function Testing and Antibody Testing

**Thyroid stimulating hormone (TSH)** is produced by the pituitary as a result of thyrotropin releasing hormone (TRH) from the hypothalamus. TSH stimulates the thyroid to produce T4 (mostly) and T3. T4 is deiodinated to T3 (active hormone), and the free hormone is active while the majority is bound to albumin and thyroxine-binding globulin. The best testing of thyroid function is the free T4 (unbound). Free T4 and TSH testing allows appropriate screening for thyroid disease.

Additionally, certain antibodies are used to screen for thyroid disease. Thyroglobulin antibodies are found in 50% of patients with Graves' disease and about 90% of those with Hashimoto's thyroiditis. Thyroid peroxidase antibodies are detected in >90% of those with Hashimoto's thyroiditis. TSH receptor antibodies (TSHR) may be either thyroid stimulating immunoglobulin (TSI) which stimulate the receptor to produce thyroid hormone (found in Graves' disease), or TSHR-blocking antibodies, which may inhibit production of thyroid hormone.

Lab values to consider include:

- **Thyroid stimulating hormone (TSH)** (0.4–6.15 mIU/L). Increase in TSH indicates hypothyroidism and decrease indicates hyperthyroidism.
- **Free thyroxine**: (FT4) (0.9–2.4 ng/dL). FT4 is used to confirm TSH abnormalities. Serum T3 (80–180 ng/dL) and T4 (4.5–11.5 mcg/dL) usually increase together, but T3 more accurately diagnoses hyperthyroidism. T3 resin uptake (25–35%) increases with hyperthyroidism and decreases with hypothyroidism.

### Additional Endocrine Function Studies

There is a wide range of endocrine function studies:

- **Pituitary:** Serum levels of pituitary hormones and hormones of target organs, dependent on stimulation by pituitary hormones, are measured to determine abnormalities.
- **Parathyroid:** Parathyroid hormone (PTH) level (10–65 ng/L) and serum calcium levels (8.5–10.2 mg/dL) both increase with hyperparathyroidism. Calcium levels decrease with hypoparathyroidism, and phosphate levels (2.5–4.5 mg/dL) increase.
- **Adrenal**: Catecholamine (urine and serum) levels: Epinephrine (<75 ng/L) and norepinephrine (<100–550 ng/mL) elevate with pheochromocytoma. Electrolyte and glucose levels.
- **ACTH** and **serum cortisol levels** and **ACTH stimulation test** to evaluate for Addison. Dexamethasone suppression test for Cushing's disease.

## Immunologic and Oncologic Diagnostics

### Frozen Sections

Frozen sections are useful in the establishment and staging of a tumor when a decision as to the optimal type of surgical procedure is pending. They also provide information about the completeness of tumor removal post-surgery. They can elucidate the type of tissue involved so that it can be evaluated further, and they can aid in diagnosis through biopsy. However, the use of frozen sections is time-consuming and costly, so they should not be utilized when other options might be more complete or specific. Examination of the sections by a pathologist also has to be taken in context, because it is virtually impossible to examine every portion of the tissue. In addition, the use of freezing can damage tissue architecture and induce distortions.

### Immunohistochemistry (IHC)

Immunohistochemistry (IHC) is a technique in which tissue antigens on frozen tissue sections are identified. The antigens are detected by the use of specific antibodies coupled to either fluorescent compounds or pigmented entities, allowing the pathologist to view these interactions on a fluoroscope or through a microscope. There are also various methods of amplifying the interactions, or enzymatically exposing masked antigens to aid in their visualization. IHC is used to distinguish between benign and malignant (antigen-positive) processes and to classify the type of tumor observed. It can also be a useful adjunct in determining the point of origin for the tumor and in identifying small areas that have metastasized. IHC can aid in the evaluation of the future aggressiveness of the tumor through the detection of characteristic nuclear antigens, and it can help predict therapeutic responses by identifying certain receptors, gene products, and proteins.

## Fine Needle Aspiration (FNA)

In fine needle aspiration (FNA), a small gauge needle is used to extract cells from a tissue area that might be malignant and then the cells are observed microscopically. The procedure is usually done before surgery and is attempted in conjunction with other tools, such as x-rays and laboratory evaluations. FNA is relatively non-invasive and inexpensive. The utility of fine needle aspiration is dependent on the nature of the mass because FNA can only broadly classify it and identify types of cells involved. Other issues, such as the architecture of the mass and its precise classification, are difficult to predict with FNA alone.

## Flow Cytometry

Flow cytometry is a method of analyzing populations of cells in suspension for various properties. The cells, such as tumor sample cells, are aspirated into the fluidic system of a machine called a flow cytometer. Here the cells are mixed with a fluid that places them in suspension and a unidirectional or laminar flow is created. As each cell flows past a laser sensor, photons emitted are picked up and intensified by photomultiplier tubes. Data is electronically converted into either histograms or dot plots that compare characteristics of the cells in the population. In addition, fluorochromes are usually injected into the mixture in order to further highlight and identify the cell populations. A fluorochrome is a fluorescent dye, i.e., a substance that absorbs light at a particular wavelength but can emit it at more than one wavelength such as fluorescein isothiocyanate (FITC).



### *Acute Leukemia*

Acute leukemia is one type of hematological neoplasia. Flow cytometry is used to establish the lineage or population from which the **leukemia cells** are derived, either myeloid or lymphoid. The most common approach is to isolate the blast cell population using a common leukocyte antigen called CD45 and then using other labeled antibodies to differentiate the cellular origin. Flow cytometry can find and count blasts, identify the phenotypes of the leukemic cells, and pinpoint molecular or cytogenetic changes. It is also useful in the detection of minimal residual disease (MRD) in the bone marrow. MRD is identified in flow cytometry by utilization of a panel of antibodies that target antigenic markers that are expressed in different patterns in leukemic and normal cells.

### *Lymphoma and Lymphoproliferative Disorders*

There is no universal gating marker for B-cell malignancies such as **lymphoma**, so the initial step in flow cytometric analysis of lymphoma tissues is the segregation of the malignant cells using a general B-cell antibody like CD19 or CD20. The technique has limitations for lymphoma identification because these cells are difficult to bring into suspension, and fine-needle aspirates are often used. For lymphoma cases, tissue immunohistochemistry is often used in conjunction with cytometry.

On the other hand, chronic **lymphoproliferative diseases** are usually easily classified using flow cytometry. For example, B-lymphocytes found in the blood or bone marrow of individuals with chronic lymphocytic leukemia (CLL) express an antigen called CD38. Further, CD38 levels are also prognostic for CLL outcome. Other B-cell disorders, such as hairy cell leukemia, MRD, and T-cell disorders can also be diagnosed by flow cytometry.

### *Solid Tumor Analysis*

At present, use of flow cytometry in analysis of **solid tumors** is not standard practice in most institutions. If utilized, the technique is used to look for DNA content in one of two ways. DNA binds to a number of fluorescent dyes. The number of chromosome sets present, or the ploidy, can affect the peak distribution on cytometry. Another way flow cytometry is utilized is to determine the proportion of cells in the S phase where DNA is synthesized. Then that population can be examined. Even so, interpretation of cytometric data for solid tumors has not been as well defined as for the lymphoid malignancies.

## Tumor Marker Assays

Tumor marker assays quantify levels of certain molecules found in serum, other body fluids, cells, and tissues that have an association with the presence of malignancy. Most of the available assays are either radioimmunoassays (RIAs) or enzyme-linked immunosorbent assays (ELISAs), which respectively use radioisotopes or enzymes linked to various substances (often specific antibodies) as detection vehicles. The value of these immunoassays depends upon their specificity (i.e., their ability to accurately detect malignancy, versus normal tissue or benign growths) and sensitivity (the capacity for early detection during screening or preliminary diagnosis). The linearity of a test is important as well, as the concentration changes must be quantifiable and directly related to changes in tumor volume or response to treatment. At present, the measurement of cancer or tumor markers is generally more useful in the monitoring of disease, rather than in the initial diagnosis.

### *Tumor Markers Currently Used in the United States*

In order for a tumor marker to be a good candidate for a screening assay, it should be both organ and cancer specific. Some markers—for example, carcinoembryonic antigen or CEA—are indicative of a malignant process, but they are not organ specific. In contrast, prostate specific antigen or total PSA is the ideal tumor marker for early detection or screening purposes because it is unique to the prostate. There is a range (4 to 10 ng/ml) where non-cancerous conditions, such as benign prostatic disease or BPH, can be picked up as well. When total PSA is combined with free PSA (which is lower in men with prostate cancer), the specificity of prostate cancer detection increases dramatically. Similarly, a carbohydrate marker called CA125 is a useful screening marker for ovarian cancer, if it is used in conjunction with other tests such as ultrasound. Thus, PSA and CA125 are valuable in screening settings, particularly if they show increases when measured sequentially. These screening assays are always serum or plasma-based.

### *Diagnostic and Prognostic Utility of Assays for Tumor Markers*

Assays for tumor markers are generally more useful for **disease diagnosis** than screening, especially if they are used in conjunction with other types of tests, such as histology. Many of these markers are good adjuncts to tumor staging. Some of the more useful markers and their associated cancers follow:

- **CA125**: Useful for ovarian cancer diagnosis and monitoring in conjunction with other testing.
- **Alpha-Fetoprotein or AFP**: Informative for distinguishing between various types of germ cell tumors, especially when used together with measurement of *B*-Human chorionic gonadotrophin (*B*-hCG).
- **Carcinoembryonic antigen (CEA)**: Can be elevated in colorectal, breast, and lung carcinomas; however, elevated levels are not tumor specific but can still be of prognostic or monitoring value.
- **Tissue estrogen and progesterone receptors**: Have prognostic utility for the treatment of breast cancer, as test-positive individuals are responsive to antiestrogen therapies.
- **Tissue HER-2/neu**: Is useful in assessment of breast cancer patients for possible treatment with Herceptin.
- **High HcG (in males)**: In conjunction with elevated AFP, may be indicative of testicular tumors.

### *Tumor Marker Assays Used for Monitoring Disease and Treatment Effectiveness*

The primary utility of most tumor marker assays is for the **monitoring of disease progression and treatment effectiveness**. After surgery, radiation, or other therapies, levels of certain markers should decrease within a few days if the treatment has significantly reduced the tumor burden. The lag time is dependent upon the half-life of the antigen in the serum and, sometimes, other factors such as renal clearance. If levels increase after treatment, then the therapy has not worked, and increasing sequential measurements indicate possible disease progression. International recommendations for monitoring intervals suggest samples be taken quarterly. If levels increase linearly, the time between samples should be lowered to every two weeks to a month.

### *Tumor Markers Useful for Monitoring Specific Malignancies*

The following serum-based tumor marker assays are useful for **monitoring the progression or remission of specific types of malignancies:**

- Prostate cancer: PSA and prostate acid phosphatase
- Breast cancer: CA15-3, CA27.29, and for patients taking Herceptin, HER-2/neu
- Ovarian cancer: CA125
- Pancreatic cancer: CA19-9
- Colorectal cancer: CEA (also some limited utility for monitoring breast and lung cancers)
- Nonseminomatous testicular cancer: AFP
- Thyroid cancer: Thyroglobulin (contraindicated if the individual has autoantibodies)



Specific values are dependent on the immunoassay performed, so sequential values must be taken using the same test.

## Imaging Methods for Cancer Detection and Staging

There are advantages and disadvantages to the use of **imaging methods for cancer detection**. One advantage is that imaging methods are non-invasive. This can provide significant benefits in burdens, costs, and time. However, a key disadvantage is that tumor masses must be large enough for visualization by the imaging technique used. This is typically about 3 to 5 millimeters in diameter. Smaller lesions may well be missed. Other detection methods are theoretically much more sensitive. Cytology, for example, can detect a single cancerous cell. Realistically, however, laboratory methods usually only sample a small portion of the overall cancerous mass, whereas imaging techniques permit the technician to look at the entire tumor. Imaging techniques are also very useful in initial staging of the tumor and evaluation of changes after treatment.

## Imaging Methods Used in Oncology

The following types of imaging methods are currently used in oncology:

- **Traditional radiographs**: Uses x-rays and development on films (or digital methods); useful for detection of bone tumors and lung cancer.
- **Mammography**: As above, but with specialized machinery to detect breast cancer.
- **Computed tomography or CT scans**: Uses a rotating source of x-rays and image digitalization for greater clarity and multiple views.
- **Angiography**: Uses a vascular introduction of iodinated contrast media while taking serial images (generally digital); similar injections can be done with CT scans.
- **Ultrasound**: Utilizes high-frequency sound waves to produce an image; it is most effective in detecting malignancies in the neck and pelvic region or in the gallbladder and liver areas.
- **Magnetic resonance imaging (MRI)**: Uses an electromagnetic field, which excites atomic nuclei, to produce a digitalized image; used primarily for detection of tumors in the brain, spinal cord, and musculoskeletal tissues.
- **Single-photon-emission computed tomography (SPECT):** Use the injection of long half-life radioisotopes (primarily $^{99m}Tc$) tracers to look at perfusion into bone or thyroid areas.
- **Positron-emission tomography (PET)**: Uses the injection of positron emitter tracers, usually coupled with agents involved with glycolytic metabolism.

### *Differences Between Imaging Methods*

Functional abilities can be picked up somewhat with modifications by use of ultrasound coupled with contrast media or MRI using spectroscopy at specific field strengths. A radiograph is the least sensitive modality in the group, and ultrasound and mammography are the least specific. Tomography techniques like SPECT and PET actually look at functional abilities rather than at anatomical features. They are very sensitive and relatively specific as well, especially PET scans. Recently, hybrid machines have been developed that can combine the functional capacities of SPECT or PET with regular computed tomography.

### *Imaging Modalities for Detection of Lung Cancer*

Benign and cancerous **nodules of the lung** are often detected by routine chest x-rays or screening CT scans. Determination of neoplastic potential of the nodules requires additional evaluation, such as comparisons to prior radiographs or scans, examination of the morphology of the nodule, uptake of contrast media on CT, and the degree of calcification, etc. PET scans using F-18 fluorodeoxyglucose (FDG) are used to determine the need for invasive procedures and to stage lung cancers; hybrid PET/CT scans are even more informative. If metastasis into the central nervous system is suspected, MRI with accompanying contrast of the brain, as well as bone scans, is usually performed. Lung cancer often metastasizes into the adrenal gland near the kidney; benign adenomas can be distinguished from malignant ones, using PET scans, by the rate of FDG uptake, which is faster in malignant tumors.

### *Imaging Modalities in the Detection of Breast Cancer*

For detection of **primary breast cancer**, mammography is the imaging method of choice. However, other imaging methods are sometimes used. For example, ultrasound is used to distinguish cystic from solid masses, and MRI with a contrast medium is used to determine the number of foci. Imaging can be particularly helpful in identifying which lymph nodes need to be removed if metastasis has occurred. For later stages, systemic metastatic involvement is usually evaluated with baseline bone scans and computed tomography of the abdominal and chest regions. PET scans might be used to look for metastases in soft tissues.

#### Mammograms

At present, about one in eight women is likely to develop breast cancer at some point. **Mammograms** or breast radiographs are recommended for all women 40 years of age or older every year or two, followed by biopsy if certain changes are observed. Areas of microcalcification and/or increases in soft tissue density on the mammogram indicate possible breast cancer. There are a number of other imaging techniques currently being evaluated as well, such as MRI, PET, digitization of the mammographic image, and scanning with radionuclides. Clinical breast examinations can also distinguish breast cancer as firm, palpable masses that have irregular shapes. Breast biopsies are usually done by one of three methods:

- Fine needle aspiration followed by cytological studies
- Needle core biopsy along with either ultrasound or stereotactic direction
- Excision

### *Imaging Modalities in Prostate Cancer Detection and Monitoring*

At present, there are no clear-cut recommendations regarding which imaging modalities should be used for **detection of prostate cancer and its metastases**. Ultrasound is often used to identify the shape of the prostate for biopsy. CT scans or MRI is sometimes done to look for the metastases. However, the predictive value and utility of any of these techniques are currently low. A radionuclide bone scan may be performed, but usually only if PSA levels are in the positive range. Levels of prostate specific antigen are more likely to be used for detection and monitoring of prostate cancer than any of the imaging methods.

### *Imaging Modalities in Colon Cancer Detection and Monitoring*

Imaging modalities are rarely used for **detection of colon cancer**. Fiberoptic colonoscopy remains the method of choice, but virtual colonoscopies using CT scanning techniques are available. Non-invasive imaging techniques are often applied during colon cancer resections or for post-surgical monitoring. For staging purposes or monitoring, evaluation of metastatic involvement commonly includes CT scanning of the abdominal and pelvic region, the bowel, and the thorax (using contrast agents). Chest radiographs are sometimes substituted for thorax CT scans. Monitoring is usually done every 6 months to a year, especially if CEA levels are increasing. In monitoring situations, PET scans are often the imaging modality of choice because of the increased sensitivity. Liver scans for metastases may also be performed using PET scans or possibly ultrasound.

### Imaging Techniques in Detection and Monitoring of Gynecologic Tumors

**Cervical carcinoma** is usually detected by a combination of physical examination, Pap smear, and possibly serum CA125 levels. Non-invasive imaging techniques, such as CT, MRI, and PET scans can be used to stage larger lesions that have been identified. Most **ovarian cancers** are not identified until they are in the later stages, although ultrasound occasionally detects tumors in earlier stages. Thus, imaging techniques in patients with ovarian cancer are used merely to evaluate the proliferation of the disease and to determine the area to remove. In such circumstances, CT scans are most useful. After surgical removal of ovarian neoplasms, imaging and laboratory tests for tumor markers are used for follow-up monitoring.

### Imaging Techniques in Patients with Lymphomas

Imaging plays an important role in the staging of lymphomas. Generally, computed tomography or PET scans of the pelvic and abdominal region are performed. After treatment, lymphomas often have lingering masses which may or may not contain tumor cells. Imaging techniques are valuable following lymphoma treatments because they can determine whether these residual bulks are actually viable. PET scans using $^{18}$flurodeoxyglucose as a tracer will show increased uptake of the FDG if malignant cells remain. Depending on the treatment interval, this increased uptake indicates either a lack of response to therapy or a poor prognosis.

### Imaging Techniques in Patients with Primary and Disseminated Melanoma

**Melanoma** usually presents as a dark pigmented tumor visible on the surface of the skin, but it can also metastasize. Lymphoscintigraphy is used to identify lymphatic drainage routes that might provide a conduit for metastatic cells. If metastatic involvement is suspected, imaging techniques are used to locate the metastatic areas as resection of them may be possible. Typically, these tests might include CT scans (chest, abdominal, and pelvic regions), MRI imaging with and without contrast media, and/or positron emission tomography with the use of FDG as a tracer.

### Imaging Techniques in Bladder and Kidney Cancers

For **bladder carcinomas**, imaging techniques are mainly used to determine the extent of the primary tumor since they often are multicentric. An intravenous pyelogram, by which dye is introduced and an x-ray taken, is often used. The sensitivity of the various methods is not maximal for minimal metastatic involvement; thus, biopsies of local lymph nodes remain common.

In the past, the algorithm for detection of kidney or renal cancers used to include an intravenous pyelogram as well. However, CT with introduction of contrast media is currently the imaging method of choice. These cancers are often detected on CT scans ordered for other reasons. In the kidney, solid masses as well as liquid-filled renal cysts can occur.

### Imaging Techniques for Head, Neck, and Brain Tumors

Imaging techniques are useful for staging and monitoring of primary **head and neck cancers** and examining any possible metastasis into the lungs. Currently, the methods of choice are CT scans with intravenous contrast media and/or PET scans with the introduction of FDG. On the other hand, if a brain tumor is suspected, usually magnetic resonance imaging is performed. This method has virtually replaced the prior use of angiography. The MRI is enhanced by the introduction of gadolinium. Even so, interpretation of the findings is limited as other pathologies may sometimes look similar to a tumor mass on the MRI, such as areas of demyelination.

### *Imaging Techniques of Choice for Pancreatic, Liver, and Other Types of Cancers*

The most common **imaging algorithms** for the remaining types of cancer are as follows:

- Pancreatic carcinoma: CT scanning with use of angiography.
- Liver cancer: CT scans, CT angiography, MRI without and with the introduction of gadolinium; for primary hepatomas, PET with FDG for metastases from colon or other cancers.
- Endocrine cancers: depends on tumor site as follows:
  - Adrenal: CT using $^{123}$I-meta-iodobenzyl guanidine.
  - Thyroid: radioiodine imaging (or PET with FDG if the tumor does not absorb radioiodine).
  - Neuroendocrine: CT with radio-tagged octreotide analogs.
- Esophageal and gastric cancers: CT to stage, endoscopic ultrasound for invasiveness.
- Sarcomas (soft tissue tumors): usually MRI.

### *Imaging Techniques Beyond Detection and Monitoring of Tumors*

Information gleaned from imaging techniques can be used to **design a therapeutic regimen**. In particular, parts of the mass that contain biologically active tumor cells can be targeted for introduction of radiation therapies. Different types of scans can be used as adjuncts during surgery to guide the surgeon. Modalities that are more functional in nature, like PET, have many potential applications, such as evaluation of the pharmacokinetics of therapeutic agents in the patient, tracking of stem cells, observation of the pathway that agents introduced follow, and the results of manipulation of these paths.

## Hematologic Diagnostics

### Red Blood Cells

Red blood cells (RBCs or erythrocytes) are biconcave disks that contain **hemoglobin** (95% of mass), which carries oxygen throughout the body. The heme portion of the cell contains **iron**, which binds to the oxygen. RBCs live about 120 days, after which they are destroyed and their hemoglobin is recycled or excreted. Normal values of **red blood cell count** vary by gender:

- Males >18 years: 4.7–6.1 million per $mm^3$
- Females >18 years: 4.2–5.4 million per $mm^3$

The most common **disorders of RBCs** are those that interfere with production, leading to various types of **anemia**:

- Blood loss
- Hemolysis
- Bone marrow failure

The **morphology** of RBCs may vary depending upon the type of anemia:

- Size: Normocytes, microcytes, macrocytes
- Shape: Spherocytes (round), poikilocytes (irregular), drepanocytes (sickled)
- Color (reflecting concentration of hemoglobin): Normochromic, hypochromic

### *Laboratory Tests*

A number of different tests are used to evaluate the condition and production of red blood cells in addition to the red blood cell count.

**Hemoglobin**: Carries oxygen and is decreased in anemia and increased in polycythemia. Normal values:

- Males >18 years: 14.0–17.46 g/dL
- Females >18 years: 12.0–16.0 g/dL

**Hematocrit**: Indicates the proportion of RBCs in a liter of blood (usually about 3 times the hemoglobin number). Normal values:

- Males >18 years: 40–50%
- Females >18 years: 35–45%

**Mean corpuscular volume (MCV)**: Indicates the size of RBCs and can differentiate types of anemia. For adults, <80 is microcytic and >100 is macrocytic. Normal values:

- Males >18 years: 84–96 $\mu m^3$
- Females >18 years: 76–96 $\mu m^3$

**Reticulocyte count**: Measures marrow production and should rise with anemia. Normal values: 0.5–1.5% of total RBCs.

## WBC Count and Differential

**White blood cell (leukocyte) count** is used as an indicator of bacterial and viral infection. WBC count is reported as the total number of all white blood cells.

- Normal WBC for adults: 4,800–10,000
- Acute infection: 10,000+; 30,000 indicates a severe infection
- Viral infection: 4,000 and below

The **differential** provides the percentage of each different type of leukocyte. An increase in the white blood cell count is usually related to an increase in one type, and often an increase in immature neutrophils (bands), referred to as a "shift to the left," is an indication of an infectious process:

- Normal immature neutrophils (bands): 1–3%, increases with infection
- Normal segmented neutrophils (segs) for adults: 50–62%, increases with acute, localized, or systemic bacterial infections
- Normal eosinophils: 0–3%, decreases with stress and acute infection
- Normal basophils: 0–1%, decreases during acute stage of infection
- Normal lymphocytes: 25–40%, increases in some viral and bacterial infections
- Normal monocytes: 3–7%, increases during recovery stage of acute infection

## C-Reactive Protein and Erythrocyte Sedimentation Rate

**C-reactive protein** is an acute-phase reactant produced by the liver in response to an inflammatory response that causes neutrophils, granulocytes, and macrophages to secrete cytokines. Thus, levels of C-reactive protein rise when there is inflammation or infection. It is helpful to measure the response to treatment for pyoderma gangrenosum ulcers:

- Normal values: <0.9 mg/dL

**Erythrocyte sedimentation rate (sed rate)** measures the distance erythrocytes fall in a vertical tube of anticoagulated blood in one hour. Because fibrinogen, which increases in response to infection, also increases the rate of the fall, the sed rate can be used as a non-specific test for inflammation when infection is suspected. The sed rate is sensitive to osteomyelitis and may be used to monitor treatment response. Values vary according to gender and age:

- <50: Males 0–15 mm/hr; females 0–20 mm/hr
- >50: Males 0–20 mm/hr; females 0–30 mm/hr

## Elements of the Coagulation Profile

The coagulation profile measures clotting mechanisms, identifies clotting disorders, screens preoperative patients, and diagnoses excessive bruising and bleeding. Values vary depending on lab:

- **Prothrombin time (PT)**: 10–14 seconds
    - Increases with anticoagulation therapy, vitamin K deficiency, decreased prothrombin, DIC, liver disease, and malignant neoplasm. Some drugs may shorten PT.
- **Partial thromboplastin time (PTT)**: 25–35 seconds
    - Increases with hemophilia A and B, von Willebrand disease, vitamin deficiency, lupus, DIC, and liver disease.
- **Activated partial thromboplastin time (aPTT)**: 21–35 seconds
    - Similar to PTT, but decreases in extensive cancer, early DIC, and after acute hemorrhage. Used to monitor heparin dosage.
- **Thrombin clotting time (TCT) or Thrombin time (TT)**: 7–12 seconds
    - Used most often to determine the dosage of heparin. Prolonged with multiple myeloma, abnormal fibrinogen, uremia, and liver disease.
- **Bleeding time**: 2.0–9.5 minutes
    - (Using the IVY method on the forearm) Increases with DIC, leukemia, renal failure, aplastic anemia, von Willebrand disease, some drugs, and alcohol.
- **Platelet count**: 150,000–400,000 per μL
    - Increased bleeding <50,000 (transfusion required) and increased clotting >750,000.

**Review Video: The Coagulation Profile**
Visit mometrix.com/academy and enter code: 423595

# Neurological Diagnostics

## LUMBAR PUNCTURE

The lumbar puncture (spinal tap) is done between the 3rd and 4th or between the 4th and 5th lumbar vertebrae. The patient is in the lateral recumbent position with knees drawn toward the chest during the procedure. A local anesthetic is applied to prevent pain when the needle is inserted into the subarachnoid space to withdraw CSF and measure CSF pressure, which should be 70–200 $mmH_2O$.

Normal values (CSF analysis):

- Clear and colorless
- Protein: 15–45 mg/dL
- Glucose: 60–80 mg/dL
- Lactic acid: <25.2 mg/dL
- Culture: Negative
- RBCs: 0
- WBCs: 0.5/mL



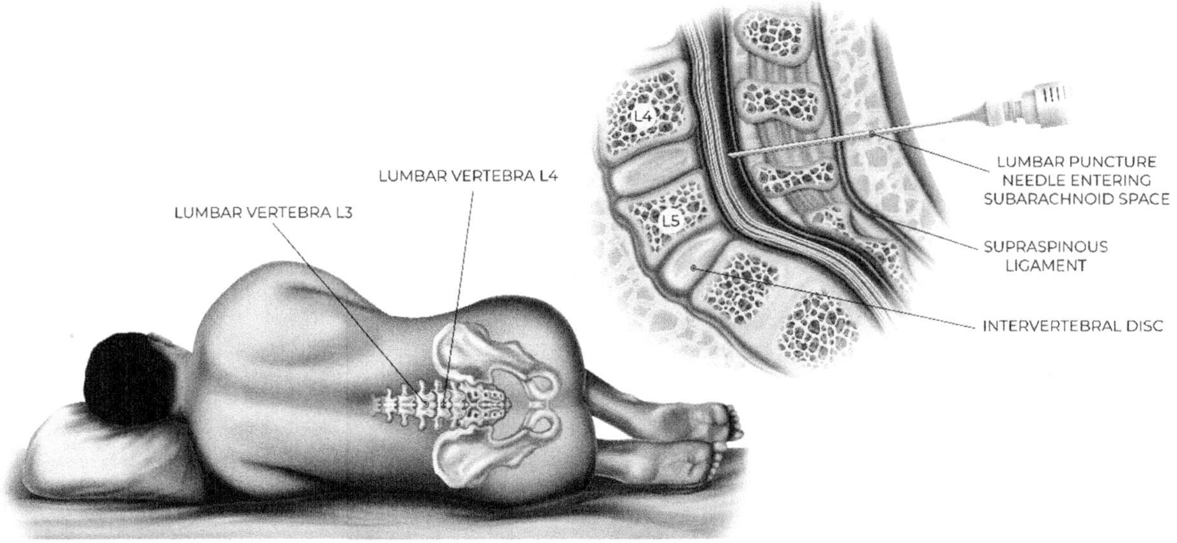


## AVOIDING COMPLICATIONS AFTER LUMBAR PUNCTURE AND EPIDURAL BLOOD PATCH

After a lumbar puncture, the patient should remain in the prone position for at least 3 hours to ensure that the needle puncture sites through the dural and arachnoid areas remain separate in order to reduce the chance of CSF leakage. If >20 mL of CSF is removed, then the patient should remain prone for 2 hours, side-lying (flat) for 2–3 hours, and supine or prone for 6 additional hours. Relieving intracranial pressure by withdrawing CSF may cause herniation of the brain, so lumbar puncture should be done with care in the presence of increased ICP. The most common complaint is of spinal headache, which may occur within a few hours or several days of the procedure. Increased fluid intake may reduce risk of headache. If headache occurs, it may be treated with analgesics, fluids, and bed rest; however, if the headache is severe or persistent, an **epidural blood patch** may be done, with venous blood withdrawn and then injected into the epidural space at the site of the puncture to seal the leaking opening.

# Gastrointestinal Diagnostics

## Liver Function Studies

Liver function studies are described below:

- **Bilirubin:** Determines the ability of the liver to conjugate and excrete bilirubin, direct 0.0–0.3 mg/dL, total 0.0–0.9 mg/dL, and urine bilirubin, which should be 0
- **Total protein:** Normal: 6.0–8.0 g/dL (Albumin: 4.0–5.5 g/dL, Globulin: 1.7–3.3 g/dL); normal albumin/globulin (A/G) ratio: 1.5:1 to 2.5:1, measured by serum protein electrophoresis
- **Prothrombin time (PT):** 100% or clot detection in 10–14 seconds; PT increases with liver disease
    - International normalized ratio (PT result/normal average): <2 for those not receiving anticoagulation, 2–3 for those receiving anticoagulation, critical value >3 in patients receiving anticoagulation therapy
- **Alkaline phosphatase:** 36–93 units/L in adults (normal values vary with method); indicates biliary tract obstruction if no bone disease
- **AST (SGOT):** 10–40 units (increases with liver cell damage)
- **ALT (SGPT):** 5–35 units (increases with liver cell damage)
- **GGT, GGTP:** 5–55 μ/L females, 5–85 μ/L males (increases with alcohol abuse)
- **LDH:** 100–200 units (increases with alcohol abuse)
- **Serum ammonia:** 150–250 mg/dL (increases with liver failure)
- **Cholesterol:** Increases with bile duct obstruction and decrease with parenchymal disease

## Nutritional Lab Monitoring

### *Total Protein and Albumin*

**Total protein** levels can be influenced by many factors, including stress and infection, but it may be monitored as part of an overall nutritional assessment. Protein is critical for general health and wound healing, and because metabolic rate increases in response to a wound, protein needs increase:

- Normal values: 6–8 g/dL
- Diet requirements for wound healing: 1.25–1.5 g/kg/day

**Albumin** is a protein that is produced by the liver and is a necessary component for cells and tissues. Levels decrease with renal disease, malnutrition, and severe burns. Albumin levels are the most common screening to determine protein levels. Albumin has a half-life of 18–20 days, so it is sensitive to long-term protein deficiencies more than short-term.

- Normal values: 3.5–5.5 g/dL
- Mild deficiency: 3.0–3.5 g/dL
- Moderate deficiency: 2.5–3.0 g/dL
- Severe deficiency: <2.5 g/dL

Levels below 3.2 correlate with increased morbidity and death. Dehydration (poor intake, diarrhea, or vomiting) elevates levels, so adequate hydration is important to ensure meaningful results.

### *Prealbumin*

Prealbumin (transthyretin) is most commonly monitored for acute changes in nutritional status because it has a half-life of only 2–3 days. Prealbumin is a protein produced in the liver, so it is often decreased with liver disease. Oral contraceptives and estrogen can also decrease levels. Levels may rise with Hodgkin's disease or the use of steroids or NSAIDS. Prealbumin is necessary for transportation of both thyroxine and vitamin A throughout the body, so if **prealbumin levels** fall, both thyroxine and vitamin A utilization are also affected:

- Normal values: 16–40 mg/dL
- Mild deficiency: 10–15 mg/dL
- Moderate deficiency: 5–9 mg/dL
- Severe deficiency: <5 mg/dL

Prealbumin is a good measurement because it quickly decreases when nutrition is inadequate and rises quickly in response to increased protein intake. Protein intake must be adequate to maintain levels of prealbumin. Death rates increase with any decrease in prealbumin levels.

### *Transferrin*

Transferrin, which transports about one-third of the body's iron, is a protein produced by the liver. It transports **iron** from the intestines to the bone marrow where it is used to produce **hemoglobin**. The half-life of transferrin is about 8–10 days. It is sometimes used as a measure of nutritional status; however, transferrin levels are sensitive to many factors. Levels rapidly decrease with protein malnutrition. Liver disease and anemia can also depress levels, but a decrease in iron, commonly found with inadequate protein, stimulates the liver to produce more transferrin, which increases transferrin levels but also decreases production of albumin and prealbumin. Transferrin levels may also increase with pregnancy, use of oral contraceptives, and polycythemia. Thus, **transferrin levels** alone are not always reliable measurements of nutritional status:

- Normal values: 200–400 mg/dL
- Mild deficiency: 150–200 mg/dL
- Moderate deficiency: 100–150 mg/dL
- Severe deficiency: <100 mg/dL

**Review Video: Transferrin**
Visit mometrix.com/academy and enter code: 267479

## EGD

**Esophagogastroduodenoscopy (EGD)** with a flexible fiberscope equipped with a lighted fiberoptic lens allows direct inspection of the mucosa of the esophagus, stomach, and duodenum. The scope has a still or video camera attached to a monitor for viewing during the procedure. The scope may be used for biopsies or therapeutically to dilate strictures or treat gastric or esophageal bleeding. The patient is positioned on the left side (head supported) to allow saliva drainage. Conscious sedation (midazolam, propofol) is commonly used along with a topical anesthetic spray or gargle to facilitate placing the lubricated tube through the mouth into the esophagus. Atropine reduces secretions. A bite guard in the mouth prevents the patient from biting the scope. The airway must be carefully monitored through the procedure (which usually takes about 30 minutes), including oximeter to measure oxygen saturation. While perforation, bleeding, or infection may occur, most complications are cardiopulmonary in nature and relate to drugs (conscious sedation) used during the procedure, so reversal agents (flumazenil, naloxone) should be available.

**Review Video: Diagnostic Procedures of the GI System**
Visit mometrix.com/academy and enter code: 645436

# Genitourinary Diagnostics

## Renal Function Studies

Renal function studies are described below:

- **Osmolality (urine):** Normal: 350–900 mOsm/kg/day. Shows early changes when the kidney has difficulty concentrating urine.
- **Osmolality (serum):** Normal: 275–295 mOsm/kg. Gives a picture of the amount of solute in the blood.
- **Uric acid:** Normal: 3.0–7.2 mg/dL. Increases with renal failure.
- **Creatinine clearance (24-hour):** Normal: 75–125 mL/min. Evaluates the amount of blood cleared of creatinine in 1 minute. Approximates the GFR.
- **Serum creatinine:** Normal: 0.6–1.2 mg/dL. Increase with decreased renal function, urinary tract obstruction, and nephritis.
- **Urine creatinine:** Normal: 11–26 mg/kg/day. Product of muscle breakdown. Increase with decreased renal function.
- **Blood urea nitrogen (BUN):** Normal: 7–8 mg/dL (8–20 mg/dL if age >60). An increase indicates impaired renal function, as urea is the end product of protein metabolism.
- **BUN/creatinine ratio:** Normal: 10:1. Increases with hypovolemia. With intrinsic kidney disease, the ratio is increased.
- **Urinalysis:** Tests various qualities of a urine sample that are reflective of kidney function and other disease processes.

### *Urinalysis*

Urinalysis components and normal findings are described below:

- **Color:** Pale yellow/amber and darkens when urine is concentrated or other substances (such as blood or bile) are present.
- **Appearance:** Clear but may be slightly cloudy.
- **Odor:** Slight. Bacteria may give urine a foul smell, depending upon the organism. Some foods, such as asparagus, change the odor.
- **Specific gravity:** Normal: 1.005–1.025. May increase if protein levels increase or if there is fever, vomiting, or dehydration.
- **pH:** Usually ranges from 4.5–8 with an average of 5–6.
- **Sediment:** Red cell casts from acute infections, broad casts from kidney disorders, and white cell casts from pyelonephritis. Leukocytes >10 per $mL^3$ are present with urinary tract infections.
- **Glucose, ketones, protein, blood, bilirubin, and nitrate:** Negative. Urine glucose may increase with infection (with normal blood glucose). Frank blood may be caused by some parasites and diseases but also by drugs, smoking, excessive exercise, and menstrual fluids. Increased red blood cells may result from lower urinary tract infections.
- **Urobilinogen:** 0.1–1.0 units.

## IVP and Radionucleotide Renal Scan

**Intravenous pyelogram (IVP)** is done to identify structural defects and tumors and to observe urinary structures. The patient is administered an IV contrast medium and may be administered antihistamine or corticosteroid before the test to minimize allergic response. Serum creatinine and BUN are done prior to the IVP to ensure that the contrast medium can be excreted. During the procedure, radiographs are taken once every minute for five minutes and then again after 15 minutes (giving the contrast medium time to pass into the bladder). A post-voiding radiograph shows how efficiently the bladder is able to empty. Fluid intake should be increased post-procedure to flush contrast.

**Radionucleotide renal scan** with dimercaptosuccinic acid (DMSA) requires IV administration of a radioactive element followed by a series of CT scans taken over 20 minutes to 4 hours. The scan is used to assess function and perfusion of the kidney and can detect lesions, atrophy, and scars and differentiate among different causes for hydronephrosis. The patient must be well-hydrated and may need to be catheterized to measure the output of urine.

### RENAL BIOPSY

Renal biopsy to remove a small segment of cortical tissue helps to identify the extent of **kidney disease** with acute renal failure, transplant rejection, glomerulopathies, and persistent hematuria or proteinuria. Preoperative coagulation studies determine the risk of bleeding. The biopsy is done percutaneously per needle biopsy (guided by fluoroscopy or ultrasound) or surgically through a small flank incision. A urine specimen must be obtained so it can be compared with a post-procedure specimen. **Post-procedure**:

- Maintain the patient in a supine position immediately after the procedure for 4–6 hours and on bed rest overnight.
- Monitor urine for hematuria and compare it with the preop specimen.
- Monitor VS every 5–15 minutes for the first hour and then less frequently. To minimize bleeding, maintain blood pressure <140/90.
- Note anorexia, vomiting, and abdominal discomfort that may suggest bleeding.
- Note pain: Severe colicky pain may indicate a clot in the ureter.
- Monitor urinalysis and CBC post-procedure.
- Maintain fluid intake at 3,000 mL/day in absence of renal insufficiency.
- Provide blood component therapy and surgical repair if bleeding occurs.



### RENAL ULTRASOUND

Renal ultrasound is a non-invasive method of viewing the **urinary structures**. Most patients that present with kidney disease of unknown origin should undergo a renal ultrasound to assess for possible obstruction. An ultrasound uses ultrasonic sound waves transmitted by a transducer, which picks up reflected sound waves that a computer converts to electronic images. An ultrasound can show fluid accumulation, the movement of blood through the kidney, masses, malformations (congenital abnormalities), changes in size of the kidney or other structures, and obstructions, such as renal calculi. An ultrasound is usually done before a renal biopsy, and may be done with a needle biopsy to guide the placement of the needle. Patient preparation includes drinking two 8-ounce glasses of water one hour before the examination to ensure that the bladder is full. The patient should be reminded not to urinate before the ultrasound. The patient usually remains in a supine position throughout the procedure but may be asked to turn to the side. No special precautions are necessary post-procedure.

## Postoperative Management

### PONV

Postoperative nausea and vomiting (PONV) varies with the type of anesthetic agent used. It occurs in about 20-30% of post-anesthesia patients and may be delayed up to 24 hours. Inhalational agents have a higher incidence of PONV than intravenous, and the incidence is lower with epidural or subarachnoid administration, although it may indicate the onset of hypotension. PONV correlates with the duration of surgery, with longer surgeries causing increased PONV. If high doses of narcotics, propofol, or nitrous oxide are used, PONV is often a problem. PONV is most common in young women and also relates to menstruation. It is also increased in those with a history of smoking or motion sickness. Some surgical procedures correlate with PONV: strabismus repair, ear surgery, laparoscopy, tonsillectomy, orchiopexy, and gynecological procedures to retrieve ova. PONV may be associated with postoperative pain, so managing pain is an important factor in preventing PONV.

**Review Video: Postoperative Care**
Visit mometrix.com/academy and enter code: 217370

## Risks for Aspiration

Risks for aspiration include:

- **Feeding tubes**: Aspiration pneumonia is a common complication, and because of reduced cough reflex there may be no obvious signs of it. Older age, cognitive impairment, poor oral hygiene, altered level of consciousness, neurological deficits, and history of GERD are all risk factors. Feedings should be given with client sitting up at least 45° if possible, and the client should remain sitting for at least an hour after feedings.
- **Sedation**: Sedation impairs the ability to swallow, increasing risk of aspiration. Risk is lower if the client has been NPO so that the stomach is empty but may still occur with gastric secretions. Oral fluids should be withheld until the client is fully alert.
- **Swallowing difficulties**: Clients with dysphagia, especially those with older age and/or stroke, Parkinson's disease, or muscular dystrophies, are at risk for aspiration. Additionally, clients with mouth sores, esophageal blockage (cancer, stenosis), or a history of radiotherapy or chemotherapy for cancers of the neck or throat are also at increased risk. Clients may need to be on a dysphagia diet, such as with soft foods and thickened liquids, and should eat with supervision while sitting upright.

## Risks for Insufficient Vascular Perfusion

Risk for insufficient vascular perfusion include the following:

- **Immobilized limb**: Usually the result of trauma, which may involve the muscles, bones, ligaments, tendons, vasculature, and nerves—all of which may result in insufficient vascular perfusion—so the limb must be assessed frequently for delayed capillary filling, pallor, edema, and sensory changes. Muscle mass may decrease rapidly even with isometric exercises, and the movement needed to promote adequate venous return is missing. In the case of extended generalized immobility, the client should be put on DVT prophylactic precautions such as a subcutaneous blood thinner (Heparin) and sequential compression devices or compression stockings to prevent clotting and promote perfusion.
- **Postoperative status**: Many conditions associated with surgical repair may result in insufficient vascular perfusion—hypoventilation, hyper- or hypovolemia, mechanical obstruction of blood flow, hypoxemia, and decreased hemoglobin resulting from bleeding. Capillary refill may exceed three seconds, and the client may exhibit dysrhythmias, dyspnea, abnormal ABGs, behavior changes, altered mental status, cooling and pallor of skin, weak/absent pulses, cyanosis, and edema as well as oliguria/anuria.
- **Diabetes**: Often associated with atherosclerosis, neuropathy, hypertension, and peripheral arterial disease, diabetes increases the risk of ulcers because of impaired perfusion.

## Indications of Output Changes from Baseline

Indications of output changes from baseline include:

- **NG tube**: Drainage per the NG tube should be light yellow/green but volume may vary so it's necessary to monitor both volume and electrolytes to determine what is normal for the client. Reddish or coffee-ground drainage may indicate bleeding, which may increase volume.
- **Emesis**: Clients should not have emesis, so the volume of any emesis must be recorded and steps taken to determine cause and treat.
- **Stool**: Fecal output may range from 3-4 occurrences daily to one every 2-3 days, so the client's normal output should be assessed through history. If diarrhea occurs, then the frequency and volume must be noted as the client may develop dehydration. Constipation lasting longer than several days can be common post-operatively or with a patient on narcotic pain medication, and may require a stool softener. This client should also be monitored for the possibility of an ileus.

- **Urine**: Normal urinary output depends on age, condition, and intake, but is typically 800-2000 mL per day with an intake of 2000 mL. Intake and output should be monitored carefully to establish an output that is normal for the client so that variations can be detected.

## PROCEDURES THAT REQUIRE SPECIFIC POSITIONING POSTOPERATIVELY

Procedures that require specific post-operative positioning to prevent complications include:

- **Angiography**: If an extremity is used, place restraint to keep the extremity straight for 6-8 hours.
- **Bronchoscopy**: Place in in semi-Fowler's position to prevent aspiration.
- **Myelogram**: With air contrast, place in Trendelenburg position; with oil contrast, place flat for 6-8 hours; with water-based contrast, place with head of bed elevated for 8 hours.
- **Liver biopsy**: Position on right side with pillow placed beneath the puncture site.
- **Arteriovenous fistula formation**: Elevate extremity.
- **Abdominal aneurysm**: Elevate head of bed to ≤45°.
- **Ear irrigation**: Position client on affected side to promote drainage.
- **Lumbar puncture**: Keep flat for 4-12 hours.
- **Appendectomy**: Place in Fowler's position.
- **Cataract removal**: Place in semi-Fowler's or Fowler's position on back or opposite side of surgery.
- **Kidney transplant**: Place in Semi-Fowler's position on back or turned to opposite side of surgery.
- **Mitral valve replacement**: Place in semi-Fowler's position.
- **Thyroidectomy**: Place in high Fowler's or semi-Fowlers.
- **Tonsillectomy**: Prone or side-lying.
- **Amputation of leg (AK, BK)**: Elevate limb for 24 hours. Place in prone position at least two times daily.
- **Insertion nasogastric tube**: Keep head elevated to at least 30°.



## INSERTION AND REMOVAL OF NG/OG TUBE

Procedure for insertion and removal of nasogastric or orogastric tube:

1. Gather PPE and equipment (stethoscope, lubricant, syringe, tape, suction if ordered, and pH strips) and carry out hand hygiene.
2. Assess nostrils for patency (if NG tube), abdomen for bowel sounds, and level of consciousness for ability to follow directions.
3. Position client at 45-90° if possible.
4. Measure NG/OG tube from tip of nose to ear and from ear to xiphoid process and mark tube.
5. Apply clean non-sterile gloves. Flush tube with water or lubricate 3-4 inches with water-soluble lubricant. Curl tube in circles around fingers and then release to ensure proper curvature.
6. Ask client to drop chin down and breathe orally if NG tube. Insert NG tube (curved side down) into nostril and guide downward. Guide OG tube along back of tongue and downward with client breathing through nose. Twist tubes slightly if resistance encountered.
7. Ask client to sip water (if allowed) or dry swallow while tube is advanced nasally or to swallow only if using OG tube.
8. Secure with tape and aspirate contents for pH testing (should be <5).
9. Verify placement with x-ray. If properly placed, measure length of NG/OG tube from where it leaves the nostril/mouth to end.

To remove NG/OG, gather supplies, carry out hand hygiene, and clear the NG/OG tube by injecting 10-20 mL of air. Then remove any tape and clips, ask the client to take and hold a deep breath, and gently pull out the tube in one steady motion.

## Maintaining Patency of Tubes

Procedures for maintaining patency of tubes include:

- **NG tube**: Flush with 30-50 mL of water or NS every 4-6 hours and before and after feeding or medications. Ensure tubing is not kinked if attached to drainage and check clamp.
- **Chest tube**: Ensure that tubes are not kinked or dislodged and that clamp is open and fluid has not collected in dependent loops. Keep chest drainage unit below level of client's chest. Ensure water levels are correct. Aggressive milking/stripping can result in negative pressure and damage to tissue and should be avoided. If clots are evident, gently squeezing and releasing the tube hand by hand along the length may prevent occlusion.
- **Percutaneous endoscopic gastrostomy tube**: Care is similar to that for the NG tube with tube flushed before and after feedings, medications, and every 4-6 hours.

## Thromboembolism

Thromboembolism includes both the formation of a thrombus (such as in the heart with A-fib and in the deep veins with immobilization) and embolism in which a clot breaks off and travels through the circulatory system. While thromboembolism may cause a heart attack or stroke, the most common presentation is a pulmonary embolism resulting from deep vein thrombosis.

**Signs and symptoms**: A thrombus is generally asymptomatic. Pain may be present at the thrombus site, which may be swollen and erythematous, typically in the lower extremity. When the patient develops pulmonary embolism, the usual presentation is acute onset of dyspnea. Some patients may have frothy sputum, cough, fever, and/or hemoptysis as well.

**Diagnosis**: Laboratory tests (CBC, troponins, D-dimer, ABGs, and BNP), ultrasound, spiral CT, pulmonary angiography, and ventilation/perfusion scanning.

**Treatment**: Anticoagulants, thrombolytic therapy, oxygen, and thrombectomy.

**Prevention**: Smoking cessation, regular exercise, discontinuation of birth control pills, early ambulation after surgery, SCDs/compression hose, control of high blood pressure, treatment for peripheral arterial disease, and avoiding prolonged sitting.

**Review Video: DVT - Prevention and Treatment**
Visit mometrix.com/academy and enter code: 234086

## Effects of Multiple Interventions on Postoperative Risk

### *General Surgery Patient with Co-Morbidities*

Multiple interventions in a patient with co-morbidities can increase the risk of postoperative complications. For example, a patient with diabetes who undergoes multiple interventions or surgical procedures may be at an increased risk for cardiac arrest; myocardial infarction; pressure sores, ulcers, or gangrene as a result of peripheral neuropathy; stroke; postoperative wound infection; wound dehiscence; contracting a hospital-acquired infection; worsening glycemic control from the stress of multiple interventions or infection; postoperative sepsis; and multi-organ failure.

### *Elderly Patients*

Many elderly patients have between two and four co-morbid conditions, all of which need to be addressed and treated. However, care must be taken to ensure that an intervention for one condition does not lead to adverse complications, particularly when prescribing multiple drugs. Common effects of multiple interventions in elderly patients with co-morbid conditions include an increased fall risk secondary to osteoarthritis and frailty, nosocomial infections secondary to decreased immune function, decubital ulcers as a result of impaired mobility or dementia, adverse medication reactions as a result of a decreased ability to metabolize medications, neurological complications, gastrointestinal bleeding, and delirium.

## Post-Procedure Complications After Cardiac Catheterization

Post-procedure complications of cardiac catheterization include:

- **Catheterization**: Dysrhythmias (ventricular arrhythmias, atrial fibrillation, conduction abnormalities, and bradycardia) may develop during or after cardiac catheterization caused by irritation of cardiac tissue. Incidence may vary depending on where the tip of the catheter lies. Risks are highest for clients with a history of congenital heart disease and a history of ECG abnormalities. In most cases, these abnormalities revert to a normal sinus rhythm, but they may require immediate intervention. Some may experience an allergic response to contrast medium.
- **Surgical/insertion site**: Bleeding (hematoma/retroperitoneal bleeding), arterial tearing (development of pseudoaneurysm), clot dislodgement (resulting in myocardial infarction or stroke), arterial occlusion (especially of radial artery), and infection (at insertion site or endocarditis) may occur at the insertion site. The surgical site should be assessed frequently (per facility protocol) for any signs of bleeding.

## Stages of Blood Loss/Hypovolemia

| Stage | Blood loss | Indications |
|---|---|---|
| 1 | 15%<br>750 mL | Client may appear pale but vital signs, urinary output, and capillary refill may remain within normal limits. |
| 2 | 15-30%<br>1500 mL | Pallor may increase with skin becoming cool and clammy. Diastolic blood pressure may increase and heart rate may increase to >100 beats per minute. The client may appear anxious. Capillary refill is delayed but urinary output remains at 20-30 mL per hour. |
| 3 | 30-40%<br>1500-2000 mL | Client becoming increasingly confused with altered mental status and diaphoresis. Systolic BP drops to below 100 and tachycardia increases to >120 beats per minute. Client is dyspneic with respirations >30 per minute. Capillary refill remains delayed but urinary output remains about 20 mL per hour. |
| 4 | >40%<br>>2000 mL | Client increasingly lethargic and may become comatose, remains diaphoretic but skin mottling may be evident. Pulse is thready at >140 beats per minutes and systolic BP falls to below 70. Respirations are very shallow and rapid. Capillary refill is absent and urinary output is negligible or absent. |

## Potential Sources of Infection for Transplant Patients

Infections pose a serious threat to **transplant patients**, especially during the first year. While opportunistic infections have decreased, nosocomial infections have increased, most related to bacterial infections. Transplant patients consistently show higher rates of infection than other patients due to their needs for immunosuppressants to prevent rejection. There are numerous potential sources:

- **Donor-infected organs** can transmit HBV, HBC, herpesvirus, HIV, and human T-cell leukemia virus type I. Additionally, donors who are immunocompromised prior to harvesting of the organs may have nosocomial bacterial or fungal infections that can be transmitted. Organs can also become infected during harvesting.
- **Health care workers** may transmit pathogens through droplets, airborne particles, or contact, frequently transmitting pathogens on their hands or clothing.

- **Blood and blood products** can transmit CMV, but transmission is rare. HCV transmission has been reduced to <1%.
- **Environmental reservoir sources** can include the water system, demolition activities, equipment, and surfaces. Some pathogens, such as MRSA and VRE, may be endemic to the hospital environment.

## Common Viral Pathogens in Transplant Patients

Several **viral infections** are more likely to occur in transplant patients due to their immunocompromised state:

- **Cytomegalovirus (CMV)**: The most common pathogen related to transplant infections, affecting 40%-90% of recipients.
- **Herpes simplex virus**: Reactivated/new; may disseminate to liver.
- **Human herpesvirus-6**: Mostly reactivation, newer strain.
- **Varicella-zoster virus**: New; may disseminate to viscera.
- **Hepatitis B and C viruses**: Causes liver failure; also affects kidney transplant patients.
- **BK virus (BKV)**: Causes renal dysfunction; transmission unknown.
- **Adenoviruses (AdV)**: Bone marrow transplant; can become systemic.

**Prevention** is as follows:

- **Serologic matching** can prevent primary transmission but the limited supply of organs may make this impractical.
- **Early diagnosis** with serum assay for targeted treatment.
- **Antiviral prophylaxis** in high-risk patients can be effective.
- **Immunization** has proven to be safe and highly effective, reducing the incidence of infection and the severity.
- **Immunoglobulin** is given to susceptible transplant patients exposed to certain viruses.
- Reduction in immunosuppressive medications if possible.
- **High-dose acyclovir** for some viruses may reduce severity of infection.
- Targeting patients at the highest risk of disease through **surveillance** and using proper transmission-based precautions are the most practical methods of infection control.

## Common Bacterial Infections After Transplant Surgery

***Staphylococcus aureus*** is the most common cause of bacterial infection in liver, heart, kidney, and pancreas transplant patients. According to the CDC, as many as 33% of individuals carry *Staphylococcus aureus* in their nares, without any other signs of illness, and approximately 5% of individuals in the hospital carry MRSA (methicillin-resistant *Staphylococcus aureus*). Because it is spread through direct contact, nosocomial infection is common. Specific risk factors for the post-transplant patient in the hospital setting include open wounds and intravenous access. Diligent hand hygiene must be performed by all health care providers and visitors.

**Vancomycin-resistant enterococci (VRE)** causes 10-15% of liver failures, according to recent studies. Nosocomial transmission occurs frequently, especially with prolonged hospitalization and ICU stay. VRE colonization puts patients at continued risk of infection and poses a reservoir for nosocomial infections.

**Nocardia** is found in soil and decaying vegetation, and transmission is through inhalation. Lung, heart, and intestinal transplants have the highest rates of infection. Mortality rates are high for those who are infected. Risk factors include high-dose cortisone, high levels of immunosuppressants, and CMV infection within six months.

**Infection control strategies** include:

- **Handwashing** and basic clean technique are still the best methods of infection control in these patients.
- **Environmental monitoring** should be used.
- **Antibiotic prophylaxis** is effective.

### Aspergillus Fungal Infection After Transplant Surgery

***Aspergillus*** infections primarily involve pneumonia and sinusitis, but 25-35% disseminate systemically, and *Aspergillus* pneumonia infections have mortality rates up to 85%. *Aspergillus* is a serious fungal infection in immunocompromised transplant patients, especially lung transplant patients with 8% infection rates within 9 months of surgery. Liver transplant patients have infection rates of 1-4% but disease occurs earlier, within 2-4 weeks. Heart transplant infection rates are 1-6% with disease within 1-2 months. *Aspergillus* affects renal transplants the least with <1% infection rates. Prophylaxis with antifungals has not proven to be effective.



**Infection control strategies** include:

- **Monitoring environment and improving air filtration** with HEPA filtration or use of laminar air flow rooms for patients at high risk.
- **Construction precautions** to prevent dust and debris from circulating in patient care areas.
- **Standard precautions** include high-resolution CT scans for early diagnosis rather than chest x-rays so treatment with voriconazole (drug of choice) can begin.

### Infection Control Strategies for Spinal Cord Injuries

Infection control strategies for neurology/spinal cord injuries target the most common types of infection:

- **Urinary tract infection***:* Patients should be monitored for fever and/or changes in spasms or voiding habits that may indicate infection. When possible, intermittent catheterization (sterile rather than clean while in the hospital) should be used rather than continuous. Antibiotic prophylaxis has not proven to be effective but bacterial interference, colonizing of the urinary tract with nonpathogenic *E. coli* 83972, has shown promising results.
- **Decubital ulcers***:* Procedures for regular monitoring of skin condition, turning patients, and avoiding friction to prevent pressure from developing are critical. Both staff and patients must be educated about prevention, skin care, and cleanliness. Nutrition and hydration must be adequate to maintain integrity of the skin.
- **Respiratory infections**: Proper use of ventilation equipment must be monitored. Assisted coughing, such as through respiratory therapy and postural drainage, can reduce infections. Prophylactic antibiotics are not recommended, but patients should receive immunizations for pneumonia.

## Chapter Quiz

Ready to see how well you retained what you just read? Scan the QR code to go directly to the chapter quiz interface for this study guide. If you're using a computer, simply visit the online resources page at **mometrix.com/resources719/nclexrn-31183** and click the Chapter Quizzes link.

# Physiological Adaptation

## Cardiovascular Pathophysiology

### Acute Coronary Syndromes

Acute coronary syndrome (ACS) is the impairment of blood flow through the coronary arteries, leading to ischemia of the cardiac muscle. Angina frequently occurs in ACS, manifesting as crushing pain substernally, radiating down the left arm or both arms. However, in females, elderly, and diabetics, symptoms may appear less acute and include nausea, shortness of breath, fatigue, pain/weakness/numbness in arms, or no pain at all (*silent ischemia*). There are multiple **classifications of angina**:

- **Stable angina**: Exercise-induced, short lived, relieved by rest or nitroglycerin. Other precipitating events include decrease in environmental temperature, heavy eating, strong emotions (such as fright or anger), or exertion, including coitus.
- **Unstable angina** (preinfarction or crescendo angina): A change in the pattern of stable angina, characterized by an increase in pain, not responding to a single nitroglycerin or rest, and persisting for >5 minutes. May cause a change in EKG, or indicate rupture of an atherosclerotic plaque or the beginning of thrombus formation. Treat as a medical emergency, indicates impending MI.
- **Variant angina** (Prinzmetal's angina): Results from spasms of the coronary arteries. Associated with or without atherosclerotic plaques and is often related to smoking, alcohol, or illicit stimulants, but can occur cyclically and at rest. Elevation of ST segments usually occurs with variant angina. Treatment is nitroglycerin or calcium channel blockers.

**Review Video: Coronary Artery Disease**
Visit mometrix.com/academy and enter code: 950720

### Myocardial Infarctions

#### *NSTEMI and STEMI*

**Non–ST-segment elevation MI (NSTEMI)**: ST elevation on the electrocardiogram (ECG) occurs in response to myocardial damage resulting from infarction or severe ischemia. The absence of ST elevation may be diagnosed as unstable angina or NSTEMI, but cardiac enzyme levels increase with NSTEMI, indicating partial blockage of coronary arteries with some damage. Symptoms are consistent with unstable angina, with chest pain or tightness, pain radiating to the neck or arm, dyspnea, anxiety, weakness, dizziness, nausea, vomiting, and heartburn. Initial treatment may include nitroglycerin, β-blockers, antiplatelet agents, or antithrombotic agents. Ongoing treatment may include β-blockers, aspirin, statins, angiotensin-converting enzyme inhibitors, angiotensin-receptor blockers, and clopidogrel. Percutaneous coronary intervention is not recommended.

**ST-segment elevation MI (STEMI)**: This more severe type of MI involves complete blockage of one or more coronary arteries with myocardial damage, resulting in ST elevation. Symptoms are those of acute MI. As necrosis occurs, Q waves often develop, indicating irreversible myocardial damage, which may result in death, so treatment involves immediate reperfusion before necrosis can occur.

**Review Video: Myocardial Infarction**
Visit mometrix.com/academy and enter code: 148923

## Q-Wave and Non-Q-Wave Myocardial Infarctions

Formerly classified as transmural or non-transmural, myocardial infarctions are now classified as Q-wave or non-Q-wave:

- **Q-Wave**
  - Characterized by a series of abnormal Q waves (wider and deeper) on ECG, especially in the early morning (related to adrenergic activity).
  - Infarction is usually prolonged and results in necrosis.
  - Coronary occlusion is complete in 80–90% of cases.
  - Q-wave MI is often, but not always, transmural.
  - Peak CK levels occur in about 27 hours.
- **Non-Q-Wave**
  - Characterized by changes in ST-T wave with ST depression (usually reversible within a few days).
  - Usually reperfusion occurs spontaneously, so infarct size is smaller. Contraction necrosis related to reperfusion is common.
  - Non-Q-wave MI is usually non-transmural.
  - Coronary occlusion is complete in only 20–30%.
  - Peak CK levels occur in 12–13 hours.
  - Reinfarction is common.

## Locations and Types

Myocardial infarctions are also classified according to their location and the extent of injury. Q-wave infarctions involve the full thickness of the heart muscle, often producing a series of Q waves on ECG. While an MI most frequently damages the left ventricle and the septum, the right ventricle may be damaged as well, depending upon the area of the occlusion:

- **Anterior** ($V_2$ to $V_4$): Occlusion in the proximal left anterior descending (LAD) or left coronary artery. Reciprocal changes found in leads II, III, $aV_F$.
- **Lateral** (I, $aV_L$, $V_5$, $V_6$): Occlusion of the circumflex coronary artery or branch of left coronary artery. Often causes damage to anterior wall as well. Reciprocal changes found in leads II, III, $aV_F$.
- **Inferior/diaphragmatic** (II, III, $aV_F$): Occlusion of the right coronary artery and causes conduction malfunctions. Reciprocal changes found in leads I and $aV_L$.
- **Right ventricular** ($V_{4R}$, $V_{5R}$, $V_{6R}$): Occlusion of the proximal section of the right coronary artery and damages in the right ventricle and the inferior wall. No reciprocal changes should be noted on an ECG.
- **Posterior** ($V_1$ to$V_4$): Occlusion in the right coronary artery or the left coronary artery or its circumflex branch and may be difficult to diagnose. Reciprocal changes found in $V_1$-$V_4$.
- **Septal** ($V_1$ and $V_2$): Occlusion of the left anterior descending (LAD) at the septal branch. T-wave inversion and absent R wave long with ST elevation.

## Clinical Manifestations and Diagnosis

Clinical manifestations of myocardial infarction may vary considerably. More than half of all patients present with acute MIs with no prior history of cardiovascular disease.

**Signs/symptoms**: Angina with pain in chest that may radiate to neck or arms, palpitations, hypertension or hypotension, dyspnea, pulmonary edema, dependent edema, nausea/vomiting, pallor, skin cold and clammy, diaphoresis, decreased urinary output, neurological/psychological disturbances: anxiety, light-headedness, headache, visual abnormalities, slurred speech, and fear.

**Diagnosis** is based on the following:

- ECG obtained immediately to monitor heart changes over time. Typical changes include T-wave inversion, elevation of ST segment, abnormal Q waves, tachycardia, bradycardia, and dysrhythmias.
- Echocardiogram: decreased ventricular function is possible, especially for transmural MI.
- Labs:
    - **Troponin**: Increases within 3–6 hours, peaks 14–20; elevated for up to 1–2 weeks.
    - **Creatinine kinase (CK-MB)**: Increases 4–8 hours and peaks at about 24 hours (earlier with thrombolytic therapy or PTCA). (Not commonly used in the US)
    - **Ischemia modified albumin (IMA)**: Increase within minutes, peak 6 hours and return to baseline; verify with other labs.
    - **Myoglobin**: Increases in 0.5–4.0 hours, peaks 6–7 hours. While an increase is not specific to an MI, a failure to increase can be used to rule out an MI.

### *Papillary Muscle Rupture*

Papillary muscle rupture is a rare but often deadly complication of myocardial ischemia/infarct. It most commonly occurs with inferior infarcts. The papillary muscles are part of the cardiac wall structure. Attached to the lower portion of the ventricles, they are responsible for the opening and closing of the tricuspid and mitral valve and preventing prolapse during systole. Rupture of the papillary muscle can occur with myocardial infarct or ischemia in the area of the heart surrounding the papillary muscle. Since the papillary muscles support the mitral valve, rupture will cause severe mitral regurgitation that may result in cardiogenic shock and subsequent death. Rupture of the papillary muscle may be partial or complete and is considered a life-threatening emergency.

**Signs/symptoms**: Acute heart failure, pulmonary edema, and cardiogenic shock (tachycardia, diaphoresis, loss of consciousness, pallor, tachypnea, mental status changes, weak or thready pulse, and decreased urinary output).

**Diagnosis**: Transesophageal echocardiography (TEE) to visualize the papillary muscles, color flow Doppler, echocardiogram, and physical assessment. In patients with papillary muscle rupture, a holosystolic murmur starting at the apex and radiating to the axilla may be present.

**Treatment**: Emergent surgical intervention to repair the mitral valve.

In the cases of complete rupture, patients often experience the rapid development of cardiogenic shock and subsequent death.

## Aortic Aneurysms

### Types

A **dissecting aortic aneurysm** occurs when the wall of the aorta is torn and blood flows between the layers of the wall, dilating and weakening it until it risks rupture (which has a 90% mortality). Aortic aneurysms are more than twice as common in males as females, but females have a higher mortality rate, possibly due to increased age at diagnosis.

**Abdominal aortic aneurysms (AAA)** are usually related to atherosclerosis, but may also result from Marfan syndrome, Ehlers-Danlos disease, and connective tissue disorders. Rupture usually does not allow time for emergent repair, so identifying and correcting before rupture is essential. Different classification systems are used to describe the type and degree of dissection. **DeBakey classification** uses anatomic location as the focal point:

- Type I (thoracic) begins in the ascending aorta but may spread to include the aortic arch and the descending aorta (60%). This is also considered a proximal lesion or Stanford type A.
- Type II (thoracic) is restricted to the ascending aorta (10–15%). This is also considered a proximal lesion or Stanford type A.
- Type III (abdominal) is restricted to the descending aorta (25–30%). This is considered a distal lesion or Stanford type B.

### Diagnosis and Treatment

Aortic aneurysms are often asymptomatic, but when symptomatic, patients present with substernal pain, back pain, dyspnea and/or stridor (from pressure on trachea), cough, distention of neck veins, palpable and pulsating abdominal mass, edema of neck and arms.

**Diagnosis**: x-ray, CT, MRI, Cardiac catheterization, TEE/transthoracic echocardiogram.

**Treatment** includes:

- **Anti-hypertensives** to reduce systolic BP, such as β-blockers (esmolol) or Alpha-β-blocker combinations (labetalol) to reduce force of blood as it leaves the ventricle to reduce pressure against the aortic wall. IV vasodilators (sodium nitroprusside) may also be needed.
- **Intubation and ventilation** may be required if the patient is hemodynamically unstable.
- **Analgesia/sedation** to control anxiety and pain.
- **Surgical repair**: Types I and II are usually repaired surgically because of the danger of rupture and cardiac tamponade. Type III (abdominal) is often followed medically and surgically only if the aneurysm is >5.5cm or rapidly expanding. There are two types of surgical repair:
  - **Open**: Patient is placed on cardiopulmonary bypass, and through an abdominal incision the damaged portion is removed, and a graft is sutured in place.
  - **Endovascular**: A stent graft is fed through the arteries to line the aorta and exclude the aneurysm.

**Complications**: Myocardial infarction, renal injury, and GI hemorrhage/ischemic bowel, which may occur up to years after surgery. Endo-leaks can occur with a stent graft, increasing risk of rupture.

## Aortic Rupture

Aortic rupture is a catastrophic breakage of the aorta, generally as the result of trauma or rupture of an aortic aneurysm. **Aortic rupture** (spontaneous) most commonly occurs in the abdominal aorta. The patient typically experiences a severe tearing pain and loses consciousness from hypovolemic shock as the blood pours out of the aorta. Tachycardia occurs and the patient may exhibit cyanosis. An ecchymotic area may appear in the flank area because of retroperitoneal pooling of blood. Diagnostic tests include ultrasound or CT. Survival depends on the size of the tear, the amount of blood loss, and the length of time until surgical repair. About 90% of patients die prior to surgery. An aortic occlusion balloon to stem bleeding may be placed temporarily in order to stabilize the patient. Surgical repair may be via an open procedure or endovascular therapy. Risk factors include male gender, older age, smoking, history of MI, family history of abdominal aortic aneurysm, peripheral arterial disease, and hypertension.

## Cardiogenic Shock

In cardiogenic shock, the heart fails to pump enough blood to provide adequate circulation and oxygen to the body. The primary cause of cardiogenic shock is acute myocardial infarction, especially an anterior wall MI. Other causes include papillary muscle/ventricular septal rupture, pericarditis/myocarditis, prolonged tachyarrhythmia, and hypotensive medications.

**Signs/symptoms**: Hypotension, altered mental status secondary to decreased cerebral circulation, oliguria, tachypnea or tachycardia, cool extremities, jugular venous distension, and pulmonary edema possible.

**Diagnosis**: ABGs: metabolic acidosis, hypoxia, hypocapnia; lactic acidosis, BNP, BUN and K elevated; EKG: arrhythmias, specifically SVT/V-tach, Sinus bradycardia, AV block and IVCDs possible; however, the EKG may be normal.

- Pulmonary artery catheter (Swan-Ganz catheter) values: CI <1.8 L/min, PCWP >18 mmHg, SBP <90, MAP <60, Increased CVP and PAP

**Treatment** includes:

- Dobutamine IV to increase cardiac contractility (used when cardiac output is low but blood pressure is stable)
- Norepinephrine IV if SBP <70
- Morphine can be given for pain; while potential for hypotension, it will decrease SNS response and decrease HR and $MVO_2$
- Treat underlying cause (e.g., papillary rupture = valve replacement, acute MI = revascularization with PCI or CABG)
- Intra-aortic balloon pump (IABP) may be indicated if re-vascularization fails (increases cardiac blood flow)

## Obstructive Shock

Obstructive shock occurs when the preload (diastolic filling of the RV) of the heart is obstructed in one or several ways. There can be obstruction to the great vessels of the heart (such as from pulmonary embolism), there can be excessive afterload because the flow of blood out of the heart is obstructed (resulting in decreased cardiac output), or there can be direct compression of the heart, which can occur when blood or air fills the pericardial sac with cardiac tamponade or tension pneumothorax. Other causes include aortic dissection, vena cava syndrome, systemic hypertension, and cardiac lesions. Obstructive shock is often categorized with cardiogenic shock because of their similarities. **Signs and symptoms** of obstructive shock may vary depending on the underlying cause but typically include:

- Decrease in oxygen saturation
- Hemodynamic instability with hypotension and tachycardia, muffled heart sounds
- Chest pain
- Neurological impairment (disorientation, confusion)
- Dyspnea
- Impaired peripheral circulation (cool extremities, pallor)
- Generalized pallor and cyanosis

**Treatment** depends on the cause and may include oxygen, pericardiocentesis, needle thoracostomy or chest tube, and fluid resuscitation.

## CARDIOMYOPATHY

### DILATED CARDIOMYOPATHY

Dilated cardiomyopathy (DCM) occurs when some precipitating factor leads to decreased cardiac perfusion. The resulting ischemic cardiac tissue is replaced with scar tissue, and the healthy cells are forced to over-compensate, causing hypertrophy and over stretching. Eventually, the muscle cells become stretched beyond compensation, and dilated and weak chamber results, unable to properly contract. This causes a decrease in stroke volume and cardiac output, with the end result being enlargement of the mitral and tricuspid valves and severe valve regurgitation. While DCM is the most common form of cardiomyopathy, causes include:

- **Vascular**: Cardiac ischemia, hypertension, atherosclerosis
- **Metabolic**: Diabetes, uremia, thyrotoxicosis, and acromegaly, muscular dystrophy
- **Genetics** (familial DCM), and childbirth (peripartum DCM)
- **Viral infections**, particularly adenovirus, Varicella zoster, HIV, and Hepatitis C may cause DCM
- **Alcohol poisoning or cocaine addiction**
- **Radiation or heavy metal poisoning**, specifically cobalt

**Signs/symptoms**: Dyspnea, SOB, tachycardia, S3/S4 heart sounds, holosystolic murmur, wheezes/crackles, pleural effusions, edema, JVD, ascites

**Diagnosis**: EKG (tachycardia/T wave changes), chest x-ray (cardiomegaly), 2D Echocardiogram (valve regurgitation/EF).

**Treatment** includes:

- Treat underlying cause if possible; supportive care
- Heart transplant if patient is a candidate and damage is permanent

### HYPERTROPHIC CARDIOMYOPATHY

Hypertrophic cardiomyopathy (HCM) is a genetic disorder that causes idiopathic thickening of the heart muscle, primarily involving the ventricular septum and portions of the left ventricle. Patients with HCM produce abnormal sarcomeres and misalignment of muscle cells (myocardial disarray). Basically, HCM is characterized by ventricular hypertrophy, an asymmetrical septum, forceful systole, cardiac dysrhythmias, and myocardial disarray. Because the abnormal cells develop over time, it is common for HCM to remain undiagnosed until middle or late adulthood.

**Signs/symptoms**: Exertional or atypical chest pain, dyspnea at rest, syncope, frequent palpitations (common due to reoccurring dysrhythmias).

**Diagnosis**: 2D echo (structure and EF), EKG (pathological Q waves and dysrhythmias), x-ray (cardiomegaly), Family history (especially cardiac death, reoccurring dysrhythmias, or myocardial hypertrophy).

**Treatment** for cases in which there is outflow tract obstruction includes the use of β-blockers and one of the following methods of septal reduction therapy:

- **Septal myectomy** (gold standard): high mortality (3–10%), but increases cardiac output and quality of life.
- **Alcohol-based septal ablation**: Ethanol 100% injected into a branch of the LAD, creating a controlled area of infarction and consequently thinning the septum.

### RESTRICTIVE CARDIOMYOPATHY

Restrictive cardiomyopathy (RCM) occurs when the ventricles become stiff and noncompliant, resulting in decreased end-diastolic cardiac refill volume. The ventricular stiffening is caused by the infiltration of fibroelastic tissue into the cardiac muscle (such as in amyloidosis or sarcoidosis). Atrial enlargement can be seen in most cases of RCM as a result of the increased effort required to push blood from the atria into the ventricles. It is not uncommon for a patient to be in atrial fibrillation secondary to atrial enlargement. In advanced cases, ventricular dysrhythmias may also be seen.

**Signs/symptoms**: Exercise intolerance/fatigue, edema, crackles, elevated CVP, S3/S4, murmur, SOB at rest

**Diagnosis**: 2D echo (enlarged atria, decreased compliance of ventricle), hemodynamic monitoring (increased right atrial pressure and pulmonary wedge pressure, and SVR), x-ray (cardiomegaly), EKG (atrial fibrillation), endomyocardial biopsy (to differentiate from constrictive pericarditis).

**Treatment** includes:

- **Medications**: β-blockers increase ventricular filling; antiarrhythmics may be ordered
- **Surgical**: Heart transplant, if patient is a candidate

## Stress (Takotsubo) Cardiomyopathy

Takotsubo cardiomyopathy, also referred to as stress cardiomyopathy or more casually as broken heart syndrome, is an acute weakening of the muscles of the heart secondary to an intensely stressful event. Stressors can be physical (extreme illness such as sepsis or shock) or emotional in nature and result in the release of stress hormones (epinephrine and norepinephrine) that are thought to be the major contributors to the ultimate weakening of the heart muscle. This produces symptoms that present similarly to a myocardial infarction (shortness of breath, chest pain, and EKG changes) without any ischemic event noted to contribute to these symptoms. Risk factors for takotsubo cardiomyopathy include:

- **Stressful events or conditions**
- **Sex**: Females have a higher risk for developing takotsubo cardiomyopathy
- **Endocrine disorders**: Pheochromocytoma and thyrotoxicosis

Treatment focuses on symptom management due to the risk for acute heart failure and cardiogenic shock. In severe cases, an intra-aortic balloon pump may be required for circulatory support until the patient is stabilized.

## Dysrhythmias

### *Sinus Bradycardia*

There are 3 primary types of **sinus node dysrhythmias**: sinus bradycardia, sinus tachycardia, and sinus arrhythmia. **Sinus bradycardia (SB)** is caused by a decreased rate of impulse from sinus node. The pulse and ECG usually appear normal except for a slower rate.

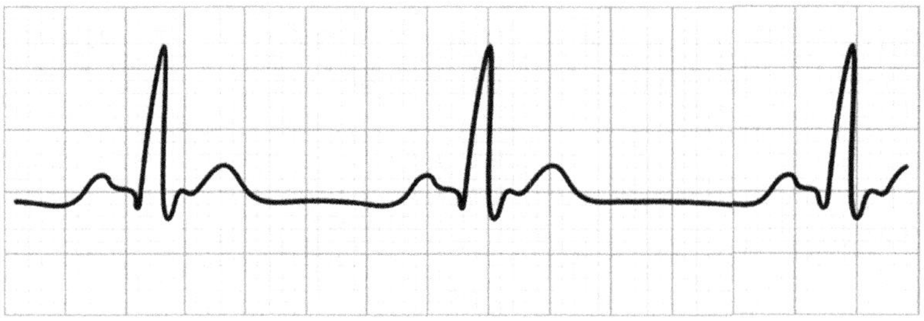

SB is characterized by a regular pulse <50–60 bpm with P waves in front of QRS, which are usually normal in shape and duration. PR interval is 0.12–0.20 seconds, QRS interval is 0.04–0.11 seconds, and P:QRS ratio of 1:1. SB may be caused by several factors:

- May be normal in athletes and older adults; generally not treated unless symptomatic
- Conditions that lower the body's metabolic needs, such as hypothermia or sleep
- Hypotension and decrease in oxygenation
- Medications such as calcium channel blockers and β-blockers
- Vagal stimulation that may result from vomiting, suctioning, defecating, or certain medical procedures (carotid stent placement, etc.)
- Increased intracranial pressure
- Myocardial infarction

**Treatment**: involves eliminating cause if possible, such as changing medications. Atropine 1 mg may be given IV to block vagal stimulation or increase rate if symptomatic.

### *Sinus Tachycardia*

Sinus tachycardia (ST) occurs when the sinus node impulse increases in frequency. ST is characterized by a regular pulse >100 with P waves before QRS but sometimes part of the preceding T wave. QRS is usually of normal shape and duration (0.04–0.11 seconds) but may have consistent irregularity. PR interval is 0.12–0.20 seconds and P:QRS ratio of 1:1.

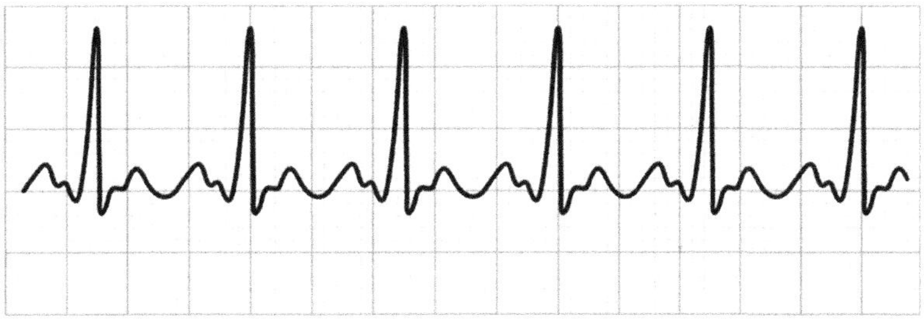

The rapid pulse decreases diastolic filling time and causes reduced cardiac output with resultant hypotension. Acute pulmonary edema may result from the decreased ventricular filling if untreated. ST may be **caused** by a number of factors:

- Acute blood loss, shock, hypovolemia, anemia
- Sinus arrhythmia, hypovolemic heart failure
- Hypermetabolic conditions, fever, infection
- Exertion/exercise, anxiety, stress
- Medications, such as sympathomimetic drugs

**Treatment**: eliminating precipitating factors, calcium channel blockers and β-blockers to reduce heart rate.

### *Supraventricular Tachycardia*

Supraventricular tachycardia (SVT) (>100 BPM) may have a sudden onset and result in congestive heart failure. Rate may increase to 200–300 BPM, which will significantly decrease cardiac output due to decreased filling time. SVT originates in the atria rather than the ventricles but is controlled by the tissue in the area of the AV node rather than the SA node. Rhythm is usually rapid but regular. The P wave is present but may not be clearly defined as it may be obscured by the preceding T wave, and the QRS complex appears normal. The PR interval is 0.12–0.20 seconds and the QRS interval is 0.04–0.11 seconds with a P:QRS ratio of 1:1.

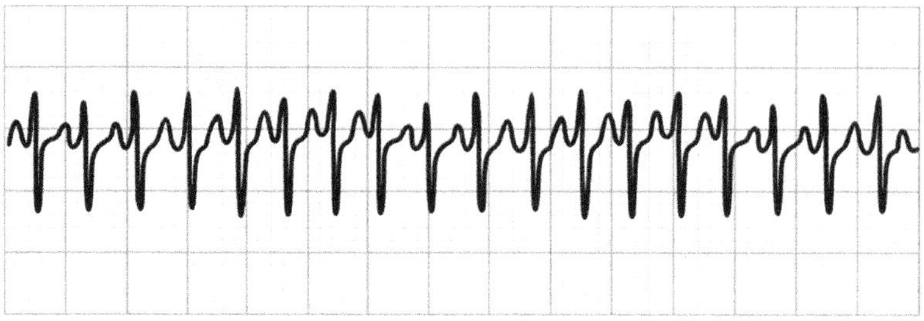

SVT may be episodic with periods of normal heart rate and rhythm between episodes of SVT, so it is often referred to as paroxysmal SVT (PSVT).

**Treatment**: Adenosine, digoxin, verapamil, vagal maneuvers, cardioversion.

### *Sinus Arrhythmia*

Sinus arrhythmia (SA) results from irregular impulses from the sinus node, often paradoxical (increasing with inspiration and decreasing with expiration) because of stimulation of the vagal nerve during inspiration and rarely causes a negative hemodynamic effect. These cyclic changes in the pulse during respiration are quite common in both children and young adults and often lesson with age but may persist in some adults. Sinus arrhythmia can, in some cases, relate to heart or valvular disease and may be increased with vagal stimulation for suctioning, vomiting, or defecating. Characteristics of SA include a regular pulse 50–100 BPM, P waves in front of QRS with duration (0.04–0.11 seconds) and shape of QRS usually normal, PR interval of 0.12–0.20 seconds, and P:QRS ratio of 1:1.

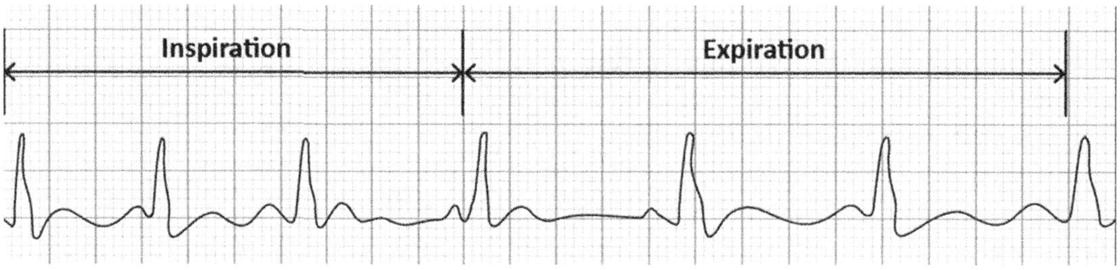


**Treatment** is usually not necessary unless it is associated with bradycardia.

## *Premature Atrial Contraction*

There are 3 primary types of **atrial dysrhythmias**: premature atrial contraction, atrial flutter, and atrial fibrillation. Premature atrial contraction (PAC) is essentially an extra beat precipitated by an electrical impulse to the atrium before the sinus node impulse. The extra beat may be caused by alcohol, caffeine, nicotine, hypervolemia, hypokalemia, hypermetabolic conditions, atrial ischemia, or infarction. Characteristics include an irregular pulse because of extra P waves, the shape and duration of QRS is usually normal (0.04–0.11 seconds) but may be abnormal, PR interval remains between 0.12–0.20, and P:QRS ratio is 1:1. Rhythm is irregular with varying P-P and R-R intervals.

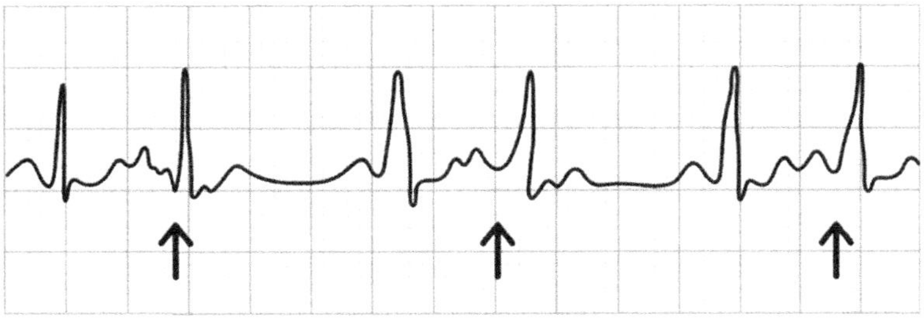

PACs can occur in an essentially healthy heart and are not usually cause for concern unless they are frequent (>6 per hr) and cause severe palpitations. In that case, atrial fibrillation should be suspected.

## *Atrial Flutter*

Atrial flutter (AF) occurs when the atrial rate is faster, usually 250–400 beats per minute, than the AV node conduction rate so not all of the beats are conducted into the ventricles. The beats are effectively blocked at the AV node, preventing ventricular fibrillation although some extra ventricular impulses may pass through. AF is caused by the same conditions that cause A-fib: coronary artery disease, valvular disease, pulmonary disease, heavy alcohol ingestion, and cardiac surgery. AF is characterized by atrial rates of 250–400 with ventricular rates of 75–150, with ventricular rate usually being regular. P waves are saw-toothed (referred to as F waves), QRS shape and duration (0.04–0.11 seconds) are usually normal, PR interval may be hard to calculate because of F waves, and the P:QRS ratio is 2:1 to 4:1. Symptoms include chest pain, dyspnea, and hypotension.

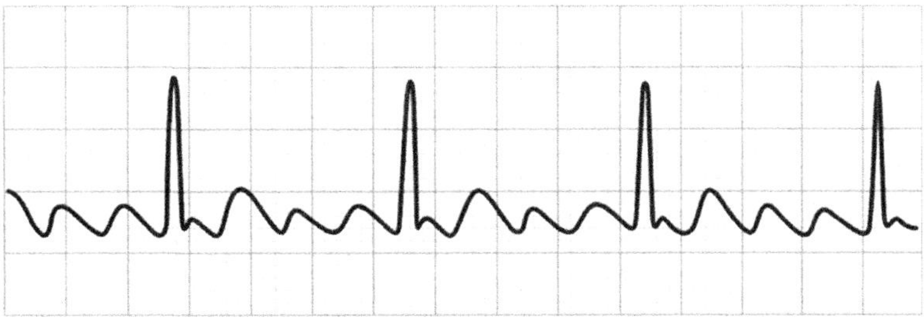

**Treatment** includes:

- Emergent cardioversion if condition is unstable
- Medications to slow ventricular rate and conduction through AV node: non-dihydropyridine calcium channel blockers (Cardizem, Calan) and beta blockers
- Medications to convert to sinus rhythm: ibutilide (Corvert), dofetilide (Tikosyn), amiodarone; also used in practice: quinidine, disopyramide (Norpace)

### ATRIAL FIBRILLATION

Atrial fibrillation (A-fib) is rapid, disorganized atrial beats that are ineffective in emptying the atria, so that blood pools in the chambers. This can lead to thrombus formation and emboli. The ventricular rate increases with a decreased stroke volume, and cardiac output decreases with increased myocardial ischemia, resulting in palpitations and fatigue. A-fib is caused by coronary artery disease, valvular disease, pulmonary disease, heavy alcohol ingestion, infection, and cardiac surgery; however, it can also be idiopathic. A-fib is characterized by a very irregular pulse with atrial rate of 300–600 and ventricular rate of 120–200, shape and duration (0.04–0.11 seconds) of QRS is usually normal. Fibrillatory (F) waves are seen instead of P waves. The PR interval cannot be measured and the P:QRS ratio is highly variable.

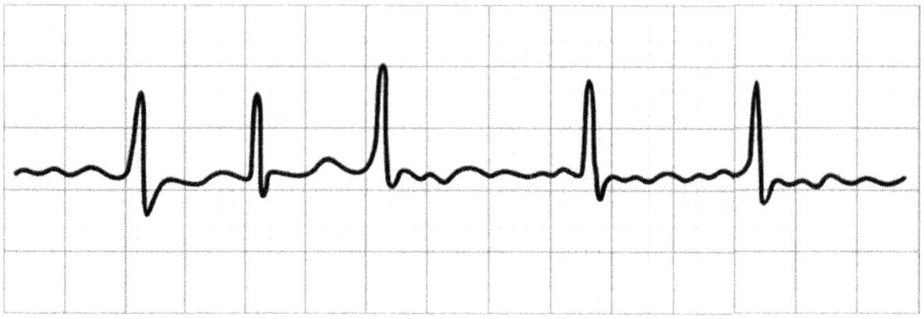

**Treatment** is the same as atrial flutter.

| **Review Video: Atrial Fibrillation and Atrial Flutter**<br>Visit mometrix.com/academy and enter code: 263842 |
|---|

### PREMATURE JUNCTIONAL CONTRACTION

The area around the AV node is the junction, and dysrhythmias that arise from that area are called junctional dysrhythmias. Premature junctional contraction (PJC) occurs when a premature impulse starts at the AV node before the next normal sinus impulse reaches the AV node. PJC is similar to premature atrial contraction (PAC) and generally requires no treatment although it may be an indication of digoxin toxicity. The ECG may appear basically normal with an early QRS complex that is normal in shape and duration (0.04–0.11 seconds). The P wave may be absent or it may precede, be part of, or follow the QRS with a PR interval of 0.12 seconds. The P:QRS ratio may vary from <1:1 to 1:1 (with inverted P wave). The underlying rhythm is usually regular at a heart rate of 60–100. Significant symptoms related to PJC are rare.

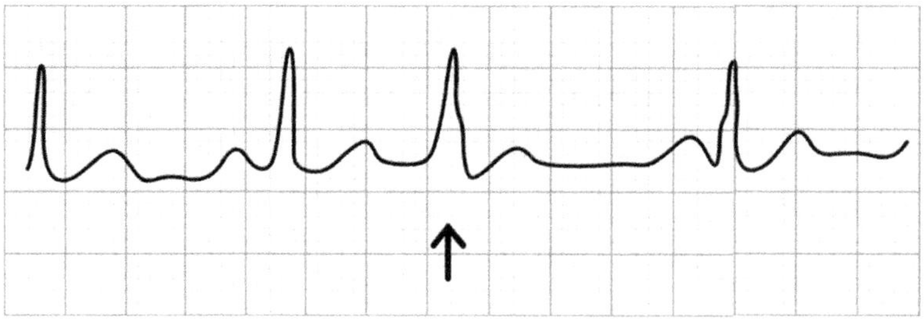

### *JUNCTIONAL RHYTHMS*

Junctional rhythms occur when the AV node becomes the pacemaker of the heart. This can happen because the sinus node is depressed from increased vagal tone or a block at the AV node prevents sinus node impulses from being transmitted. While the sinus node normally sends impulses 60–100 beats per minute, the AV node junction usually sends impulses at 40–60 beats per minute. The QRS complex is of usual shape and duration (0.04–0.11 seconds). The P wave may be inverted and may be absent, hidden or after the QRS. If the P wave precedes the QRS, the PR interval is <0.12 seconds. The P:QRS ratio is <1:1 or 1:1. The junctional escape rhythm is a protective mechanism preventing asystole with failure of the sinus node. An **accelerated junctional rhythm** is similar, but the heart rate is 60–100. **Junctional tachycardia** occurs with heart rate of >100.

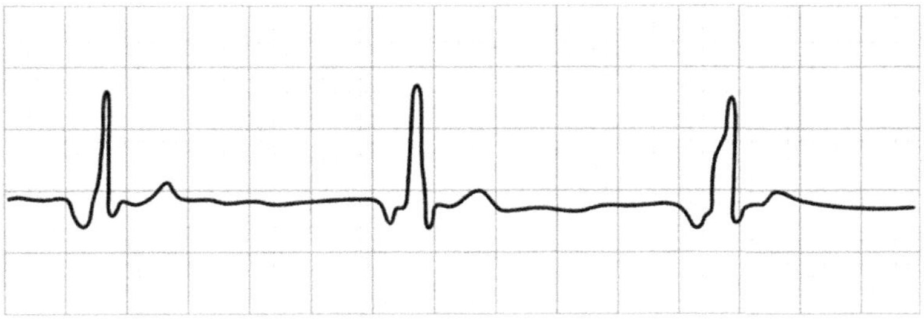

### *AV NODAL REENTRY TACHYCARDIA*

AV nodal reentry tachycardia occurs when an impulse conducts to the area of the AV node and is then sent in a rapidly repeating cycle back to the same area and to the ventricles, resulting in a fast ventricular rate. The onset and cessation are usually rapid. AV nodal reentry tachycardia (also known as paroxysmal atrial tachycardia or supraventricular tachycardia if there are no P waves) is characterized by atrial rate of 150–250 with ventricular rate of 75–250, P wave that is difficult to see or absent, QRS complex that is usually normal and a PR interval of <0.12 if a P wave is present. The P:QRS ratio is 1–2:1. Precipitating factors include nicotine, caffeine, hypoxemia, anxiety, underlying coronary artery disease and cardiomyopathy. Cardiac output may be decreased with a rapid heart rate, causing dyspnea, chest pain, and hypotension.

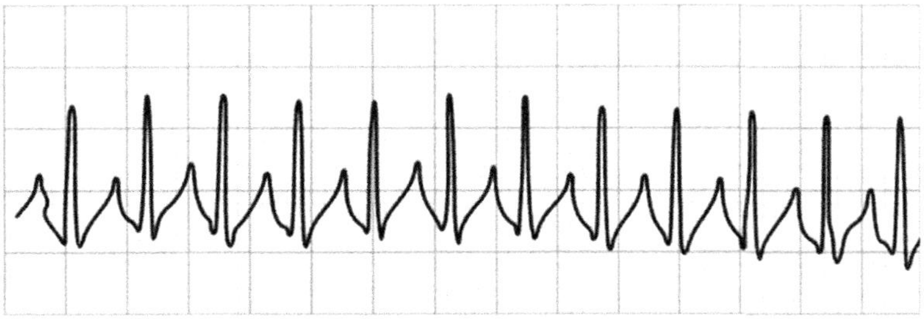

**Treatment** includes:

- Vagal maneuvers (carotid sinus massage, gag reflex, holding breath/bearing down)
- Medications (adenosine, verapamil, or diltiazem)
- Cardioversion if other methods unsuccessful

### *Premature Ventricular Contractions*

Premature ventricular contractions (PVCs) are those in which the impulse begins in the ventricles and conducts through them prior to the next sinus impulse. The ectopic QRS complexes may vary in shape, depending upon whether there is one site (unifocal) or more (multifocal) that stimulates the ectopic beats. PVCs usually cause no morbidity unless there is underlying cardiac disease or an acute MI. PVCs are characterized by an irregular heartbeat, QRS that is ≥0.12 seconds and oddly shaped. PVCs are often not treated in otherwise healthy people. PVCs may be precipitated by electrolyte imbalances, caffeine, nicotine, or alcohol. Because PVCs may occur with any supraventricular dysrhythmia, the underlying rhythm must be noted as well as the PVCs. If there are more than six PVCs in an hour, that is a risk factor for developing ventricular tachycardia.

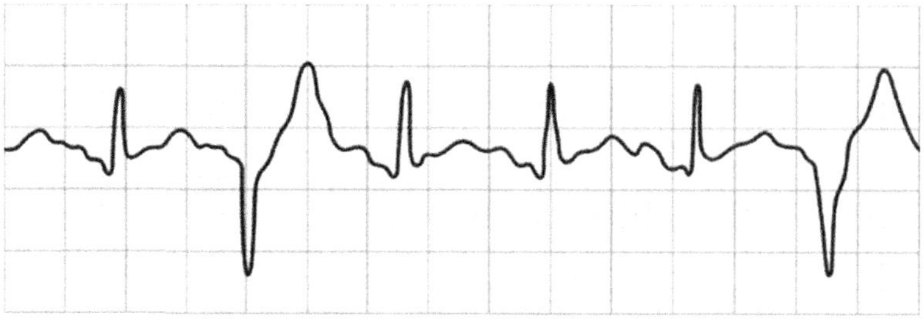

**Bigeminy** is a rhythm where every other beat is a PVC. **Trigeminy** is a rhythm where every third beat is a PVC.

**Ventricular bigeminy** is a rhythm where every other beat is a PVC. **Ventricular trigeminy** is a rhythm where every third beat is a PVC.

**Treatment**: Lidocaine (affects the ventricles, may cause CNS toxicity with nausea and vomiting), procainamide (affects the atria and ventricles and may cause decreased BP and widening of QRS and QT); treat underlying cause.

### *Ventricular Tachycardia*

Ventricular tachycardia (VT) is greater than 3 PVCs in a row with a ventricular rate of 100–200 beats per minute. Ventricular tachycardia may be triggered by the same factors as PVCs and often is related to underlying coronary artery disease. The rapid rate of contractions makes VT dangerous as the ineffective beats may render the person unconscious with no palpable pulse. A detectable rate is usually regular and the QRS complex is ≥0.12 seconds and is usually abnormally shaped. The P wave may be undetectable with an irregular PR interval if P wave is present. The P:QRS ratio is often difficult to ascertain because of the absence of P waves.

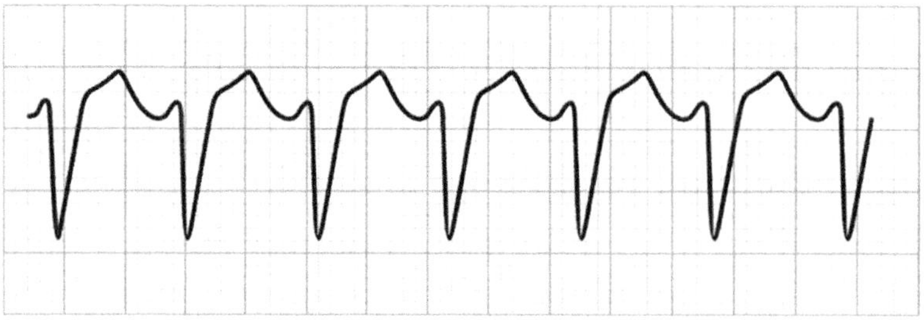

**Treatment** is as follows:

- With pulse: Synchronized cardioversion, adenosine
- No pulse: Same as ventricular fibrillation

## NARROW COMPLEX AND WIDE COMPLEX TACHYCARDIAS

Tachycardias are classified as narrow complex or wide complex. Wide and narrow refer to the configuration of the QRS complex.

- **Wide complex tachycardia (WCT)**: About 80% of cases of WCT are caused by ventricular tachycardia. WCT originates at some point below the AV node and may be associated with palpitations, dyspnea, anxiety, diaphoresis, and cardiac arrest. Wide complex tachycardia is diagnosed with more than 3 consecutive beats at a heart rate >100 BPM and QRS duration ≥0.12 seconds.

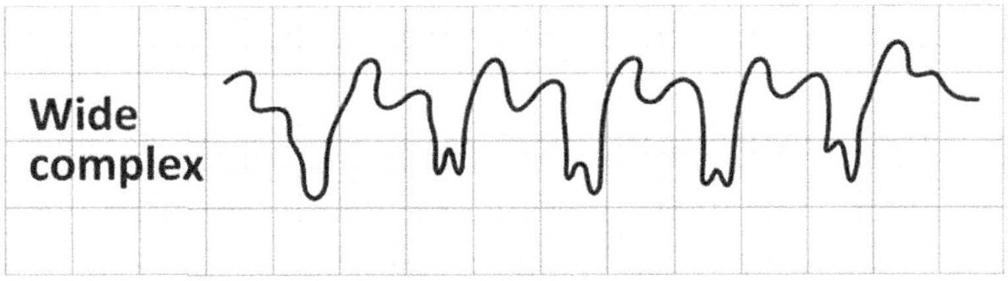


- **Narrow complex tachycardia (NCT)**: NCT is associated with palpitations, dyspnea, and peripheral edema. NCT is generally supraventricular in origin. Narrow complex tachycardia is diagnosed with ≥3 consecutive beats at heart rate of >100 BPM and QRS duration of <0.12 seconds.

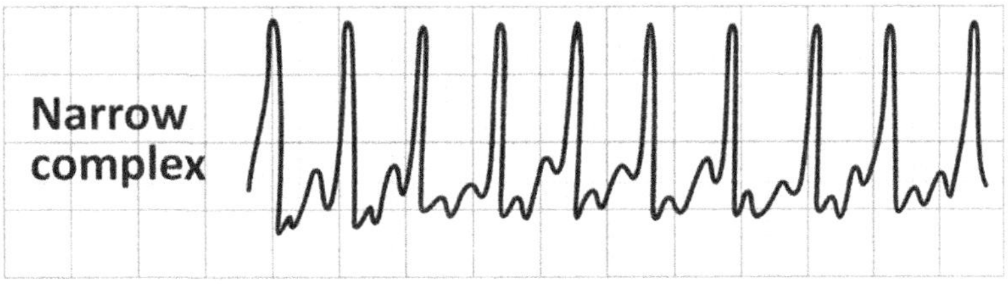


### *VENTRICULAR FIBRILLATION*

Ventricular fibrillation (VF) is a rapid, very irregular ventricular rate >300 beats per minute with no atrial activity observable on the ECG, caused by disorganized electrical activity in the ventricles. The QRS complex is not recognizable as ECG shows irregular undulations. The causes are the same as for ventricular tachycardia and asystole. VF is accompanied by lack of palpable pulse, audible pulse, and respirations and is immediately life threatening without defibrillation.

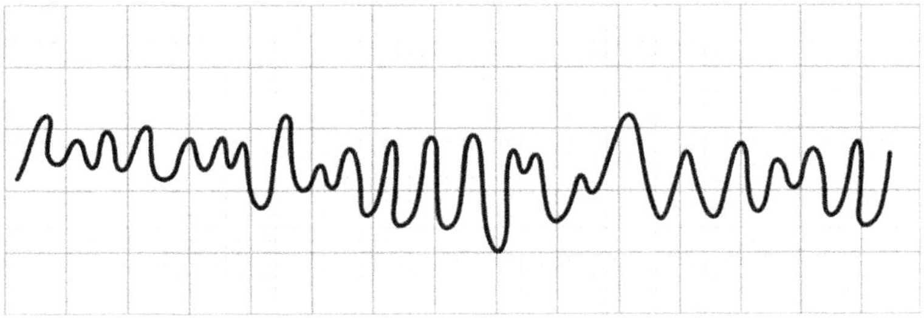

**Treatment** includes:

- Emergency defibrillation, the cause should be identified and treated
- Epinephrine 1 mg q 3–5 minutes then amiodarone 300 mg (2nd dose: 150 mg) IV push

**Review Video: Ventricular Arrythmias**
Visit mometrix.com/academy and enter code: 933152

Physiological Adaptation

### *Idioventricular Rhythm*

Ventricular escape rhythm (idioventricular) occurs when the Purkinje fibers below the AV node create an impulse. This may occur if the sinus node fails to fire or if there is blockage at the AV node so that the impulse does not go through. Idioventricular rhythm is characterized by a regular ventricular rate of 20–40 BPM. Rates >40 BPM are called accelerated idioventricular rhythm. The P wave is missing and the QRS complex has a very bizarre and abnormal shape with duration of ≥0.12 seconds. The low ventricular rate may cause a decrease in cardiac output, often making the patient lose consciousness. In other patients, the idioventricular rhythm may not be associated with reduced cardiac output.

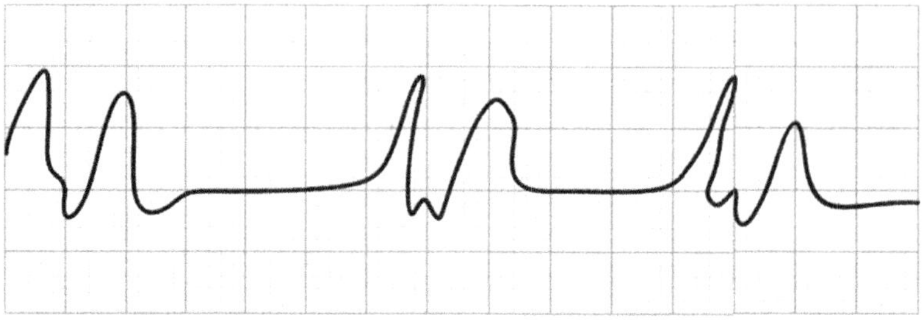

### *Ventricular Asystole*

Ventricular asystole is the absence of audible heartbeat, palpable pulse, and respirations, a condition often referred to as "cardiac arrest." While the ECG may show some P waves initially, the QRS complex is absent although there may be an occasional QRS "escape beat" (agonal rhythm). Cardiopulmonary resuscitation is required with intubation for ventilation and establishment of an intravenous line for fluids. Without immediate treatment, the patient will suffer from severe hypoxia and brain death within minutes. Identifying the cause is critical for the patient's survival. Consider the "Hs & Ts": hypovolemia, hypoxia, hydrogen ions (acidosis), hypo/hyperkalemia, hypothermia, tension pneumothorax, tamponade (cardiac), toxins, and thrombosis (pulmonary or coronary). Even with immediate treatment, the prognosis is poor and ventricular asystole is often a sign of impending death.

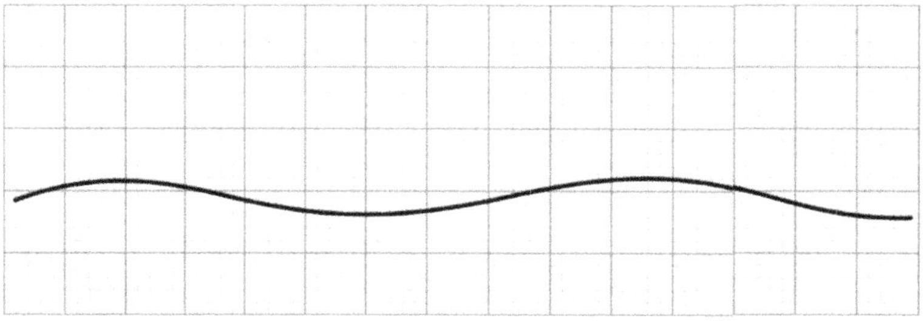

**Treatment** includes:

- CPR only; Asystole is not a shockable rhythm therefore defibrillation is not indicated
- Epinephrine 1 mg q 3–5 minutes

### SINUS PAUSE

Sinus pause occurs when the sinus node fails to function properly to stimulate heart contractions, so there is a pause on the ECG recording that may persist for a few seconds to minutes, depending on the severity of the dysfunction. A prolonged pause may be difficult to differentiate from cardiac arrest. During the sinus pause, the P wave, QRS complex and PR and QRS intervals are all absent. P:QRS ratio is 1:1 and the rhythm is irregular. The pulse rate may vary widely, usually 60–100 BPM. Patients with frequent pauses may complain of dizziness or syncope. The patient may need to undergo an electrophysiology study and medication reconciliation to determine the cause. If measures such as decreasing medication are not effective, a pacemaker is usually indicated (if symptomatic).

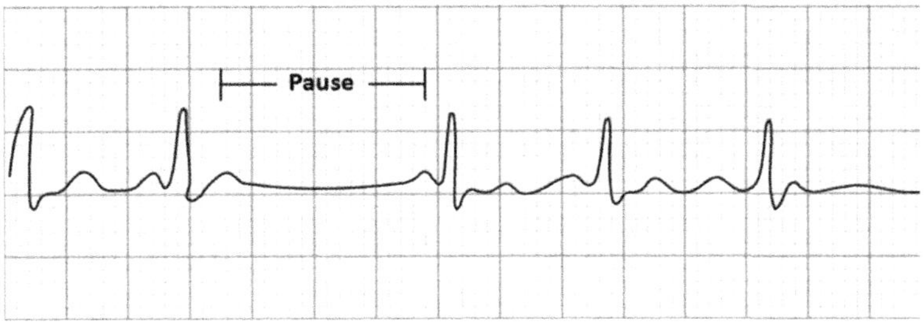


### FIRST-DEGREE AV BLOCK

First-degree AV block occurs when the atrial impulses are conducted through the AV node to the ventricles at a rate that is slower than normal. While the P and QRS are usually normal, the PR interval is >0.20 seconds, and the P:QRS ratio is 1:1. A narrow QRS complex indicates a conduction abnormality only in the AV node, but a widened QRS indicates associated damage to the bundle branches as well. *Chronic* first-degree block may be caused by fibrosis/sclerosis of the conduction system related to coronary artery disease, valvular disease, cardiac myopathies and carries little morbidity, thus is often left untreated. *Acute* first-degree block, on the other hand, is of much more concern and may be related to digoxin toxicity, β-blockers, amiodarone, myocardial infarction, hyperkalemia, or edema related to valvular surgery.

**Treatment**: involves eliminating cause if possible, such as changing medications. Atropine 1 mg may be given IV if rate falls.

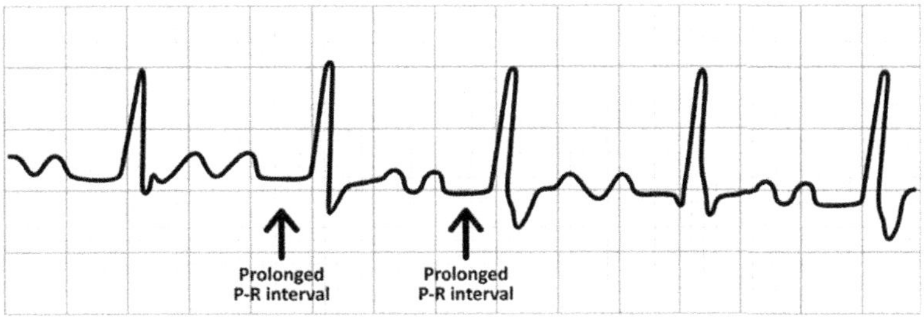

### *Second-Degree AV Block*

Second-degree AV block occurs when some of the atrial beats are blocked. Second-degree AV block is further subdivided according to the patterns of block.

#### Type I

Mobitz type I block (Wenckebach) occurs when each atrial impulse in a group of beats is conducted at a lengthened interval until one fails to conduct (the PR interval progressively increases), so there are more P waves than QRS complexes, but the QRS complex is usually of normal shape and duration. The sinus node functions at a regular rate, so the P-P interval is regular, but the R-R interval usually shortens with each impulse. The P:QRS ratio varies, such as 3:2, 4:3, 5:4. This type of block by itself usually does not cause significant morbidity unless associated with an inferior wall myocardial infarction.

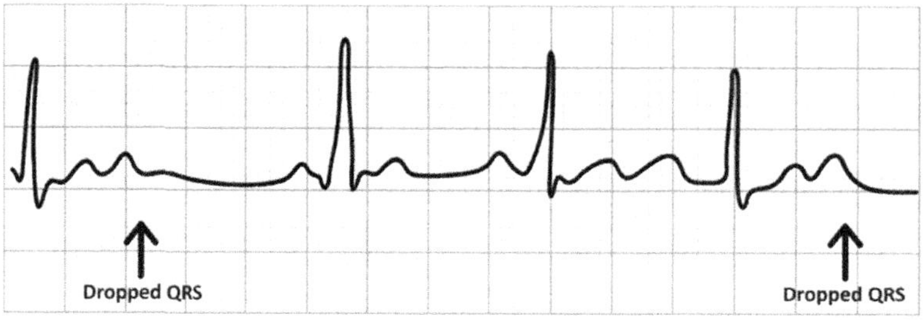


#### Type II

In Mobitz type II, only some of the atrial impulses are conducted unpredictably through the AV node to the ventricles, and the block always occurs below the AV node in the bundle of His, the bundle branches, or the Purkinje fibers. The PR intervals are the same if impulses are conducted, and the QRS complex is usually widened. The P:QRS ratio varies 2:1, 3:1, and 4:1. Type II block is more dangerous than Type I because it may progress to complete AV block and may produce Stokes-Adams syncope (fainting induced by insufficient perfusion of the brain secondary to a dysfunctional rhythm). Additionally, if the block is at the Purkinje fibers, there is no escape impulse. Usually, a transcutaneous cardiac pacemaker and defibrillator should be at the patient's bedside. **Symptoms** may include chest pain if the heart block is precipitated by myocarditis or myocardial ischemia.

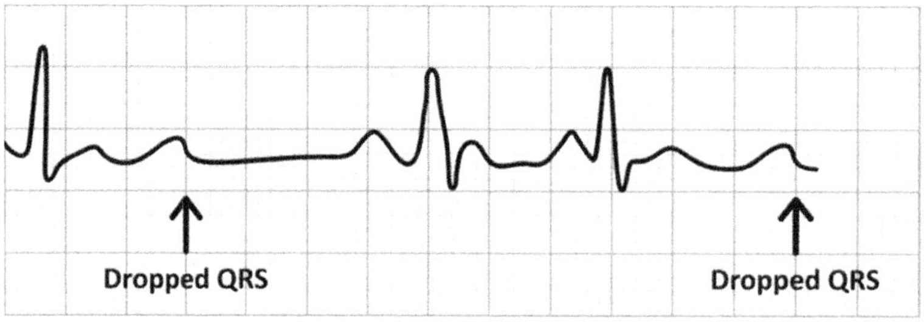

### *Third-Degree AV Block*

With third-degree AV block, there are more P waves than QRS complexes, with no clear relationship between them. The atrial rate is 2–3 times the pulse rate, so the PR interval is irregular. If the SA node malfunctions, the AV node fires at a lower rate, and if the AV node malfunctions, the pacemaker site in the ventricles takes over at a bradycardic rate; thus, with complete AV block, the heart still contracts, but often ineffectually. With this type of block, the atrial P (sinus rhythm or atrial fibrillation) and the ventricular QRS (ventricular escape rhythm) are stimulated by different impulses, so there is AV dissociation.

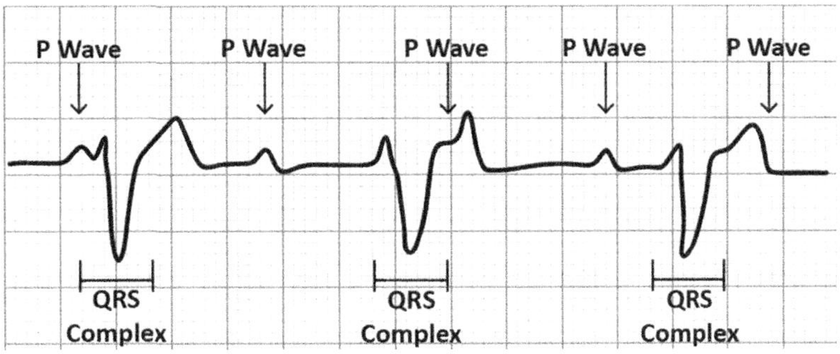


The heart may compensate at rest but can't keep pace with exertion. The resultant bradycardia may cause congestive heart failure, fainting, or even sudden death, and usually conduction abnormalities slowly worsen. **Symptoms** include dyspnea, chest pain, and hypotension, which are treated with IV atropine. Stokes-Adams syncope may occur. Transcutaneous pacing may be needed. Complete persistent AV block normally requires implanted pacemakers, usually dual chamber.

**Review Video: AV Heart Blocks**
Visit mometrix.com/academy and enter code: 487004

### *Bundle Branch Blocks*

A **right bundle branch block (RBBB)** occurs when conduction is blocked in the right bundle branch that carries impulses from the Bundle of His to the right ventricle. The impulse travels through the left ventricle instead, and then reaches the right ventricle, but this causes a slight delay in contraction of the right ventricle. A RBBB is characterized by normal P waves (as the right atrium still contracts appropriately), but the QRS complex is widened and notched (referred to as an "RSR pattern" that resembles the letter "M") in lead V1, which is a reflection of the asynchronous ventricular contraction. The PR interval is normal or prolonged, and the QRS interval is > 0.12 seconds. P:QRS ratio remains 1:1 with regular rhythms.

A **left bundle branch block (LBBB)** occurs when there is a delay in conduction between the left atrium and left ventricle. It is also characterized by normal or inverted P waves, but the QRS complex may be widened with a deep S wave and an interval of >0.12 seconds (in lead V1) that resembles a "W." The PR interval may be normal or prolonged. The P:QRS ratio is 1:1 and the rhythm is regular.

**RBBB** **LBBB**

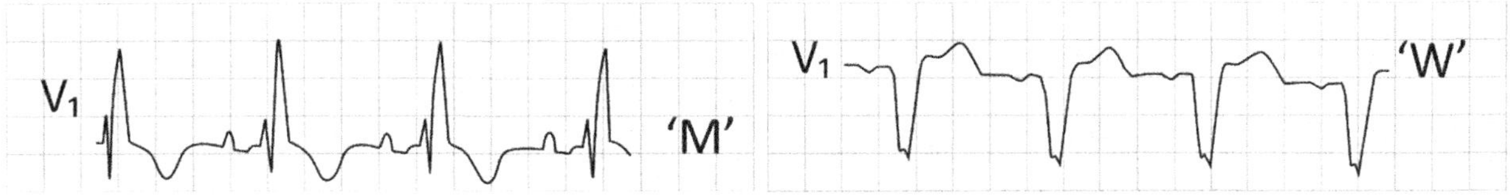

## Heart Failure

Heart failure (formerly congestive heart failure) is a cardiac disease that includes disorders of contractions (systolic dysfunction) or filling (diastolic dysfunction) or both and may include pulmonary, peripheral, or systemic edema. The most common causes are coronary artery disease, systemic or pulmonary hypertension, cardiomyopathy, and valvular disorders. The incidence of chronic heart failure correlates with age. The 2 main types of HF are systolic and diastolic. HF is classified according to symptoms and prognosis:

- **Class I**: The patient is essentially asymptomatic during normal activities with no pulmonary congestion or peripheral hypotension. There is no restriction on activities, and prognosis is good.
- **Class II**: Symptoms appear with physical exertion but are usually absent at rest, resulting in some limitations of activities of daily living (ADLs). Slight pulmonary edema may be evident by basilar rales. Prognosis is good.
- **Class III**: Obvious limitations of ADLs and discomfort on any exertion. Prognosis is fair.
- **Class IV**: Symptoms at rest. Prognosis is poor.

**Treatment** may include:

- Careful monitoring of **fluid balance** and **weight** to determine changes in fluid retention
- **Low sodium diet**
- **Restriction of activity**
- **Medications** may include diuretics, vasodilators, or ACE inhibitors to decrease the heart's workload, digoxin may be given to increase contractibility
- **Anticoagulant therapy** if distended atria, enlarged ventricles, or atrial fibrillation to decrease the danger of thromboembolic

**Review Video: Congestive Heart Failure**
Visit mometrix.com/academy and enter code: 924118

### *Systolic Heart Failure*

Systolic heart failure is the typical "left-sided" failure and reduces the amount of blood ejected from the ventricles during contraction (decreased ejection fraction). This stimulates the SNS to produce catecholamines to support the myocardium, which eventually causes down regulation, the destruction of beta and adrenergic receptor sites, and ultimately further myocardial damage. Because of reduced perfusion, the R-A-A pathway (renin, angiotensin I&II, aldosterone) is initiated by the kidneys, causing sodium and fluid retention. The end result of these processes is increased preload and afterload, thus increased workload on the ventricles. They begin to lose contractibility and blood begins to pool inside, stretching the myocardium (ventricular remodeling). The heart compensates by thickening the muscle (hypertrophy) without an adequate increase in capillary blood supply, leading to ischemia.

**Symptoms**: Activity intolerance, dyspnea/orthopnea (sleeping in a recliner is a classic symptom), cough (frothy sputum), edema, heart sounds S3 and S4, hepatomegaly, JVD, LOC changes, and tachycardia.

**Treatment** includes:

- Medication (most commonly β-blockers, diuretics, ACE inhibitors, or digoxin)
- **Surgery**: Heart transplant (if a candidate)
- **Lifestyle modification**: Low-sodium diet, supplemental oxygen, daily weights (report >3 lb/day or 5 lb/week weight gain to physician)

### Diastolic Heart Failure

Diastolic heart failure may be difficult to differentiate from systolic heart failure based on clinical symptoms, which are similar. With diastolic heart failure, the myocardium is unable to sufficiently relax to facilitate filling of the ventricles. This may be the end result of systolic heart failure as myocardial hypertrophy stiffens the muscles, and the causes are similar. Diastolic heart failure is more common in females >75. Typically, intracardiac pressures at rest are within normal range but increase markedly on exertion. Because the relaxation of the heart is delayed, the ventricles do not expand enough for the fill-volume, and the heart cannot increase stroke volume during exercise, so symptoms (dyspnea, fatigue, pulmonary edema) are often pronounced on exertion. Ejection fractions are usually >40–50% with increase in left ventricular end-diastolic pressure (LVEDP) and decrease in left ventricular end-diastolic volume (LVEDV).

The major goal with all types of heart failure is to prevent further damage and remodeling, prevent exacerbations, and improve the patient's long-term prognosis.

### Acute Heart Failure

Acute decompensated heart failure occurs when the body cannot compensate for the heart's inability to provide adequate perfusion. Cardiac output is no longer sufficient to meet the metabolic demands of the body. Acute heart failure occurs suddenly and can be precipitated by dysrhythmias, illness, noncompliance with medications, acute ischemia, fluid overload or hypertensive crisis. Acute heart failure is most commonly related to left ventricular systolic or diastolic dysfunction. It requires immediate treatment to restore adequate perfusion and is often life-threatening.

**Signs/symptoms**: Dyspnea, cough, edema, ascites and elevated jugular venous pressure, fatigue, cool extremities, hypotension and altered mental status

**Diagnostic testing**: Chest x-ray, electrocardiogram, physical exam; labs—basic metabolic panel, BUN, creatinine, and B-natriuretic peptide (BNP)

**Treatment**: Rapid assessment and stabilization of the patient. The physical assessment should include a thorough evaluation of the patient's respiratory status and supplemental oxygen and potentially ventilator support may be necessary. Medications: Diuretics to decrease fluid volume; vasodilators to decrease pulmonary congestion. Cardiac monitoring, urine output monitoring, sodium restriction, and venous thromboembolism prophylaxis may also be utilized.

### Acute Cardiac-Related Pulmonary Edema

Acute cardiac-related pulmonary edema occurs when heart failure results in fluid overload, leading to third-spacing of fluid into the interstitial spaces of the lungs. Pulmonary edema may result from MI, chronic HF, volume overload, ischemia, or mitral stenosis.

**Symptoms** include severe dyspnea, cough with blood-tinged frothy sputum, wheezing/rales/crackles on auscultation, cyanosis, and diaphoresis.

**Diagnosis**: Auscultation, chest x-ray, and echocardiogram.

**Treatment** includes:

- Sitting position with 100% oxygen by mask to achieve $PO_2$ >60%
- Non-invasive pressure support ventilation (BiPAP) or endotracheal intubation and mechanical ventilation
- Morphine sulfate 2–8 mg (IV for severe cases), repeated every 2–4 hours as needed—decreases pre-load and anxiety
- IV diuretics (furosemide ≥40 mg or bumetanide ≥1 mg) to provide venous dilation and diuresis
- Nitrates as a bolus with an infusion—decreases pre-load
- Inhaled β-adrenergic agonists or aminophylline for bronchospasm
- Digoxin IV for tachycardia
- ACE inhibitors, nitroprusside to reduce afterload

## Endocarditis

Endocarditis is an infection of the lining of the heart that covers the heart valves and contains Purkinje fibers, known as the endocardium. Risk factors include being over 60 years of age, being male, IV drug use, and dental infections. *Staphylococcal aureus* is the most common cause of infective endocarditis. Etiology includes subacute bacterial endocarditis (often related to dental procedures), prosthetic valvular endocarditis (following valve replacement), and right sided endocarditis (often related to catheter infections and IV drug use). Organisms enter the bloodstream from portals of entry (surgery, catheterization, IV drug abuse) and migrate to the heart, growing on the endothelial tissue and forming vegetations (verrucae), collagen deposits, and platelet thrombi. With endocarditis, the valves frequently become deformed, but the pathogenic agents may also invade other tissues, such as the chordae tendineae. The lesions may invade adjacent tissue and break off, becoming emboli. The mitral valve is the most common valve affected, followed by aortic, tricuspid, and the pulmonary valve being the least often affected. Positive blood cultures, widened pulse pressures, ECG, murmurs, and vegetations seen on a transesophageal echocardiogram are used to make the diagnosis. After diagnosis is made, antibiotics are used for treatment, and when unsuccessful or when heart failure is present, valve repair may be warranted. Serious complications from endocarditis include emboli, sepsis, and heart failure. Untreated endocarditis is fatal.

### *Diagnosis and Treatment*

Diagnosis of endocarditis is made on the basis of clinical presentation and **diagnostic procedures** that may include:

- **Blood cultures** should be done with 3 sets for both aerobic and anaerobic bacteria. Diagnosis is definitive if 2 cultures are positive, but a negative culture does not preclude bacterial endocarditis.
- **Echocardiogram** may identify vegetation on valves or increasing heart failure
- **ECG** may demonstrate prolonged PR interval
- **Anemia** (normochromic, normocytic)
- Elevated **white blood cell count**
- Elevated **erythrocyte sedimentation rate** (ESR) and **C-reactive protein** (CRP)

**Treatment** includes general management of symptoms and the following:

- **Antimicrobials** specific to the pathogenic organism, usually administered IV for 4–6 weeks
- **Surgical replacement** of aortic and/or mitral valves may be necessary (in 30–40% of cases) if there is no response to treatment and/or after infection is controlled if there are severe symptoms related to valve damage

### *Clinical Symptoms*

Clinical symptoms of endocarditis usually relate to the response to infection, the underlying heart disease, emboli, or immunological response. Typical **symptoms** include:

- Slow onset with unexplained low-grade and often intermittent **fever**
- **Anorexia** and weight loss, difficulty feeding
- General **lassitude** and malaise
- **Splenomegaly** present in 60% of patients; **hepatomegaly** may also be present
- **Anemia** is present in almost all patients
- Sudden **aortic valve insufficiency** or mitral valve insufficiency
- **Cyanosis** with clubbing of fingers
- **Embolism** of other body organs (brain, liver, bones)
- **Congestive heart failure**
- **Dysrhythmias**
- New or change in **heart murmur**
- **Immunological responses**
- **Janeway lesions**: painless areas of hemorrhage on palms of hands and soles of feet
- **Splinter hemorrhages**: thin, brown-black lines on nails of fingers and toes
- **Petechiae**: pinpoint-sized hemorrhages on oral mucous membranes, as well as hands and trunk
- **Roth spots**: retinal hemorrhagic lesions caused by emboli on nerve fibers
- **Glomerulonephritis**: microscopic hematuria



## Myocarditis

Myocarditis is inflammation of the cardiac myocardium (muscle tissue), usually triggered by a viral infection, such as the influenza virus, Coxsackie virus, and HIV. Myocarditis can also be caused by bacteria, fungi, or parasites, or an allergic response to medications. In some cases, it is also a complication of endocarditis. It may also be triggered by chemotherapy drugs and some antibiotics. Myocarditis can result in dilation of the heart, development of thrombi on the heart walls (known as mural thrombi), and infiltration of blood cells around the coronary vessels and between muscle fibers, causing further degeneration of the muscle tissue. The heart may become enlarged and weak, as the ability to pump blood is impaired, leading to congestive heart failure. Symptoms depend upon the extent of damage but may include fatigue, dyspnea, pressure and discomfort in chest or epigastric area, and palpitations.

### *Diagnosis and Treatment*

Diagnosis of myocarditis depends upon the clinical picture, as there is no test specific for myocarditis, although a number of tests may be done to verify the **clinical diagnosis**:

- **Chest radiograph** may indicate cardiomegaly or pulmonary edema.
- **ECG** may show nonspecific changes.
- **Echocardiogram** may indicate cardiomegaly and demonstrate defects in functioning.
- **Cardiac catheterization** and **cardiac biopsy** will yield confirmation in 65% of cases, but not all of the heart muscle may be affected, so a negative finding does not rule out myocarditis.
- **Viral cultures** of nasopharynx and rectal may help to identify organism.
- **Viral titers** may increase as disease progresses.
- **Polymerase chain reaction** (PCR) of biopsy specimen may be most effective for diagnosis.

**Treatment**:

- As indicated for underlying cause (such as antibiotics)
- Restriction of activities
- Careful **monitoring** for heart failure and medical treatment as indicated (e.g., diuretics, digoxin)
- **Oxygen** as needed to maintain normal oxygen saturation
- **IV gamma globulin** for acute stage

## Acute Pericarditis

Pericarditis is inflammation of the pericardial sac with or without increased pericardial fluid. It may be an isolated process or the effect of an underlying disease. If the underlying cause is autoimmune or related to malignancy of some sort, the patient usually presents with symptoms that relate to that disorder. However, most cases are related to a viral etiology, and therefore usually present with flu-like symptoms. Patients that have idiopathic pericarditis or viral pericarditis have a good prognosis with medication alone.

**Signs/symptoms**: Sharp chest pain, worsened with inspiration and relieved by leaning forward or sitting up, pericardial effusion, respiratory distress, auscultated friction rub, ST elevation/PR depression (progresses to flattened T, inverted T, then return to normal); risk of pericardial effusion.

**Diagnosis**: Echocardiogram, ECG, pericardiocentesis or pericardial biopsy, cardiac enzymes (may be mildly elevated), WBC/ESR/CRP all elevated.

**Treatment** includes:

- **Medications**: NSAIDs for pain/inflammation, Colchicine 0.5 mg twice a day for six months is often prescribed in adjunct to NSAID therapy, as it decreases the incidence of recurrence
- **Surgery**: Pericardiectomy only in extreme cases

## Mitral Stenosis

Mitral stenosis is a narrowing of the mitral valve that allows blood to flow from the left atrium to the left ventricle. Pressure in the left atrium increases to overcome resistance, resulting in enlargement of the left atrium and increased pressure in the pulmonary veins and capillaries of the lung (pulmonary hypertension). Mitral stenosis can be caused by infective endocarditis, calcifications, or tumors in the left atrium.

**Signs/symptoms**: Exertional dyspnea, orthopnea/nocturnal dyspnea, right-sided heart failure, loud $S_1$ and $S_2$, and mid-diastolic murmur.

**Diagnosis**: Cardiac catheterization, chest x-ray, echocardiogram, ECG.

**Treatment** includes:

- **Medications**: Antiarrhythmic, anticoagulant, and antihypertensive medications
- **Surgical**: Open/closed commissurotomy, balloon valvuloplasty, and mitral valve replacement

## Mitral Valve Insufficiency

Mitral valve insufficiency occurs when the mitral valve fails to close completely so that there is backflow into the left atrium from the left ventricle during systole, decreasing cardiac output. It may occur with mitral stenosis or independently. Mitral valve insufficiency can result from damage caused by rheumatic fever, myxomatous degeneration, infective endocarditis, collagen vascular disease (Marfan's syndrome), or cardiomyopathy/left heart failure. There are **three phases** of the disease:

- **Acute**: May occur with rupture of a chordae tendineae or papillary muscle causing sudden left ventricular flooding and overload.
- **Chronic compensated**: Enlargement of the left atrium to decrease filling pressure, and hypertrophy of the left ventricle.
- **Chronic decompensated**: Left ventricle fails to compensate for the volume overload; decreased stroke volume and increased cardiac output.

**Symptoms**: Orthopnea/dyspnea, split $S_2/S_3/S_4$ heart sounds, systolic murmur, palpitations, right-sided heart failure, fatigue, angina (rare).

**Diagnosis**: Cardiac catheterization, chest x-ray, echocardiogram, ECG.

**Treatment** includes:

- **Medications**: Antiarrhythmic, anticoagulant, and antihypertensive medications.
- **Surgical**: Annuloplasty or valvuloplasty, and mitral valve replacement.

## Aortic Stenosis

Aortic stenosis is a stricture (narrowing) of the aortic valve that controls the flow of blood from the left ventricle. This causes the left ventricular wall to thicken as it increases pressure to overcome the valvular resistance, increasing afterload and increasing the need for blood supply from the coronary arteries. This condition may result from a birth defect or childhood rheumatic fever, and tends to worsen over the years as the heart grows.

**Symptoms**: Angina, exercise intolerance, dyspnea, split $S_1$ and $S_2$, systolic murmur at base of carotids, hypotension on exertion, syncope, left-sided heart failure; sudden death can occur.

**Diagnosis**: Cardiac catheterization, chest x-ray, echocardiogram, ECG.

**Treatment** includes:

- **Medications**: Antiarrhythmic, anticoagulant, and antihypertensive medications
- **Surgical**: Balloon valvuloplasty, and aortic valve replacement

## Pulmonic Stenosis

Pulmonic stenosis is a stricture of the pulmonary blood that controls the flow of blood from the right ventricle to the lungs, resulting in right ventricular hypertrophy as the pressure increases in the right ventricle and decreased pulmonary blood flow. The condition may be asymptomatic or symptoms may not be evident until adulthood, depending upon the severity of the defect. Pulmonic stenosis may be associated with a number of other heart defects.

**Symptoms**: May be asymptomatic; dyspnea on exertion, systolic heart murmur, right-sided heart failure.

**Diagnosis**: Cardiac catheterization, chest x-ray, echocardiogram, ECG.

**Treatment** includes:

- **Medications**: Antiarrhythmic, anticoagulant, and antihypertensive medications
- **Surgical**: Balloon valvuloplasty, valvotomy, valvectomy with or without transannular patch, and pulmonary valve replacement

## Blunt Cardiac Trauma and Traumatic Injury to the Great Vessels

Blunt cardiac trauma most often occurs as the result of motor vehicle accidents, falls, or other blows to the chest. This can result in respiratory distress, rupture of the great vessels, and cardiac tamponade/increasing intrathoracic pressure. The right atrium and right ventricle are the most commonly injured because they are anterior to the rest of the heart. While not definitive, echocardiogram in conjunction with CPK MB levels is useful in predicting complications. Because diagnosis is challenging until complications appear, every patient with suspected blunt chest trauma should receive an ECG upon admission/STAT. If abnormalities are present, continuous cardiac monitoring should be done for 24–48 hours. Decreased cerebral perfusion/anoxia may result in severe agitation with combative behavior.

Traumatic injuries to the great vessels most commonly result from severe decelerating blunt force or penetrating injuries, with aortic trauma the most common. If the aorta is torn, it will result in almost instant death, but in some cases, there is an incomplete laceration to the intimal lining (innermost membrane) of the aorta, causing an aortic hematoma or bulging. This lining, the adventitia, is quite strong and often will contain the rupture long enough to allow surgical repair.

**Diagnosis**: Chest x-ray or CT; transesophageal echocardiogram to verify

**Treatment**: STAT surgical repair to avoid eventual rupture, during which other vessels are examined for clotting or internal injuries

## Penetrating Cardiac Injuries

The incidence of penetrating cardiac injuries has been on the rise, primarily associated with gunshot injuries and stabbings. The extent of damage caused by a stab wound is often easier to assess than gunshot wounds, which may be multiple and often result in unpredictable and widespread damage not only to the heart but other structures. Mortality rates are very high in the first hour after a penetrating cardiac injury, so it is imperative that the patient be taken immediately to a trauma center rather than attempts be made to stabilize the person at the site. NEVER attempt to remove the object in the field/without a physician present.

The primary **complications**:

- **Exsanguination** is frequently related to gunshot wounds, and prognosis is very poor. This may lead to hemothorax and hemorrhagic shock.
- **Cardiac tamponade** is more common with knife wounds, but prognosis is fairly good with surgical repair. Cardiac tamponade often presents with three classic symptoms, known as Beck's triad that should be quickly recognized: muffled heart sounds, low arterial blood pressure, and jugular vein distention.
- **Pneumothorax**: Deviated trachea, increasing SVR, tachypnea and anxiety all may indicate tension pneumothorax, which is a medical emergency. It is treated by emergent insertion of a chest tube or needle aspiration of trapped air. Open wounds can be emergently dressed with a three-sided dressing until a chest tube can be inserted to create a "flutter valve" effect and allow trapped air to escape.

**Nursing considerations**: Management includes controlling bleeding, giving fluids and vasopressors for blood pressure, preparing patient for surgery, and monitoring for the above-mentioned complications.

## Carotid Artery Stenosis

The common carotid artery branches from the subclavian artery and then bifurcates into the external carotid and internal carotid arteries. This point of bifurcation is a common site for the development of plaques, causing **carotid artery stenosis** that interferes with cranial blood flow. When stenosis develops slowly, collateral vessels may form to aid circulation, but sudden occlusion can cause permanent brain damage and death. Most stenosis is caused by atherosclerosis, with increasing incidence with age. Most ischemia relates to an embolism or thrombus formation.

**Symptoms** of occlusion are often asymptomatic; however, they include severe pain, anxiety, and those symptoms common to brain attacks (hemiparesis, confusion, aphasia, and diplopia).

**Diagnosis**: Duplex ultrasound (combining conventional ultrasound with Doppler, determines blood flow and obstruction), CT scan, MRA or angiogram (will indicate degree of blockage).

**Treatment** may include:

- Medications: Anticoagulants and thrombolytics.
- Carotid endarterectomy (recommended if stenosis >60%): poses the danger of a post-procedure stroke due to plaque dislodgement or increased blood flow to narrowed vessels, so the benefits must be carefully weighed.
- Carotid stents/angioplasty (newer non-invasive approaches).

## Cardiac Tamponade

Cardiac tamponade occurs with pericardial effusion, causing pressure against the heart. It may be a complication of trauma, pericarditis, cardiac surgery, pneumothorax, or heart failure. About 50 mL of fluid normally circulates in the pericardial area to reduce friction, and a sudden increase in this volume or air in the pericardial sac can compress the heart, causing a number of cardiac responses such as:

- Increased end-diastolic pressure in both ventricles
- Decrease in venous return
- Decrease in ventricular filling

Symptoms may include pressure or pain in the chest, dyspnea, and pulsus paradoxus >10 mmHg. Beck's triad (increased CVP, distended neck veins, muffled heart sounds, and hypotension) is common. A sudden decrease in chest tube drainage can occur as fluid and clots accumulate in the pericardial sac, preventing the blood from filling the ventricles and decreasing cardiac output and perfusion of the body, including the kidneys (resulting in decreased urinary output). X-ray may show change in cardiac silhouette and mediastinal shift (in 20%). Treatment includes pericardiocentesis with large bore needle or surgical repair to control bleeding and relieve cardiac compression. Risk factors include cardiac surgery, cardiac tumors, MI, and chest trauma.

**Review Video: Cardiac Tamponade**
Visit mometrix.com/academy and enter code: 920182

## Hypertensive Crises

Hypertensive crises are marked elevations in blood pressure that can cause severe organ damage if left untreated. Hypertensive crises may be caused by endocrine/renal disorders (pheochromocytoma), dissection of an aortic aneurysm, pulmonary edema, subarachnoid hemorrhage, stroke, eclampsia, and medication noncompliance. There are two **classifications**:

- **Hypertensive emergency** occurs when acute hypertension, usually >220 systolic and 120 mmHg diastolic, must be treated immediately to lower blood pressure in order to prevent damage to vital organs.
- **Hypertensive urgency** occurs when acute hypertension must be treated within a few hours but the vital organs are not in immediate danger. Blood pressure is lowered more slowly to avoid hypotension, ischemia of vital organs, or failure of autoregulation. To avoid these complications, guidelines recommend not lowering the blood pressure by more than 30% in the first few hours.

**Symptoms**: Basilar HA, blurred vision, chest pain, N/V, SOB, seizures, ruddy pallor, and anxiety

**Diagnostics**: ECG, Chest x-ray, CBC, BMP, Urinalysis (+ blood and casts)

**Treatment** includes:

- Medications: Vasodilators (Cardene, Nitro, etc.) and diuretics
- Nursing Interventions: Raise HOB to 90°, supplemental $O_2$, frequent neuro checks, teach concerning medication compliance

## Congenital Heart Defects Seen in Adulthood

Congenital heart defects are often identified in infancy or early childhood; however, diagnosis may be delayed until adulthood due to the lack of signs and symptoms. Atrial septal and ventricular septal defects are common congenital anomalies that can present at any age. An atrial septal defect occurs when part of the atrial septum does not form properly, leaving a hole in the septum. A ventricular septal defect results from a hole in the septum separating the ventricles. Patent ductus arteriosus, coarctation of the aorta and Ebstein's anomaly are other types of congenital defects that are less commonly diagnosed in adulthood.

**Signs/symptoms**: Murmurs, cyanosis, clubbing of the fingernails, shortness of breath, fatigue, syncope, palpitations, and edema. Heart failure and endocarditis may also occur.

**Diagnosis**: Physical assessment, EKG, Chest x-ray, transesophageal echocardiogram, CT, and MRI.

**Treatment**: Treatment options depend on the size and location of the defect. Most commonly the anomaly will be corrected by open surgical repair; however percutaneous intervention may be an option in some patients.

## Peripheral Arterial and Venous Insufficiency

Characteristics of peripheral arterial and venous insufficiency are listed below:

- **Arterial insufficiency**
  - **Pain**: Ranging from intermittent claudication to severe and constant shooting pain
  - **Pulses**: Weak or absent
  - **Skin**: Rubor on dependency, but pallor of foot on elevation; pale, shiny, and cool skin with loss of hair on toes and foot; nails thick and ridged
  - **Ulcers**: Painful, deep, circular, often necrotic ulcers on toe tips, toe webs, heels, or other pressure areas
  - **Edema**: Minimal

- **Venous insufficiency**
  - **Pain**: Aching/cramping
  - **Pulses**: Strong/present
  - **Skin**: Brownish discoloration around ankles and anterior tibial area
  - **Ulcers**: Varying degrees of pain in superficial, irregular ulcers on medial or lateral malleolus and sometimes the anterior tibial area
  - **Edema**: Moderate to severe

## Acute Peripheral Vascular Insufficiency

Acute peripheral arterial insufficiency can occur when sudden occlusion of a blood vessel causes tissue ischemia, ultimately leading to cellular death and necrosis. This can occur as a result of traumatic injury or non-traumatic events such as arterial thrombus or embolism, vasospasm, or severe swelling (compartment syndrome). Risk factors for acute peripheral arterial insufficiency include age, tobacco use, diabetes mellitus, hyperlipidemia, and hypertension.

- **Signs/symptoms**: Classic 6 P's: Pain (extreme, unrelieved by narcotics), pallor, pulselessness, poikilothermia (the inability to regulate body temperature; extremity is room temperature), paresthesias, and paralysis (late).
- **Diagnosis**: Ultrasound, angiography, and physical exam; labs—coagulation studies, CBC, BMP, creatinine phosphokinase
- **Treatment**: Re-establishment of blood flow to the affected area
- **Arterial thrombus or embolism**: Mechanical thrombolysis may be performed to remove the clot occluding the vessel.
  - **Trauma**: Surgical repair of the severed/injured vessels. Fasciotomy may be performed in the event of compartment syndrome to relieve pressure.
  - **Other treatment options**: Hyperbaric oxygen therapy, anti-platelet therapy for the prevention of arterial thrombosis and anti-coagulant therapy for the prevention of venous thrombosis



## Acute Venous Thromboembolism

Acute venous thromboembolism (VTE) is a condition that includes both deep vein thrombosis (DVT) and pulmonary emboli (PE). VTE may be precipitated by invasive procedures, lack of mobility, and inflammation, so it is a common complication in critical care units. **Virchow's triad** comprises common risk factors: blood stasis, injury to endothelium, and hypercoagulability. Some patients may be initially asymptomatic, but **symptoms** may include:

- Aching or throbbing pain
- Positive Homan's sign (pain in calf when foot is dorsiflexed)
- Unilateral erythema and edema
- Dilation of vessels
- Cyanosis

**Diagnosis**: ultrasound and/or D-dimer test, which tests the serum for cross-linked fibrin derivatives. A CT scan, pulmonary angiogram, and ventilation-perfusion lung scan may be used to diagnose pulmonary emboli.

**Treatment** includes:

- Medications: IV heparin, tPA, or other anticoagulation; analgesia for pain
- Surgical: May have to surgically remove clot if large
- Bed rest, elevation of affected limb; stockings on ambulation

**Prevention**: Use of sequential compression devices (SCDs) or foot pumps, routine anticoagulant use for those at highest risk (Heparin SQ), early and frequent ambulation

Review Video: DVT Prevention and Treatment
Visit mometrix.com/academy and enter code: 234086

# Cardiovascular Procedures and Interventions

## Cardioversion

Cardioversion sends a timed electrical stimulation to the heart to convert a tachydysrhythmia (such as atrial fibrillation) to a normal sinus rhythm. Usually, anticoagulation therapy is done for at least 3 weeks prior to elective cardioversion to reduce the risk of emboli, and digoxin is discontinued for at least 48 hours prior. During the procedure, the patient is usually sedated and/or anesthetized. Electrodes in the form of gel-covered paddles or pads are placed in the anteroposterior position and then connected by leads to a computerized ECG and cardiac monitor with a defibrillator. The defibrillator is synchronized with the ECG so that the electrical current is delivered during ventricular depolarization (QRS). The timing must be precise in order to prevent ventricular tachycardia or ventricular fibrillation. Sometimes, drug therapy is used in conjunction with cardioversion; for example, antiarrhythmics (Cardizem, Cordarone) may be given before the procedure to slow the heart rate.

| Arrhythmia | Beginning Monophasic Shock | Beginning Biphasic Shock |
|---|---|---|
| Atrial Fibrillation | 100 J | 70 J |
| Atrial Flutter | 50–100 J | 50 J |
| Ventricular Tachycardia | 100 J | 75 J |

## Emergency Defibrillation

Emergency defibrillation delivers a non-synchronized shock that is given to treat acute ventricular fibrillation, pulseless ventricular tachycardia, or polymorphic ventricular tachycardia with a rapid rate and decompensating hemodynamics. **Defibrillation** can be given at any point in the cardiac cycle. It causes depolarization of myocardial cells, which can then repolarize to regain a normal sinus rhythm. Defibrillation delivers an electrical discharge through pads/paddles. In an acute care setting, the preferred position to place the pads is the anteroposterior position. In this position, one pad is placed to the right of the sternum about the second to third intercostal space, and the other pad is placed between the left scapula and the spinal column. This decreases the chances of damaging implanted devices, such as pacemakers, and this positioning has also been shown to be more effective for external cardioversion (if indicated at some point during resuscitation). There are two main types of defibrillator shock waveforms: monophasic and biphasic. Biphasic defibrillators deliver a shock in one direction for half of the shock, and then in the return direction for the other half, making them more effective and able to be used at lower energy levels. Monophasic defibrillation is given at 200–360 J and biphasic defibrillation is given at 100–200 J.

## Pericardiocentesis

Pericardiocentesis is done with ultrasound guidance to diagnose pericardial effusion or with ECG and ultrasound guidance to relieve cardiac tamponade. **Pericardiocentesis** may be done as treatment for cardiac arrest or with presentation of PEA with increased jugular venous pressure. Non-hemorrhagic tamponade may be relieved in 60–90% of cases, but hemorrhagic tamponade requires thoracotomy, as blood will continue to accumulate until the cause of the hemorrhage is corrected. Resuscitation equipment must be available, including a defibrillator, intravenous line in place, and cardiac monitoring.

The **procedure** is as follows:

- Elevate the chest 45° to bring the heart closer to the chest wall, pre-medicate with atropine, and insert a nasogastric tube if indicated.
- Cleanse the skin with chlorhexidine or another appropriate cleanser.

- After insertion of the needle using ultrasound guidance, remove the obturator and attach a syringe for aspiration.
- The needle can often be replaced with a catheter after removal for drainage.
- A post-procedure chest x-ray should be done to check for pneumothorax.

**Possible complications:** Pneumo/hemothorax, coronary artery rupture, hepatic injury, dysrhythmias, and false negative/positive aspiration.

## PACEMAKERS

Pacemakers are used to stimulate the heart when the normal conduction system of the heart is defective. **Pacemakers** may be used temporarily or be permanently implanted. Temporary pacemakers for external cardiac pacing are commonly used in the emergency setting. Temporary pacemakers may be used prophylactically or therapeutically to treat a cardiac abnormality. Clinical uses include:

- To treat persistent **dysrhythmias** not responsive to medications
- To increase **cardiac output** with bradydysrhythmia by increasing rate
- To decrease **ventricular or supraventricular tachycardia** by "overdrive" stimulation of contractions
- To treat **secondary heart block** caused by myocardial infarction, ischemia, and drug toxicity
- To improve **cardiac output** after cardiac surgery
- To provide **diagnostic information** through electrophysiology studies, which induce dysrhythmias for purposes of evaluation
- To provide **pacing** when a permanent pacemaker malfunctions

**Review Video: Pacemaker Care**
Visit mometrix.com/academy and enter code: 979075



### *TRANSCUTANEOUS PACING*

Transcutaneous pacing is used temporarily in an emergency situation to treat symptomatic bradydysrhythmias that don't respond to medications (atropine) and result in hemodynamic instability. Generally, the patient is provided oxygen and some sort of mild sedation before the pacing. The placement of pacing pads is usually one pacing pad (negative) on the left chest, inferior to the clavicle, and the other (positive) on the left back, inferior to the scapula, so the heart is sandwiched between the two. Lead wires attach the pads to the monitor. The rate of pacing is usually set around 80 bpm. The current is increased slowly until capture occurs—a spiking followed by QRS sequence—then the current is readjusted downward if possible just to maintain capture, keeping it 5–10 mA above the pacing threshold. Both demand and fixed modes are available, but demand mode is preferred. The patient should be warned that the shocks may induce pain.

### *EPICARDIAL PACING*

Epicardial pacing wires may be attached directly to the exterior atria, ventricles, or both at the conclusion of surgery for CPB or valve repair in the event that postoperative pacing support is required or for those with risk of AV block because of medications used to control atrial fibrillation. Cold cardioplegia may precipitate the transient sinus node or AV node dysfunction. While some surgeons avoid placing epicardial pacing wires because of concerns about bleeding and cardiac tamponade on removal, recommendations include placing at least one ventricular pacing wire. A typical configuration for pacing wires is atrial pacing wires placed in a plastic disk that is sutured low on the right atrium. The two ventricular wires are attached over the right ventricular wall. Atrial pacing wires may be used to record atrial activity and, and with standard ECG, can help to distinguish atrial and junctional arrhythmias and ventricular arrhythmias. Pacing wires can also be used therapeutically to increase the heart rate to about 90 bpm in order to achieve optimal hemodynamics. The epicardial leads are intended for use of 7 days or less and may be less reliable if used for extended periods. The wires are removed by applying gentle traction.

## *Temporary Transvenous Pacemakers*

Transvenous pacemakers, comprised of a catheter with a lead at the end, may be used prophylactically or therapeutically on a temporary basis to treat symptomatic bradycardias or heart blocks when other methods have failed. The catheter has a balloon tip that must be checked for leaks prior to insertion—this is usually done by inflating the catheter tip while submersed in normal saline and checking for bubbles. After the balloon's integrity is verified, the catheter is inserted through the femoral or jugular vein and the balloon is inflated. The catheter is then attached to an external pulse generator, and the settings are adjusted to achieve capture. The balloon is then deflated, and placement can be verified via ultrasound or chest x-ray.

Complications are similar to those of PCI and permanent pacemaker insertion, including infection, hemorrhage, catheter migration, perforation, embolism, thrombosis, and pacemaker syndrome.

### Transvenous Pacer Settings

Temporary transvenous pacing utilizes bipolar leads with two tails, positive/proximal and negative/distal, and these must be connected properly to the pulse generator, with the distal end of the pacing lead to the negative terminal and the proximal end to the positive terminal. Once the transvenous pacing wire is inserted and the leads are connected to the pulse generator, it must be set to the patient's needs:

- **Rate**: The beats per minute are usually set between 70 and 80 (allowable range is generally 50–90), but this may vary according to individual needs.
- **Sensitivity**: The myocardial voltage needed for the pacing electrode to detect P or R waves. The sensitivity is usually set at 2 mV and then adjusted as needed to ensure capture. Most pacemakers can sense 0.3–10.0 mV from the atria and 0.8–29.0 mV from the ventricles, but setting it relatively low prevents oversensing.
- **Output**: The current or pulse produced by the pulse generator is usually set at 5 mA. The current is delivered rapidly, in about 0.6 ms.

### Problems Related to Transvenous Pacing

With transvenous pacing (usually per a pulse generator connected to a pacing cable and a pacing wire, which is inserted into the right internal jugular to the right ventricle for ventricular pacing and right atrium for atrial pacing), sensing refers to the ability to detect electrical activity of the heart. Capture occurs when an artificial stimulus (the pulse generator) depolarizes the heart, indicated by a pacer spike followed by the QRS complex. **Problems** include:

| | |
|---|---|
| 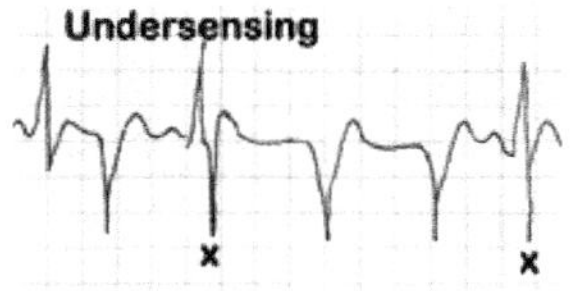 | **Undersensing**:<br>The sensitivity is too low to detect cardiac depolarizations, and triggers unneeded contractions, competing with the patient's native rhythm. This may be related to the dislodging of the lead, incorrect positioning of the lead, or a low-amplitude cardiac signal. |
| 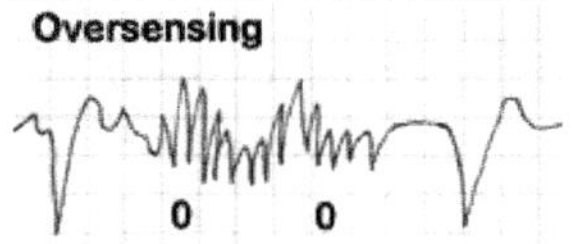 | **Oversensing**:<br>The sensitivity is too high and misinterprets artifacts (such as muscle contractions) and non-depolarization events as contractions and fails to trigger, resulting in decreased cardiac output because of the interruption in contractions. This may result from damage or disconnection of the lead. |
| 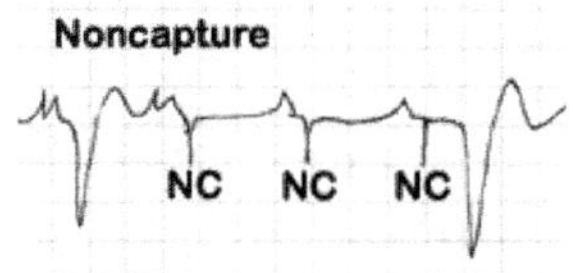 | **Noncapture**:<br>The pacemaker does not trigger contractions. This may be related to settings, lead disconnection, low battery, or metabolic changes. |

### PACEMAKER COMPLICATIONS

Pacemakers, transvenous and permanent, are invasive foreign bodies and, as such, can cause a number of different **complications**:

- Infection, bleeding, or hematoma may occur at the entry site of leads for temporary pacemakers or at the subcutaneous area of implantation for permanent generators.
- Puncture of the subclavian vein or internal mammary artery may cause a hemothorax.
- The endocardial electrode may irritate the ventricular wall, causing ectopic beats or tachycardia.
- Dislodgement of the transvenous lead may lead to malfunction or perforation of the myocardium. This is one of the most common early complications.
- Dislocation of leads may result in phrenic nerve or muscle stimulation (which may be evidenced by hiccupping).
- Cardiac tamponade may result when the epicardial wires of temporary pacing are removed.
- General malfunctioning of the pacemaker may indicate dislodgement, dislocation, interference caused by electromagnetic fields, and the need for new batteries or a new generator.
- Pacemaker syndrome

### PACEMAKER SYNDROME

Pacemaker syndrome can occur with any type of pacemaker if there is inadequate synchronicity between the contractions of the atria and ventricles, resulting in a decrease in cardiac output and inadequate atrial contribution to the filling of the ventricles. Total peripheral vascular resistance may increase to maintain blood pressure, but hypotension occurs after decompensation.

- **Mild**:
  - Pulsations evident in the neck and abdomen
  - Cardiac palpitations
  - Headache and feeling of anxiety
  - General malaise and unexplained weakness
  - Pain or feeling of fullness in jaw and/or chest
- **Moderate**:
  - Increasing dyspnea on exertion with accompanying orthopnea
  - Dizziness, vertigo, and increasing confusion
  - Feeling of choking
- **Severe**:
  - Increasing pulmonary edema with dyspnea even at rest
  - Crackling rales
  - Syncope
  - Heart failure

## AUTOMATIC ICD

The **automatic implantable cardioverter-defibrillator (AICD)** is similar to the pacemaker and is implanted in the same way, with one or more leads to the ventricular myocardium or the epicardium, but it is used to control tachycardia and/or fibrillation. Most AICDs consist of a pacing/sensing electrode, a pulse generator, and defibrillation electrodes. Severe tachycardia may be related to electrical disturbances, cardiomyopathy, or postoperative response to the repair of congenital disease. In some cases, it is not responsive to medications. When the pulse reaches a certain preset rate, then the device automatically provides a small electrical impulse to the atrial or ventricular myocardium to slow the heart. If fibrillation occurs, a higher energy shock is delivered. It takes 5–15 seconds for the device to detect abnormalities in the pulse rate, and more than one shock may be required so fainting can occur. Contemporary devices can function as both a pacemaker and an ICD, which is especially important for those who have episodes of both bradycardia and tachycardia. The use of adjunctive antiarrhythmics or ablation is important to prevent AICD shocks.

## CLOSURE DEVICES WITH PCI

**Percutaneous coronary intervention (PCI)** is often the treatment choice for patients with symptomatic coronary artery disease. Percutaneous transluminal coronary angioplasty (PTCA), arthrectomy, and stent insertion are common types of PCI procedures. While historically, manual compression has been utilized to achieve hemostasis after PCI, different types of devices exist to assist in achieving hemostasis post-procedure. Passive devices such as hemostasis pads and compression devices help to enhance hemostasis. Active devices are used at the femoral access site after the sheath used for the procedure is removed. There are different types of active devices, including percutaneous suture mediated devices, that use needles and sutures to suture the artery closed after the procedure. Collagen plugs are another type of closure, where collagen is injected into the supra-arterial space until hemostasis is achieved. These devices may be used independently or in combination. Clip devices such as implantable clips can be used to pull the edges of the arteriotomy together for closure. Active devices shorten the time to achieve hemostasis as well as the time the patient must remain hospitalized post-procedure.

**Complications**: Persistent coronary artery spasms, dissection of the coronary artery, thrombosis, bleeding, and hematoma formation. Other complications may arise depending on the type of closure device utilized. For example, the use of clip devices may result in arterial laceration, occlusion of the artery, or arterial stenosis.

## PTCA AND STENT INSERTION

**Percutaneous transluminal coronary angioplasty (PTCA)** is a procedure done to reperfuse coronary arteries blocked by plaque or an embolus. Cardiac catheterization is done with a hollow catheter (sheath), usually inserted into the femoral vein or artery and fed through the vessels to the coronary arteries. When the atheroma is verified by fluoroscopy, a balloon-tipped catheter is fed over the sheath and the balloon is inflated with a contrast agent to a specified pressure to compress the atheroma. The balloon may be inflated a number of times to ensure that residual stenosis is <20%. Laser angioplasty using the excimer laser is also used to vaporize plaque. **Stents** may be inserted during the angioplasty to maintain patency. Stents may be flexible plastic or wire mesh and are typically placed over the catheter, which is inflated to expand the stent against the arterial wall. All patients with a stent must be discharged on aspirin, an antiplatelet, and a statin.

**Complications** include:

- **Intraoperative**: Perforation/dissection of the coronary artery, arrythmias, and vasospasm
- **Postoperative**: Hemorrhage/hematoma at insertion site, thrombus/embolus, arteriovenous fistula/pseudoaneurysm, retroperitoneal bleed, and failure of angioplasty

### Carotid Endarterectomy

A carotid endarterectomy involves clamping the carotids, opening the occluded artery, and removing the plaque that is occluding the artery. A shunt may be inserted during the procedure to ensure blood supply to the brain. Postoperative **complications** may include:

- **Hematoma:** May obstruct respiration; watch closely for increased respiratory effort and swelling near the airway.
- **Hypertension:** Especially in the first 48 postoperative hours, may increase risk of neurologic impairment and hematoma.
- **Hypotension:** Usually resolves in 24–48 hours, but may indicate myocardial infarction.
- **Hyperperfusion syndrome:** Caused by inadequate vasoconstriction of vessels dilated from long-term diminished blood flow. It can cause hemorrhage and edema, usually identified by severe unilateral headache relieved by raising the head.
- **Hemorrhage:** May be fatal or cause severe impairment.
- **Stroke:** Risk of plaque dislodging and forming an embolus; frequent neurological checks are crucial.

## CABG

**Coronary artery bypass graft (CABG)** is a surgical procedure for the treatment of angina that does not respond to medical treatment, unstable angina, blockage of >60% in the left main coronary artery, blockage of multiple coronary arteries that include the proximal left anterior descending artery, left ventricular dysfunction, and previous unsuccessful PCIs. The surgery is performed through a midsternal incision that exposes the heart, which is chilled and placed on cardiopulmonary bypass with blood going from the right atrium to the machine and back to the body while the aorta is clamped to keep the surgical field free of blood. Bypass grafts are sutured into place to bypass areas of occluded coronary arteries. Grafts may be obtained from various sites: gastroepiploic artery, internal mammary artery, radial artery, or saphenous vein (commonly used, especially for emergency procedures).

**Complications:** Arrhythmias, infection, cardiac tamponade, cardiogenic shock, embolus/stroke, and renal or pulmonary dysfunction

### *MIDCAB and Port Access Coronary Artery Bypass Graft*

**Minimally-invasive direct coronary artery bypass (MIDCAB)** applies a bypass graft through a 10 cm incision in the mid-chest without using cardiopulmonary bypass. Because the incision must be over the bypass area, this procedure is suitable only for bypass of one or two coronary arteries, usually on the left side of the heart. A small portion of rib is removed to allow access to the heart, and the internal mammary artery is used for grafting. Special instruments, such as a heart stabilizer, are used to limit movement of the heart during suturing. Surgery usually takes 2–3 hours and recovery time is decreased as patients have less pain. Because anastomosis is difficult on a beating heart, complications such as ischemia may occur during surgery, so a cardiopulmonary bypass machine must be available.

**Port access coronary artery bypass graft** is an alternative form of CABG that utilizes a number of small incisions (ports) along with cardiopulmonary bypass (CPB) and cardioplegia to do a video-assisted surgical repair. Usually, 3 or more incisions are required, with one in the femoral area to allow access to the femoral artery for a multipurpose catheter that is threaded through to the ascending aorta to return blood from the CPB, block the aorta with a balloon, provide a cardioplegic solution, and vent air. Another catheter is threaded through the femoral vein to the right atrium to carry blood to the CPB. An incision is also needed for access to the jugular vein for catheters to the pulmonary artery and the coronary sinus. One to three thoracotomy incisions are made for the insertion of video imaging equipment and instruments. While the midsternal incision is avoided, multiple incisions pose the potential for possible increased morbidity.

## Cardiac Surgical Options for Repair of Cardiac Valves

There are a number of different surgical options for the repair of cardiac valves:

- **Valvotomy/Valvuloplasty** is usually done through cardiac catheterization. A valvotomy/valvuloplasty involves releasing valve leaflet adhesions or opening a stenosed valve. In balloon valvuloplasty, a catheter with an inflatable balloon is positioned in the stenotic valve and inflated and deflated a number of times to dilate the opening. Risks include stroke from a broken-off calcified valve and worsened valvular insufficiency/rupture.
- **Aortic valve replacement** is an open-heart procedure with cardiopulmonary bypass. Aortic valves are tricuspid (3 leaflets) and repair is usually not possible, so defective valves must be replaced with either mechanical (metal, plastic, or pyrolytic carbon) or biological (porcine or bovine) grafts.
- **Aortic homograft** uses part of a donor's aorta with the aortic valve attached to replace the recipient's faulty aortic valve and part of the ascending aorta.
- **Ross procedure** uses the patient's pulmonary artery with the pulmonary valve to replace the aortic valve and part of the aorta and then uses a donor graft to replace the pulmonary artery.

### *TAVR*

**Transcatheter aortic valve replacement (TAVR)** is usually reserved for patients with advanced symptomatic stenosis of the aortic valve who are unable to tolerate open-heart surgery or are at high risk with the procedure. Symptoms of aortic stenosis include chest pain, peripheral edema, dyspnea, fainting, weakness, and heart failure. With a TAVR, patients generally receive a general anesthesia, and a catheter is inserted, usually transfemoral (most common), transaortic, or transapical. Two types of replacement valves are available in the US: a balloon-expandable valve (Sapien XT) or a self-expanding valve (CoreValue). Once the catheter with a balloon device and the replacement valve attached is in place in the aortic valve, the balloon is inflated to secure the replacement valve, then the balloon is deflated and the catheter is removed. With the self-expanding valve, the valve is attached to the catheter and expanded when it is in place in the stenotic valve and the catheter is removed.

## Postoperative Care for Cardiac Surgery

The **recovery period** is discussed below:

- 2:1 nursing ratio; monitor hemodynamics closely (check vitals every 5–15 minutes).
- Warm patient according to policy; monitor ECG closely for arrhythmias during rewarming.
- Maintain MAP between 70–110 mmHg to prevent inadequate perfusion or graft rupture/hemorrhage; urine output should be >30 mL/hr.
- The patient will have multiple chest tubes; ensure output is not excessive (>200 mL/hr = hemorrhage) and does not suddenly stop/decrease.
- Auscultate heart sounds and evaluate extremities frequently to assess perfusion; hourly urine output should be 30 mL/hr OR 1 mL/kg/hr (gold standard).
- Monitor ABGS (every 2–4 hr during recovery) and adjust ventilator settings accordingly.
- Close blood sugar control (will probably be on insulin drip) and prophylactic cephalosporin to prevent infection.
- Monitor CMP and replace electrolyte imbalances as ordered.

**Monitor for the following complications:**

- Cardiac Tamponade: bleeding from graft sites into the pericardial sac
- Hypotension/shock: decreased cardiac output
- Arrhythmias: due to blood flow changes and cardioplegic solution – be prepared for epicardial pacing and defibrillation if needed
- Stroke (clots from grafts), infection (surgical site), etc.

**Nursing considerations** are as follows:

- Educate patient: recovery, possibility of Dressler's Syndrome and postoperative depression; adequate pain management and splinting.

## Arterial Line Insertion

Indications for an **arterial line** include hemodynamic instability, frequent ABG monitoring, placement of IABP, monitoring arterial pressure, and medication administration when venous access cannot be obtained. Sterile technique is utilized for arterial line insertion. Insertions sites include radial (most common), femoral (second choice), brachial, or dorsalis pedis arteries.

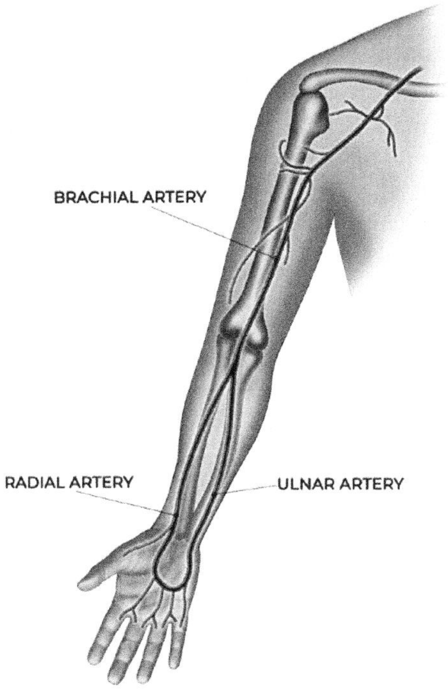


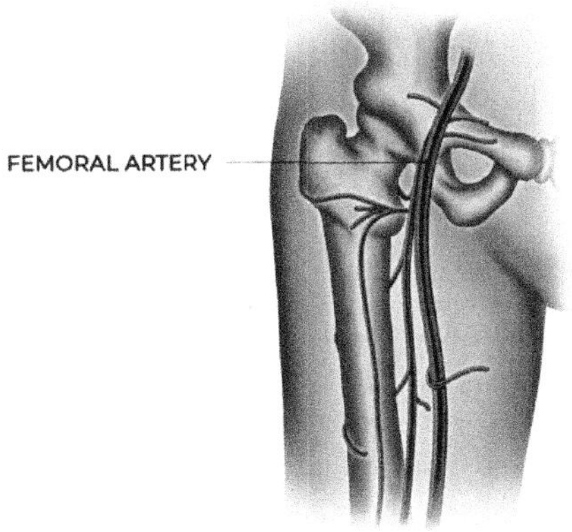


**Procedure:**

- Verify adequate perfusion and position.
  - Radial: Perform modified Allen test and position wrist in dorsiflexion with an arm board.
  - Femoral: Place the patient in a supine position with the leg on the insertion side slightly abducted and extended.
- Prep and drape. Apply 1% lidocaine if the patient is conscious.
- Insert needle.
  - Over-the-needle catheter insertion: Needle is inserted at a 30–45° degree angle and decreased to a 10–15° angle when blood returns, catheter advanced into vessel, needle removed, and catheter connected to transducer.
  - Over-wire catheter insertion: Needle is inserted into the artery at a 30–45° angle until blood returns. A wire is then inserted and advanced through the needle, and needle removed, leaving the wire in place. A catheter is then advanced over the wire, wire removed, and catheter connected to transducer system.
- A small incision is made at insertion site and catheter sutured into place.

**Complications** include bleeding, coagulopathy, thrombosis (especially with larger catheters or smaller arteries), advanced atherosclerosis, and infection.

**Review Video: Nursing Care of Arterial Lines**
Visit mometrix.com/academy and enter code: 561047

## Central Line Insertion

Central lines allow rapid administration of large volumes of fluid, blood testing, and CVP measuring. Central lines may be placed into the internal jugular vein (right preferred), subclavian vein, or femoral vein (usually avoided). The insertion site is located through an ultrasound. The patient is positioned, supine Trendelenburg (or legs elevated) for interior jugular, using sterile technique. Following skin prep, the CVC kit is placed on a sterile field and opened, the equipment is prepared, and the insertion site is again verified by a probe (covered with sterile cover). Topical anesthetic (lidocaine) is administered and the needle inserted with the triangulation or spear method, always pulling back on the plunger of the syringe so that blood returns when entering the vein. The syringe is removed and the guidewire inserted into needle ≤20 cm. The needle is then removed and the wire position verified with ultrasound. A small incision is made at the insertion site, and a dilator is applied over the wire and inserted about 2.5–3.5 cm. The catheter is placed over the wire and advanced into the vein (13–17 cm). The wire is then removed, the lines are flushed, and the catheter is sutured in place and dressing is applied. Long (24-inch) PICCs may be inserted in the basilic or cephalic veins and advanced into central circulation.

## Intraosseous Infusion

Intraosseous (IO) infusion is an alternative to IV access for neonates, pediatric emergencies, and adult emergencies when rapid temporary access is necessary or when peripheral or vascular access can't be achieved. It is often used in pediatric cardiac arrest. Because yellow marrow replaces red marrow, access in those older than 5 is more difficult. Preferred sites are based on age, though across all ages, the **proximal tibia is preferred**. Additional sites include:

- 0–1: Distal femur
- 1–12: Distal tibia or fibula
- 12–18: Distal tibia or fibula, sternum
- 18 and older: Distal tibia or fibula, proximal humerus, sternum

IO infusion is used to administer fluids and anesthesia and to obtain blood samples. Equipment requires a special needle (13–20 gauge) as standard needles may bend. The bone injection gun (BIG) with a loaded spring facilitates insertion. The FAST needle is intended for use in the sternum of adults and prevents accidental puncture of the thoracic cavity. Knowledge of bony landmarks and correct insertion angle and site is important. The position is confirmed by aspiration of 5–10 mL of blood and marrow before infusion.

## Vascular Interventions

Vascular interventions are required when a patient has a condition that is decreasing blood flow to the limbs, causing ischemia-related damage. Conditions that require a vascular intervention include acute occlusion (embolus), severe unresponsive vascular disease, ruptured/dissecting aneurysm, damaged vessels, or congenital defect.

- **Bypass grafts:** The MD uses a harvested vein from another part of the body (saphenous usually) or synthetic graft to bypass the occlusion. Because veins have valves, they must be reversed or stripped of valves prior to attachment; however, synthetic grafts have a higher failure rate. A common peripheral bypass is the femoropopliteal (Fem-pop) bypass, extending from the femoral artery around the blockage to the popliteal artery.

- **Embolectomy:** A catheter is inserted into the blocked artery and threaded through the thrombus. Then a balloon on the tip is inflated, and the physician removes the catheter, removing the clot with it.
- **Aortic aneurysm repair:** This is an intense procedure, requiring an open incision and the patient to be placed on cardiopulmonary bypass. The affected area is resected and replaced with a vascular or Dacron graft.

**Nursing considerations:** Monitor and control blood pressure carefully to protect the patency and integrity of the grafts. Neurologic and renal function should also be carefully monitored, as emboli could block the renal or cerebral artery. Frequent neuro, urine output, vascular, and dressing checks.

**Possible complications:** Pulmonary infection, graft-site infection, renal dysfunction, occlusion, hemorrhage, and embolus/thrombus.

## Peripheral Stents

**Peripheral vascular stenting** may be utilized as an intervention in the treatment of peripheral vascular insufficiency. Often performed in interventional radiology, the interventionalist uses balloon angioplasty to unblock the vessel under fluoroscopic guidance. A small balloon attached to a catheter is inserted into the occluded vessel and inflated to expand the arterial wall and compress the blockage. A small metal tube (stent) is then placed to support the vessel and maintain its patency. Stents are primarily made of stainless steel or a metal alloy. This intervention helps to restore circulation to the affected area and prevent restenosis of the vessel. There are different types of stents available based on the type of vessel affected and the type of lesion. Stenting may be used in both peripheral and coronary arteries.

- **Indications**: Stenting may be the initial choice of intervention in patients with iliac, renal, subclavian, or carotid stenosis. Stenting may be indicated in patients with severe claudication, non-healing ulcers of the extremities, ischemic pain with rest, and in patients who have a high operative risk. Peripheral stenting often results in shorter hospital stays and shorter recovery times in comparison with surgical intervention.
- **Complications**: Complications that may occur in patients undergoing peripheral stenting include bleeding, infection, arterial spasm or rupture, dissection of the vessel, restenosis or thrombus formation within the vessel, and intravascular fracture of the stent.

## Fem-Pop Bypass

**Femoropopliteal (Fem-Pop) bypass** is used for femoral artery disease in order to bypass an occluded femoral artery above or below the knee. Either a man-made or a vein graft (such as the saphenous vein) is used and is sewn above the blocked area to the femoral artery and below to the popliteal artery, allowing the blood to bypass the occluded area. In addition to the incisions in the affected leg, if a vein graft is obtained from the other leg, the patient may also have a long incision where the vein was removed. Edema in the surgical sites is common and may persist for up to 3 months. Femoral popliteal bypass surgery is indicated for peripheral vascular insufficiency that does not respond to medical treatment, causes severe intermittent claudication and/or ischemic resting pain, and results in gangrene or other non-healing wounds, especially if the limb is at risk for amputation because of impaired oxygenation. The limb(s) must be monitored carefully in the postoperative period for color, sensation, warmth, and ability to move.

# Respiratory Pathophysiology

## Acute Pulmonary Embolism

Acute pulmonary embolism occurs when a pulmonary artery or arteriole is blocked, cutting off blood supply to the pulmonary vessels and subsequent oxygenation of the blood. While most pulmonary emboli are from thrombus formation, they can also be caused by air, fat, or septic embolus (from bacterial invasion of a thrombus). Common originating sites for thrombus formation are the deep veins in the legs, the pelvic veins, and the right atrium. Causes include stasis related to damage to endothelial wall and changes in blood coagulation factors. Atrial fibrillation poses a serious risk because blood pools in the right atrium, forming clots that travel directly through the right ventricle to the lungs. The obstruction of the artery/arteriole causes an increase in alveolar dead space in which there is ventilation but impairment of gas exchange because of the ventilation/perfusion mismatching or intrapulmonary shunting. This results in hypoxia, hypercapnia, and the release of mediators that cause bronchoconstriction. If more than 50% of the vascular bed becomes excluded, pulmonary hypertension occurs.

### *Symptoms and Diagnosis*

Clinical manifestations of acute pulmonary embolism (PE) vary according to the size of the embolus and the area of occlusion.

**Symptoms** include:

- Dyspnea with tachypnea
- Cyanosis; may turn grey or blue from nipple line up (massive PE)
- Anxiety and restlessness, feeling of doom
- Chest pain, tachycardia, may progress to arrhythmias (PEA)
- Fever
- Rales
- Cough (sometimes with hemoptysis)
- Hemodynamic instability

**Diagnostic tests** are as follows:

- ABG analysis may show hypoxemia (decreased $PaO_2$), hypocarbia (decreased $PaCO_2$) and respiratory alkalosis (increased pH).
- D-dimer will show elevation with PE but is not definitively diagnostic without a CT scan.
- ECG may show sinus tachycardia or other abnormalities.
- Echocardiogram can show emboli in the central arteries and can assess the hemodynamic status of the right side of the heart.
- Spiral CT may provide definitive diagnosis.
- V/Q scintigraphy can confirm diagnosis.
- Pulmonary angiograms also can confirm diagnosis.

### *Medical Management*

Medical management of pulmonary embolism starts with preventive measures for those at risk, including leg exercises, elastic compression stockings, and anticoagulation therapy. Most pulmonary emboli present as medical emergencies, so the immediate task is to stabilize the patient. **Medical management** may include:

- **Oxygen** to relieve hypoxemia
- **Intravenous infusions:** Dobutamine (Dobutrex) or dopamine (Intropin) to relieve hypotension
- **Cardiac monitoring** for dysrhythmias and issues due to right sided heart failure
- **Medications** as indicated: digitalis glycosides, diuretic, and antiarrhythmics
- Intubation and mechanical ventilation may be required

- **Analgesics** (such as morphine sulfate) or sedation to relieve anxiety
- **Anticoagulants** to prevent recurrence (although it will not dissolve clots already present), including heparin and warfarin (Coumadin)
- **Placement of percutaneous venous filter** (Greenfield) in the inferior vena cava to prevent further emboli from entering the lungs, if anticoagulation therapy is contraindicated
- **Thrombolytic therapy,** recombinant tissue-type plasminogen activator (rt-PA) or streptokinase, for those severely compromised, but these treatments have limited success and pose the danger of bleeding

## Acute Lung Injury and Acute Respiratory Distress Syndrome

Acute lung injury (ALI) comprises a syndrome of respiratory distress culminating in acute respiratory distress syndrome (ARDS). ARDS is a dangerous, potentially fatal respiratory condition, always caused by an illness or injury to the lungs. Lung injury causes fluid to leak into the spaces between the alveoli and capillaries, increasing pressure on the alveoli, causing them to collapse. With increased fluid accumulation in the lungs, the ability of the lungs to move oxygen into the blood is decreased, resulting in hypoxemia. Lung injury also causes a release of cytokines, a type of inflammatory protein, which then brings neutrophils to the lung. These proteins and cells leak into nearby blood vessels and cause inflammation throughout the body. This immune response, in combination with low levels of blood oxygen, can lead to organ failure. Symptoms are characterized by respiratory distress within 72 hours of surgery or a serious injury to a person with otherwise normal lungs and no cardiac disorder. Untreated, the condition results in respiratory failure, MODS, and a mortality rate of 5–30%.

**Symptoms** include:

- Refractory hypoxemia (hypoxemia not responding to increasing levels of oxygen)
- Crackling rales/wheezing in lungs
- Decrease in pulmonary compliance which results in increased tachypnea with expiratory grunting
- Cyanosis/skin mottling
- Hypotension and tachycardia
- Symptoms associated with volume overload are missing (3rd heart sound or JVD)
- Respiratory alkalosis initially but, as the disease progresses, replaced with hypercarbia and respiratory acidosis
- Normal x-ray initially but then diffuse infiltrates in both lungs, while the heart and vessels appear normal

### *Management*

The management of acute respiratory distress syndrome (ARDS) involves providing adequate gas exchange and preventing further damage to the lung from forced ventilation.

**Treatment** includes:

- Mechanical ventilation to maintain oxygenation and ventilation
- Corticosteroids (may increase mortality rates in some patient populations, though this is the most commonly given treatment), nitrous oxide, inhaled surfactant, and anti-inflammatory medications
- Treatment of the underlying condition is the only proven treatment, especially identifying and treating an infection with appropriate antibiotics, as sepsis is most common etiology for ARDS, but prophylactic antibiotics are not indicated.
- Conservative fluid management is indicated to reduce days on the ventilator, but does not reduce overall mortality.

**Pharmacologic preventive care**: Enoxaparin 40 mg subcutaneously QD, sucralfate 1 g NGT four times daily or omeprazole 40 mg IV QD, and enteral nutrition support within 24 hours of ICU admission or intubation.

### *Ventilation Management*

Ventilation management in ARDS consists of the following:

- $O_2$ therapy by nasal prongs, cannula, or mask may be sufficient in very mild cases to maintain oxygen saturation above 90%. Oxygen should be administered at 95–100% because of the mismatch between ventilation (V) and perfusion (Q), which can result in hypoxia on position change.
- ARDS oxygenation goal is $PaO_2$ 55–80 mmHg or $SpO_2$ 88–95%.
- Endotracheal intubation may be needed if $SpO_2$ falls or $CO_2$ levels rise.
- The ARDS Network recommends low tidal volumes (6 mL/kg) and a PEEP based on the $FiO_2$ required to maintain oxygenation goals. High PEEPs may be required to start.
- The low tidal volume ventilation described above is referred to as lung protective ventilation, and it has been shown to reduce mortality in patients with ARDS.
- Placing patients with severe ARDS in prone position for 18–24 hours per day with chest and pelvis supported and abdomen unsupported allows the diaphragm to move posteriorly, increasing functional residual capacity (FRC) in many patients.

## Acute Respiratory Failure

### *Cardinal Signs*

The cardinal signs of respiratory failure include:

- Tachypnea
- Tachycardia
- Anxiety and restlessness
- Diaphoresis

**Symptoms** may vary according to the cause. An obstruction may cause more obvious respiratory symptoms than other disorders.

- Early signs may include changes in the depth and pattern of respirations with flaring nares, sternal retractions, expiratory grunting, wheezing, and extended expiration as the body tries to compensate for hypoxemia and increasing levels of carbon dioxide.
- Cyanosis may be evident.
- Central nervous depression, with alterations in consciousness occurs with decreased perfusion to the brain.
- As the hypoxemia worsens, cardiac arrhythmias, including bradycardia, may occur with either hypotension or hypertension.
- Dyspnea becomes more pronounced with depressed respirations.
- Eventually stupor, coma, and death can occur if the condition is not reversed.

### *Hypoxemic and Hypercapnic Respiratory Failure*

**Hypoxemic respiratory failure** occurs suddenly when gaseous exchange of oxygen for carbon dioxide cannot keep up with demand for oxygen or production of carbon dioxide:

- $PaO_2$ <60 mmHg
- $PaCO_2$ >40 mmHg
- Arterial pH <7.35

Hypoxemic respiratory failure can be the result of low inhaled oxygen, as at high elevations or with smoke inhalation. The following ventilatory mechanisms may be involved:

- Alveolar hypotension
- Ventilation-perfusion mismatch (the most common cause)

- Intrapulmonary shunts
- Diffusion impairment

**Hypercapnic respiratory failure** results from an increase in $PaCO_2$ >45–50 mmHg associated with respiratory acidosis and may include:

- Reduction in minute ventilation, total volume of gas ventilated in one minute (often related to neurological, muscle, or chest wall disorders, drug overdoses, or obstruction of upper airway)
- Increased dead space with wasted ventilation (related to lung disease or disorders of chest wall, such as scoliosis)
- Increased production of $CO_2$ (usually related to infection, burns, or other causes of hypermetabolism)
- Oxygen saturation normal or below normal

### *UNDERLYING CAUSES*

There are a number of underlying causes for respiratory failure:

- **Airway obstruction:** Obstruction may result from an inhaled object or from an underlying disease process, such as cystic fibrosis, asthma, pulmonary edema, or infection.
- **Inadequate respirations:** This is a common cause among adults, especially related to obesity and sleep apnea. It may also be induced by an overdose of sedation medications such as opioids.
- **Neuromuscular disorders:** Those disorders that interfere with the neuromuscular functioning of the lungs or the chest wall, such as muscular dystrophy or spinal cord injuries can prevent adequate ventilation.
- **Pulmonary abnormalities:** Those abnormalities of the lung tissue, found in pulmonary fibrosis, burns, ARDS, and reactions to drugs, can lead to failure.
- **Chest wall abnormalities:** Disorders that impact lung parenchyma, such as severe scoliosis or chest wounds can interfere with lung functioning.

**Nursing interventions** to help prevent respiratory issues:

- Turn, position, and ambulate the patient.
- Have the patient cough and breathe deeply.
- Use vibration and percussion treatments.
- Hydrate the patient to help hydrate the airway secretions, and incentive spirometry.

### *MANAGEMENT*

Respiratory failure must be **treated** immediately before severe hypoxemia causes irreversible damage to vital organs.

- **Identifying and treating** the underlying cause should be done immediately because emergency medications or surgery may be indicated. Medical treatments will vary widely depending upon the cause; for example, cardiopulmonary structural defects may require surgical repair, pulmonary edema may require diuresis, inhaled objects may require surgical removal, and infections may require aggressive antimicrobials.
- **Intravenous lines/central lines** are inserted for testing, fluids, and medications.
- **Oxygen therapy** should be initiated to attempt to reverse hypoxemia; however, if refractory hypoxemia occurs, then oxygen therapy alone will not suffice. Oxygen levels must be titrated carefully.
- **Intubation and mechanical ventilation** are frequently required to maintain adequate ventilation and oxygenation. Positive end expiratory pressure (PEEP) may be necessary with refractory hypoxemia and collapsed alveoli.
- **Respiratory status** must be monitored constantly, including arterial blood gases and vital signs.

## PNEUMONIA

Pneumonia is inflammation of the lung parenchyma, filling the alveoli with exudate. It is common throughout childhood and adulthood. Pneumonia may be a primary disease or may occur secondary to another infection or disease, such as lung cancer. Pneumonia may be caused by bacteria, viruses, parasites, or fungi. Common causes for community-acquired pneumonia (CAP) include:

- *Streptococcus pneumoniae*
- *Legionella* species
- *Haemophilus influenzae*
- *Staphylococcus aureus*
- *Mycoplasma pneumoniae*
- Viruses

Pneumonia may also be caused by chemical damage. Pneumonia is characterized by **location**:

- **Lobar** involves one or more lobes of the lungs. If lobes in both lungs are affected, it is referred to as bilateral or double pneumonia.
- **Bronchial/lobular** involves the terminal bronchioles, and exudate can involve the adjacent lobules. Usually, the pneumonia occurs in scattered patches throughout the lungs.
- **Interstitial** involves primarily the interstitium and alveoli where white blood cells and plasma fill the alveoli, generating inflammation and creating fibrotic tissue as the alveoli are destroyed.

**Review Video: Pneumonia**
Visit mometrix.com/academy and enter code: 628264

### *HOSPITAL-ACQUIRED PNEUMONIA*

Hospital-acquired pneumonia (HAP) is defined as pneumonia that did not appear to be present on admission that occurs at least 48 hours after admission to a hospital. **Healthcare-associated pneumonia (HCAP)** is defined as pneumonia that occurs in a patient within 90 days of being hospitalized for 2 or more days at an acute care hospital or LTAC. **Ventilator-associated pneumonia (VAP)** is one type of hospital acquired pneumonia that a patient acquires more than 48 hours after having an ETT placed. The most common way that the patient is infected is via aspiration of bacteria that is colonized in the upper respiratory tract Critically ill individuals are highly susceptible to colonization with multidrug resistant bacteria within 48 hours of entering an ICU. Aspiration occurs at a higher rate in those patients with HAP, HCAP, and VAP. The frequency of patients developing these types of pneumonia is increasing, with those at highest risk being those with immunosuppression, septic shock, currently hospitalized for more than five days, and those who have had antibiotics for another infection within the previous three months. These types of pneumonia should be considered if a patient already hospitalized has purulent sputum or a change in respiratory status such as deoxygenating, in combination with a worsening or new chest x-ray infiltrate.

**Treatment** includes:

- Antibiotic therapy
- Using appropriate isolation and precautions with infected patients
- Preventive measures including maintaining ventilated patients in 30° upright positions, frequent oral care for vent patients, and changing ventilator circuits as per protocol

Antibiotic treatment options for HAP, HCAP, and VAP should take into account many factors, including culture data (when available), patient's comorbidities, flora in the unit, any recent antibiotics by the patient, and whether the patient is at high risk for having multidrug resistant bacteria. As most critical care patients are at high risk, due to factors such as being in an ICU setting, ventilators, and comorbidities, antibiotic recommendations to follow are for coverage for patients with risk factors for multidrug resistant bacteria.

**Only one** of the following:

- Ceftazidime 2 g every 8 hours IV
- Cefepime 2 g every 8 hours IV
- Imipenem 500 mg every 6 hours IV
- Piperacillin-tazobactam 4.5 g every 6 hours IV

If the patient has a positive MRSA swab or risk of MRSA, add **only one** of the following:

- Vancomycin 15–20 mg/kg every 8–12 hours IV
- Linezolid 600 mg every 12 hours IV

### *Aspiration Pneumonitis/Pneumonia*

Aspiration pneumonitis/pneumonia may occur as the result of any type of aspiration, including foreign objects. The aspirated material creates an inflammatory response, with the irritated mucous membrane at high risk for bacterial infection secondary to the aspiration, causing pneumonia. Gastric contents and oropharyngeal bacteria are commonly aspirated. Gastric contents can cause a severe chemical pneumonitis with hypoxemia, especially if the pH is <2.5. Acidic food particles can cause severe reactions. With acidic damage, bronchospasm and atelectasis occur rapidly with tracheal irritation, bronchitis, and alveolar damage with interstitial edema and hemorrhage. Intrapulmonary shunting and V/Q mismatch may occur. Pulmonary artery pressure increases. Non-acidic liquids and food particles are less damaging, and symptoms may clear within 4 hours of liquid aspiration or granuloma may form about food particles in 1–5 days. Depending upon the type of aspiration, pneumonitis may clear within a week, ARDS or pneumonia may develop, or progressive acute respiratory failure may lead to death.

There are a number of risk factors that can lead to **aspiration pneumonitis/pneumonia:**

- Altered level of consciousness related to illness or sedation
- Depression of gag, swallowing reflex
- Intubation or feeding tubes
- Ileus or gastric distention
- Gastrointestinal disorders, such as gastroesophageal reflux disorders (GERD)

**Diagnosis** is based on clinical findings, ABGs showing hypoxemia, infiltrates observed on x-ray, and elevated WBC if infection is present.

**Symptoms:** Similar to other pneumonias:

- Cough often with copious sputum
- Respiratory distress, dyspnea
- Cyanosis
- Tachycardia
- Hypotension

**Treatment** includes:

- Suctioning as needed to clear upper airway
- Supplemental oxygen
- Antibiotic therapy as indicated after 48 hours if symptoms not resolving
- Symptomatic respiratory support

### *Foreign Body Aspiration*

Foreign body aspiration can cause obstruction of the pharynx, larynx, or trachea, leading to acute dyspnea or asphyxiation, and the object may also be drawn distally into the bronchial tree. With adults, most foreign bodies migrate more readily down the right bronchus. Food is the most frequently aspirated, but other small objects, such as coins or needles, may also be aspirated. Sometimes the object causes swelling, ulceration, and general inflammation that hampers removal.

**Symptoms** include:

- **Initial**: Severe coughing, gagging, sternal retraction, wheezing. Objects in the larynx may cause inability to breathe or speak and lead to respiratory arrest. Objects in the bronchus cause cough, dyspnea, and wheezing.
- **Delayed**: Hours, days, or weeks later, an undetected aspirant may cause an infection distal to the aspirated material. Symptoms depend on the area and extent of the infection.

**Treatment** includes:

- Removal with laryngoscopy or bronchoscopy (rigid is often better than flexible)
- Antibiotic therapy for secondary infection
- Surgical bronchotomy (rarely required)
- Symptomatic support

## Chronic Bronchitis

Chronic bronchitis is a pulmonary airway disease characterized by severe cough with sputum production for at least 3 months a year for at least 2 consecutive years. Irritation of the airways (often from smoke or pollutants) causes an inflammatory response, increasing the number of mucus-secreting glands and goblet cells while ciliary function decreases so that the extra mucus plugs the airways. Additionally, the bronchial walls thicken, alveoli near the inflamed bronchioles become fibrotic, and alveolar macrophages cannot function properly, increasing susceptibility to infections. Chronic bronchitis is most common in those >45 years old and occurs twice as frequently in females as males.

**Symptoms** include:

- Persistent cough with increasing sputum
- Dyspnea
- Frequent respiratory infections

**Treatment** includes:

- Bronchodilators
- Long term continuous oxygen therapy or supplemental oxygen during exercise
- Pulmonary rehabilitation to improve exercise and breathing
- Antibiotics during infections
- Corticosteroids for acute episodes

## Emphysema

Emphysema, the primary component of COPD, is characterized by abnormal distention of air spaces at the ends of the terminal bronchioles, with destruction of alveolar walls so that there is less and less gaseous exchange and increasing dead space with resultant hypoxemia, hypercapnia, and respiratory acidosis. The capillary bed is damaged as well, altering pulmonary blood flow and raising pressure in the right atrium (cor pulmonale) and pulmonary artery, leading to cardiac failure. Complications include respiratory insufficiency and failure. There are two primary types of emphysema (and both forms may be present):

- **Centrilobular** (the most common form) involves the central portion of the respiratory lobule, sparing distal alveoli, and usually affects the upper lobes. Typical symptoms include abnormal ventilation-perfusion ratios, hypoxemia, hypercapnia, and polycythemia with right-sided heart failure.
- **Panlobular** involves enlargement of all air spaces, including the bronchiole, alveolar duct, and alveoli, but there is minimal inflammatory disease. Typical symptoms include hyperextended rigid barrel chest, marked dyspnea, weight loss, and active expiration.

## COPD

### *Stages*

Functional dyspnea, body mass index (BMI), and spirometry are used to assess the **stages of chronic obstructive pulmonary disease (COPD)**. Spirometry measures used are the ratio of forced expiratory volume in the first second of expiration ($FEV_1$) after full inhalation to total forced vital capacity (FVC). Normal lung function decreases after age 35; so normal values are adjusted for height, weight, gender, and age:

- **Stage I** (mild): Minimal dyspnea with or without cough and sputum. $FEV_1$ is ≥80% of predicted rate and $FEV_1$:FVC <70%.
- **Stage 2** (moderate): Moderate to severe chronic exertional dyspnea with or without cough and sputum. $FEV_1$ is 50–80% of predicted rate and $FEV_1$:FVC <70%.
- **Stage 3** (severe): Same as stage 2 but with repeated episodes with increased exertional dyspnea and condition impacting quality of life. $FEV_1$ is 30–50% of predicted rate and $FEV_1$:FVC <70%.
- **Stage 4** (very severe): Severe dyspnea and life-threatening episodes that severely impact quality of life. $FEV_1$ is 30% of predicted rate or <50% with chronic respiratory failure and $FEV_1$:FVC <70%.



### *Management*

COPD is not reversible, so management aims at slowing its progression, relieving symptoms, and improving quality of life:

- Smoking cessation is the primary means to slow progression and may require smoking cessation support in the form of classes or medications, such as bupropion, nicotine patches or gum, clonidine, or nortriptyline.
- Bronchodilators, such as albuterol and salmeterol, relieve bronchospasm and airway obstruction.
- Corticosteroids, both inhaled (budesonide, beclomethasone) and oral (prednisone) may improve symptoms but are used mostly for associated asthma.
- Oxygen therapy may be long term continuous or used during exertion.
- Bullectomy (for bullous emphysema) to remove bullae (enlarged airspaces that do not ventilate).
- Lung volume reduction surgery may be done if involvement in the lung is limited; however, mortality rates are high.
- Lung transplantation is a definitive high-risk option.
- Pulmonary rehabilitation includes breathing exercises, muscle training, activity pacing, and modification of activities.

**Review Video: Respiratory Diseases**
Visit mometrix.com/academy and enter code: 973392

## Chronic Ventilatory Failure

Chronic ventilatory failure occurs when alveolar ventilation fails to increase in response to increasing levels of carbon dioxide, usually associated with chronic pulmonary diseases, such as asthma and COPD, drug overdoses, or diseases that impair respiratory effort, such as Guillain-Barré and myasthenia gravis. Normally, the ventilatory system is able to maintain $PCO_2$ and pH levels within narrow limits, even though $PO_2$ levels may be more variable, but with ventilatory failure, the body is not able to compensate for the resultant hypercapnia and pH falls, resulting in respiratory acidosis. Symptoms include increasing dyspnea with tachypnea, gasping respirations, and use of accessory muscles. Patients may become confused as hypercapnia causes increased intracranial pressure. If pH is <7.2, cardiac arrhythmias, hyperkalemia, and hypotension can occur as pulmonary arteries constrict and the peripheral vascular system dilates. Diagnosis is per symptoms, ABGs consistent with respiratory acidosis ($PCO_2$ >50 and pH <7.35), pulse oximetry, and chest x-ray. Treatment can include non-invasive PPV (BiPAP), endotracheal mechanical ventilation, corticosteroids, and bronchodilators.

## Chronic Asthma

The three primary symptoms of chronic asthma are cough, wheezing, and dyspnea. In cough-variant asthma, a severe cough may be the only symptom, at least initially. Chronic asthma is characterized by recurring bronchospasm and inflammation of the airways resulting in airway obstruction. Asthma affects the bronchi and not the alveoli. While no longer considered part of COPD because airway obstruction is not constant and is responsive to treatment, over time fibrotic changes in the airways can result in permanent obstruction, especially if asthma is not treated adequately. **Symptoms** of chronic asthma include nighttime coughing, exertional dyspnea, tightness in the chest, and cough. Acute exacerbations may occur, sometimes related to triggers, such as allergies, resulting in increased dyspnea, wheezing, cough, tachycardia, bronchospasm, and rhonchi. **Treatment** of chronic asthma includes chest hygiene, identification and avoidance of triggers, prompt treatment of infections, bronchodilators, long-acting β-2 agonists, and inhaled glucocorticoids.

## Status Asthmaticus

### *Pathophysiology*

Status asthmaticus is a severe acute attack of asthma that does not respond to conventional therapy. An acute attack of asthma is precipitated by some stimulus, such as an antigen that triggers an allergic response, resulting in an inflammatory cascade that causes edema of the mucous membranes (swollen airway), contraction of smooth muscles (bronchospasm), increased mucus production (cough and obstruction), and hyperinflation of airways (decreased ventilation and shunting). Mast cells and T lymphocytes produce cytokines, which continue the inflammatory response through increased blood flow coupled with vasoconstriction and bronchoconstriction, resulting in fluid leakage from the vasculature. Epithelial cells and cilia are destroyed, exposing nerves and causing hypersensitivity. Sympathetic nervous system receptors in the bronchi stimulate bronchodilation.

### *Clinical Symptoms*

The person with status asthmaticus will often present in acute distress, non-responsive to inhaled bronchodilators. **Symptoms** include:

- Signs of airway obstruction
- Sternal and intercostal retractions
- Tachypnea and dyspnea with increasing cyanosis
- Forced prolonged expirations
- Cardiac decompensation with increased left ventricular afterload and increased pulmonary edema resulting from alveolar-capillary permeability. Hypoxia may trigger an increase in pulmonary vascular resistance with increased right ventricular afterload.
- Pulsus paradoxus (decreased pulse on inspiration and increased on expiration) with extra beats on inspiration detected through auscultation but not detected radially. Blood pressure normally decreases slightly during inspiration, but this response is exaggerated. Pulsus paradoxus indicates increasing severity of asthma.
- Hypoxemia (with impending respiratory failure)
- Hypocapnia followed by hypercapnia (with impending respiratory failure)
- Metabolic acidosis

### *Indications for Mechanical Ventilation for Status Asthmaticus*

Mechanical ventilation (MV) for status asthmaticus should be avoided, if possible, because of the danger of increased bronchospasm as well as barotrauma and decreased circulation. However, there are some absolute indications for the use of intubation and ventilation and a number of other indications that are evaluated on an individual basis.

The following are **absolute indications for MV:**

- Cardiac and/or pulmonary arrest
- Markedly depressed mental status (obtundation)
- Severe hypoxia and/or apnea

The following are **relative indications for MV:**

- Exhaustion/muscle fatigue from exertion of breathing
- Sharply diminished breath sounds and no audible wheezing
- Pulse paradoxus >20–40 mmHg; absent = imminent respiratory arrest
- $PaO_2$ <70 mmHg on 100% oxygen
- Dysphonia
- Central cyanosis
- Increased hypercapnia
- Metabolic/respiratory acidosis: pH <7.20

In this patient population, ventilator goal is to minimize airway pressures while oxygenating the patient. Vent settings include: low tidal volume (6–8 mL/kg), low respiratory rate (10–14 respirations/minute), and high inspiratory flow rate (80–100 L/min).

**Review Video: Mechanical Ventilation**
Visit mometrix.com/academy and enter code: 679637

### Air Leak Syndromes

Air leak syndromes may result in significant respiratory distress. Leaks may occur spontaneously or secondary to some type of trauma (accidental, mechanical, iatrogenic) or disease. As pressure increases inside the alveoli, the alveolar wall pulls away from the perivascular sheath and subsequent alveolar rupture allows air to follow the perivascular planes and flow into adjacent areas. There are two categories:

- **Pneumothorax:**
  - Air in the pleural space causes a lung to collapse.
- **Barotrauma/volutrauma** with air in the interstitial space (usually resolve over time):
  - Pneumoperitoneum is air in the peritoneal area, including the abdomen and occasionally the scrotal sac of male infants.
  - Pneumomediastinum is air in the mediastinal area between the lungs.
  - Pneumopericardium is air in the pericardial sac that surrounds the heart.
  - Subcutaneous emphysema is air in the subcutaneous tissue planes of the chest wall.
  - Pulmonary interstitial emphysema (PIE) is air trapped in the interstitium between the alveoli.

### PNEUMOTHORAX

Pneumothorax occurs when there is a leak of air into the pleural space, resulting in complete or partial collapse of a lung.

**PNEUMOTHORAX**

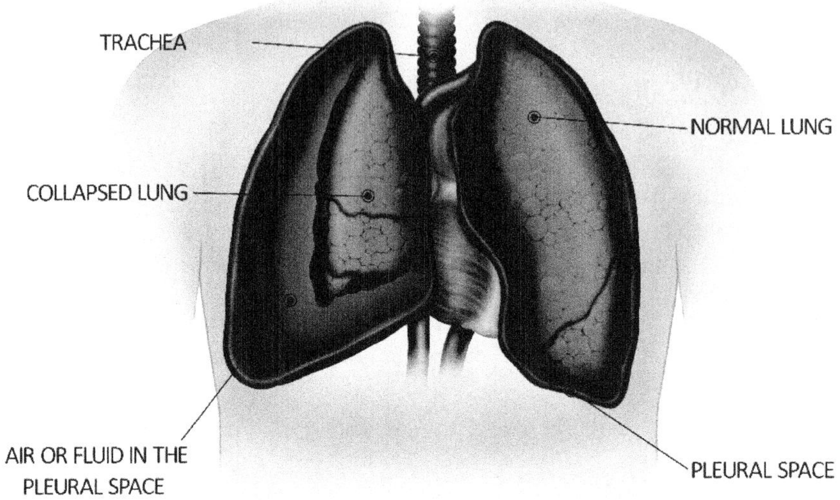


**Symptoms:** Vary widely depending on the cause and degree of the pneumothorax and whether or not there is an underlying disease. Symptoms include acute pleuritic pain (95%), usually on the affected side, and decreased breath sounds. In a *tension pneumothorax,* symptoms include tracheal deviation and hemodynamic compromise.

**Diagnosis:** Clinical findings; radiograph: 6-foot upright posterior-anterior; ultrasound may detect traumatic pneumothorax.

**Treatment:** Chest-tube thoracostomy with underwater seal drainage is the most common treatment for all types of pneumothorax.

- Tension pneumothorax: Immediate needle decompression and chest tube thoracostomy
- Small pneumothorax, patient stable: Oxygen administration and observation for 3–6 hours. If no increase is shown on repeat x-ray, patient may be discharged with another x-ray in 24 hours.
- Primary spontaneous pneumothorax: Catheter aspiration or chest tube thoracostomy

**Review Video: Pneumothorax**
Visit mometrix.com/academy and enter code: 186841

### PLEURAL EFFUSION AND EMPYEMA

**Pleural effusion** is the accumulation of fluid in the pleural space, usually secondary to other disease processes, such as heart failure, TB, neoplasms, nephrotic syndrome, and viral respiratory infections. The fluid may be serous, bloody, or purulent (empyema) and transudative or exudative. Signs and symptoms depend on underlying condition but includes dyspnea, from mild to severe. Tracheal deviation away from the affected side may be evident. Diagnosis includes chest x-ray, lateral decubitus x-ray, CT, thoracentesis, and pleural biopsy. Treatment includes treating underlying cause, thoracentesis to remove fluid, insertion of chest tube, pleurodesis, or pleurectomy or pleuroperitoneal shunt (primarily with malignancy).

**Review Video: Pleural Effusions**
Visit mometrix.com/academy and enter code: 145719

**Empyema** is a pleural effusion in which the collection of pleural fluid is thick and purulent, usually as a result of bacterial pneumonia or penetrating chest trauma. Empyema may also occur as a complication of thoracentesis or thoracic surgery. Signs and symptoms include acute illness with fever, chills, pain, cough, and dyspnea. Diagnosis is per chest CT and thoracentesis with culture and sensitivity. Treatment includes antibiotics and drainage of pleural space per needle aspiration, tube thoracostomy, or open chest drainage with thoracotomy.

## Pulmonary Fibrosis

Pulmonary fibrosis is a progressive disease of the lungs in which scarring of the tissue causes the lining of the lungs to thicken. This thickening prevents adequate oxygen exchange from occurring. The cause of pulmonary fibrosis is unknown, however environmental toxins such as asbestos, infections, smoking and occupational exposure to wood or metal dust may be contributing factors. The disease is more prevalent in males and the average age at the time of diagnosis is between 40 and 70. There may also be a genetic predisposition in the development of pulmonary fibrosis. The median survival for patients diagnosed with pulmonary fibrosis is less than five years.

**Signs/symptoms**: Shortness of breath, dry cough, fatigue, weight loss, and clubbing of the finger tips and nails.

**Diagnosis**: Physical assessment, chest x-ray and/or computed tomography, pulmonary function tests, arterial blood gases and lung biopsy.

**Treatment**: There is no cure for pulmonary fibrosis and treatment options are minimal. Anti-inflammatory medications such as corticosteroids may be used for symptom management as well as supplemental oxygen therapy. Lung transplantation may be an option for some patients based on age and advancement of disease. Some patients may be eligible for participation in a clinical trial, as there are research efforts focused on treatment options to halt the progression of the disease.

## Pulmonary Hypertension and Pulmonary Arterial Hypertension

Pulmonary arterial hypertension (PAH) is a progressive disease of the pulmonary arteries that can severely compromise cardiovascular patients. It may involve multiple processes. Usually, the pulmonary vasculature adjusts easily to accommodate blood volume from the right ventricle. If there is increased blood flow, the low resistance causes vasodilation and vice versa. However, sometimes the pulmonary vascular bed is damaged or obstructed, and this can impair the ability to handle changing volumes of blood. In that case, an increase in flow will increase the pulmonary arterial pressure, increasing pulmonary vascular resistance (PVR). This in turn, increases pressure on the right ventricle (RV) with increased RV workload and eventually causes RV hypertrophy with displacement of the intraventricular septum and tricuspid regurgitation (cor pulmonale). Over time, this leads to right heart failure and death. Pulmonary hypertension is usually diagnosed by right-sided heart catheterization and is indicated by systolic pulmonary artery pressure >30 mmHg and mean pulmonary artery pressure >25 mmHg. Non-invasive testing may include echocardiogram to look for cardiac changes.

### *Types*

Pulmonary hypertension or pulmonary arterial hypertension (PAH) may be classified as primary (idiopathic) or secondary.

- **Primary (idiopathic) PAH** may result from changes in immune responses, pulmonary emboli, sickle cell disease, collagen diseases, Raynaud's, and the use of contraceptives. The cause may be unknown or genetic.
- **Secondary PAH** may result from pulmonary vasoconstriction brought on by hypoxemia related to COPD, sleep-disordered breathing, kyphoscoliosis, obesity, smoke inhalation, altitude sickness, interstitial pneumonia, and neuromuscular disorders. It may also be caused by a decrease in pulmonary vascular bed of 50–75%, which may result from pulmonary emboli, vasculitis, tumor emboli, and interstitial lung disease, such as sarcoidosis. Primary cardiac disease, such as congenital defects in infants, and acquired disorders, such as rheumatic valve disease, mitral stenosis, and left ventricular failure may also contribute to PAH.

### *Treatment Options for PAH*

Medical treatment for pulmonary arterial hypertension (PAH) aims to identify and treat any underlying cardiac or pulmonary disease, control symptoms, and prevent complications:

- **Oxygen therapy** may be needed, especially supplemental oxygen during exercise.
- **Calcium channel blockers** may provide vasodilation for some patients.
- **Pulmonary vascular dilators**, such as IV epoprostenol (Flolan) and subcutaneous treprostinil sodium (Remodulin) and oral bosentan (Tracleer) help to control symptoms and prolong life.
- **Anticoagulants**, such as warfarin (Coumadin) are an important part of therapy because of recurrent pulmonary emboli. Studies have shown that anticoagulation increases survival rates.
- **Diuretics**, such as furosemide (Lasix) may be needed to relieve edema and restrict fluids, especially with right ventricular hypertrophy.

In some patients who cannot be managed adequately through medical treatment, a heart-lung transplant may be considered as the only effective treatment for long-term survival.

## Management of Pulmonary and Thoracic Trauma

### *Pulmonary Hemorrhage*

Pulmonary hemorrhage is an acute life-threatening injury that often results in death prior to arrival at the hospital; however, those presenting with traumatic pulmonary hemorrhage, as from a blunt or penetrating injury, require immediate surgical repair. Even with immediate surgery, survival after serious injury to a major pulmonary vessel is rare. It is important that a large bore IV be immediately inserted and fluid replacement begun while blood is typed and cross matched. The patient should be evaluated for shock and treatment, including colloid solutions, crystalloids, or blood, provided as indicated. Pulmonary hemorrhage may result in hemothorax. In some cases, pneumothorax may also be present, resulting in mediastinal shift that increases the difficulty of identifying and repairing the bleeding vessel. If the patient is stabilized, computed tomography may provide accurate diagnosis to isolate the area of hemorrhage.

### *Tracheal Perforation/Injury*

Tracheal perforation/injury may result from external injury, such as from trauma from a vehicle accident or from an assault, such as a gunshot or knife wound, or in some cases a laceration as a complication of percutaneous dilation tracheostomy (PDT) or other endotracheal tubes. In some cases, an inhaled foreign object may become lodged in the trachea and eventually erode the tissue. If the injury is severe, respiratory failure may cause death in a very short period of time, so rapid diagnosis and treatment is critical.

**Symptoms** include:

- Severe respiratory distress
- Hemoptysis
- Strider with progressive dysphonia
- Pneumothorax, pneumomediastinum
- Subcutaneous emphysema from air leaking from the pleural space into the tissues of the chest wall, neck, face, and even into the upper extremities

**Treatment** includes:

- Intubation and non-surgical healing for small lacerations
- Surgical repair for larger wounds or severe respiratory distress

### *Pulmonary Contusion*

Pulmonary contusion is the result of direct force to the lung, resulting in parenchymal injury, bleeding, and edema that impact the capillary-alveoli juncture, resulting in intrapulmonary shunting as the alveoli and interstitium fill with fluid. Parenchymal injury reduces compliance and impairs ventilation. **Diagnosis** may be more difficult if other injuries, such as fractured ribs or pneumothorax, are also present because they may all contribute to respiratory distress. CT scans provide the best diagnostic tool.

**Symptoms** vary widely depending upon the degree of injury:

- Mild dyspnea
- Severe progressive dyspnea
- Hemoptysis
- Acute respiratory failure

**Treatment** varies according to the injury:

- Close monitoring of arterial blood gases and respiratory status
- Supplemental oxygen
- Intubation and mechanical ventilation with positive-end expiratory pressure (PEEP) for more severe respiratory distress
- Fluid management and diuretics to control pulmonary edema
- Respiratory physiotherapy to clear secretions

### *Fractured Ribs*

Fractured ribs are usually the result of severe trauma, such as blunt force from a motor vehicle accident or physical abuse. Underlying injuries should be expected according to the area of fractures:

- Upper 2 ribs: Injuries to trachea, bronchi, or great vessels
- Right-sided ≥ rib 8: Trauma to liver
- Left-sided ≥ rib 8: Trauma to spleen

Pain, often localized or experienced on respirations or compression of chest way may be the primary symptom of rib fractures, resulting in shallow breathing that can lead to atelectasis or pneumonia.

**Diagnosis**: Chest x-ray or CT scan.

**Treatment** is primarily supportive as rib fractures usually heal in about 6 weeks: however, preventing pulmonary complications (pneumothorax, hemothorax) often necessitates adequate pain control. Underlying injuries are treated according to the type and degree of injury:

- Supplemental oxygen
- Analgesia may include NSAIDs, intercostal nerve blocks, and narcotics
- Pulmonary physiotherapy
- Rib belts
- Surgical fixation (ORIF) only in those requiring thoracotomy for underlying injuries
- Splinting

### *Flail Chest*

Flail chest is a more common injury in adults and older teens than children. It occurs when at least 3 adjacent ribs are fractured, both anteriorly and posteriorly, so that they float free of the rib cage. There may be variations, such as the sternum floating with ribs fractured on both sides. Flail chest results in a failure of the chest wall to support changes in intrathoracic pressure so that paradoxical respirations occur with the flail area contracting on inspiration and expanding on expiration. The lungs are not able to expand properly, decreasing ventilation, but the degree of respiratory distress may relate to injury to underlying structures more than the flail chest alone. **Treatment**:

- Initial stabilization with tape, one side only, don't wrap chest
- Give analgesia for pain relief
- Respiratory physiotherapy is done to prevent atelectasis
- Mechanical ventilation is usually not indicated unless needed for underlying injuries
- Surgical fixation is usually done only in those who require thoracotomy for underlying injuries

### *Hemothorax*

Hemothorax occurs with bleeding into the pleural space, usually from major vascular injury such as tears in intercostal vessels, lacerations of great vessels, or trauma to lung parenchyma. A small bleed may be self-limiting and seal, but a tear in a large vessel can result in massive bleeding, followed quickly by hypovolemic shock. The pressure from the blood may result in the inability of the lung to ventilate and a mediastinal shift. Often a hemothorax occurs with a pneumothorax, especially in severe chest trauma. Further symptoms include severe respiratory distress, decreased breath sounds, and dullness on auscultation.

**Treatment** includes placement of a chest tube to drain the hemothorax, but with large volumes, the pressure may be preventing exsanguination, which can occur abruptly as the blood drains and the pressure is reduced, so a large bore intravenous line should be in place before placement of the chest tube and typed and cross-matched blood immediately available. Autotransfusion may be used, but it is contraindicated if the wound is older than three hours and has the possibility of bowel/stomach contamination, liver failure, and malignancy. Thoracotomy may be indicated after chest tube insertion if there is still hemodynamic instability, tension hemothorax, more than 1500 mL blood initially on insertion, or bleeding continues at a rate of >300 mL/hr.

# Respiratory Procedures and Interventions

## Non-Invasive Ventilation

### *Nasal Cannula*

A nasal cannula can be used to deliver supplemental oxygen to a patient, but it is only useful for flow rates ≤6 L/min as higher rates are drying of the nasal passages. As it is not an airtight system, some ambient air is breathed in as well so oxygen concentration ranges from about 24–44%. The nasal cannula does not allow for control of respiratory rate, so the patient must be able to breathe independently.

### *Non-Rebreather Mask*

A non-rebreather mask can be used to deliver higher concentrations (60–90%) of oxygen to those patients who are able to breathe independently. The mask fits over the nose and mouth and is secured by an elastic strap. A 1.5 L reservoir bag is attached and connects to an oxygen source. The bag is inflated to about 1 liter at a rate of 8–15 L/min before the mask is applied as the patient breathes from this reservoir. A one-way exhalation valve prevents most exhaled air from being rebreathed.

### *Non-Invasive Positive Pressure Ventilators*

Non-invasive positive pressure ventilators provide air through a tight-fitting nasal or face mask, usually pressure cycled, avoiding the need for intubation and reducing the danger of hospital-acquired infection and mortality rates. It can be used for acute respiratory failure and pulmonary edema. There are 2 types of non-invasive positive pressure ventilators:

- **CPAP (Continuous positive airway pressure)** provides a steady stream of pressurized air throughout both inspiration and expiration. CPAP improves breathing by decreasing preload for patients with congestive heart failure. It reduces the effort required for breathing by increasing residual volume and improving gas exchange.
- **Bi-PAP (Bi-level positive airway pressure)** provides a steady stream of pressurized air as CPAP but it senses inspiratory effort and increases pressure during inspiration. Bi-PAP pressures for inspiration and expiration can be set independently. Machines can be programmed with a backup rate to ensure a set number of respirations per minute.

**NEVER place a patient in wrist restraints while wearing these devices. If the patient vomits, they need to be able to remove the mask to prevent aspiration.*

### *Face Mask*

Ensuring that a face mask (Ambu bag) is the correct fit and type is important for adequate ventilation, oxygenation, and prevention of aspiration. Difficulties in management of face mask ventilation relate to risk factors: >55 years, obesity, beard, edentulous, and history of snoring. In some cases, if dentures are adhered well, they may be left in place during induction. The face mask is applied by lifting the mandible (jaw thrust) to the mask and avoiding pressure on soft tissue. Oral or nasal airways may be used, ensuring that the distal end is at the angle of the mandible. There are a number of steps to prevent mask airway leaks:

- Increasing or decreasing the amount of air to the mask to allow better seal
- Securing the mask with both hands while another person ventilates
- Accommodating a large nose by using the mask upside down
- Utilizing a laryngeal mask airway if excessive beard prevents seal

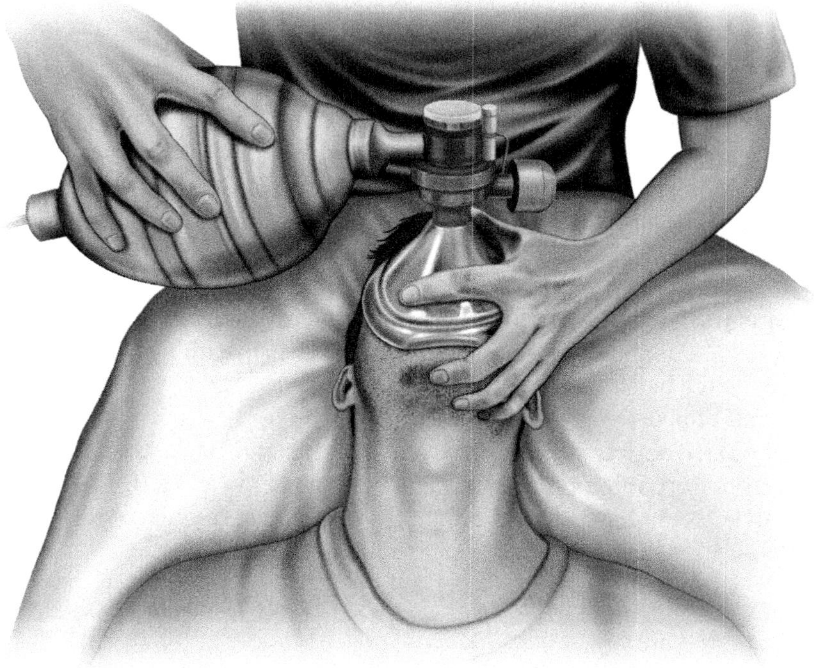

### *High and Low Flow Oxygen Delivery*

**High flow** oxygen delivery devices provide oxygen at flow rates higher than the patient's inspiratory flow rate at specific medium to high $FiO_2$, up to 100%. The actual amount of oxygen received depends on the type of interface or mask. Additionally, the flow rate is actually less than the inspiratory flow rate upon actual delivery. High flow oxygen delivery is usually not used in the sleep center. Humidification is usually required because the high flow is drying.

**Low flow** oxygen delivery devices provide 100% oxygen at flow rates lower than the patient's inspiratory flow rate, but the oxygen mixes with room air, so the $FiO_2$ varies. Humidification is usually only required if flow rate is >3L/min. Much oxygen is wasted with exhalation, so a number of different devices to conserve oxygen are available. Interfaces include transtracheal catheters and cannulae with reservoirs.

## Airway Devices

### *Oropharyngeal, Nasopharyngeal, and Tracheostomy Tubes*

**Airways** are used to establish a patent airway and facilitate respirations:

- **Oropharyngeal**: This plastic airway curves over the tongue and creates space between the mouth and the posterior pharynx. It is used for anesthetized or unconscious patients to keep tongue and epiglottis from blocking the airway.

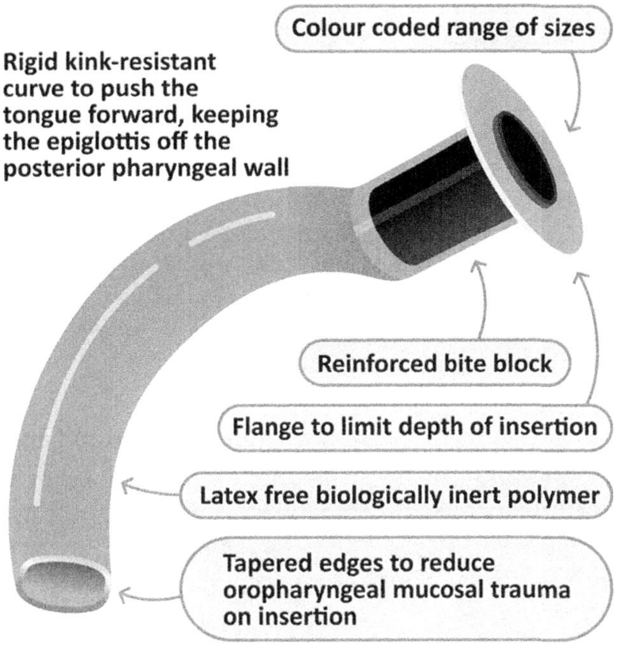


- **Nasopharyngeal** (trumpet): This smaller flexible airway is more commonly used in conscious patients and is inserted through one nostril, extending to the nasopharynx. It is commonly utilized in patients who need frequent suctioning.

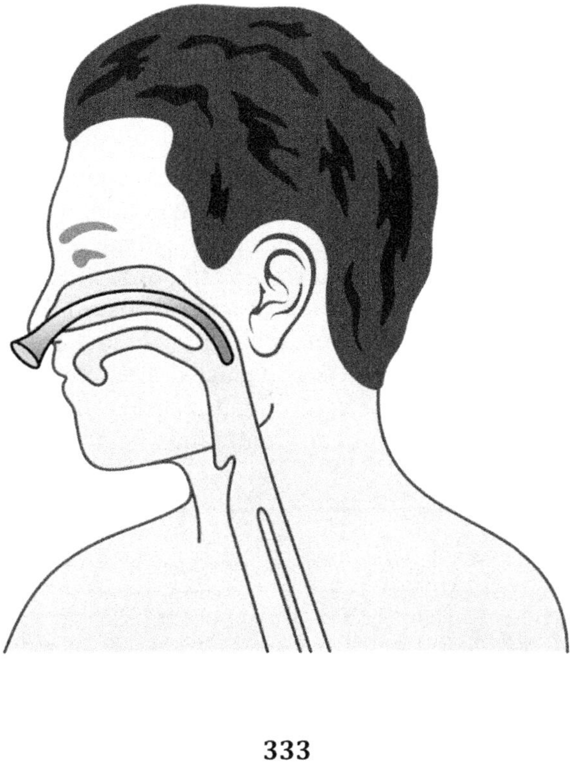

- **Tracheostomy tubes**: Tracheostomy may be utilized for mechanical ventilation. Tubes are inserted into the opening in the trachea to provide a conduit and maintain the opening. The tube is secured with ties around the neck. Because the air entering the lungs through the tracheostomy bypasses the warming and moistening effects of the upper airway, air is humidified through a room humidifier or through the delivery of humidified air through a special mask or mechanical ventilation. If the tracheostomy is going to be long-term, eventually a stoma will form at the site, and the tube can be removed.

### *Laryngeal Mask Airway*

The laryngeal-mask airway (LMA) is an intermediate airway allowing ventilation but not complete respiratory control. The LMA consists of an inflatable cuff (the mask) with a connecting tube. It may be used temporarily before tracheal intubation or when tracheal intubation can't be done. It can also be a conduit for later blind insertion of an endotracheal tube. The head and neck must be in neutral position for insertion of the LMA. If the patient has a gag reflex, conscious sedation or topical anesthesia (deep oropharyngeal) is required. The LMA is inserted by sliding along the hard palate, using the finger as a guide, into the pharynx, and the ring is inflated to create a seal about the opening to the larynx, allowing ventilation with mild positive-pressure. The ProSeal LMA has a modified cuff that extends onto the back of the mask to improve seal. LMA is contraindicated in morbid obesity, obstructions or abnormalities of oropharynx, and non-fasting patients, as some aspiration is possible even with the cuff seal inflated.

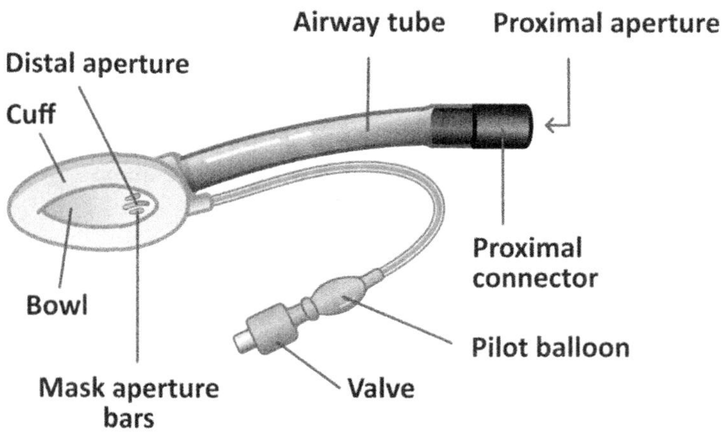


### *Esophageal-Tracheal Combitube*

The esophageal tracheal Combitube (ETC) is an intermediate airway that contains two lumens and can be inserted into either the trachea or the esophagus (≤91%). The twin-lumen tube has a proximal cuff providing a seal of the oropharynx and a distal cuff providing a seal about the distal tube. Prior to insertion, the Combitube cuffs should be checked for leaks (15 mL of air into distal and 85 mL of air into proximal). The patient should be non-responsive and with absent gag reflex with head in neutral position. The tube is passed along the tongue and into the pharynx, utilizing markings on the tube (black guidelines) to determine depth by aligning the ETC with the upper incisors or alveolar ridge. Once in place the distal cuff is inflated (10–15 mL) and then placement in the trachea or esophagus should be determined, so the proper lumen for ventilation can be used. The proximal cuff is inflated (usually to 50–75 mL) and ventilation begun. A capnogram should be used to confirm ventilation.

## MECHANICAL VENTILATION

### ENDOTRACHEAL INTUBATION

Endotracheal intubation is often necessary with respiratory failure for control of hypoxemia, hypercapnia, hypoventilation, and/or obstructed airway. Equipment should be assembled and tubes and connections checked for air leaks with a 10 mL syringe. The mouth and/or nose should be cleaned of secretions and suctioned if necessary. The patient should be supine with the patient's head level with the lower sternum of the clinician. With orotracheal/endotracheal intubation, the clinician holds the laryngoscope (in left hand) and inserts it into right corner of mouth, the epiglottis is lifted and the larynx exposed. A thin flexible intubation stylet may be used and the endotracheal tube (ETT) (in right hand) is inserted through the vocal cords and into the trachea, cuff inflated to minimal air leak (10 mL initially until patient stabilizes), and placement confirmed through capnometry or esophageal detection devices. While insertion depths vary, the generally accepted depth for males is 23 cm and for females is 21 cm. This acts as a starting point from which minor adjustments can be made. After insertion, the tube is secured.

**Review Video: Mechanical Ventilation**
Visit mometrix.com/academy and enter code: 679637

### RAPID SEQUENCE INTUBATION (RSI)

Rapid sequence intubation (RSI) is the simultaneous giving of a sedative and a paralytic in order to facilitate emergency intubation and is considered to be the standard of care for emergency airway management (except in patients with anticipated difficult intubation or in those with contraindications to sedatives/paralytics).

Initial preparation includes inserting 2 IV lines and establishing cardiac monitoring, oximetry, and capnography. The patient should be preoxygenated (100%) for at least 3 minutes, but without pressure ventilation that may cause aspiration of stomach contents. Procedure includes:

- **Induction agent**: Ketamine, etomidate, propofol
- **Paralysis**: Succinylcholine, rocuronium, other NMBAs
- **Sellick's maneuver** (pressure applied externally with thumb and index finger to cricoid) to close off the esophagus and prevent aspiration
- **Suction** to clear mouth if necessary
- **Laryngoscopy** to visual vocal cords
- **EET** inserted, cuff inflated, and ETT secured

Proper placement verified by capnometer or capnograph. Breath sounds should be auscultated. Post intubation chest x-ray to assess depth of tube and check for any trauma or issue. Induction agents and use of additional sedation may vary from one institution to another, but the primary goal is to safely anesthetize and intubate while preventing regurgitation of stomach contents.

### CONFIRMING CORRECT PLACEMENT OF ENDOTRACHEAL TUBES

There are a number of methods to **confirm correct placement** of endotracheal tubes. Clinical assessment alone is not adequate.

- **Capnometry** utilizes an end-tidal $CO_2$ ($ETCO_2$) detector that measures the concentration of $CO_2$ in expired air, usually through pH sensitive paper that changes color (commonly purple to yellow). The capnometer is attached to the ETT and a bag-valve-mask (BVM) ventilator is also attached. The patient is provided 6 ventilations and the $CO_2$ concentration is checked.
- **Capnography** is attached to the ETT and provides a waveform graph, showing the varying concentrations of $CO_2$ in real time throughout each ventilation (with increased $CO_2$ on expiration) and can indicate changes in respiratory status.

- **Esophageal detection devices** fit over the end of the ETT so that a large syringe can be used to attempt to aspirate. If the ETT is in the esophagus, the walls collapse on aspiration and resistance occurs, whereas the syringe fills with air if the ETT is in the trachea. A self-inflating bulb (Ellik device) may also be used.
- **Chest x-ray** provides visual confirmation of placement.

### *Ventilator Management*

There are many types of ventilators now in use, and the specific directions for each type must be followed carefully, but there are general principles that apply to all **ventilator management**. The following should be monitored:

- **Type of ventilation:** Volume-cycled, pressure-cycled, negative-pressure, HFJV, HFOV, CPAP, Bi-PAP
- **Control mode**: Controlled ventilation, assisted ventilation, synchronized intermittent mandatory (allows spontaneous breaths between ventilator-controlled inhalation/exhalation), positive end-expiratory pressure (PEEP), CPAP, Bi-PAP
- **Tidal volume** (TV) range should be set in relation to respiratory rate
- **Inspiratory-expiratory ratio** (I:E) usually ranges from 1:2–1:5, but may vary
- **Respiratory rate** will depend upon TV and $PaCO_2$ target
- **Fraction of inspired oxygen** ($FiO_2$) [percentage of oxygen in the inspired air], usually ranging from 21–100%, usually maintained <40% to avoid toxicity
- **Sensitivity** determines the effort needed to trigger inspiration
- **Pressure** controls the pressure exerted in delivering TV
- **Rate of flow** controls the L/min speed of TV

### *Tracheostomy*

Tracheostomy, surgical tracheal opening, may be utilized for mechanical ventilation. Tracheostomy tubes are inserted directly into an opening in the trachea to provide a conduit and maintain the opening. Tracheostomy tubes are usually silastic or plastic, and may have permanent or disposable inner cannulas. The tube is secured with ties around the neck. Because the air entering the lungs through the tracheostomy bypasses the warming and moistening effects of the upper airway, air is humidified through a room humidifier or through delivery of humidified air through a special mask or mechanical ventilation. The patient with a tracheostomy must have continuous monitoring of vital signs and respiratory status to ensure patency of tracheostomy. The inner cannula should be cleaned/replaced regularly (every 8–24 hours and PRN). Regular suctioning is needed, especially initially, to remove secretions:

- Suction catheter should be 50% the size of the tracheostomy tube to allow ventilation during suctioning
- Vacuum pressure: 80–100 mmHg
- Catheter should only be inserted ≤0.5 cm beyond tube to avoid damage to tissues or perforation
- Catheter should be inserted without suction and intermittent suction on withdrawal

### *Ventilation-Induced Lung Injury*

Ventilation-induced lung injury (VILI) is damage caused by mechanical ventilation. It is common in acute distress syndrome (ARDS) but can affect any mechanically ventilated patient. VILI comprises four interrelated elements:

- **Barotrauma**: Damage to the lung caused by excessive pressure
- **Volutrauma**: Alveolar damage related to high tidal volume ventilation
- **Atelectotrauma**: Injury caused by repetitive forced opening and closing of alveoli
- **Biotrauma**: Inflammatory response

In VILI, essentially the increased pressure and tidal volume over-distends the alveoli, which rupture, and air moves into the interstitial tissue resulting in pulmonary interstitial emphysema. With continued ventilation, the air in the interstitium moves into the subcutaneous tissue and may result in pneumopericardium and pneumomediastinum, or rupture the pleural sac which can cause tension pneumothorax and mediastinal shift, which can cause respiratory failure and cardiac arrest. VILI has caused a change in ventilation procedures with lower tidal volumes and pressures used as well as newer forms of ventilation, HFJV and HFOV, preferred to traditional mechanical ventilation for many patients.

### *PREVENTING COMPLICATIONS FROM VENTILATORS*

Methods to prevent complications from mechanical ventilation ("ventilator bundle") include:

- Elevate patient's head and chest to 30° to prevent aspiration and ventilation-associated pneumonia.
- Reposition patient every 2 hours.
- Provide DVT prophylaxis, such as external compression support and/or heparin (5000 u sq 2–3 times daily).
- Administer famotidine or pantoprazole PO/IV daily to prevent gastrointestinal stress-ulcers/bleeding.
- Decrease and eliminate sedation/analgesia as soon as possible—regular sedation vacations to assess neurological status.
- Follow careful protocols for pressure settings to prevent barotrauma. Tidal volumes are usually maintained at 8–12 mL/kg PBW (per AACN guidelines), but in incidences of high probability of ARDS, volumes should be less (6 mL/kg) to avoid lung injury.
- Monitor for pneumothorax or evidence of barotrauma.
- Conduct nutritional assessment (including lab tests) to prevent malnutrition.
- Monitor intake and output carefully and administer IV fluids to prevent dehydration.
- Do daily spontaneous breathing trials and discontinue ventilation as soon as possible.



### *VENTILATOR WEANING*

Ventilator weaning has three phases: Changing settings of the ventilator to allow the patient to demonstrate the ability to breath on their own (standby mode), extubation, and finally removal of supportive oxygen. Criteria for ventilator weaning may include some or all of the following, depending on facility guidelines:

- Vital capacity 10–15 mL/kg
- Maximum (negative) inspiratory pressure of at least -20 $cmH_2O$
- Tidal volume (TV) of 7–9 mL/kg
- Minute ventilation of about 6L/min (Respiratory rate x TV)
- Rapid shallow breathing index <100 breaths/min/L
- $PaO_2$ >60 mmHg
- $FiO_2$ <40%
- pH >7.25
- Hemodynamic stability (minimal to no dependence on vasopressors for blood pressure maintenance)

If these criteria are met and the patient passes a spontaneous breathing trial (SBT), then extubation can be done. Various protocols are followed in weaning patients off of ventilators, including the use of intermittent mandatory ventilation (IMV) and synchronized intermittent mandatory ventilation (SIMV), which can be used with pressure support ventilation (PSV).

**Criteria for oxygen weaning**:

- $FiO_2$ reduced until $PaO_2$ 70–100 mmHg on room air
- Supplemental $O_2$ necessary with $PaO_2$<70 mmHg (Medicare requires $PaO_2$ 55 mmHg for reimbursement for home oxygen use)

### *Spontaneous Breathing Trial as Preparation for Extubation*

A spontaneous breathing trial (SBT) is when a patient is taken off mechanical ventilation while remaining intubated (usually by changing the ventilator settings to CPAP) for a short period of time (30–120 minutes) to assess readiness to extubate. SBTs are often performed daily to ensure extubation possibility is identified as early as possible. SBT should be used prior to extubating a patient if the patient is not agitated and has no evidence of myocardial ischemia or increased ICP. The patient should exhibit some spontaneous triggering of respirations and should not be receiving large doses of vasopressor or inotropic agent. $SpO_2$ should be ≥88% with $FiO_2$ of 0.50 and PEEP at 7.5 $cmH_2O$ prior to the SBT. The SBT should be done in the morning for a prescribed period (usually 30–120 minutes). The ventilator rate is adjusted to 0 and pressure support decreased to 0–7. The SBT should be discontinued if the following occur:

- Respiratory rate >35 or <8 for at least 5 minutes
- Mental status changes
- $SpO_2$ <88% for >15 minutes
- Respiratory distress (HR >130 BPM or <60 BPM, marked dyspnea, diaphoresis, increased use of accessory respiratory muscles, respiratory arrest)

Patients who pass the SBT have an 85–90% chance of breathing successfully after extubation. Patients who repeatedly fail daily SBT may require tracheostomy.

### *Failure to Wean from Mechanical Ventilation*

Failure to wean from mechanical ventilation can occur in approximately 20–30% of ventilated patients. Many factors affect a patient's ability to wean from mechanical ventilation including physical, psychological, and situational factors. Before discontinuation of ventilation can be considered, the patient must be able to protect his/her airway, be hemodynamically stable and have resolution of the clinical problem that initiated the need for mechanical ventilation. Weaning protocols use clinical criteria such as oxygen saturation, blood pressure, respiratory rate, and tidal volume to determine the patient's tolerance of lessening mechanical ventilator support. Failure to wean is demonstrated by multiple daily spontaneous breathing trial failures or the need for reintubation within 48 hours of extubation. Failure to resolve the clinical problem(s) that initiated mechanical ventilation, insufficient ventilator drive, respiratory muscle weakness, co-morbidities, and/or the development of new clinical problems (e.g., infection) may contribute to the inability to wean.

**Signs/symptoms**: Decreased tidal volume, increased respiratory rate, increased $PaCO_2$, oxygen desaturation, anxiety, diaphoresis, fatigue, changes in blood pressure or heart rate, mental status changes, and hemodynamic changes.

**Treatment**: The initial treatment strategy for patients who experience a dysfunctional ventilator weaning response is identification and treatment of the underlying cause(s) of the weaning failure. In addition, other treatment strategies may include psychological preparation of the patient for further weaning attempts, readiness testing and respiratory muscle training.

## Sedation/Analgesia with Mechanical Ventilation

Patients intubated for mechanical ventilation are usually given **sedation and/or analgesia** initially, but medications should be reduced and given in boluses rather than with continuous IV drip with a goal of stopping sedation as it prolongs ventilation time. Typical sedatives include midazolam, propofol, and lorazepam. Narcotic analgesics include fentanyl and morphine sulfate. Uses of sedation include:

- Controlling agitation and excessive movement that may interfere with ventilation
- Reduce pain and discomfort associated with ventilation
- Control respiratory distress

Triglyceride levels must be checked periodically if propofol is administered for more than 24–48 hours. Neuromuscular blocking agents are rarely used because they may cause long-term weakness and increase length of ventilation although they may be indicated in some cases, such as with excessive shivering or cardiac arrest. Many patients are able to tolerate mechanical ventilation without sedation, and sedation should always be decreased to the minimal amount necessary as excess sedation may delay extubation. An ideal level of sedation will keep the patient calm and compliant with the ventilator but still alert and able to follow commands.

### CONSCIOUS SEDATION

Conscious sedation is used to decrease sensations of pain and awareness caused by a surgical or invasive procedure, such a biopsy, chest tube insertion, fracture repair, and endoscopy. It is also used during presurgical preparations, such as insertion of central lines, catheters, and use of cooling blankets. Conscious sedation uses a combination of analgesia and sedation so that patients can remain responsive and follow verbal cues but have a brief amnesia preventing recall of the procedures. The patient must be monitored carefully, including pulse oximetry, during this type of sedation. The most commonly used drugs include:

- Midazolam (Versed): This is a short-acting water-soluble sedative, with onset of 1–5 minutes, peaking in 30, and duration usually about 1 hour (up to 6 hours).
- Fentanyl: This is a short-acting opioid with immediate onset, peaking in 10–15 minutes and with a duration of about 20–45 minutes. Monitor respiratory function.

The fentanyl/midazolam combination provides both sedation and pain control. Conscious sedation usually requires 6 hours fasting prior to administration.

### THERAPEUTIC GASES

**Carbon dioxide** is a potent stimulator of respirations, but it is rarely used therapeutically because it can depress respirations if hypercarbia or respiratory acidosis is present. $CO_2$ may be administered at times as part of anesthesia, but it is most commonly used for insufflation for laparoscopic/endoscopic procedures.

**Nitric oxide** (NO) is used as a pulmonary vessel dilator to improve oxygenation by decreasing pulmonary artery pressure and pulmonary vascular resistance. NO is FDA-approved for use for neonatal PPH but is sometimes used for adults with pulmonary arterial hypertension (PAH) who require acute vasodilator testing prior to initiating additional therapies. NO is an effective drug to use when testing acute vasoreactivity. During acute vasodilator testing, inhaled NO is administered at 10–80 ppm for 5–10 minutes during which hemodynamics are measured and monitored. Studies have not shown it to be an effective treatment for ARDS. Toxic reactions include methemoglobinemia and platelet inhibition with resultant bleeding.

**Heliox** is helium mixed with oxygen that is used to reduce airway resistance during mechanical ventilation and for pulmonary function tests. Heliox may also be used to treat respiratory obstruction and is used during laser surgery on the airway because it readily conducts heat away from the surgical site, reducing tissue damage. Heliox is sometimes used for COPD patients as it increases hyperventilation and reduces carbon dioxide levels.

## THORACENTESIS

A thoracentesis (aspiration of fluid or air from pleural space) is done to make a diagnosis, relieve pressure on the lung caused by pleural effusion, or instill medications. A chest x-ray is done prior to the procedure. A sedative may be given. The patient is in a sitting position, leaning onto a padded bedside stand, straddling a chair with head supported on the back of the chair, or lying on the opposite side with the head of the bed elevated 30–45° to ensure that fluid remains at the base. The patient should avoid coughing or moving during the procedure. The chest x-ray or ultrasound determines needle placement. After a local anesthetic is administered, a needle (with an attached 20-mL syringe and 3-way stopcock with tubing and a receptacle) is advanced intercostally into the pleural space. Fluid is drained, collected, examined, and measured. The needle is removed and a pressure dressing applied. A chest x-ray is done to ensure there is no pneumothorax. The patient is monitored for cough, dyspnea, and hypoxemia.

**Review Video: Thoracentesis**
Visit mometrix.com/academy and enter code: 321111

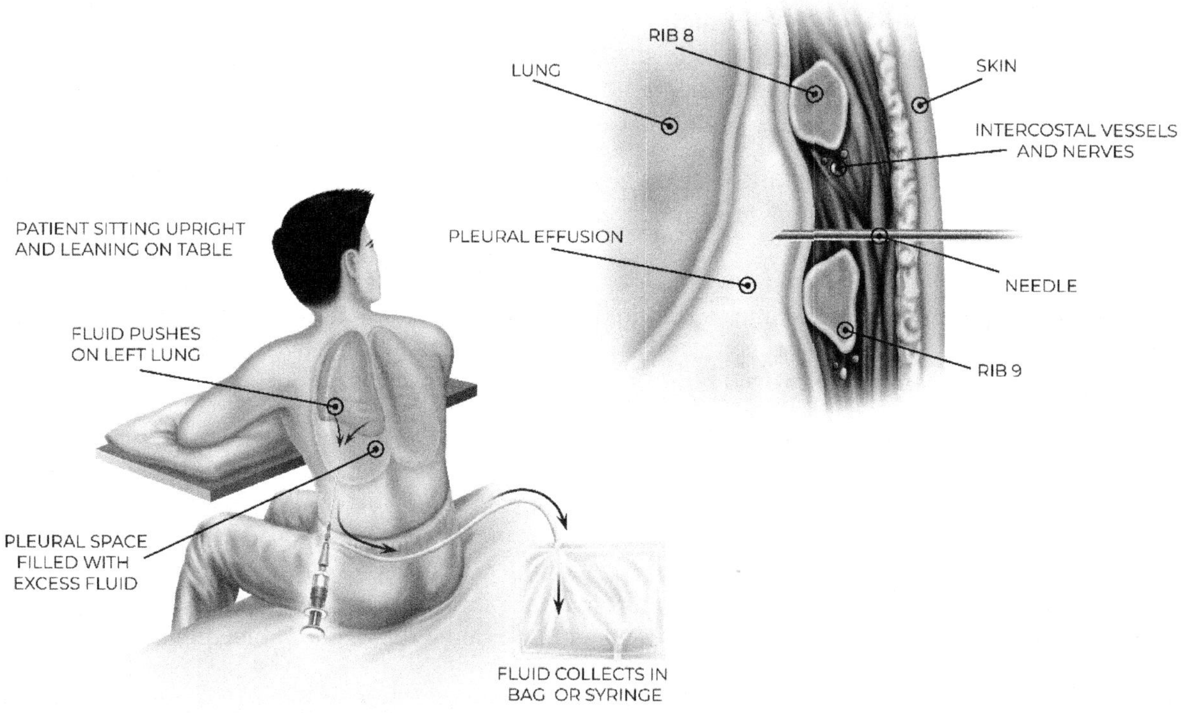

### Bronchoscopy

Bronchoscopy utilizes a thin, flexible fiberoptic bronchoscope to inspect the larynx, trachea, and bronchi for diagnostic purposes. It is also used to collect specimens, obtain biopsies, remove foreign bodies or secretions, treat atelectasis, and to excise lesions. The patient is in supine position during the procedure. The Mallampati classification may be used to determine difficulty of airway. The patient receives local anesthesia to the nares (lidocaine gel) and oropharynx (lidocaine gel, spray, or nebulizer), and usually receives a benzodiazepine (commonly midazolam or lorazepam), an opioid (fentanyl or meperidine), or propofol. Medications are usually given in small incremental doses throughout the procedure and may be combined. Over-sedation may cause physiologic depression, but undersedation may result in recall and agitation with sympathetic activation. The tube is advanced through the nares and down the trachea to the bronchi. Airway patency, respiratory rate, and oxygen saturation must be constantly monitored. Complications can include bleeding, arrhythmias, obstruction, laryngospasm, and respiratory failure.

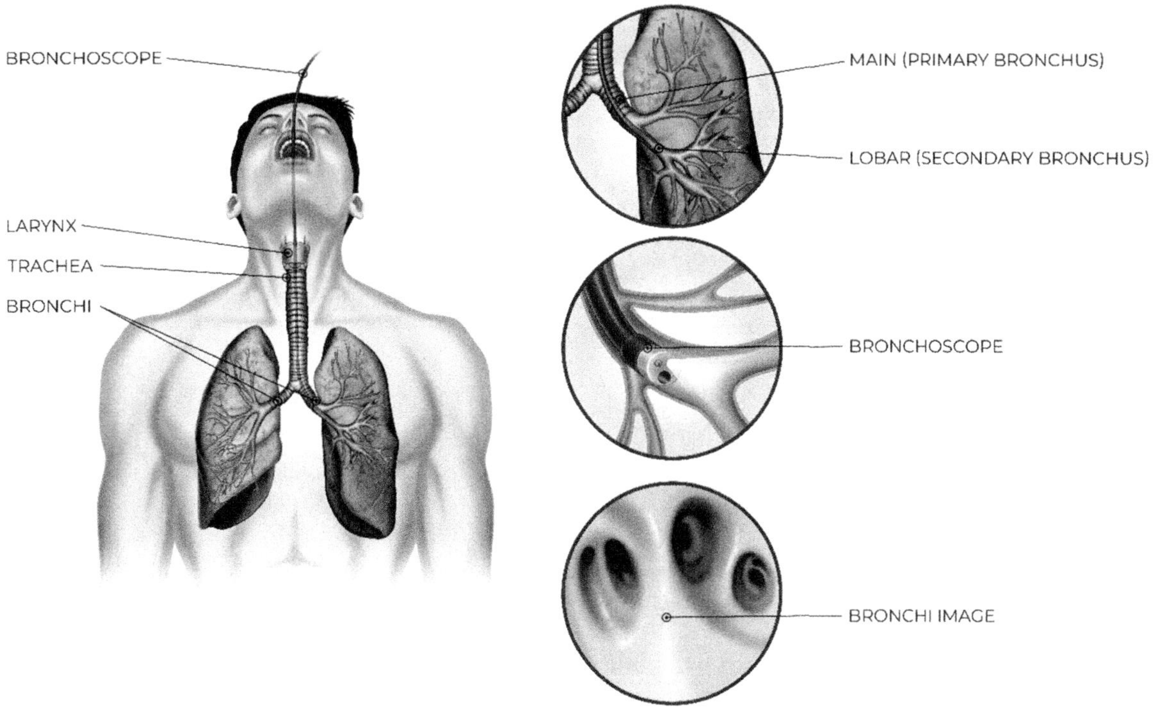


### Chest Tubes

Chest tubes with a closed drainage system are usually left in place after thoracic surgery or pneumothorax to drain air or fluid. Nursing interventions during insertion include ensuring the patient receives adequate pain control, attending to sterile technique, assisting the physician with suturing as needed, attaching the tube to the chest tube drainage device, placing an occlusive dressing, and confirming placement.

Chest tube drainage systems have three major parts: suction control, water seal, and a chamber for collection. The system should have no bubbling in the water seal area (such would indicate a leak), but a subtle rise and fall of the water seal corresponding with respirations, and gentle bubbling in the suction control chamber.

Physiological Adaptation

Nursing interventions after chest tube is in place: in most circumstances, report drainage >100 mL/hr, assess tubing after position changes for occlusion, maintain sterile dressing, avoid stripping the tubing, and assessing the insertion site for drainage or crepitus, the tubing, the patency of the entire system, and the output (including color, amount, and any other traits). The nurse should be knowledgeable about specimen collection, replacing the system, and dealing with clots.

**Review Video: Chest Tubes**
Visit mometrix.com/academy and enter code: 696975

# Neurological Pathophysiology

## Encephalopathies

### *Hypertensive Encephalopathy with Cerebral Edema*

Hypertensive encephalopathy can occur as part of a hypertensive crisis. With chronic hypertension, the brain adapts to higher pressures to regulate blood flow, but in a hypertensive crisis, autoregulation of the blood-brain barrier is overwhelmed and the capillaries leak fluid into the tissue and vasodilation takes place with resultant cerebral edema. Damage to arterioles occurs, causing increasing neurological deficits and papilledema. Hypertensive encephalopathy is relatively rare, but carries a high mortality rate and is most common in middle-aged males with long-standing hypertension. **Symptoms** usually develop over 1–2 days and include:

- Non-specific neurological deficits, such as weakness and visual abnormalities
- Alterations in mental status, including confusion
- Headache, often constant
- Nausea and vomiting
- Seizures
- Coma

### *Treatment for Hypertensive Encephalopathy with Cerebral Edema*

Hypertensive encephalopathy with cerebral edema requires prompt treatment in order to prevent neurological damage.

**Treatment** includes identifying and treating the underlying causes for the hypertensive crisis and taking steps to lower the blood pressure:

- **Nitroprusside sodium** is usually used initially to lower BP. However, caution must be used not to lower the blood pressure too quickly, as this can lead to cerebral ischemia. Other antihypertensive medications used include clevidipine, nicardipine, fenoldopam, and labetalol.
- **Positioning** of the patient to prevent obstruction of venous return from the head
- **Monitoring blood gas** and maintaining $PaCO_2$ at 33–37 mmHg to facilitate vasoconstriction of cerebral arteries
- **Preventing hyperthermia** with antipyretics and cooling devices
- **BP monitoring** and maintenance
- **Seizure control** with phenobarbital and/or phenytoin
- **Lidocaine** through endotracheal tube or intravenously prior to nasotracheal suctioning
- **Diuretics**, such as osmotic agents (mannitol) and loop diuretics (furosemide) to control fluid volume
- **Controlling metabolic demand** by measures to increase pain control and reduce stimulation
- **Barbiturates** (pentobarbital, thiopental) in high doses may be used if other treatments fail to decrease intracranial pressure

### *Hypoxic Encephalopathy*

Cerebral hypoxia (hypoxic encephalopathy) occurs when the oxygen supply to the brain is decreased. If hypoxia is mild, the brain compensates by increasing cerebral blood flow, but it can only double in volume and cannot compensate for severe hypoxic conditions. Hypoxia may be the result of insufficient oxygen in the environment, inadequate exchange at the alveolar level of the lungs, or inadequate circulation to the brain. Brain cells may begin dying within 5 minutes if deprived of adequate oxygenation, so any condition or trauma that interferes with oxygenation can result in brain damage:

- Near-drowning
- Asphyxia
- Cardiac arrest
- High altitude sickness
- Carbon monoxide
- Diseases that interfere with respiration, such as myasthenia gravis and amyotrophic lateral sclerosis
- Anesthesia complications

**Symptoms** include increasing neurological deficits, depending upon the degree and area of damage, with changes in mentation that range from confusion to coma. Prompt identification of the cause and increase in perfusion to the brain is critical for survival.

### *Metabolic Encephalopathy*

Metabolic encephalopathy (hepatic encephalopathy) is damage to the brain resulting from a disturbance in metabolism, primarily hepatic failure to remove toxins from the blood. There may be impairment in cerebral blood flow, cerebral edema, or increased intracranial pressure. It can occur as the result of the ingestion of drugs or toxins which can have a direct toxic effect on neurons, but it can also occur with liver disease, especially when stressed by co-morbidities, such as hemorrhage, hypoxemia, surgery, trauma, renal failure with dialysis, or electrolyte imbalances.

**Symptoms** may vary:

- Irritability and agitation
- Alterations in consciousness
- Dysphonia
- Lack of coordination, spasticity
- Seizures are common and may be the presenting symptom
- Disorientation progressing to coma

Prompt diagnosis is important because the condition may be reversible if underlying causes are identified and treated before permanent neuronal damage occurs.

**Treatment** varies according to the underlying cause.

### *Infectious Encephalopathy*

Infectious encephalopathy is an encompassing term describing encephalopathies caused by a wide range of bacteria, viruses, or prions. Common to all infections are altered brain function that results in alterations in consciousness and personality, cognitive impairment, and lethargy. A wide range of neurological symptoms may occur: myoclonus, seizures, dysphagia, and dysphonia, neuromuscular impairment with muscle atrophy and tremors or spasticity. **Treatment** depends on the underlying cause and response to treatment. Prion infections are not treatable, but bacterial infections may respond to antibiotic therapy, and viral infections may be self-limiting. HIV-related encephalopathy results from opportunistic infections as immune responses decrease, usually indicated by CD4 counts $<50$. Aggressive antiretroviral treatment and treatment of the infection may reverse symptoms if permanent damage has not occurred for HIV-related encephalopathy.

Treatment for other infectious encephalopathies varies according to the type of infection and underlying causes.

## Cerebral Aneurysms

Cerebral aneurysms, the weakening and dilation of a cerebral artery, are usually congenital (90%) while the remaining (10%) result from direct trauma or infection. Aneurysms are usually 2–7 mm in size and occur in the Circle of Willis at the base of the brain.

Circle of Willis

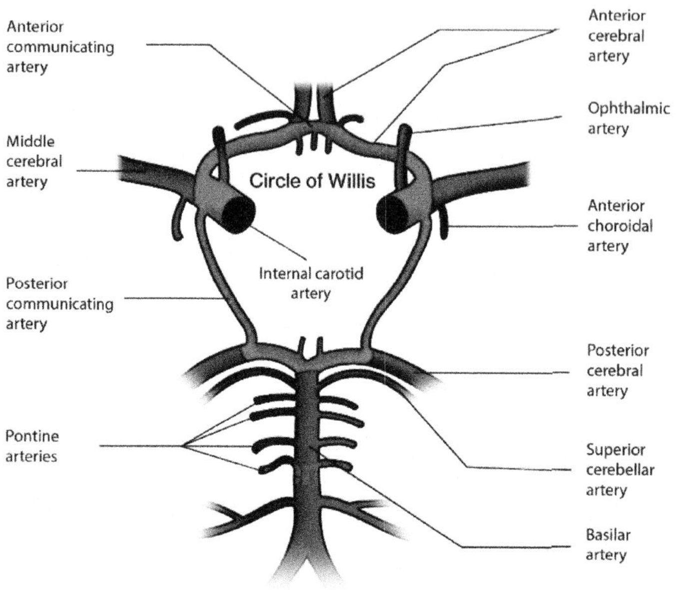


A rupturing aneurysm may decrease perfusion as well as increasing pressure on surrounding brain tissue. Cerebral aneurysms are classified as follows:

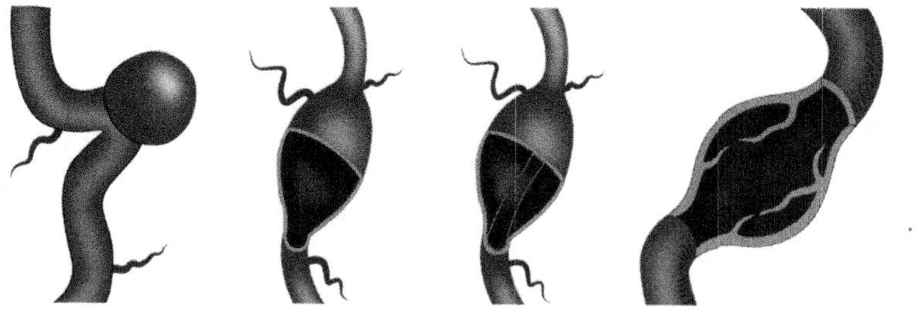

Saccular Fusiform Dissecting Mycotic

- **Berry/saccular:** The most common congenital type occurs at a bifurcation and grows from the base on a stem, usually at the Circle of Willis.
- **Fusiform**: Large and irregular (>2.5 cm) and rarely ruptures but causes increased intracranial pressure. Usually involves the internal carotid or vertebrobasilar artery.
- **Mycotic**: Rare type that occurs secondary to bacterial infection and aseptic emboli.
- **Dissecting**: Wall is torn apart and blood enters layers. This may occur during angiography or secondary to trauma or disease.
- **Traumatic Charcot-Bouchard (pseudoaneurysm):** Small lesion resulting from chronic hypertension.

## Arteriovenous Malformation

Arteriovenous malformation (AVM) is a congenital abnormality within the brain consisting of a tangle of dilated arteries and veins without a capillary bed. AVMs can occur anywhere in the brain and may cause no significant problems. Usually the AVM is "fed" by one or more cerebral arteries, which enlarge over time, shunting more blood through the AVM. The veins also enlarge in response to increased arterial blood flow because of the lack of a capillary bridge between the two. Because vein walls are thinner and lack the muscle layer of an artery, the veins tend to rupture as the AVM becomes larger, causing a subarachnoid hemorrhage. Chronic ischemia that may be related to the AVM can result in cerebral atrophy. Sometimes small leaks, usually accompanied by headache and nausea and vomiting, may occur before rupture. AVMs may cause a wide range of neurological symptoms, including changes in mentation, dizziness, sensory abnormalities, confusion, increasing ICP, and dementia.

**ARTERIOVENOUS MALFORMATION**

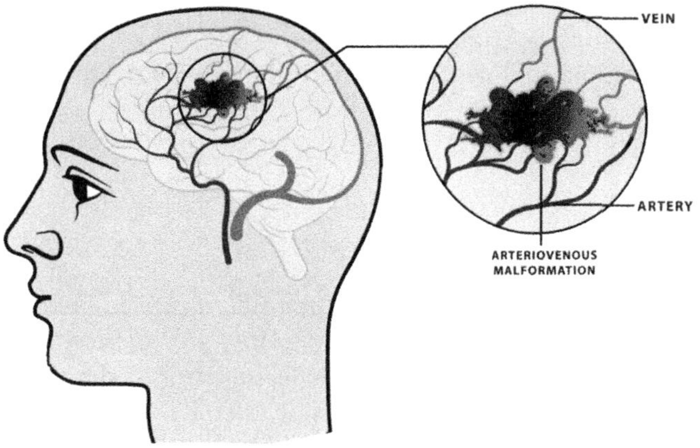




**Treatment** includes:

- Supportive management of symptoms
- Surgical repair or focused irradiation (definitive treatments)

## Intracranial/Intraventricular Hemorrhage

### *Epidural and Subdural*

**Epidural hemorrhage** is bleeding between the dura and the skull that pushes the brain downward and inward. The hemorrhage is usually caused by arterial tears, so bleeding is often rapid, leading to severe neurological deficits and respiratory arrest.

**Subdural hemorrhage** is bleeding between the dura and the cerebrum, usually from tears in the cortical veins of the subdural space. It tends to develop more slowly than epidural hemorrhage and can result in a subdural hematoma. If the bleeding is acute and develops within minutes or hours of injury, the prognosis is poor. Subacute hematomas that develop more slowly cause varying degrees of injury. Subdural hemorrhage is a common injury related to trauma but it can also result from coagulopathies or aneurysms. Symptoms of acute injury may occur within 24–48 hours, but subacute bleeding may not be evident for up to 2 weeks after injury. Chronic hemorrhage occurs primarily in the elderly. Symptoms vary and may include bradycardia, tachycardia, hypertension, and alterations in consciousness. Older children and adults usually require surgical evacuation of the hematoma.

### *Subarachnoid*

**Subarachnoid hemorrhage (SAH)** may occur after trauma but is a common result of rupture of a berry aneurysm or an arteriovenous malformation (AVM). However, there are a number of disorders that may be implicated: neoplasms, sickle cell disease, infection, hemophilia, and leukemia. The first presenting symptom may be complaints of severe headache, nausea and vomiting, nuchal rigidity, palsy related to cranial nerve compression, retinal hemorrhages, and papilledema. Late complications include hyponatremia and hydrocephalus. **Symptoms** worsen as intracranial pressure rises. SAH from aneurysm is classified as follows:

- **Grade I**: No symptoms or slight headache and nuchal rigidity
- **Grade II**: Moderate to severe headache with nuchal rigidity and cranial nerve palsy
- **Grade III**: Drowsy, progressing to confusion or mild focal deficits
- **Grade IV**: Stupor, with hemiparesis (moderate to severe), early decerebrate rigidity, and vegetative disturbances
- **Grade V**: Coma state with decerebrate rigidity

**Treatment** includes:

- Identifying and treating underlying cause
- Observing for re-bleeding
- Anti-seizure medications (such as levetiracetam or phenytoin) to control seizures
- Antihypertensives
- Surgical repair if indicated

## Hydrocephalus

### *Communicating and Noncommunicating*

The ventricular system produces and circulates cerebrospinal fluid (CSF). The right and left lateral ventricles open into the third ventricle at the interventricular foramen (foramen of Monro). The aqueduct of Sylvius connects the third and fourth ventricles. The fourth ventricle, anterior to the cerebellum, supplies CSF to the subarachnoid space and the spinal cord (dorsal surface). The CSF circulates and then returns to the brain and is absorbed in the arachnoid villi. **Hydrocephalus** occurs when there is an imbalance between production and absorption of cerebrospinal fluid in the ventricles, resulting from impaired absorption or obstruction, which may be congenital or acquired. There are two common types of hydrocephalus:

- **Communicating:** CSF flows (communicates) between the ventricles but is not absorbed in the subarachnoid space (arachnoid villi).
- **Noncommunicating:** CSF is obstructed (non-communicating) between the ventricles, with the obstruction most often due to stenosis of the aqueduct of Sylvius.

### *Symptoms*

**Symptoms** of hydrocephalus depend on the age of onset. In *early infancy*, before closure of cranial sutures, head enlargement is the most common presentation, but in adults with less elasticity in the skull, neurological symptoms usually relate to increasing pressure on structures of the brain. Hydrocephalus may occur at any age, but the type that occurs in *young/middle-aged adults* is different than that common in children or those >50. Hydrocephalus in young and middle-aged adults may result from a congenital defect, hydrocephalus of infancy with shunt failure, or trauma and is characterized by:

- Headache relieved by vomiting
- Papilledema
- Lack of bladder control
- Strabismus and other visual disorders
- Ataxia
- Irritability
- Lethargy
- Confusion and impairment of cognitive abilities

With **adult-onset normal pressure hydrocephalus** (>50) cerebrospinal fluid increases and dilates the ventricles, but frequently without increasing intracranial pressure. The cause is often unclear. Symptoms include gait disturbance, bladder control issues, and mild dementia

### *Treatment*

Hydrocephalus is diagnosed through CT and MRI scans, which help to determine the cause. **Treatment** may vary somewhat depending upon the underlying disorder. For example, if obstruction is caused by a tumor, surgical excision to directly remove the obstruction is required. Generally, however, most hydrocephalus is treated with shunts:

- **Ventricular-peritoneal shunt:** This procedure is the most common and consists of placing a ventricular catheter directly into the ventricles (usually lateral) at one end with the other end in the peritoneal area to drain away excess CSF. There is a one-way valve near the proximal end that prevents backflow but opens when pressure rises to drain fluid. In some cases, the distal end drains into the right atrium.
- **Third ventriculostomy:** A small opening is made in the base of the third ventricle so CSF can bypass an obstruction. This procedure is not common and is done with a small endoscope.

## Neurologic Infectious Disease

### *Bacterial Meningitis*

Bacterial meningitis may be caused by a wide range of bacteria, including *Streptococcus pneumoniae* and *Neisseria meningitidis.* Bacteria can enter the CNS from distant infection, surgical wounds, invasive devices, nasal colonization, or penetrating trauma. The infective process includes inflammation, exudates, WBC accumulation, and brain tissue damage with hyperemia and edema. Purulent exudate covers the brain and invades and blocks the ventricles, obstructing CSF and leading to increased intracranial pressure. **Symptoms** include abrupt onset, fever, chills, severe headache, nuchal rigidity, and alterations of consciousness with seizures, agitation, and irritability. Antibodies specific to bacteria don't cross the blood brain barrier, so immune response is poor. Some may have photophobia, hallucinations, and/or aggressive behavior or may become stuporous and lapse into coma. Nuchal rigidity may progress to opisthotonos. Reflexes are variable but Kernig and Brudzinski signs are often positive. Signs may relate to particular bacteria, such as rashes, sore joints, or a draining ear. **Diagnosis** is usually based on lumbar puncture examination of cerebrospinal fluid and symptoms. **Treatment** includes IV antibiotics and supportive care: fluids, a dark and calm environment, measures to reduce ICP, etc.



### *Fungal Meningitis*

Fungal meningitis is the least common cause of meningitis. It occurs when a fungal organism enters into the subarachnoid space, cerebral spinal fluid, and meninges. Immune deficient patients such as those with HIV, cancer, or immunodeficiency syndromes are most at risk for the development of fungal meningitis. The most common organisms causing fungal meningitis are candida albicans and Cryptococcus neoformans. Fungal meningitis caused by candida may occur in immunosuppressed patients, in those who have had a ventricular shunt placed, or in those that have had a lumbar puncture performed. Cryptococcus is a fungus found in soil throughout the world and does not usually affect people with a healthy immune system. Cryptococcal meningitis is most commonly seen in patients with HIV/AIDS and is one of the leading causes of death in HIV/AIDS patients in certain parts of Africa.

**Signs/symptoms**: Headache, fever, nausea and vomiting, stiff neck, photophobia, and mental status changes.

**Diagnosis**: Lumbar puncture with subsequent culture of cerebral spinal fluid. In addition, blood cultures may be obtained as well as a CT of the head.

**Treatment**: The treatment of fungal meningitis involves a long course of anti-fungal medications, including Amphotericin B, flucytosine, and fluconazole. Anticonvulsants may be administered for seizure control.

**Review Video: Meningitis**
Visit mometrix.com/academy and enter code: 277418

### *Viral Infections That Can Impact the Neurological System*

Many different types of viral infections can impact the neurological system either by direct infection transmitted through the bloodstream or by spreading along the nerve pathways (such as rabies). Common viral infections affecting the neurological system include:

- **Viral encephalitis**: Arboviral infections are transmitted from an animal host to an arthropod (typically a mosquito or tick) to humans, who are typically dead-end hosts. Arboviral infections include western equine encephalitis, eastern equine encephalitis, St. Louis encephalitis, Powassan encephalitis, Colorado tick fever and La Crosse encephalitis. West Nile virus may also invade the CNS and cause encephalitis.
- **Viral meningitis**: Viral meningitis is usually self-limiting within 7–10 days and is less severe than bacterial meningitis.
- **Herpes virus**: Herpes simplex virus can invade the nervous system and cause herpes simplex encephalitis, which has a high mortality rate.
- **HIV**: Inflammation may affect the CNS and interfere with neuronal functions.

## Neuromuscular Disorders

### *Multiple Sclerosis*

Multiple sclerosis is an autoimmune disorder of the CNS in which the myelin sheath around the nerves is damaged and replaced by scar tissue that prevents conduction of nerve impulses.

**Symptoms** vary widely and can include problems with balance and coordination, tremors, slurring of speech, cognitive impairment, vision impairment, nystagmus, pain, and bladder and bowel dysfunction. Symptoms may be relapsing-remitting, progressive, or a combination. Onset is usually at 20–30 years of age, with incidence higher in females. Patient may initially present with problems walking or falling or optic neuritis (30%) causing loss of central vision. Males may complain of sexual dysfunction as an early symptom. Others have dysuria with urinary retention.

**Diagnosis** is based on clinical and neurological examination and MRI. **Treatment** is symptomatic and includes treatment to shorten duration of episodes and slow progress.

- **Glucocorticoids**: Methylprednisolone
- **Immunomodulator**: Interferon beta, glatiramer acetate, natalizumab
- **Immunosuppressant**: Mitoxantrone
- **Hormone**: Estriol (for females)

**Review Video: Multiple Sclerosis (MS)**
Visit mometrix.com/academy and enter code: 417355

### *ALS*

Amyotrophic lateral sclerosis (ALS) is a progressive degenerative disease of the upper and lower motor neurons, resulting in progressively severe symptoms such as spasticity, hyperreflexia, muscle weakness, and paralysis that can cause dysphagia, cramping, muscular atrophy, and respiratory dysfunction. ALS may be sporadic or familial (rare). Speech may become monotone; however, cognitive functioning usually remains intact. Eventually, patients become immobile and cannot breathe independently.

**Diagnosis** is based on history, electromyography, nerve conduction studies, and MRI. Treatment includes riluzole to delay progression of the disease. Patients in the ED usually have been diagnosed and have developed an acute complication, such as acute respiratory failure, aspiration pneumonia, or other trauma.

**Treatment** includes:

- Nebulizer treatments with bronchodilators and steroids
- Antibiotics for infection
- Mechanical ventilation

If **ventilatory assistance** is needed, it is important to determine if the patient has a living will expressing the wish to be ventilated or not or has assigned power of attorney for health matters to someone to make this decision.

**Review Video: Amyotrophic Lateral Sclerosis (ALS)**
Visit mometrix.com/academy and enter code: 178603

### *Parkinson's Disease*

Parkinson's disease (PD) is an extrapyramidal movement motor system disorder caused by loss of brain cells that produce dopamine. Typical symptoms include tremor of face and extremities, rigidity, bradykinesia, akinesia, poor posture, and a lack of balance and coordination causing increasing problems with mobility, talking, and swallowing. Some may suffer depression and mood changes. Tremors usually present unilaterally in an upper extremity.

**Diagnosis** includes:

- **Cogwheel rigidity test**: The extremity is put through passive range of motion, which causes increased muscle tone and ratchet-like movements.
- **Physical and neurological exam**
- **Complete history** to rule out drug-induced Parkinson akinesia

**Treatment** includes:

- Symptomatic support
- Dopaminergic therapy: Levodopa, amantadine, and carbidopa
- Anticholinergics: Trihexyphenidyl, benztropine
- For drug-induced Parkinson's, terminate drugs

Drug therapy tends to decrease in effectiveness over time, and patients may present with a marked increase in symptoms. Discontinuing the drugs for 1 week may exacerbate symptoms initially, but functioning may improve when drugs are reintroduced.

### *Guillain-Barré Syndrome*

Guillain-Barré syndrome (GBS) is an autoimmune disorder of the myelinated motor peripheral nervous system, causing ascending and descending paralysis. GBS is often triggered by a viral infection, but may be idiopathic in origin. Diagnosis is by history, clinical symptoms, and lumbar puncture, which often show increased protein with normal glucose and cell count although protein may not increase for a week or more.

**Review Video: Guillain-Barre Syndrome**
Visit mometrix.com/academy and enter code: 742900

**Symptoms** include:

- Numbness and tingling with increasing weakness of lower extremities that may become generalized, sometimes resulting in complete paralysis and inability to breathe without ventilatory support.
- Deep tendon reflexes are typically absent and some people experience facial weakness and ophthalmoplegia (paralysis of muscles controlling movement of eyes).

**Treatment** includes:

- Supportive: Fluids, physical therapy, and antibiotics for infections
- Patients should be hospitalized for observation and placed on ventilator support if forced vital capacity is reduced.
- While there is no definitive treatment, plasma exchange or IV immunoglobulin may shorten the duration of symptoms.

### *Muscular Dystrophy*

Muscular dystrophies are genetic disorders with gradual degeneration of muscle fibers and progressive weakness and atrophy of skeletal muscles and loss of mobility. **Pseudohypertrophic (Duchenne) muscular dystrophy** is the most common form and the most severe. It is an X-linked disorder in about 50% of the cases with the rest sporadic mutations, affecting males almost exclusively. Children typically have some delay in motor development with difficulty walking and have evidence of muscle weakness by about age 3. Pseudohypertrophic refers to enlargement of muscles by fatty infiltration associated with muscular atrophy, which causes contractures and deformities of joints. Abnormal bone development results in spinal and other skeletal deformities. The disease progresses rapidly, and most children are wheelchair bound by about 12 years of age. As the disease progresses, it involves the muscles of the diaphragm and other muscles needed for respiration. Mild to frank mental deficiency is common. Facial, oropharyngeal, and respiratory muscles weaken late in the disease. Cardiomegaly commonly occurs. Death most often relates to respiratory infection or cardiac failure by age 25. Treatment is supportive.

### *Cerebral Palsy*

Cerebral palsy (CP) is a non-progressive motor dysfunction related to CNS damage associated with congenital, hypoxic, or traumatic injury before, during, or ≤2 years after birth. It may include visual defects, speech impairment, seizures, and intellectual disability. There are four **types of motor dysfunction:**

- **Spastic**: Damage to the cerebral cortex or pyramidal tract. Constant hypertonia and rigidity lead to contractures and curvature of the spine.
- **Dyskinetic**: Damage to the extrapyramidal, basal ganglia. Tremors and twisting with exaggerated posturing and impairment of voluntary muscle control.
- **Ataxic**: Damage to the extrapyramidal cerebellum. Atonic muscles in infancy with lack of balance, instability of muscles, and poor gait.
- **Mixed**: Combinations of all three types with multiple areas of damage.

**Characteristics** of CP include:

- Hypotonia or hypertonia with rigidity and spasticity
- Athetosis (constant writhing motions)
- Ataxia
- Hemiplegia (one-sided involvement, more severe in upper extremities)
- Diplegia (all extremities involved, but more severe in lower extremities)
- Quadriplegia (all extremities involved with arms flexed and legs extended)

### *Myasthenia Gravis*

Myasthenia gravis is an autoimmune disorder that results in sporadic, progressive weakness of striated (skeletal) muscles because of impaired transmission of nerve impulses. Myasthenia gravis usually affects muscles controlled by the cranial nerves although any muscle group may be affected. Many patients also have thymomas.

**Signs/symptoms** include weakness and fatigue that worsens throughout the day. Patients often exhibit ptosis and diplopia. They may have trouble chewing and swallowing and often appear to have masklike facies. If respiratory muscles are involved, patients may exhibit signs of respiratory failure. Myasthenic crisis occurs when patients can no longer breathe independently.

**Diagnosis** includes electromyography and the Tensilon test (an IV injection of edrophonium or neostigmine, which improves function if the patient has myasthenia gravis, but does not improve function if the symptoms are from a different cause). CT or MRI to diagnose thymoma.

**Treatment** includes anticholinesterase drugs (neostigmine, pyridostigmine) to relieve some muscle weakness, but these drugs lose effectiveness as the disease progresses. Corticosteroids may be used. Thymectomy is performed if thymoma is present. Tracheotomy and mechanical ventilation may be needed for myasthenic crisis.

**Review Video: Myasthenia Gravis**
Visit mometrix.com/academy and enter code: 162510

## Seizure Disorders

### *Partial Seizures*

Partial seizures are caused by electrical discharges to a localized area of the cerebral cortex, such as the frontals, temporal, or parietal lobes with seizure characteristics related to the area of involvement. They may begin in a focal area and become generalized, often preceded by an aura.

- **Simple partial:** Unilateral motor symptoms including somatosensory, psychic, and autonomic
  - Aversive: Eyes and head turned away from focal side
  - Sylvan (usually during sleep): Tonic-clonic movements of the face, salivation, and arrested speech
- **Special sensory:** Various sensations (numbness, tingling, prickling, or pain) spreading from one area. May include visual sensations, posturing or hypertonia.
- **Complex (psychomotor):** No loss of consciousness, but altered consciousness and non-responsive with amnesia. May involve complex sensorium with bad tastes, auditory or visual hallucinations, feeling of déjà vu, strong fear. May carry out repetitive activities, such as walking, running, smacking lips, chewing, or drawling. Rarely aggressive. Seizure usually followed by prolonged drowsiness and confusion. Most common ages 3 through adolescence.

### *Generalized Seizures*

Generalized seizures lack a focal onset and appear to involve both hemispheres, usually presenting with loss of consciousness and no preceding aura.

- **Tonic-clonic (Grand Mal)**: Occurs without warning
  - Tonic period (10–30 seconds): Eyes roll upward with loss of consciousness, arms flexed; stiffen in symmetric tonic contraction of body, apneic with cyanosis and salivating
  - Clonic period (10 seconds to 30 minutes, but usually 30 seconds). Violent rhythmic jerking with contraction and relaxation. May be incontinent of urine and feces. Contractions slow and then stop.

Following seizures, there may be confusion, disorientation, and impairment of motor activity, speech, and vision for several hours. Headache, nausea, and vomiting may occur. Person often falls asleep and awakens more lucid.

- **Absence (Petit Mal):** Onset is at ages 4–12 and usually ends in puberty. Onset is abrupt with brief loss of consciousness for 5–10 seconds and slight loss of muscle tone but often appears to be daydreaming. Lip smacking or eye twitching may occur.

### *Epilepsy*

Epilepsy is diagnosed based on a history of seizure activity as well as supporting EEG findings. Treatment is individualized. First line treatments include antiepileptic medications for partial and generalized tonic-clonic seizures. Usually, treatment is started with one medication, but this may need to be changed, adjusted, or an additional medication added until the seizures are under control or to avoid adverse effects, which include allergic reactions, especially skin irritations and acute or chronic toxicity. Milder reactions often subside with time or adjustment in doses. Toxic reactions may vary considerably, depending upon the medication and duration of use, so close monitoring is essential. Severe rash and hepatotoxicity are common toxic reactions that occur with many of the antiepileptic drugs. Dosages of drugs may need to be adjusted to avoid breakthrough seizures during times of stress, such as during illness or surgery. Alcohol/drug abuse and sleep deprivation may also cause breakthrough seizures. Most anticonvulsant drugs are teratogenic.

### *Status Epilepticus*

Status epilepticus (SE) is usually generalized tonic-clonic seizures that are characterized by a series of seizures with intervening time too short for regaining of consciousness. The constant assault and periods of apnea can lead to exhaustion, respiratory failure with hypoxemia and hypercapnia, cardiac failure, and death.

**Causes:** Uncontrolled epilepsy or non-compliance with anticonvulsants, infections such as encephalitis, encephalopathy or stroke, drug toxicity (isoniazid), brain trauma, neoplasms, and metabolic disorders.

**Treatment** includes:

- Anticonvulsants usually beginning with a fast-acting benzodiazepine (lorazepam), often in steps, with administration of medication every 5 minutes until seizures subside.
- If cause is undetermined, acyclovir and ceftriaxone may be administered.
- If there is no response to the first 2 doses of anticonvulsants (refractory SE), rapid sequence intubation (RSI), which involves sedation and paralytic anesthesia, may be done while therapy continues. Combining phenobarbital and benzodiazepine can cause apnea, so intubation may be necessary.
- Antiepileptic medications are added.

**Review Video: Seizures**
Visit mometrix.com/academy and enter code: 977061

## Brain Tumors

Any type of brain tumor can occur in adults. Brain tumors may be primary, arising within the brain, or secondary as a result of metastasis:

- **Astrocytoma**: This arises from astrocytes, which are glial cells. It is the most common type of tumor, occurring throughout the brain. There are many types of astrocytomas, and most are slow growing. Some are operable while others are not. Radiation may be given after removal. Astrocytomas include glioblastomas, aggressively malignant tumors occurring most often in adults 45–70.
- **Glioblastoma**: This is the most common and most malignant adult brain tumor/astrocytoma. Treatment includes surgery, radiation, and chemotherapy, but survival rates are very low.
- **Brain stem glioma**: This may be fast or slow growing but is generally not operable because of location, although it may be treated with radiation or chemotherapy.
- **Craniopharyngioma**: This is a congenital, slow-growing, recurrent (especially if >5 cm) and benign cystic tumor that is difficult to resect and is treated with surgery and radiation.
- **Meningioma**: Slow growing recurrent tumors are usually benign and most often occur in women, ages 40–70; however, they can cause severe impairment/death, depending on size and location. Meningiomas are surgically removed if causing symptoms.
- **Ganglioglioma**: This can occur anywhere in the brain and is usually slow growing and benign.

- **Medulloblastoma**: There are many types of medulloblastoma, most arising in the cerebellum, malignant, and fast growing. Surgical excision is often followed by radiation and chemotherapy although recent studies show using just chemotherapy controls recurrence with less neurological damage.
- **Oligodendroglioma**: This tumor most often occurs in the cerebrum, primarily the frontal or temporal lobes, involving the myelin sheath of the neurons. It is slow growing and most common in those age 40–60.
- **Optical nerve glioma**: This slow growing tumor of the optic nerve is usually a form of astrocytoma. Optic nerve glioma is often associated with neurofibromatosis type I (NF1), occurring in 15–40% of patients with NF1. Despite surgical, chemotherapy, or radiotherapy treatment, it is usually fatal.

## Brain Space-Occupying Cysts

Brain space-occupying cysts are fluid-filled or semisolid sacs within the brain. Most cysts are congenital. Common cysts include:

- **Arachnoid cysts** (most common): Occur most often in the temporal or posterior fossa and contain cerebrospinal fluid (CSF).
- **Colloid cysts** (mucous-like): Usually occur in the third ventricle and can obstruct the flow of CSF if large, resulting in hydrocephalus. May cause a sudden life-threatening decline ("drop attack") if the flow of CSF is blocked and the intracranial pressure (ICP) rapidly increases.
- **Epidermal/dermoid cysts**: Slow growing but can compress the cranial nerves.
- **Parasitic cysts** (Neurocysticercosis): Usually multiple cysts occur and can cause seizures.

Symptoms of brain space-occupying cysts include headache, vision changes, nausea and vomiting, irritability, seizures, gait disturbance, and focal deficits. **Diagnostic procedures** include computed tomography scans, magnetic resonance imaging, electroencephalogram (when seizures are noted or suspected), and ICP monitoring. **Treatment** varies according to the type, size, and effects of the cyst but may include surgical removal, watch and wait, fenestration, seizure prophylaxis, ventriculoperitoneal shunt, and antiparasitic therapy (e.g., albendazole and steroids). Nursing priorities include monitoring for signs of ICP, neurological assessment (e.g., Glasgow Coma Scale, pupils, limb strength/drift, speech, orientation, and level of consciousness), and seizure activity.



## Strokes

### *Hemorrhagic Strokes*

Hemorrhagic strokes account for about 20% of all strokes and result from a ruptured cerebral artery, causing not only a lack of oxygen and nutrients but also edema that causes widespread pressure and damage:

- **Intracerebral** is bleeding into the substance of the brain from an artery in the central lobes, basal ganglia, pons, or cerebellum. Intracerebral hemorrhage usually results from atherosclerotic degenerative changes, hypertension, brain tumors, anticoagulation therapy, or use of illicit drugs, such as cocaine.
- **Intracranial aneurysm** occurs with ballooning cerebral artery ruptures, most commonly at the Circle of Willis.
- **Arteriovenous malformation**. Rupture of AVMs can cause brain attack in young adults.
- **Subarachnoid hemorrhage** is bleeding in the space between the meninges and brain, resulting from aneurysm, AVM, or trauma. This type of hemorrhage compresses brain tissue.

**Treatment includes:** The patient may need airway protection/artificial ventilation if neurologic compromise is severe. Blood pressure is lowered to control rate of bleeding but with caution to avoid hypotension and resulting cerebral ischemia (Goal – CPP >70). Sedation can lower ICP and blood pressure, and seizure prophylaxis will be indicated as blood irritates the cerebral cells. An intraventricular catheter may be used in ICP management; correct any clotting disorders if identified.

### *Ischemia Strokes*

Strokes (brain attacks, cerebrovascular accidents) result when there is interruption of the blood flow to an area of the brain. The two basic types are ischemic and hemorrhagic. About 80% are **ischemic**, resulting from blockage of an artery supplying the brain:

- **Thrombosis** in a large artery, usually resulting from atherosclerosis, may block circulation to a large area of the brain. It is most common in the elderly and may occur suddenly or after episodes of transient ischemic attacks.
- **Lacunar infarct** (a penetrating thrombosis in a small artery) is most common in those with diabetes mellitus and/or hypertension.
- **Embolism** travels through the arterial system and lodges in the brain, most commonly in the left middle cerebral artery. An embolism may be cardiogenic, resulting from cardiac arrhythmia or surgery. An embolism usually occurs rapidly with no warning signs.
- **Cryptogenic** has no identifiable cause.

**Medical management** of ischemic strokes with tissue plasminogen activator (tPA) or tenecteplase, the primary treatment, should be initiated within 3 hours (or up to 4.5 hours if inclusion criteria are met):

- **Thrombolytic,** such as tPA or tenecteplase, which is produced by recombinant DNA and is used to dissolve fibrin clots. It is given intravenously (0.9 mg/kg up to 90 mg) with 10% injected as an initial bolus and the rest over the next hour.
- **Antihypertensives** if MAP >130 mmHg or systolic BP >220
- **Cooling** to reduce hyperthermia
- **Osmotic diuretics** (mannitol), hypertonic saline, loop diuretics (Lasix), and/or corticosteroids (dexamethasone) to decrease cerebral edema and intracranial pressure
- **Aspirin/anticoagulation** may be used with embolism
- Monitor and treat hyperglycemia
- **Surgical Intervention:** Used when other treatment fails, may go in through artery and manually remove the clot

### *Symptoms of Brain Attacks in Relation to Area of Brain Affected*

Brain attacks most commonly occur in the right or left hemisphere, but the exact location and the extent of brain damage from a brain attack affects the type of presenting symptoms. If the frontal area of either side is involved, there tends to be memory and learning deficits. Some symptoms are common to specific areas and help to identify the area involved:

- **Right hemisphere**: This results in left paralysis or paresis and a left visual field deficit that may cause spatial and perceptual disturbances, so people may have difficulty judging distance. Fine motor skills may be impacted, resulting in trouble dressing or handling tools. People may become impulsive and exhibit poor judgment, often denying impairment. Left-sided neglect (lack of perception of things on the left side) may occur. Difficulty following directions, short-term memory loss, and depression are also common. Language skills usually remain intact.
- **Left hemisphere**: Results in right paralysis or paresis and a right visual field defect. Depression is common and people often exhibit slow, cautious behavior, requiring repeated instruction and reinforcement for simple tasks. Short-term memory loss and difficulty learning new material or understanding generalizations is common. Difficulty with mathematics, reading, writing, and reasoning may occur. Aphasia (expressive, receptive, or global) is common.
- **Brain stem**: Because the brain stem controls respiration and cardiac function, a brain attack in the brain stem frequently causes death, but those who survive may have a number of problems, including respiratory and cardiac abnormalities. Strokes may involve motor or sensory impairment or both.
- **Cerebellum**: This area controls balance and coordination. Brain attacks in the cerebellum are rare but may result in ataxia, nausea and vomiting, and headaches and dizziness or vertigo.

## *TIA*

Transient ischemic attacks (TIAs) from small clots cause similar but short-lived (minutes to hours) symptoms. Emergent treatment includes placing patient in semi-Fowlers or Fowler's position and administering oxygen. The patient may require oral suctioning if secretions pool. The patient's circulation, airway, and breathing should be assessed and IV access line placed. Thrombolytic therapy to dissolve blood clots should be administered within 1–3 hours. While a patient can recover fully from a TIA, they should be educated, because having a TIA increases an individual's risk for a stroke.

**Review Video: Overview of Strokes**
Visit mometrix.com/academy and enter code: 310572

## Acute Spinal Cord Injury

**Spinal cord injuries** may result from blunt trauma (such as automobile accidents), falls from a significant height, sports injuries, and penetrating trauma (such as gunshot or knife wounds). Damage results from mechanical injury and secondary responses resulting from hemorrhage, edema, and ischemia. The type of symptoms relates to the area and degree of injury. About 50% of spinal cord injuries involve the cervical spine between C4 and C7 with a 20% mortality rate, and 50% of injuries result in quadriplegia. Neurogenic shock may occur with injury above T6, with bradycardia, hypotension, and autonomic instability. Patients may develop hypoxia because of respiratory dysfunction. With high injuries, up to 70% of patients will require a tracheostomy (especially at or above C3). Patients with paralysis are at high risk for pressure sores, urinary tract infections (from catheterization), and constipation and impaction. Management varies according to the level of injury but may include mobilization, mechanical ventilation, support surfaces, ROM, assisted mobility, rehabilitation therapy, analgesia, psychological counseling, bowel training, and skin care.

## Spinal Surgeries

Common spinal surgeries include the following:

- **Artificial disc replacement**: The damaged intervertebral disc is replaced with an implant made of metal, plastic, or another material. Retains movement.
- **Discectomy**: The damaged part of the intervertebral disc is removed to relieve compression of a nerve root or the spinal cord. Indications include herniated disc with radiculopathy (such as sciatic nerve pain).
- **Foraminotomy**: Each vertebra contains a right and a left foramen, an opening through which the nerves pass. The foraminotomy enlarges these foramina when they become obstructed to relieve pressure on the nerve roots.
- **Laminectomy**: The laminae form the back wall of the spinal canal, with each vertebra having a lamina on each side. A laminectomy removes the laminae or other structures, such as bone spurs and ligaments, to enlarge the opening of the spinal canal and relieve pressure on the spinal cord. Indications include spinal stenosis and bone spurs.
- **Spinal fusion**: Two or more vertebrae are fused to form a single, solid bone. Indications include spondylolisthesis and degenerative disc disease, but movement is restricted.
- **Vertebroplasty/kyphoplasty**: Liquid bone cement is injected into spinal compression fracture to stabilize the fracture and relieve pain. With kyphoplasty, a balloon is inserted and filled with the cement to stabilize and restore height.

## Head Trauma

### Blunt Head Trauma

Head trauma can occur as the result of intentional or unintentional blunt or penetrating trauma, such as from falls, automobile accidents, sports injuries, or violence. The degree of injury correlates with the impact force. The skull provides protection to the brain, but a severe blow can cause significant neurological damage. **Blunt trauma** can include:

- **Acceleration-deceleration injuries** are those in which a blow to the stationary head causes the elastic skull to change shape, pushing against the brain, which moves sharply backward in response, striking against the skull.
- **Bruising** can occur at the point of impact (*coup*) and the point where the brain hits the skull (*contrecoup*). So, a blow to the frontal area can cause damage to the occipital region.

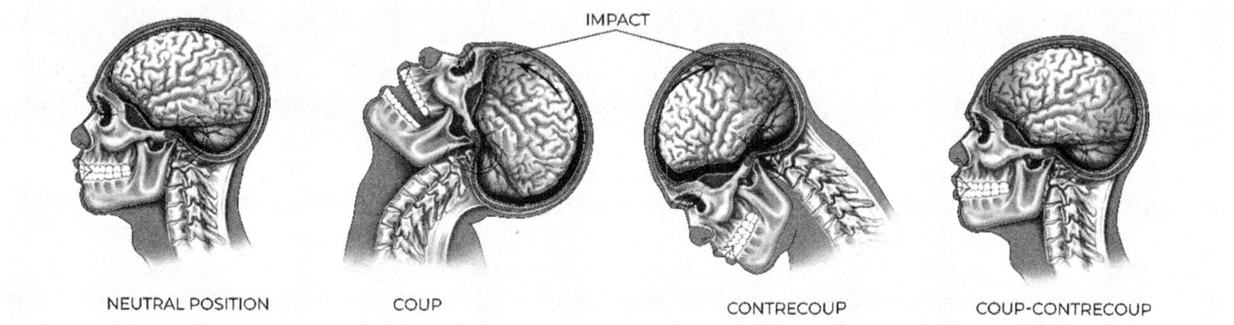


- **Shear injuries,** where vessels are torn, result from sudden movement of the brain.
- **Severe compression** may force the brain through the tentorial opening, damaging the brainstem.

### Cerebral Edema and Increased ICP Secondary to Head Trauma

Head injuries that occur at the time of trauma include fractures, contusions, hematomas, and diffuse cerebral and vascular injury. These injuries may result in hypoxia, increased intracranial pressure, and cerebral edema. Open injuries may result in infection. Patients often suffer initial hypertension, which increases intracranial pressure, decreasing perfusion. Often the primary problem with head trauma is a significant increase in swelling, which also interferes with perfusion, causing hypoxia and hypercapnia, which trigger increased blood flow. This increased volume at a time when injury impairs auto-regulation increases cerebral edema, which increases intracranial pressure and results in a further decrease in perfusion with resultant ischemia. If pressure continues to rise, the brain may herniate. Concomitant hypotension may result in hypoventilation, further complicating treatment. **Treatments** include:

- Monitoring ICP and CCP
- Providing oxygen
- Elevating the head of the bed and maintaining proper body alignment
- Giving medications: Analgesics, anticonvulsants, and anesthetics
- Providing blood/fluids to stabilize hemodynamics
- Managing airway, providing mechanical ventilation if needed
- Providing osmotic agents, such as mannitol and hypertonic saline solution, to reduce cerebral edema

### CONCUSSIONS, CONTUSIONS, AND LACERATIONS

A variety of different injuries can occur as a result of head trauma:

- **Concussions** are diffuse areas of bleeding in the brain and one of the most common injuries. They are usually relatively transient, causing no permanent neurological damage. They may result in confusion, disorientation, and mild amnesia, which last only minutes or hours.
- **Contusions/lacerations** are bruising and tears of cerebral tissue. There may be petechial areas at the impact site (coup) or larger bruising. Contrecoup injuries are less common in children than in adults. Areas most impacted by contusions and lacerations are the occipital, frontal, and temporal lobes. The degree of injury relates to the amount of vascular damage, but initial symptoms are similar to a concussion; however, symptoms persist and may progress, depending upon the degree of injury. Lacerations are often caused by fractures.

### SKULL FRACTURES

Skull fractures are a common mechanism of penetrating wounds causing cerebral lacerations. Open fractures are those in which the dura is torn, and closed fractures are those in which the dura remain intact. While fractures by themselves do not cause neurological damage, force is needed to fracture the skull, often causing damage to underlying structures. Meningeal arteries lie in grooves on the underside of the skull, and a fracture can cause an arterial tear and hemorrhage. **Skull fractures** include:

- **Basilar**: Occurs in bones at the base of the brain and can cause severe brainstem damage. May see bruising around the ear ("Battles sign") and leaking of CSF from nose and ears ("Halo sign"—bloody fluid will develop a ring of clear fluid when placed on gauze or linens).
- **Comminuted**: Skull fractures into small pieces.
- **Compound**: Surface laceration extends to include a skull fracture.
- **Depressed**: Pieces of the skull are depressed inward on the brain tissue, often producing dural tears.
- **Linear/hairline:** Skull fracture forms a thin line without any splintering.

### TRAUMATIC BRAIN INJURY

Traumatic brain injury (TBI) occurs when an external force damages the brain, thereby causing an alteration in its function. TBIs can be classified as mild, moderate, or severe. Common causes of traumatic brain injury include falls, motor vehicle accidents, and assaults. Traumatic brain injuries are more common in males than females.

**Signs/symptoms**: May not be immediately present, depending on the severity of the injury. Symptoms may be subtle initially and then worsen. Symptoms include: loss of consciousness, headache, blurred vision, confusion, nausea, vomiting, fatigue, somnolence, dizziness, loss of balance or coordination, seizures, tinnitus, slurred speech, and photosensitivity.

**Diagnosis**: X-rays of the spine, CT and MRI of the head and angiography if penetrating injury occurred. The Glasgow coma scale is most commonly used to assess neurologic status in the TBI patient.

**Treatment**: Treatment of TBI includes frequent monitoring of vital signs, fluid balance and neurologic status. Intracranial pressure may also be monitored. Mannitol and hypertonic saline may be administered to decrease intracranial pressure and cerebral edema. Antiepileptic medications may be utilized to prevent or minimize seizure activity. In cases of severe injury, decompressive craniotomy and initiation of a hypothermia protocol may be used to reduce intracranial pressure, cerebral edema, and cell death.

## Neurological Storming

Neurological storming (i.e., neurostorming, paroxysmal sympathetic hyperactivity) is a condition that can result from a severe brain injury, such as stroke, traumatic brain injury, intracranial hemorrhage, or hypoxic injury. When the brain injury occurs, the sympathetic nervous system responds, but this autonomic response may become dysregulated because the inhibitory pathways are damaged, resulting in paroxysmal episodes of physiologic arousal: tachycardia (>130 bpm), hypertension, tachypnea (i.e., a respiratory rate of >40 breaths per minute), fever (>101 °F [38.5 °C]), dystonia, diaphoresis, dilated pupils, muscular rigidity, agitation, tremors, flushing, and posturing (i.e., decerebrate, decorticate) may occur. Energy needs increase markedly during episodes, which can result in a loss of weight and muscle mass.

While neurological storming may occur spontaneously, triggers can include environmental stimulation (e.g., alarms, lights, noises), suctioning, pain, urinary retention, constipation, medication changes, and repositioning. Treatment includes reducing external stimuli; ensuring an adequate airway; controlling hyperthermia; preventing injury; and administering medications such as opioids, anesthetics (e.g., propofol), β-adrenergic blockers (e.g., propranolol, metoprolol), α2-agonists (e.g., clonidine, dexmedetomidine), benzodiazepines (e.g., diazepam, lorazepam), and neuromodulators (e.g., gabapentin, baclofen). Patients should be weaned off medications slowly to avoid triggering a reaction.

## Brain Death

While each state has its own laws that describe the legal definition of **brain death,** most include some variation of this description:

- Brain death has occurred if the person has "sustained irreversible cessation of circulatory and respiratory functions; or has sustained irreversible cessation of all functions of the entire brain, including the brain stem."

Some states specify the number of physicians that must make the determination and others simply say the decision must be made in accordance with accepted medical practice. Criteria for determination of brain death include coma or lack of responsiveness, apnea (without ventilation), and absence of brainstem reflexes. In many states, findings must be confirmed by at least 2 physicians. **Tests used to confirm brain death** include:

- Cerebral angiograms: Delayed intracerebral filling or obstruction
- EEG: Lack of response to auditory, visual, or somatic stimuli
- Ultrasound (transcranial): Abnormal/lack of flow
- Cerebral scintigrams: Static images at preset time intervals
- Absence of oculocephalic reflex ("Doll's eyes"): patients eyes stay fixed when head is turned side to side
- Absence of oculovestibular reflex ("cold caloric"): When ice cold water is injected into the ear, the patient's eyes exhibit no response. The patient's HOB must be at least 20° for this test to be accurate

## Delirium

Delirium is an acute, sudden, and fluctuating change in consciousness. Delirium occurs in 10–40% of hospitalized older adults and about 80% of patients who are terminally ill. Delirium may result from drugs, infections, hypoxia, trauma, dementia, depression, vision and hearing loss, surgery, alcoholism, untreated pain, fluid/electrolyte imbalance, and malnutrition. If left untreated, delirium greatly increases the risk of morbidity and death.

**Signs/symptoms:** Reduced ability to focus/sustain attention, language and memory disturbances, disorientation, confusion, audiovisual hallucinations, sleep disturbance, and psychomotor activity disorder.

**Diagnosis:** Patient interview, history/chart/medication review, and possible blood tests to identify electrolyte imbalance/abnormalities.

**Treatment** includes:

- **Medications**: Trazodone, lorazepam, haloperidol—though these may make confusion worse in elderly patients
- **Procedures**: Provide a sitter to ensure safety, decreasing dosage of hypnotics and psychotropics, correct underlying cause

**Prevention**: Reorient patient frequently, ensure adequate rest/nutrition, monitor response to medications, and treat infections and dehydration/malnutrition early.

## AGITATION

Agitation is a common occurrence in the critically ill patient. Factors contributing to the development of agitation include drug or alcohol withdrawal, sleep deprivation, hypoxemia, electrolyte or metabolic imbalance, anxiety, pain, and adverse drug reactions. Delirium may also include agitation as a manifestation.

**Diagnosis**: The physiologic effects of agitation may include increases in heart rate, respiratory rate, blood pressure, intracranial pressure, and oxygen consumption. In addition, agitation can contribute to the self-removal of lines or tubes and combative behavior that may result in patient harm.

**Treatment**: Treatment of agitation involves the identification and correction of causative factors. The use of pharmacologic agents to manage pain, anxiety, and agitation are often utilized. Non-pharmacologic interventions including verbal de-escalation (when possible). The promotion of normal sleep patterns and relaxation techniques may also be effective. Early identification of signs and symptoms is also critical in the successful management of agitation.

## DEMENTIA

Dementia is a chronic condition in which there is progressive and irreversible loss of memory and function. There are many types of dementia a nurse may encounter:

- **Creutzfeldt-Jakob disease**: Rapidly progressive dementia with impaired memory, behavioral changes, and incoordination
- **Dementia with Lewy Bodies**: Similar to Alzheimer's, but symptoms may fluctuate frequently; may also include visual hallucinations, muscle rigidity, and tremors
- **Frontotemporal dementia**: Causes marked changes in personality and behavior; characterized by difficulty using and understanding language
- **Mixed dementia**: Combination of different types of dementia
- **Normal pressure hydrocephalus**: Characterized by ataxia, memory loss, and urinary incontinence
- **Parkinson dementia**: Involves impaired decision making and difficulty concentrating, learning new material, understanding complex language, and sequencing
- **Vascular dementia**: Memory loss less pronounced than that common to Alzheimer's, but symptoms are similar

**Nursing considerations**: Distraction is usually the best course of action to deter the patient with dementia. Reorient frequently, but do not argue with the patient. Avoid restraints or sedatives, which worsen confusion.

# Neurological Procedures and Interventions

## EVACUATION OF HEMATOMAS

Evacuation of hematomas can be done in a number of different ways, including burr holes, needle aspiration, direct surgical craniotomy, or endoscopic craniotomy, but evacuation can pose considerable risks:

- **Epidural hematomas** are usually arterial but may be venous (20%) and are always medical emergencies and require craniotomy with evacuation before compression damage to the brain occurs. Prognosis is good if corrected early because underlying brain damage is rarely severe.
- **Subdural hematomas**, often from acceleration-deceleration accidents or abuse, involve damage to the brain tissue. Evacuation may be done if the hematoma is large and causing compression, but the brain tissue beneath hematomas is often extremely swollen. If the dura is opened, suddenly relieving the pressure may cause the brain to herniate through the opening, so aggressive therapy to reduce swelling preoperatively and careful surgical planning are necessary.

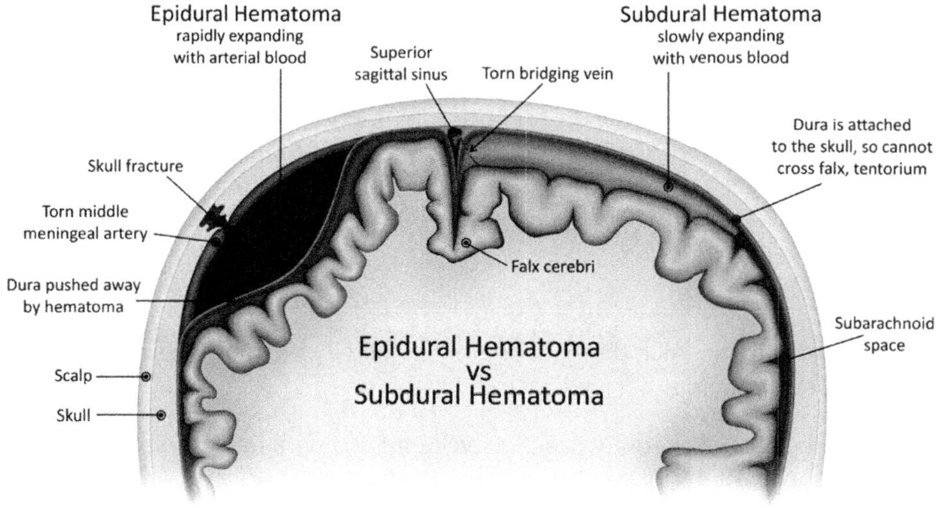


## CRANIOTOMIES

Craniotomies for tumors or other surgical repair (AVMs, aneurysms) are increasingly done with micro-endoscopic equipment, but the surgical opening must be large enough to allow access and the use of necessary instruments. Procedures vary widely according to the reason for craniotomy, the type of tumor, and the age and condition of the patient. Direct craniotomies through the skull are needed in some instances, but newer approaches, including transnasal and transsphenoidal endoscopy are used when possible. Some areas of the brain are not accessible with craniotomy, but may be accessible through stereotactic radiosurgery with Gamma Knife or CyberKnife. Stereotactic radiosurgery is often used as a secondary treatment after primary removal of tumor for regrowth or residual tumor. Radiosurgery may be fractionated and given in a series of treatments. These non-invasive treatments are usually done while adults are awake.

### *POSTOPERATIVE CARE FOR CRANIOTOMY PATIENTS*

In the post-operative period immediately following a craniotomy, the patient must be observed carefully for any **complications** or changes in condition:

- Monitor intracranial pressure
- Position the head in a midline, neutral position. HOB is elevated 30–45° for supratentorial surgery and is flat or only slightly elevated for infratentorial surgery
- Initiate anti-thromboembolism measures: Compression stockings or intermittent pneumatic compression device

- Monitor fluid balance (intake and output)
- Observe surgical wound for swelling and drainage; empty and measure drainage devices (usually bulb drains)
- Monitor oxygen saturation and ABGs to ensure proper oxygenation
- Monitor thermoregulation and prevent hyperthermia
- Administer analgesics and antiemetics routinely to maintain comfort and prevent stress or increased ICP from vomiting
- Administer corticosteroids to reduce postoperative swelling
- Administer anticoagulants (heparin) to prevent clotting
- Monitor laboratory status:
  - Complete blood count to observe for blood loss/infection
  - Electrolyte levels, especially observing for hyponatremia and/or hyperkalemia
  - Blood glucose level (may elevate with corticosteroids)

## VENTRICULAR DRAINS

Ventricular drains are inserted into one of the **brain's lateral ventricles** (usually on the right to prevent damage to the language center) to drain cerebrospinal fluid associated with hydrocephalus. The catheter is tunneled under the skin and sutured in place with an occlusive dressing covering the insertion site. The catheter drains into a collection chamber, which is separated from a drainage bag by a stopcock that can be opened or closed. A pressure scale (which should be leveled with zero at the tragus of the ear) is at the same level as the collection chamber. The target pressure should be determined by the neurosurgeon. The dressing should be changed only if soiled, and any indication of CSF leakage or blood in the CSF should be immediately reported. The CSF output should be measured and recorded hourly (after which the collection chamber is emptied into the drainage bag) and VS and neurological assessment at least every 4 hours. The catheter should be checked when the collection chamber is emptied to ensure it is patent and not kinked. During straining or activities that involve moving the patient, the drainage should be stopped, but for short periods only. Over drainage may result in headache.

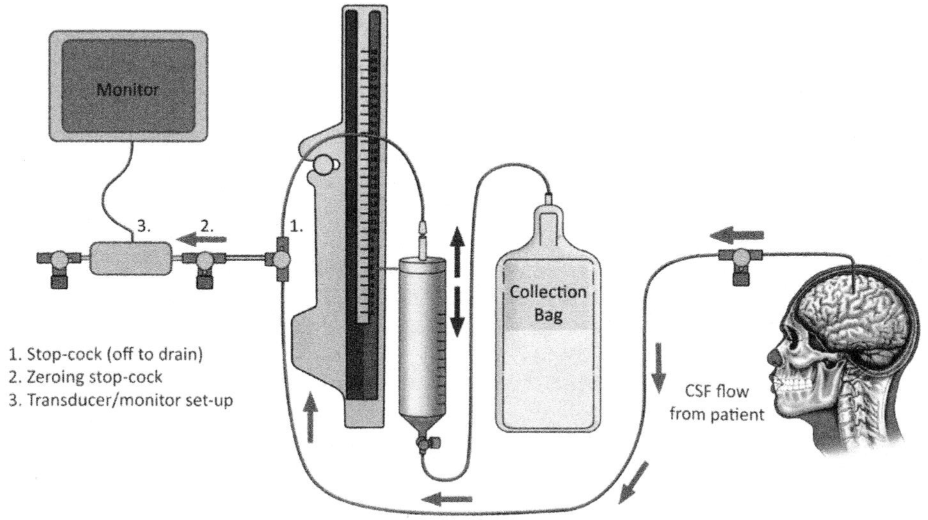


Ventricular-peritoneal shunts may become occluded or disconnected, the catheter may be positioned incorrectly, and the valve pressure may not be adequate. If the shunt does not function properly, signs of hydrocephalus and increased intracranial pressure can occur. If there is a flush valve, this may relieve the obstruction, but obstruction may be difficult to assess with radiography, so a neurosurgical consult may be indicated for revision of the shunt.

### LUMBAR DRAINS

A lumbar drain is inserted in the lumbar region (usually L3-L4 or L4-L5) into the arachnoid space in order to drain cerebrospinal fluid. Indications for a lumbar drain include shunt infection, increased intracranial pressure, hydrocephalus, thoracoabdominal aortic aneurysm repair, and dural fistula (traumatic/postoperative). The patient should be positioned with the head of the bed elevated to 30 degrees and the transducer leveled to the phlebostatic axis or to the right atrium. The cerebrospinal fluid pressure should be monitored continuously and recorded at least every hour for the first 72 hours as well as the volume of drainage, which should be prescribed by the neurosurgeon. Over-drainage may cause a sudden decline in ICP and subarachnoid hemorrhage. Vital signs, neuromuscular and neurovascular checks should be carried out at least every hour for 24 hours. Systolic BP should be maintained ≥140 mmHg and fluid bolus administered for hypotension. After 24 hours, the patient may sit in a chair if stable, but CSF should not be drained while the patient is out of bed. Any sign of blood in CSF should be immediately reported to the neurosurgeon. Hemoglobin should be maintained at >9 mg/dL.

## Endocrine Pathophysiology

### DIABETES MELLITUS TYPES 1 AND 2

Diabetes mellitus is the most common metabolic disorder. Over 6% of adults have diabetes, but only 4% of adults are diagnosed. Insulin resistance tends to increase in older adults, so there is less ability to handle glucose. Type II is more common in older adults, with incidence increasing with age.

- **Type I:** Immune-mediated form with insufficient insulin production because of the destruction of pancreatic beta cells
  - **Symptoms** include pronounced polyuria and polydipsia, short onset, obesity or recent weight loss, and ketoacidosis present on diagnosis.
  - **Treatment** includes insulin as needed to control blood sugar, glucose monitoring 1–4 times daily, diet with carbohydrate control, and exercise.
- **Type II:** Insulin resistant form with defect in insulin secretion
  - **Symptoms** include long onset, obesity with no weight loss or significant weight loss, mild or absent polyuria and polydipsia, ketoacidosis or glycosuria without ketonuria, androgen-mediated problems such as hirsutism and acne (adolescents), and hypertension.
  - **Treatment** includes diet and exercise, glucose monitoring, and oral medications.

**Review Video: Diabetes Mellitus**
Visit mometrix.com/academy and enter code: 501396

**Review Video: Diet, Exercise, and Medications for Diabetes**
Visit mometrix.com/academy and enter code: 774388

**Review Video: Complications of Diabetes**
Visit mometrix.com/academy and enter code: 996788

### DIABETIC KETOACIDOSIS

Diabetic ketoacidosis is a complication of type 1 diabetes mellitus, usually related to noncompliance with treatment, stress, illness, or lack of awareness of having diabetes (this event often being the first time that diabetes is diagnosed). Inadequate production of insulin results in glucose being unavailable for metabolism, so lipolysis (breakdown of fat) produces free fatty acids (FFAs) as an alternate fuel source. Glycerol is converted to ketone bodies which are used for cellular metabolism less efficiently than glucose. Excess ketone bodies are excreted in the urine (ketonuria) or exhalations. Acidosis of any type causes potassium in cells to shift to the serum. The ketone bodies lower serum pH, leading to ketoacidosis.

**Symptoms** include:

- Kussmaul respirations: "Ketone breath," or fruity smelling breath; progresses to CNS depression with loss of airway
- Fluid imbalance, including loss of potassium and other electrolytes from cellular death resulting in dehydration and diuresis with excess thirst
- Dangerous cardiac arrhythmias, related to potassium loss; hypotension, chest pain, tachycardia
- GI: Nausea/vomiting, abdominal pain, loss of appetite
- Neurological: malaise, confusion/lethargy progressing to coma

**Diagnosis** is based on:

- Labs: Blood glucose >250 mg/dL, lower Na and elevated K (switches after treatment), elevated beta-hydroxybutyrate (byproduct of ketones)
- ABG: pH <7.3, $HCO_3$ <18 mEq/L
- Urine: positive for glucose and ketones

### *Treatment and Potential Complications*

**Treatment** of DKA:

- **Fluids**: Priority is fluid resuscitation with 1–2 liters of isotonic fluids given in the first hour, up to 8 liters in the first 24 hours. Potassium will be added to the fluids when levels begin to fall.
- **Insulin**: Continuous drip IV, with/without loading dose. Will usually begin at 0.1 unit/kg/ hour (5–7 units an hour generally), with a goal of decreasing blood glucose 50–75 mg/dL an hour. Blood glucose is checked every hour, and when levels are < 200 mg/dL, add dextrose to IV fluids to prevent rebound hypoglycemia.
- **Potassium**: Watch carefully, as fluids and insulin will cause rapid fall in serum levels. When K <5 mEq/L, it should be added to the IV fluids (Per liter: 20 mEq for K 4–5, 40 mEq for K 3–4). If potassium falls below 3, stop insulin drip and give 10–20 an hour until >3.5.
- **Sodium and Magnesium**: Na has an inverse relationship with potassium, and will increase as potassium falls. If sodium levels rise above 150 mEq, switch fluids to 0.45 NS. Low magnesium levels prevent potassium uptake, so replace as necessary.
- **Electrolytes**: Continue to monitor electrolytes and anion gap during ICU stay. When ABG and electrolytes normalized, transition to SQ insulin.

**Potential complications** include:

- Sudden electrolyte shifts (potassium) leading to catastrophic arrythmias, cerebral edema, and other complications
- Vomiting and decreased LOC leading to aspiration/ARDS
- Mechanical ventilation stops respiratory alkalosis and increases acidosis

## HHNK

Hyperglycemic hyperosmolar nonketotic syndrome (HHNK), also referred to as hyperosmolar hyperglycemic state (HHS), occurs in people without history of diabetes or with mild type 2 diabetes, resulting in persistent hyperglycemia leading to osmotic diuresis. Fluid shifts from intracellular to extracellular spaces to maintain osmotic equilibrium, but the increased glucosuria and dehydration results in hypernatremia and increased osmolarity. This condition is most common in those 50–70 years old and often is precipitated by an acute illness, such as a stroke, medications (thiazides), or dialysis treatments. HHNK differs from ketoacidosis because, while the insulin level is not adequate, it is high enough to prevent the breakdown of fat. Onset of symptoms often occurs over a few days. Glucose levels are often higher than those in DKA due to the gradual increase over time (often greater than 600), and the body living in a state of hyperglycemia, therefore the individual is not symptomatic until the blood glucose level is at an extreme high.

**Symptoms:** Polyuria, dehydration, hypotension, tachycardia, changes in mental status, seizures, hemiparesis.

**Diagnosis:** Increased glucose, Na, osmolality (urine and serum), BUN/Creatinine.

**Treatment** is similar to that for ketoacidosis:

- Insulin drip with frequent (hourly) blood sugar monitoring.
- Intravenous fluids and electrolytes.
- Correct blood glucose and other labs.

## Acute Hypoglycemia

Acute hypoglycemia (hyperinsulinism) may result from pancreatic islet tumors or hyperplasia, increasing insulin production, or from the use of insulin to control diabetes mellitus. Hyperinsulinism can cause damage to the central nervous and cardiopulmonary systems, interfering with functioning of the brain and causing neurological impairment. Other causes may include: genetic defects (chromosome 11: short arm), severe infections, and toxic ingestion of alcohol or drugs (salicylates).

**Symptoms** include:

- Blood glucose <50–60 mg/dL
- Central nervous system: seizures, altered consciousness, lethargy, and poor feeding with vomiting, myoclonus, respiratory distress, diaphoresis, hypothermia, and cyanosis
- Adrenergic system: diaphoresis, tremor, tachycardia, palpitation, hunger, and anxiety

**Diagnosis:** Blood work, patient history, presentation.

**Treatment** depends on underlying cause:

- Glucose/Glucagon administration to elevate blood glucose levels
- Diazoxide to inhibit release of insulin
- Somatostatin to suppress insulin production
- Careful monitoring

## Diabetes Insipidus

Diabetes insipidus (DI) is caused by a deficiency of the antidiuretic hormone (ADH), or vasopressin. DI may develop secondary to head trauma, primary brain tumor, meningitis, encephalitis, or surgical ablation or irradiation of the pituitary gland, or metastatic tumors. This is different from congenital nephrogenic diabetes insipidus, in which production of ADH is normal but the renal tubules do not respond.

**Symptoms:**

- Polydipsia—enormous quantities of fluid may be ingested (3–30 L/day)
- Polyuria—large volumes of very dilute urine is excreted (3–30 L/day); nocturia almost always occurs
- Dehydration and hypovolemia can develop quickly if urinary losses are not continuously replaced

**Diagnosis:** A water restriction test is the most reliable diagnostic test, but should only be done while the patient is under constant supervision. The test measures urine production, blood electrolyte levels, and weight over about 12 hours, during which the person is not allowed to drink. At the end of the 12 hours, vasopressin is given and a diagnosis of DI is confirmed if the person's excessive urination stops, BP rises to normal, and HR is normal.

**Treatment** includes:

- **Hormonal drugs**—Desmopressin, a synthetic analog of vasopressin, has prolonged antidiuretic activity, lasting 12–24 hours in most patients, and may be given intranasally, SQ, IV, or orally. Overdosage can lead to water intoxication, so monitor neurological status.
- **Nonhormonal drugs**—Three groups of nonhormonal drugs can reduce polyuria:
  - Diuretics, primarily thiazides (hydrochlorothiazide)
  - Vasopressin-releasing drugs (chlorpropamide or carbamazepine)
  - Prostaglandin inhibitors (indomethacin)

## SIADH

Syndrome of inappropriate secretion of antidiuretic hormone (SIADH) is related to hypersecretion of the posterior pituitary gland. This causes the kidneys to reabsorb fluids, resulting in fluid retention, and triggers a decrease in sodium levels (dilutional hyponatremia), resulting in production of overly concentrated urine. This syndrome may result from central nervous system disorders, such as brain trauma, surgery, or tumors. It may also be triggered by other disorders, such as tumors of various organs, pneumothorax, acute pneumonia, and other lung disorders. Some medications (vincristine, phenothiazines, tricyclic antidepressants, and thiazide diuretics) may also trigger SIADH.

**Symptoms:** Edema, dyspnea, crackles on auscultation, anorexia with nausea and vomiting, irritability, stomach cramps, alterations of personality, stupor, and seizures (related to progressive sodium depletion).

**Diagnosis:** Increased urine specific gravity, decreased Na and serum osmolality.

**Treatment** includes: (treat underlying cause)

- Correct fluid volume excess and electrolytes.
- Monitor urine output continuously: <0.5 mL/kg/hour is cause for concern.
- Seizure precautions.
- With SIADH expect low serum sodium and serum osmolality with high urine osmolality.

## Chronic Adrenal Insufficiency (Addison Disease)

Adrenal/Adrenocortical insufficiency (Addison disease) is caused by damage to the adrenal cortex related to a variety of causes, such as autoimmune disease or genetic disorders, but it may relate to destructive lesions or neoplasms. Without treatment the condition is life threatening.

**Symptoms** may be vague and the condition undiagnosed until 80–90% of the adrenal cortex has been destroyed:

- Chronic weakness and fatigue
- Abdominal distress with nausea and vomiting
- Salt or licorice craving as a result of aldosterone deficiency
- Pigmentary changes in skin and mucous membranes, hyperpigmentation
- Hypotension
- Hypoglycemia
- Recurrent seizures (more common in children)

**Treatment** includes hormone replacement therapy with glucocorticoids (cortisol) and mineralocorticoids (aldosterone), which may be taken orally or by monthly parenteral injections. Androgen replacement is sometimes recommended for women.

**Note:** During times of stress or illness, the demand for glucocorticoids may increase, and dosages up to 3 times the normal dosage may be needed to prevent an acute crisis.

**Review Video: Addison Disease**
Visit mometrix.com/academy and enter code: 813552

## Acute Adrenal Insufficiency (Adrenal Crisis)

Acute adrenal insufficiency (adrenal crisis) is a sudden, life-threatening condition resulting from an exacerbation of primary chronic adrenal insufficiency (Addison disease), often precipitated by sepsis, surgical stress, adrenal hemorrhage related to septicemia, anticoagulation complications, and cortisone withdrawal related to a decreased or inadequate dose to compensate for stress. Acute adrenal insufficiency may occur in those who do not have Addison disease, such as those who have received cortisone for various reasons, usually a minimum of 20 mg daily for at least 5 days.

**Symptoms**:

- Fever
- Nausea and vomiting
- Abdominal pain
- Weakness and general fatigue
- Disorientation, confusion
- Hypotensive shock
- Dehydration
- Electrolyte imbalance with hyperkalemia, hypercalcemia, hypoglycemia, and hyponatremia

**Treatment**:

- IV fluids in large volume
- Glucocorticoid
- 50% dextrose if indicated (hypoglycemia)
- Mineralocorticoid may be needed after intravenous solutions
- The precipitating cause must be identified and treated as well

## Hyperthyroidism

Hyperthyroidism (thyrotoxicosis) usually results from excess production of thyroid hormones (Graves' disease) from immunoglobulins providing abnormal stimulation of the thyroid gland. Other causes include thyroiditis and excess thyroid medications.

**Review Video: Hyperthyroidism**
Visit mometrix.com/academy and enter code: 923159

**Review Video: Graves' Disease**
Visit mometrix.com/academy and enter code: 516655

**Review Video: An Overview of Thyroid and Antithyroid Drugs**
Visit mometrix.com/academy and enter code: 666133

**Symptoms** vary and may be non-specific, especially in the elderly:

- Hyperexcitability
- Tachycardia (100–160) and atrial fibrillation
- Increased systolic (but not diastolic) BP
- Poor heat tolerance, skin flushed and diaphoretic

- Dry skin and pruritus (especially in the elderly)
- Hand tremor, progressive muscular weakness
- Exophthalmos (bulging eyes)
- Increased appetite and intake but weight loss

**Treatment** includes:

- Radioactive iodine to destroy the thyroid gland. Propranolol may be used to prevent thyroid storm. Thyroid hormones are given for resultant hypothyroidism.
- Antithyroid medications, such as methimazole (recommended) to block the synthesis of T3 or propylthiouracil to block conversion of T4 to T3.
- Surgical removal of thyroid is used if patients cannot tolerate other treatments or in special circumstances, such as large goiter. Usually one-sixth of the thyroid is left in place and antithyroid medications are given before surgery.

## THYROTOXIC STORM

Thyrotoxic storm is a severe type of hyperthyroidism with sudden onset, precipitated by stress such as injury or surgery, in those un-treated or inadequately treated for hyperthyroidism. If not promptly diagnosed and treated, it is fatal. Incidence has decreased with the use of antithyroid medications but can still occur with medical emergencies or pregnancy. Diagnostic findings are similar to hyperthyroidism and include increased T3 uptake and decreased TSH.

**Symptoms**:

- Increase in symptoms of hyperthyroidism
- Increased temperature >38.5 °C
- Tachycardia >130 with atrial fibrillation and heart failure
- Gastrointestinal disorders such as nausea, vomiting, diarrhea, and abdominal discomfort
- Altered mental status with delirium progressing to coma

**Treatment**:

- Controlling production of thyroid hormone through antithyroid medications such as propylthiouracil and methimazole
- Inhibiting release of thyroid hormone with iodine therapy (or lithium)
- Controlling peripheral activity of thyroid hormone with propranolol
- Fluid and electrolyte replacement
- Glucocorticoids, such as dexamethasone
- Cooling blankets
- Treatment of arrhythmias as needed with antiarrhythmics and anticoagulation

## HYPOTHYROIDISM

Hypothyroidism occurs when the thyroid produces inadequate levels of thyroid hormones. Conditions may range from mild to severe myxedema. There are a number of **causes**:

- Chronic lymphocytic thyroiditis (Hashimoto's thyroiditis)
- Excessive treatment for hyperthyroidism
- Atrophy of thyroid
- Medications such as lithium and iodine compounds
- Radiation to the area of the thyroid
- Diseases that affect the thyroid such as scleroderma
- Iodine imbalances

**Symptoms** may include chronic fatigue, menstrual disturbances, hoarseness, subnormal temperature, low pulse rate, weight gain, thinning hair, thickening skin. Some dementia may occur with advanced conditions. Clinical findings may include increased cholesterol with associated atherosclerosis and coronary artery disease. Myxedema may be characterized by changes in respiration with hypoventilation and $CO_2$ retention resulting in coma.

**Treatment** involves hormone replacement with synthetic levothyroxine (Synthroid) based on TSH levels, but this increases the oxygen demand of the body, so careful monitoring of cardiac status must be done during early treatment to avoid myocardial infarction while reaching euthyroid (normal) level.

## Hyperparathyroidism

Hyperparathyroidism occurs when there is **overproduction of parathyroid hormone (PTH)**. Normal range is 10–55 pg/mL. This occurs more often in women and those over 50 years old. Hypercalcemia (total $Ca^{++}$ >10.4 mg/dL) is the most common finding in hyperparathyroidism. Patients may complain about signs of hypercalcemia which can be easily remembered with bones, stones, groans, and moans. This includes **bone pain** due to demineralization, **kidney stones**, **abdominal groans** (nausea, vomiting, constipation, loss of appetite), and **psychiatric moans** (nervous system issues: muscle weakness, fatigue, lethargy, depression, confusion). Polyuria can occur with renal failure. Cardiac arrhythmias, hypertension, and even coma can occur. $Ca^{++}$ levels >12 mg/dL may be due to cancer, and therefore cancer must be ruled out, especially if $Ca^{++}$ levels rise rapidly. Hyperparathyroidism is treated with parathyroidectomy of affected glands.

## Hypoparathyroidism

Hypoparathyroidism is the **deficiency of PTH**. This is more common in women and is usually due to accidental damage during thyroid/neck surgery, radioactive iodine treatment for hyperthyroidism, radiation, or due to autoimmune causes. As $Ca^{++}$ levels drop, patients may complain of paresthesia of the fingers, toes, and perioral area. Patients will show other signs of neuromuscular irritability with muscle aches, hyperreflexia, carpopedal spasm (tetany), laryngospasm, and facial grimacing. A positive Chvostek sign (unilateral spasm of the facial muscles when the facial nerve is tapped) and a positive Trousseau sign (carpal spasm when upper arm is compressed with a blood pressure cuff) may be present. Irritability, confusion, fatigue, seizures, brittle hair and nails, and personality changes may occur. Diagnose with an ionized $Ca^{++}$ level (<4.7 mg/dL), reduced PTH, and elevated phosphate. Treat with $Ca^{++}$ and vitamin D supplements. Patients with renal failure must also reduce the amount of phosphate in their diet. Patients with tetany are treated with IV calcium gluconate.

## Cushing Syndrome and Cushing's Disease

Cushing syndrome results when **cortisol levels** are increased. Most commonly, this is due to steroid treatment with **prednisone**. Endogenous causes include a pituitary adenoma producing excess amounts of adrenocorticotropic hormone (ACTH) which leads to elevated cortisol (termed **Cushing's disease**) or a primary tumor of the adrenal gland causing increased cortisol secretion. Forms of cancer (e.g., lung, carcinoid) can present with ectopic sources of ACTH secretion. Patients will develop proximal muscle weakness, muscular atrophy, truncal obesity with thin arms and legs, round facies, buffalo hump, and purple striae usually across the abdomen. Patients may bruise easily, have non-healing sores, and women may be affected with hirsutism and oligomenorrhea/amenorrhea. Osteoporosis can occur as can glucose intolerance. For diagnosis a patient should be screened with one of the following: 24-hour urine free cortisol x3, low dose (1 mg) dexamethasone suppression test, midnight serum or salivary cortisol. Once Cushing syndrome is established, determine the cause using an ACTH and simultaneous cortisol measurement (elevated = adrenal adenoma or carcinoma) or a high-dose (8 mg overnight, or 2-day) dexamethasone suppression test (differentiates between pituitary cause and ectopic ACTH cause). Patients should be weaned off prednisone if possible. Removal of a pituitary adenoma can decrease ACTH production. Removal of an adrenal adenoma or other ectopic source of hormone secretion can decrease cortisol levels. Complications include hypertension, CV disease, DM, osteoporosis, risk of adrenal crisis, and psychosis.

## HYPERALDOSTERONISM

Hyperaldosteronism leads to hypokalemia and hypernatremia (and often resulting hypertension). In fact, patients with untreated hypertension and potassium <2.8meq/dL often have primary hyperaldosteronism:

- **Aldosterone-producing adenoma** (Conn's syndrome) accounts for most primary hyperaldosteronism and affects women more often than men.
- **Idiopathic hyperaldosteronism** accounts for about 30% of primary hyperaldosteronism and has no identifiable changes on imaging.
- **Glucocorticoid suppressible hyperaldosteronism** is familial and rare.
- **Aldosterone-producing adrenocortical carcinoma** is another rare cause and presents with hyperandrogenism.

**Diagnosis** of hyperaldosteronism requires diastolic hypertension without edema, low renin levels that do not respond to volume depletion, and high aldosterone levels that fail to drop with saline boluses. An adrenal CT scan is performed to distinguish between Conn's syndrome and idiopathic hyperaldosteronism. **Treatment** includes spironolactone or eplerenone to block the mineralocorticoid receptor, normalizing potassium and improving blood pressure. Adrenalectomy is indicated for unilateral hyperplasia or Conn's syndrome.

## PHEOCHROMOCYTOMA

Pheochromocytoma is a rare tumor of chromaffin tissue. Ninety percent of these occur in the adrenal medulla, 10% are bilateral, and 10% are malignant. These tumors produce epinephrine and norepinephrine, leading to episodic symptoms of headaches, chest pain, palpitations, diaphoresis, tremor, nausea, vomiting, weight loss, and constipation. Initial diagnosis requires a 24-hour urine test to check for metanephrine, VMA, and catecholamines. These are always elevated with pheochromocytoma. If associated with a multiple endocrine neoplasia (MEN) syndrome, then one must check serum free metanephrine. Then one should begin imaging with CT or MRI scanning of the adrenals. If the adrenals appear normal, a radiolabeled iodine (called MIBG-metaiodobenzylguanidine scintigraphy) scan can localize extra-adrenal pheochromocytoma tissue or metastases. This scan uses a compound that concentrates in the adrenals to highlight the pheochromocytoma tissue. **Treatment** is surgical. But first, phenoxybenzamines are used to block the catecholamines, and then beta-blockers are used to control heart rate. Surgery has a 90% cure rate. Urinary catecholamines should be followed for at least 10 years.



## PAGET'S DISEASE

Paget's disease is a disease of high bone turnover and disorganized osteoid formation. It is most prevalent in patients in the northeast US or of European descent and in older patients. The disease is usually asymptomatic, being detected on radiographs. However, it may present with bone pain, fractures, and bony deformities. Commonly involved bones include the skull, femur, tibia, pelvis, and humerus. Specifically, with skull involvement, the patient may note frequent headaches and increasing hat size, sometimes associated with deafness. Examination findings include frontal bossing, bowed legs, and superficial erythema and warmth, due to the increased vascularity of the bones. This disease is **diagnosed** with increased alkaline phosphatase, and elevated urinary hydroxyproline. Calcium and phosphorous are often normal. Imaging reveals hyperdense and enlarged bones in some regions and erosions in others. Bone scanning reveals increased uptake in certain areas. **Treatment** includes bisphosphonate and management of complications, including CHF, spinal cord compression, or nerve entrapment.

# Immunologic and Oncologic Pathophysiology

## Lung Cancer

### *SCLC*

Small cell lung cancer (SCLC) is a rapidly-growing variant of lung cancer found in about 15% of new cases. Its origin is in the bronchi and this type of lung cancer occurs predominantly in smokers. At the time of diagnosis, the disease is usually symptomatic and metastases have generally already occurred. There are 3 subtypes of SCLC: oat cell or small-cell carcinoma, intermediate cell, and small cell combined with squamous cell carcinoma or adenocarcinoma. Differential diagnosis includes tests to distinguish it from slower-growing non-small cell lung cancer, lymphoma, sarcoidosis, metastases due to other primary tumors, or infectious processes. In addition to routine procedures like history, physical examination, and laboratory tests, SCLC is generally staged using imaging tests. In particular, a CT scan with contrast is done to assess the involvement in the lung and other sites, and an MRI of the brain and/or a bone scan may also be done to look for metastases. A bone marrow biopsy may also be indicated.

### *NSCLC*

Non-small cell lung cancer (NSCLC) is a blanket term for several histological types of lung cancer not classified as SCLC. The major histological variants are adenocarcinoma, squamous cell carcinoma, and large cell. The large cell type is anaplastic, which means the cells are relatively undifferentiated. Diagnosis of NSCLCs includes exclusion of small cell lung carcinoma, metastatic lung lesions from other primary sources, sarcoidosis, and infections. The clinician generally stages the disease through use of history, physical examination, and laboratory tests. Imaging studies usually include not only CT scans but also positron emission tomography (PET) and, if metastases are suspected, a brain MRI and possibly a bone scan. Mediastinal node biopsies are generally performed if the PET scan indicates later stage disease; various types of incisions can be made, such as those into the sternum or mediastinum.

## Breast Cancer

### *Staging*

The American Joint Committee on Cancer **TNM Staging** has recently developed a complex staging classification for breast cancer. In general, however, early invasive breast cancer would be Stage I or II (IIA or IIB). In these stages, there is either no lymph node involvement or only same-side axillary region lymph node involvement with no distant metastases. Nevertheless, diagnostic tests should include bilateral mammography (and possibly other imaging techniques), blood profiles, hepatic and renal function tests, serum alkaline phosphatase levels, and lymph node biopsy or mapping. Assays for prognostic factors like high levels of HER2 or hormone receptors may also be done. Management is surgery that either conserves the breast or a modified radical mastectomy in which the pectoral muscles are not removed. If there is nodal involvement or other factors exist (such as positive hormone receptors or large tumor size), adjuvant chemotherapy or endocrine treatment is added.

### *Locally Advanced or Recurrent Breast Cancer or Distant Metastases*

Locally advanced stage III breast cancer is a comprehensive term for a highly heterogeneous grouping. All Stage III patients have either some sort of nodal involvement and/or their tumor has extended into the chest wall or skin. They do not have distant metastases. Once the disease has reached this stage, multiple treatment strategies are needed, including chemotherapy (and endocrine therapy in receptor-positive women), surgery, and radiation. Locally recurrent breast cancer, on the other hand, is generally due to insufficient removal of the primary lesion (such as with breast conservation surgery); it can often be managed with further surgery, although other modalities may be needed if there has been nodal or metastatic spread. Once there is metastatic involvement, therapies are merely palliative and the prognosis is poor.

## Prostate Cancer

At present, about one out of nine men will develop **prostate cancer** at some point, and approximately 2-3% of those will die of the disease. There are familial groupings of prostate cancer; for example, mutations in the RNASEL and MSR1 loci coding for host response to infection appear to predispose a man to prostate cancer. Diet affects susceptibility to prostate cancer; in particular, consumption of red meat cooked at high temperature to release aromatic compounds is highly correlated to development of the cancer. Ethnicity may play a role, as African Americans in the U. S. have an especially high rate of prostate cancer, but this may be due in part to diet.

### *Mechanisms That Contribute to Development of Prostate Cancer*

Germline mutations in the RNASEL and MSR1 genes have been associated with an increased risk of developing prostate cancer. There is some evidence that inflammation and infection may play a role in the progression of the disease, and development of lesions termed proliferate inflammatory atrophy (PIA) may predispose a man to later prostate intraepithelial neoplasia and prostate cancer. Molecular changes have also been closely associated with disease progression. These include somatic inactivation of the GSTP1 gene, which fosters susceptibility to oxidant and electron-accepting carcinogens and depression of various functions caused by gene mutations, such as the PTEN tumor-suppressor gene, NKA3.1, and CDKN1B. As discussed previously, screening tests include serum prostate-specific antigen (PSA) levels and digital rectal examination. Diagnosis is generally confirmed by core needle biopsy.

### *Staging and Grading*

There are two **staging systems** that are commonly used for prostate cancer.

- The **TNM system**, which is adapted to many types of cancer, defines the primary tumor (T) when observable as T1 (identified only by histology or needle biopsy), T2 (limited to the prostate), T3 (reaches through the prostate capsule) or T4 (invasion of adjacent structures). The TMN system also expresses regional lymph node involvement from N1 to N3 and distant metastases as M1 if present. An *X* after the T, N, or M indicates inability to assess and a zero means no evidence of presence.
- The **American Urological Association or AUA staging system** classifies prostate cancer in four stages. These stages are fairly similar to the primary tumor staging of the TMN program. Basically, Stage A is disease that is not clinically observable. Stage B is a tumor confined within the prostate gland. Stage C involves malignancy that extends outside the prostate capsule but remains within the area. Stage D is malignancy with metastatic involvement. A Gleason score is a combined measurement of histological grading of the two most prevalent differentiation patterns; a lower score reflects a higher amount of differentiation and each component can be graded from 1 to 5.

## Colon Cancer

The factor most closely associated with development of **colon cancer** is age, with about 9 out 10 cases identified after age 50. The vast majority of cases have not been correlated to any heritable gene mutation. However, there is a several-fold increase in risk of development of the disease when a close relative is affected, and there are several familial syndromes related to colon cancer (most notably familial adenomatous polyposis or FAP and HNPCC or hereditary nonpolyposis colon cancer). Risk of colon cancer has been associated with certain dietary practices, including high intake of low fiber and high fat foods. It has also been associated with environmental influences, such as exposure to tobacco. The disease often develops through mutations attributable to either chromosomal instability or to a lesser extent microsatellite (repetitive DNA sequence) instability. The genetic change most often found in patients with both precursor adenomatous polyps or actual colon cancer is a defective APC tumor suppressor locus.

### *Procedures for Prevention, Diagnosis, and Staging of Colon Cancer*

Identification of individuals with familial syndromes or known genetic changes associated with colon cancer is theoretically a means of preventing colon cancer. Realistically, at present this is rarely done. COX-2 inhibitors, which are basically anti-inflammatory agents, are sometimes used as chemo preventive drugs. Patients usually present with symptoms like anemia, fatigue, weight loss, or changes in bowel habits. A small portion of them have other cancers and up to 40% have polyps in addition to the primary tumor. Colonoscopy is suggested as a diagnostic procedure every 10 years beginning at age 50, and it involves inspection of the entire large intestine using a flexible fiberoptic endoscope. Benign polyps, possible cancer precursors, can be immediately excised. Other diagnostic probes include sigmoidoscopy and virtual colonoscopy. Staging is usually done utilizing imaging techniques like CT scans, MRIs, or PET scans. Liver metastases, common in conjunction with colorectal cancers, can be best visualized using intraoperative ultrasound.

### *Staging*

There are several classification systems for **staging** colorectal cancers. The most common scheme utilized is the Astler-Coller modified Duke's system. The emphasis of this classification scheme is the depth of tumor invasion into the colon wall. The modified Astler-Coller (MAC), the traditional Duke, and the American Joint Committee on Cancer or AJCC (based on TMN) classification schemes are interrelated. According to Astler-Coller, MAC A is comprised of lesions limited to the mucosa or sub mucosa; MAC B1 and B2 involve extension into or through the muscularis propria; MAC C1, 2, or 3 imply nodal involvement along with extension into or through the bowel wall; MAC D means evidence of distant metastases. These correspond roughly to Duke's A, B, C and D. The AJCC or TMN classification defines stages 0 (carcinoma in situ) through IV.

## Skin Cancer

### *Melanomas*

The severity of melanoma is primarily related to the thickness of the primary lesion and to the presence of histologic ulceration. The American Joint Commission on Cancer's Stage Grouping for melanoma reflects these parameters. The T or tumor size component for identifiable melanomas is up to 1.0 mm thick for T1, 1.01 to 2.0 mm for T2, 2.01 to 4.0 mm for T3, and greater than 4.0 mm thick for T4. Within each of these groups for cases of melanoma in situ, an *a* is added for no ulceration and a *b* is added to indicate ulceration. Regional lymph node involvement is described by an N followed by a 1, 2 or 3 (for 1, 2-3, or 4 or more involved lymph nodes) and an *a* or *b* to indicate either micro- or macrometastases. Distant metastases, if present, are classified as M1a, b, or c, depending on the site. As with other schemes, an *X* after the letter indicates inability to assess, and a zero means no evidence. Staging is from 0 (in situ) to stage IV (distant metastases). Stages I and II have no nodal or metastatic involvement, and stage III means regional lymph node presence. Within each stage (I, II, and III) there are various subgroups, and the presence of ulceration can put a thinner melanoma in the same stage with a thicker but non-ulcerated lesion.

### *Basic Features of Nonmelanoma Skin Cancers*

About four out of every five cases of nonmelanoma skin cancer are **basal cell carcinoma** (BCC), which usually presents as either a reddish ulcerated bump on the skin or as a lighter hardened plaque. Most other nonmelanoma skin cancers are **squamous cell carcinomas** (SCC), which usually appear as raised areas that are either red or skin-toned and have ulcerations and patchy areas of hard horny tissue called keratoses.

Organ transplant patients are prone to develop SCC. Patients with SCC are more likely to develop metastases than those with BCC, although the latter can reoccur at the primary site. Lack of differentiation in either type can portend a more clinically aggressive tumor. There are other generally rare and often more aggressive malignancies that can emulate BCC or SCC that should be excluded via differential diagnosis such as sebaceous gland carcinoma and Merkel cell carcinoma.

## LEUKEMIA

Leukemia is a condition in which the proliferating cells compete with normal cells for nutrition. Leukemia affects all cells because the abnormal cells in the bone marrow depress the formation of all elements, resulting in several consequences, regardless of the type of leukemia:

- Decrease in production of **erythrocytes** (RBCs), resulting in anemia
- Decrease in **neutrophils**, resulting in increased risk of infection
- Decrease in **platelets**, with subsequent decrease in clotting factors and increased bleeding
- Increased risk of **physiological fractures** because of invasion of bone marrow that weakens the periosteum
- Infiltration of **liver, spleen, and lymph glands**, resulting in enlargement and fibrosis
- Infiltration of the **CNS**, resulting in increased intracranial pressure, ventricular dilation, and meningeal irritation with headaches, vomiting, papilledema, nuchal rigidity, and coma progressing to death
- **Hypermetabolism** that deprives cells of nutrients, resulting in anorexia, weight loss, muscle atrophy, and fatigue

**Review Video: Leukemia**
Visit mometrix.com/academy and enter code: 940024

### *RELATIONSHIP OF LEUKOCYTOSIS TO LEUKEMIA*

Leukemia occurs when one type of WBC proliferates with immature cells, with the defect occurring in the hematopoietic stem cell, either lymphoid or myeloid. Usually, leukemias classified as blast cell or stem cell refer to lymphoid defects. With acute leukemia, WBC count remains low because the cells are halted at the blast stage and the disease progresses rapidly. Chronic leukemia progresses more slowly and most cells are mature.

## TUMOR LYSIS SYNDROME

Tumor lysis syndrome occurs when intracellular contents are released from tumor cells, leading to electrolyte imbalances (hyperkalemia, hyperphosphatemia, hypocalcemia, and hyperuricemia) when the kidneys are unable to excrete the large volume of metabolites. **Tumor lysis syndrome** is most common after treatment of hematologic malignancies but can occur due to any type of tumor that is sensitive to chemotherapy. The primary goals of therapy for tumor lysis syndrome are to increase urine production through IV hydration in order to prevent renal failure and to decrease uric acid concentration, usually with administration of allopurinol. The urine pH should be maintained at 7 or higher. Electrolyte levels should be closely monitored, as hyperkalemia is a risk. Patients at moderate risk (intermediate grade lymphomas, acute leukemias) should begin prophylactic allopurinol before chemotherapy, and those at higher risk (high grade lymphomas or acute leukemias with WBC count >50,000) should begin rasburicase.

## CANCER-SPECIFIC TREATMENT

### *LEUKEMIA TREATMENT*

Leukemia treatment depends upon the protocol established for each type of leukemia. Combined drugs are usually more effective than any single drug. Chemotherapy usually includes three stages:

- **Induction therapy**: The purpose is to induce remission to the point that the bone marrow is clear of disease and blood cell counts are normal. Chemotherapy is usually given for about 4-6 weeks, followed by transplantation or the next stage of chemotherapy. The chemotherapy is potent and suppresses blood elements, leaving the body at risk for serious infections and hemorrhage, so supportive care is critical.
- **Consolidation therapy**: The goal is to kill any cells that may have escaped the induction stage. This stage lasts 4-8 months. Intrathecal chemotherapy may be co-administered as a prophylaxis to prevent CNS involvement.

- **Maintenance therapy**: Treatment may continue for another 2-3 years, but with less intense chemotherapy to maintain remission. Weekly blood cell counts monitor progress and side effects.

Sometimes after the three stages of chemotherapy are completed, the patient will relapse and leukemic cells return. In that case, **reinduction** is carried out, usually using a different arsenal of drugs. Many drugs in use now, especially for relapses, are those in clinical trials. Clinical trials are ongoing for many chemotherapeutic agents to determine the best combination of drugs and duration of treatment. Other treatments may be instituted, depending on the severity of the disease:

- **Intrathecal chemotherapy** is administered into the spinal fluid for treatment of infiltration of the CNS.
- **Radiation** to the brain may be indicated in addition to intrathecal chemotherapy with severe disease but poses danger to brain development.
- **Bone marrow or cord blood transplant**, also known as hematopoietic stem cell transplantation (HCST), may be done if chemotherapy fails or after the first remission for AML, which has a lower cure rate.

### *Lung Cancer Treatment*

Since SCLC is an aggressive disease, surgical procedures are not useful and not generally performed. If the cancer is relatively limited, chemotherapy and irradiation of both the chest and brain (to prevent brain metastases) are done. Otherwise, several cycles of combination or multi-agent chemotherapy are tried but the prognosis is poor.

For NSCLC, surgical resection is usually effective for the early stages I and II. For stages IIIA and IIIB, indicating metastatic involvement, chemotherapy possibly combined with radiation is generally used either before surgery (IIIA) or as the treatment modality. If the latter patients also have a malignant pleural effusion, they are treated as stage IV. Stage IV patients are given combination chemotherapy, mainly to improve their quality of life. Individuals with recurrent NSCLC are also treated with combination chemotherapy.

### *Management of Localized Versus Advanced Prostate Cancer*

**Localized prostate cancer** would be defined as falling into the TMN categories of T1 or T2. Usually, these individuals also have serum PSA levels of ≤10 ng/mL and a Gleason score in the range of 2 to 6. Patients falling into these categories are often just watched carefully, but a radical retropubic prostatectomy may be performed or radiation (either external beam or brachytherapy) may be used. Androgen deprivation has also been used as an adjunct to external beam radiation treatment. Radiation therapy can be utilized after prostatectomy if the disease recurs, usually monitored by looking for rising PSA levels. More **advanced stages of prostate cancer** are generally managed primarily through suppression of androgens by luteinizing hormone-releasing (LHRH) agonists and possibly antiandrogens. However, if the disease progresses (usually indicated by rising PSA levels) systemic chemotherapy may be initiated. Other modalities are under investigation as well. Any of these approaches can produce side effects related to sexual function or pleasure or urinary function, and the androgen deprivation can lead to loss of muscle mass or bone density.

### *Colon Cancer Treatment*

Standard **treatment** for colorectal cancer is radical surgical resection followed by anastomosis of the remaining colon, including elimination of lymphatic drainage portals. The bowel must be cleared of fecal matter through liquid diet, hydration, and the use of salt solutions and lavage before the surgery. The most suitable surgical option for management of obstructive colon cancers is a subtotal colectomy. After surgery, recommendations for surveillance are physical examination every three months for two years tapering to twice yearly, quarterly monitoring by CEA levels and CT scans, and colonoscopy a year later with follow-up every three to five years. Most cases of recurrence happen within the first few years and many can be successfully surgically removed. Systemic chemotherapy (such as 5-fluorouracil combined with leucovorin) is also administered to most patients in an attempt to eliminate possible micrometastases. Similar chemotherapeutic regimens, possibly in conjunction with additional agents, are used to manage metastatic disease. The liver is the most common site of disease spread.

### *Procedures for Primary or Salvage Therapy of Melanomas*

Primary melanomas are surgically excised. The margin around the site required is ascertained by the thickness of the melanoma and the area where it is located. A thicker lesion requires a larger excision margin, and some sites such as the fingers, toes, soles of the foot or ears may necessitate other surgical procedures in conjunction. Sentinel nodes are often biopsied if regional lymph node involvement is not clinically evident. If regional nodes are metastatic, they are dissected. Patients who have large primary lesions or nodal involvement are generally also given interferon alpha or dacarbazine (DTIC), the only currently approved agents, or they may be enrolled in other clinical trials. These systemic adjuvants mainly alleviate symptoms. Once metastatic disease becomes systemic, patient survival is typically only about six to nine months.

### *Treatment of Nonmelanoma Skin Cancers*

Primary basal cell or squamous cell carcinomas are generally surgically excised. A procedure called Mohs surgery is used in more aggressive or indistinct cases. Other approaches include radiation treatment, obliteration of the lesion by physical means, and administration of interferons or their activators. Once metastasis has occurred, treatment is generally multimodal, including surgery, radiation, and chemotherapy. Most people with nonmelanoma skin cancers have a much better chance of survival than those who present with melanoma. The prognosis for patients with either BCC or SCC is usually excellent, but if metastases develop in SCC cases, the individual has a less than 50% chance of surviving 5 years. The rarer skin cancers are associated with greater severity. Most skin cancers are associated with exposure to ultraviolet radiation, and there are available potential chemopreventive agents such as retinoids and COX-2 inhibitors.



# Hematologic Pathophysiology

## Anemia

Anemia occurs when there is an insufficient number of red blood cells to sufficiently oxygenate the body. As a result of the decreased level of oxygen being supplied to the organs, the body will attempt to compensate by increasing cardiac output and redistributing blood to the brain and heart. In return, the blood supply to the skin, abdominal organs, and kidneys is decreased. Anemia can occur from blood loss, increased destruction of red blood cells (hemolytic anemia), or as a result of a decreased production in red blood cells.

**Signs/symptoms**: Pallor, fatigue, hypotension, weakness, and mental status changes. As perfusion decreases and the body attempts to compensate for the lack of oxygenation, tachycardia, chest pain, and shortness of breath may occur. In hemolytic anemias, jaundice and splenomegaly may occur as the result of the breakdown of red blood cells and the excretion of bilirubin.

**Diagnosis**: A complete blood count, reticulocyte count, and iron studies may be used to diagnose anemia.

**Treatment**: The treatment of anemia is focused on treating the underlying cause. Parenteral iron may be given for patients with iron deficiency anemias caused from chronic blood loss, or inadequate iron intake or absorption. Blood transfusions are used to treat patients with active bleeding as well as those patients who are displaying significant clinical symptoms. Erythropoietin stimulating proteins may also be utilized to decrease the need for a transfusion.

## Sickle Cell Disease

Sickle cell disease is a recessive genetic disorder of chromosome 11, causing hemoglobin to be defective so that red blood cells (RBCs) are sickle-shaped and inflexible, resulting in their accumulating in small vessels and causing painful blockage. While normal RBCs survive 120 days, sickled cells may survive only 10–20 days, stressing the bone marrow that cannot produce fast enough and resulting in severe anemia. There are 5 variations of sickle cell disease, with sickle cell anemia the most severe. Different types of crises occur (aplastic, hemolytic, vaso-occlusive, and sequestrating), which can cause infarctions in organs, severe pain, damage to organs, and rapid enlargement of liver and spleen. Complications include anemia, acute chest syndrome, congestive heart failure, strokes, delayed growth, infections, pulmonary hypertension, liver and kidney disorders, retinopathy, seizures, and osteonecrosis. Sickle cell disease occurs almost exclusively in African Americans in the United States, with 8–10% carriers.

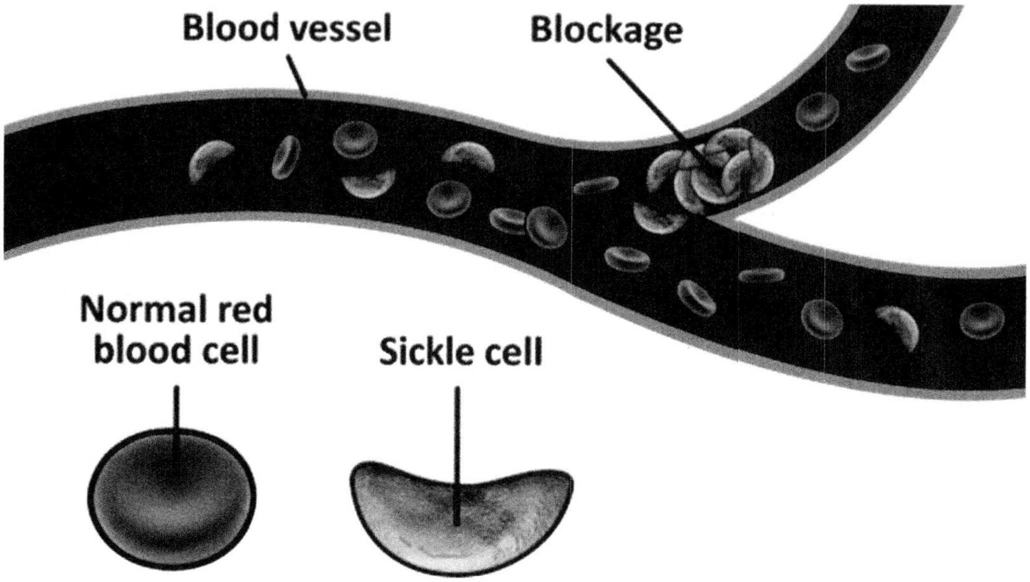


**Review Video: Sickle Cell Disease**
Visit mometrix.com/academy and enter code: 603869

### *TREATMENT*

Treatment for sickle cell disease includes:

- **Prophylactic penicillin** for children from 2 months to 5 years to prevent pneumonia
- **Hydroxyurea** for long-term management of sickle cell disease in individuals ages 6 months and older. This medication has been shown to decrease the complications from sickle cell disease, increase life expectancy, and improve overall quality of life.
- **IV fluids** to prevent dehydration
- **Analgesics** (morphine) during painful crises
- **Folic acid** for anemia
- **Oxygen** for congestive heart failure or pulmonary disease
- **Blood transfusions** with chelation therapy to remove excess iron OR erythropheresis, in which red cells are removed and replaced with healthy cells, either autologous or from a donor
- **Hematopoietic stem cells transplantation** is the only curative treatment, but immunosuppressive drugs must be used and success rates are only about 85%, so the procedure is only used on those at high risk. It requires ablation of bone marrow, placing the patient at increased risk.
- **Partial chimerism** uses a mixture of the donor and the recipient's bone marrow stem cells and does not require ablation of bone marrow. It is showing good success.

## Polycythemia Vera

Polycythemia vera is a condition in which there is abnormal production of blood cells in the bone marrow. Erythrocytes (red blood cells) are primarily affected. The disease is more common in men older than 40 years. Polycythemia may be primary or secondary, related to conditions causing hypoxia. The blood increases in viscosity, resulting in a number of **symptoms**:

- Dizziness, headache, weakness, and fatigue
- Dyspnea, especially when supine
- Flushing of skin, blue-tinged skin discoloration, and red lesions
- Itching after warm bath
- Left upper abdominal fullness and splenomegaly
- Phlebitis from blood clots
- Vision disturbances
- Complications include stroke, hemorrhage, and heart failure

**Diagnosis** includes CBC with differential, chemistry panel, bone marrow biopsy, and Vitamin $B_{12}$ level. Red cell mass will be more than 25% above normal.

**Treatment** includes:

- **Phlebotomy** to remove 500 mL (lesser amounts for children) of blood to decrease blood viscosity, repeated weekly until hematocrit stable (less than 45%)
- Referral for **chemotherapy** (hydroxyurea) to suppress marrow production
- **Interferon** to decrease need for phlebotomy

## Von Willebrand Disease

Von Willebrand disease is a group of congenital bleeding disorders (inherited from either parent) affecting 1–2% of the population, associated with deficiency or lack of von Willebrand factor (vWF), a glycoprotein that is synthesized, stored, and secreted by vascular endothelial cells. This protein interacts with thrombocytes to create a clot and prevent hemorrhage; however, with von Willebrand disease, this clotting mechanism is impaired. There are three types:

- **Type I**: Low levels of vWF and also sometimes factor VIII (dominant inheritance)
- **Type II**: Abnormal vWF (subtypes a, b) may increase or decrease clotting (dominant inheritance)
- **Type III**: Absence of vWF and less than 10% factor VIII (recessive inheritance)

**Symptoms** vary in severity and include bruising, menorrhagia, recurrent epistaxis, and hemorrhage.

**Treatment** includes:

- Avoiding aspirin, ibuprofen, and other NSAIDs
- **Desmopressin acetate** parenterally or nasally to stimulate production of clotting factor (mild cases)
- **Severe bleeding**: factor VIII concentrates with vWF, such as Humate-P

## Hemophilia

Hemophilia is an inherited disorder in which the person lacks adequate clotting factors. There are three types:

- **Type A**: lack of clotting factor VIII (90% of cases)
- **Type B**: lack of clotting factor IX
- **Type C**: lack of clotting factor XI (affects both sexes, rarely occurs in the United States)

Both Type A and B are usually X-linked disorders, affecting only males. The severity of the disease depends on the amount of clotting factor in the blood.

**Symptoms**:

- Bleeding with severe trauma or stress (mild cases)
- Unexplained bruises, bleeding, swelling, joint pain
- Spontaneous hemorrhage (severe cases), often in the joints but can be anywhere in the body
- Epistaxis, mucosal bleeding
- First symptoms often occur during infancy when the child becomes active, resulting in frequent bruises

**Treatment**:

- Desmopressin acetate parenterally or nasally to stimulate production of clotting factor (mild cases)
- Infusions of clotting factor from donated blood or recombinant clotting factors (genetically engineered), utilizing guidelines for dosing
- Infusions of plasma (Type C)

## Disseminated Intravascular Coagulation

### *Pathology*

Disseminated intravascular coagulation (DIC) (consumption coagulopathy) is a secondary disorder that is triggered by another disorder such as trauma, congenital heart disease, necrotizing enterocolitis, sepsis, and severe viral infections. DIC triggers both coagulation and hemorrhage through a complex series of events. Trauma causes tissue factor (transmembrane glycoprotein) to enter the circulation and bind with coagulation factors, triggering the coagulation cascade. This stimulates thrombin to convert fibrinogen to fibrin, causing aggregation and destruction of platelets and forming clots that can be disseminated throughout the intravascular system. These clots increase in size as platelets adhere to the clots, causing blockage of both the microvascular systems and larger vessels, which can result in ischemia and necrosis. Clot formation triggers fibrinolysis and plasmin to breakdown fibrin and fibrinogen, causing the destruction of clotting factors and resulting in hemorrhage. Both processes, clotting and hemorrhage, continue at the same time, placing the patient at high risk for death, even with treatment.

### *Symptoms and Treatment*

The onset of symptoms of DIC may be very rapid or be a slower chronic progression from a disease. Those who develop the chronic manifestation of the disease usually have fewer acute symptoms and may slowly develop ecchymosis or bleeding wounds.

**Symptoms** include:

- Bleeding from surgical or venous puncture sites
- Evidence of GI bleeding with distention, bloody diarrhea
- Hypotension and acute symptoms of shock
- Petechiae and purpura with extensive bleeding into the tissues
- Laboratory abnormalities:
  - Prolonged prothrombin and partial prothrombin times
  - Decreased platelet counts and fragmented RBCs
  - Decreased fibrinogen

**Treatment** includes:

- Identifying and treating underlying cause
- Massive blood transfusion protocol; replacement of blood products, such as platelets and fresh frozen plasma
- Anticoagulation therapy (heparin) to increase clotting time
- Cryoprecipitate to increase fibrinogen levels
- Coagulation inhibitors and coagulation factors

## THROMBOCYTOPENIA

Thrombocytopenia is a deficiency of circulating platelets in the blood. It can be caused by a decrease in the production of platelets from the bone marrow or an increase in destruction of platelets. Thrombocytopenia may also be caused from the use of heparin. Heparin induced thrombocytopenia can occur after heparin therapy (average 4–14 days post therapy) and is characterized by a decrease in platelet count to less than 50% of baseline or the occurrence of an unexplained thrombolytic event. A decreased production of platelets within the bone marrow can occur as a result of malignancy, bone marrow failure, infection, alcohol abuse, or a nutritional deficiency. An increase in the destruction of platelets may occur in disseminated intravascular coagulation, vasculitis, thrombotic thrombocytopenic purpura, sepsis, or idiopathic thrombocytopenic purpura.

**Signs/symptoms**: Petechiae, ecchymosis, bleeding from the mouth or gums, epistaxis, pallor, weakness, fatigue, splenomegaly, blood in the urine or stool, and jaundice.

**Diagnosis**: Physical exam and lab studies including complete blood count, partial thromboplastin time and prothrombin time may be used to diagnosis thrombocytopenia. A bone marrow biopsy may be indicated to determine the cause of the decreased production of platelets.

**Treatment**: Treatment of thrombocytopenia involves identifying and treating the underlying cause. Medications that decrease the platelet count should be held. Platelet transfusions may be administered to patients with extremely low counts (less than 50,000) or if spontaneous bleeding occurs. Platelet transfusions are contraindicated in patients with thrombotic thrombocytopenia purpura.

## ITP

The autoimmune disorder **idiopathic thrombocytopenic purpura (ITP)** causes an immune response to platelets, resulting in decreased platelet counts. ITP affects primarily children and young women although it can occur at any age. The acute form primarily occurs in children, but the chronic form affects primarily adults. Platelet counts are usually 150,000–400,000 per mcL. With ITP, platelet levels are less than 100,000. Maintaining a platelet count of at least 30,000 is necessary to prevent intracranial hemorrhage, the primary concern. The cause of ITP is unclear and may be precipitated by viral infection, sulfa drugs, and conditions, such as lupus erythematosus. ITP is usually not life threatening and can be controlled. **Symptoms** include:

- Bruising and petechiae with hematoma in some cases
- Epistaxis
- Increased menstrual flow in post-puberty females

**Treatment** includes:

- Corticosteroids to depress immune response and increase platelet count
- Splenectomy may be indicated for chronic conditions
- Platelet transfusions
- Avoiding aspirin, ibuprofen, or other NSAIDs

## HITTS

**Heparin-induced thrombocytopenia and thrombosis syndrome** (HITTS) occurs in patients receiving heparin for anticoagulation. There are two types:

- **Type I** is a transient condition occurring within a few days and causing depletion of platelets (<100,000 $mm^3$), but heparin may be continued as the condition usually resolves without intervention.
- **Type II** is an autoimmune reaction to heparin that occurs in 3–5% of those receiving unfractionated heparin and also occurs with low-molecular-weight heparin. It is characterized by low platelets (<50,000 $mm^3$) that are ≥50% below baseline. Onset is 5–14 days but can occur within hours of heparinization. Death rates are <30%. Heparin-antibody complexes form and release platelet factor 4 (PF4), which attracts heparin molecules and adheres to platelets and endothelial lining, stimulating thrombin and platelet clumping. This puts the patient at risk for thrombosis and vessel occlusion rather than hemorrhage, causing stroke, myocardial infarction, and limb ischemia with symptoms associated with the site of thrombosis. Treatment includes:
    - Discontinuation of heparin
    - Direct thrombin inhibitors (lepirudin, argatroban)
    - Monitor for signs/symptoms of thrombus/embolus

# Immunologic Pathophysiology

## Immune Deficiencies

There are multiple disorders that fall into the category of **primary immunodeficiency diseases.** These disorders are genetic or inherited disorders in which the body's immune system does not function properly. These disorders may involve low levels of antibodies, defects in the antibodies, or defects in cells that make up the immune system (T-cells, B-cells). Common variable immune deficiency is a common immune deficiency diagnosed in adulthood. This disorder is characterized by low levels of serum immunoglobins and antibodies, which substantially increases the risk of infection.

- **Signs/symptoms**: Recurrent infections are the hallmark sign of immune deficiency disorders. Recurrent infections most often involve the ears, sinuses, bronchi, and lungs. Lymphadenopathy may occur as well as splenomegaly. GI symptoms may include abdominal pain, nausea, vomiting, diarrhea, and weight loss. Some patients may experience polyarthritis. Granulomas are also common and may occur in the lungs, lymph nodes, liver, and skin.
- **Diagnosis**: A physical assessment and patient history are used to diagnose immune deficiency disorders. Since immune deficiency disorders are genetic or inherited, family history should also be evaluated. Lab tests such as serum antibodies, serum immunoglobin levels and a complete blood count may also be used to assist in the diagnosis of immune deficiency disorders.
- **Treatment**: Patients with immune deficiency disorders often receive immunoglobulin replacement. Long term antibiotics may also be administered for recurrent infections. Educate patients to frequently wash hands, cook foods thoroughly, avoid large crowds, and other infection prevention techniques.

### *Congenital Immunodeficiencies*

Congenital immunodeficiencies include:

- **Common variable immunodeficiency** is primarily an IgG deficiency due to absent plasma cells and B cell differentiation. These patients have increased susceptibility to encapsulated organisms and are more likely to develop bronchiectasis from the recurrent damage. They are also at higher risk for B cell neoplasms, GI malignancy, and autoimmune disease. Test is with functional antibody response and treatment with IVIG.
- **Congenital Agammaglobulinemia** (Bruton's, x-linked) usually leads to a susceptibility to recurrent pyogenic infections and low IgG and no IgA, IgM, IgE, IgD, or B cells.

- **Selective IgA deficiency** is the most common Ig deficiency and leads to recurrent sinopulmonary infections. It has association with recurrent giardiasis, GI malignancy, and autoimmune disorders, including celiac sprue. One should withhold IVIG due to possible anaphylactic reaction to IgA.
- **Wiskott-Aldrich syndrome** is the combination of thrombocytopenia, eczema, and immunodeficiency. It has associated low IgM and elevated IgA and IgE. BMT treats this successfully.

### *Complement Deficiencies*

There are deficiencies of all parts of the complement pathway, including the following:

- **Classical deficiency** may include C1 (q, r, s), C2, and C4. This leads to immune complex syndromes and pyogenic infection, such as recurrent sinopulmonary infections with encapsulated bacteria. There is an association with SLE and other rheumatoid diseases. C2 is the most common deficiency in Caucasians in the US.
- **C3 and alternative complement deficiency** may lead to immune complex syndromes and recurrent infections, such as severe pyogenic infections. It may also be associated with HUS.
- **Membrane attack complex (MAC) deficiency** is also known as terminal complement deficiency. This is associated with recurrent Neisseria infections (which can cause meningitis and sepsis) and immune complex diseases. The CH50 assay must be checked to determine the activity of the classical pathway. CH50 may also be used to follow disease activity in SLE.

## Autoimmune System Disorders

**Allergic interstitial/tubulointerstitial nephritis** is inflammation and edema of the interstitial areas of the kidneys. Up to 92% of cases caused by allergic reaction to medications, such as antibiotics (B-lactams, fluoroquinolones, macrolides, and anti-tuberculin drugs), antivirals, NSAIDs, PPIs, antiepileptics, diuretics, chemotherapy, and allopurinol. **Symptoms** include fever, rash, and renal enlargement as well as fatigue, nausea, vomiting, and weight loss. **Diagnosis** is by renal biopsy. Urine tests may show eosinophils, blood, RBC casts and sterile pyuria. Increased protein may be seen in response to NSAIDs. **Treatment** is primarily supportive but requires stopping the triggering medication.

**Eosinophilic esophagitis** is the accumulation of eosinophils in the esophagus, resulting in chronic inflammation. Damage from proteins produced in esophageal tissue causes scarring and narrowing, resulting in dysphagia, vomiting, choking, GERD, upper abdominal pain, heartburn, and regurgitation. **Causes** include allergic reaction to pollens or foods. **Risk factors** include cold/dry climate, male gender, family history, allergies, and asthma. **Diagnosis** is per endoscopy with biopsy. Blood tests may help confirm allergic reactions. **Treatment** may include dietary limitations, PPIs, and topical steroids. Some may require dilation of the esophagus.

**Churg-Strauss syndrome** (AKA **eosinophilic granulomatosis with polyangiitis**) is an idiopathic form of pulmonary vasculitis that can affect multiple systems (skin and lungs most often) as well as affecting small- and medium-sized arteries in those with asthma. **Symptoms** include dyspnea, chest pain, skin rash, myopathy, arthropathy, rhinitis, sinusitis, abdominal pain, blood in stools, and paresthesia (from the involvement of nerves). The syndrome is characterized by eosinophilia >1500 cells/mcL or >10% of peripheral total WBC count. X-rays or CTs may show transient opacities or multiple nodules. Tissue biopsies typically show allergic granulomas. **Treatment** usually begins with corticosteroids but other immunosuppressive drugs (cyclophosphamide, methotrexate, azathioprine) may be used, especially if critical organs are involved. The goal of treatment is remission, but patients usually need to take drugs at least 2 years before they are tapered off of the drugs. Up to 50% of patients have relapses.

### *LUPUS ERYTHEMATOSUS*

Lupus erythematosus is an autoimmune inflammatory disease that can involve multiple body systems, manifesting with the following symptoms:

| | |
|---|---|
| **Cardiopulmonary** | Pneumonitis, pleural effusion, Raynaud's phenomenon, myocarditis, endocarditis, pericarditis |
| **Gastrointestinal** | Pain, diarrhea, dysphagia, nausea, and vomiting |
| **Hematologic** | Lymphadenopathy, splenomegaly, anemia, leukopenia, thrombocytopenia |
| **Integumentary** | Malar (butterfly) rash, alopecia, discoid and palmar erythema, mucosal ulcers, photosensitivity |
| **Musculoskeletal** | Arthritis, synovitis, myositis |
| **Neurologic** | Stroke, seizures, psychoses, neuropathy, cognitive impairment |
| **Reproductive** | Increased risk of pregnancy complications |
| **Urologic** | Glomerulonephritis, cystitis, kidney failure, proteinuria |

**Diagnosis** of lupus erythematosus is based on symptoms, signs of inflammation, low blood counts, kidney disorders, positive antinuclear antibody test (a required criterion for diagnosis with other signs/symptoms), and the presence of abnormal antibodies, including anti-dsDNA, anti-Sm, anti-U1RNP, anti-Ro/SSA and anti-La/SSB.

**Treatment** includes hydroxychloroquine (first line), glucocorticoids, immunosuppressive agents (e.g., methotrexate, azathioprine, mycophenolate mofetil, cyclophosphamide), monoclonal antibodies (e.g., anifrolumab, belimumab, rituximab), sun protection, smoking cessation, and vaccinations.

**Complications** include lupus flare (i.e., worsening of symptoms in one or more systems, ranging from mild to severe), which may be triggered by stress, exposure to sunlight, infection, and failure to adhere to a prescribed medication regimen. Common symptoms include increased fatigue; skin rash; mouth sores; peripheral edema; fever (unrelated to infection); and swollen, painful joints. Patients often experience periods of remission between flares.

## NEUTROPENIA

Neutropenia is identified as an **absolute neutrophil count** equal to or less than 500/mL. **Chronic neutropenia** is a sustained condition of minimal neutrophils lasting 3 or more months. Neutropenia may occur from a decreased production of **white blood cells** (e.g., from chemotherapy or radiation therapy). It may also occur from a loss of white blood cells from autoimmune disease processes. Neutropenia is silent but dangerous. It leaves essentially no neutrophils to fight any threat of infection. Neutrophils make up as much as 70% of the white blood cells circulating in the blood. Neutropenia can be the cause of a septic situation, which can be life-threatening. Up to 70% of patients experiencing a fever while in a neutropenic state will die within 48 hours if not treated aggressively.

## LEUKOPENIA

Leukopenia is defined as a decrease in white blood cells. Neutropenia is defined as a low number of neutrophils and is often used interchangeably with the term leukopenia. With a decrease in the number of circulating white blood cells, the patient is at an increased risk for the development of an infection. Leukopenia and neutropenia can occur from either a decrease in the production of white blood cells or an increase in their destruction. Infections, malignancy, autoimmune disorders, medications (including chemotherapy) and a history of radiation therapy may contribute to the development of leukopenia/neutropenia.

**Signs/symptoms**: Malaise, fever, chills, night sweats, shortness of breath, headache, cough, abdominal pain, tachycardia, and hypotension. A patient with neutropenia/leukopenia is at risk for the development of infections including pneumonia, skin infections, urinary tract infections and gastrointestinal infections. In addition, the patient is at an increased risk for sepsis.

**Diagnosis**: Complete blood count including an absolute neutrophil count. In addition, a bone marrow biopsy may be performed to determine the cause of the decrease in neutrophils.

**Treatment**: Supportive therapy is used in the treatment of leukopenia including the aggressive treatment of infections that may develop. Precautions should be taken to protect the patient from additional infections, including strict adherence to sterile technique and infection control procedures. Hematopoietic growth factors may also be given to stimulate the production of neutrophils.

### LYMPHEDEMA

Lymphedema results from untreated or incurable **edema**. It is a chronic condition marked by swelling and accumulated fluids within the tissue. This accumulation is a result of lymphatic drainage failure, inadequate lymph transport capacity, an increased lymph production, or a combination of these. Primary disease is a result of **inadequately developed lymphatic pathways**, while the secondary disease process is due to **damage outside of the pathways**. The process is worsened and complicated as **macrophages** are released to control inflammation caused by the increased release of fibroblasts and keratinocytes. There is a gradual increase in adipose tissue and leakage of lymph through the skin. The skin and tissues gradually thicken and change in color, texture, tone, and temperature. It begins to blister and produce hyperkeratosis, warts, papillomatosis, and elephantiasis. There is an ever-increasing risk of infection and further complications.

## HIV/AIDS

**AIDS** is a progression of infection with **human immunodeficiency virus** (HIV). AIDS is diagnosed when the following criteria are met:

- HIV infection
- CD4 count less than 200 cells/$mm^3$
- AIDS defining condition, such as opportunistic infections (cytomegalovirus, tuberculosis), wasting syndrome, neoplasms (Kaposi sarcoma), or AIDS dementia complex

Because there is such a wide range of AIDS defining conditions, the patient may present with many types of **symptoms**, depending upon the diagnosis, but more than half of AIDS patients exhibit:

- Fever
- Lymphadenopathy
- Pharyngitis
- Rash
- Myalgia/arthralgia
- It is important to review the following:
  - CD4 counts to determine immune status
  - WBC and differential for signs of infection
  - Cultures to help identify any infective agents
  - CBC to evaluate for signs of bleeding or thrombocytopenia

Treatment aims to cure or manage opportunistic conditions and control underlying HIV infection through highly active anti-retroviral therapy (HAART), 3 or more drugs used concurrently.

# Hematological Procedures and Interventions

## Transfusion Components

**Blood components** that are commonly used for transfusions include:

- **Packed red blood cells:** RBCs (250–300 mL per unit) should be warmed >30 °C (optimal 37 °C) before administration to prevent hypothermia and may be reconstituted in 50–100 mL of normal saline to facilitate administration. RBCs are necessary if blood loss is about 30% (1,500–2,000 mL lost; Hgb ≤7). Above 30% blood loss, whole blood may be more effective. RBCs are most frequently used for transfusions.
- **Platelet concentrates:** Transfusions of platelets are used if the platelet count is <50,000 cells/mm$^3$. One unit increases the platelet count by 5,000–10,000 cells/mm$^3$. Platelet concentrates pose a risk for sensitization reactions and infectious diseases. Platelet concentrate is stored at a higher temperature (20–24 °C) than RBCs. This contributes to bacterial growth, so it is more prone to bacterial contamination than other blood products and may cause sepsis. Temperature increase within 6 hours should be considered an indication of possible sepsis. ABO compatibility should be observed but is not required.
- **Fresh frozen plasma** (FFP) (obtained from a unit of whole blood frozen ≤6 hours after collection) includes all clotting factors and plasma proteins, so each unit administered increases clotting factors by 2–3%. FFP may be used for deficiencies of isolated factors, excess warfarin therapy, and liver-disease-related coagulopathy. It may be used for patients who have received extensive blood transfusions but continue to hemorrhage. It is also helpful for those with antithrombin III deficiency. FFP should be warmed to 37 °C prior to administration to avoid hypothermia. ABO compatibility should be observed if possible, but it is not required. Some patients may become sensitized to plasma proteins.
- **Cryoprecipitate** is the precipitate that forms when FFP is thawed. It contains fibrinogen, factor VIII, von Willebrand, and factor XIII. This component may be used to treat hemophilia A and hypofibrinogenemia.

## Transfusion Administration

Prior to the transfusion of any blood component, the nurse should obtain the patient's transfusion history along with a consent form. A type and crossmatch must be completed on the patient's blood and an IV in place for administration. An 18-gauge catheter is standard, but 20- to 22-gauge can also be used at a slower rate. Baseline vital signs need to be taken prior to starting the infusion, and then the patient should be under direct observation for at least the first 15 minutes. Vital signs should be monitored at 5 minutes, 15 minutes, and then at least every 30 minutes during the transfusion and one hour post-transfusion.

## Transfusion-Related Complications

There are a number of transfusion-related complications, which is the reason that transfusions are given only when necessary. Complications include:

- **Infection**: Bacterial contamination of blood, especially platelets, can result in severe sepsis. A number of infective agents (viral, bacterial, and parasitic) can be transmitted, although increased testing of blood has decreased rates of infection markedly. Infective agents include HIV, hepatitis C and B, human T-cell lymphotropic virus, CMV, WNV, malaria, Chagas' disease, and variant Creutzfeldt-Jacob disease (from contact with mad cow disease).
- **Transfusion-related acute lung injury (TRALI):** This respiratory distress syndrome occurs ≤6 hours after transfusion. The cause is believed to be antileukocytic or anti-HLA antibodies in the transfusion. It is characterized by non-cardiogenic pulmonary edema (high protein level) with severe dyspnea and arterial hypoxemia. Transfusion must be stopped immediately and the blood bank notified. TRALI may result in fatality but usually resolves in 12–48 hours with supportive care.

- **Graft vs. host disease:** Lymphocytes cause an immune response in immunocompromised individuals. Lymphocytes may be inactivated by irradiation, as leukocyte filters are not reliable.
- **Post-transfusion purpura:** Platelet antibodies develop and destroy the patient's platelets, so the platelet count decreases about 1 week after transfusion.
- **Transfusion-related immunosuppression:** Cell-mediated immunity is suppressed, so the patient is at increased risk of infection, and in cancer patients, transfusions may correlate with tumor recurrence. This condition relates to transfusions that include leukocytes. RBCs cause a less pronounced immunosuppression, suggesting a causative agent is in the plasma. Leukoreduction is becoming more common to reduce transmission of leukocyte-related viruses.
- **Hypothermia**: This may occur if blood products are not heated. Oxygen utilization is halved for each 10 °C decrease in normal body temperature.

## Autotransfusion

Autotransfusion (autologous blood transfusion) is collecting of the patient's blood and re-infusing it. This is life-saving if another donor's blood is not available. Blood in trauma cases is usually collected from a body cavity, such as pleural (hemothorax with ≥1,500 mL blood) or peritoneal space (rare). **Autotransfusion** is contraindicated if malignant lesions are present in the area of blood loss, contamination of pooled blood, or wounds more than 4–6 hours old. Commercial collection/transfusion kits (Pleur-Evac, Thora-Klex) are available, but blood can be collected through the chest tube into a sterile bottle, which is then disconnected and connected to IV tubing for infusion, or the blood in the bottle may be transferred to a blood collection bag for use. Commercial kits use either a chest tube or suction tube to withdraw blood and provide specific procedures. Blood is filtered. Heparin is not routinely used, but citrate phosphate dextrose (CPD) (25–70 mL per 500 mL blood) is often added to the aspirant to prevent clotting. Complications from autotransfusion are rare.

## Plasmapheresis

With plasmapheresis, whole blood is removed from the body, anticoagulant is added, cellular components are separated from the plasma (which is removed), and cellular components are suspended in saline, albumin (most common), or another substitute for plasma. This is reinfused into the patient. The purpose is to remove harmful antibodies found in plasma. ACE inhibitors increase risk of hypotension and should be withheld for 24 hours before the procedure. Machine settings may vary. Typically, the patient's height and weight are entered into the automated system to aid in calculating the plasma volume. The patient must be carefully monitored during the procedure for signs of hypocalcemia (perioral/fingertip tingling, alterations in mental status, VT), which requires the administration of calcium; hypomagnesemia (confusion, headaches, dizziness, twitching), which requires administration of magnesium; and hypotension, which requires saline bolus. If the patient shows indications of transfusion reaction, the infusion must be discontinued and medications (diphenhydramine, corticosteroids) administered. The patient should be kept warm to avoid hypothermia. Post-procedure, the patient may experience thrombocytopenia and hypofibrinogenemia, so the patient must be observed for signs of bleeding.

## Exchange Transfusion

Exchange transfusions replace a person's blood with donor blood to remove sickled blood for sickle cell anemia or to remove toxins. The exchange may be complete or partial. An automated machine is generally used, and the time on the machine ranges from 1–4 hours. (If done manually, removal and replacement are done in cycles with blood first removed followed by replacement.) A catheter is inserted (usually in the arm) to drain the blood and another, usually in the femoral area (under local or moderate sedation), to administer donor blood, plasma, or another substitute for plasma. During the exchange, the patient's VS must be carefully monitored. If the patient exhibits signs of hypocalcemia (perioral/finger tingling) then calcium is administered. Some may receive calcium routinely during administration. Blood may be taken from the femoral line for testing after the exchange. When the femoral catheter is removed, pressure must be applied to the area for at least 5 minutes and the patient instructed to lie flat for at least 30 minutes to prevent bleeding.

## Leukocyte Depletion

Red blood cell and platelet transfusions typically contain some leukocytes, which are recognized as foreign by the immune system of a patient receiving the transfusion. This can lead to adverse reactions, especially in patients who are immunocompromised. **Leukocyte depletion** is carried out by various processes, including filtration. One disadvantage to leukodepletion of RBCs is that the process results in the loss of about 10% of the RBCs, and some hemolysis may occur. Leukocyte depleted RBCs are given in volumes of 200–250 mL within a 4-hour time period.

## Blood Conservation

Blood conservation includes methods to:

- **Minimize the loss of blood during surgical procedures**: May include regional anesthesia instead of general, positioning to reduce blood loss, cell salvage, autotransfusion, non-invasive monitoring (BP, pulse oximetry), limited blood draws, normovolemic hemodilution, and medications to reduce bleeding (vitamin K, tranexamic acid, desmopressin, somatostatin, vasopressin, recombinant factor VIIa).
- **Lower the threshold for receiving transfusions**: Transfusion threshold lowered from 10 g/dL to 7 g/dL.
- **Maintain the hematocrit at acceptable levels**: Administration of oral or parenteral iron therapy to increase tolerance for blood loss. Erythropoietin alpha may also be administered perioperatively to stimulate the production of RBCs.
- **Ensure optimal oxygenation of tissue**: Hyperoxic ventilation during surgery, crystalloid/colloid volume replacement, and utilizing techniques to minimize consumption of oxygen.

Blood conservation includes a commitment to bloodless surgery as much as possible, especially through the utilization of minimally-invasive procedures.

## Massive Transfusion Protocol

A massive transfusion protocol (MTP) is a proactive standardized protocol used during an uncontrolled hemorrhage, designed to ensure effective management of massive blood loss and to improve patient outcome.

Indications for activation of **massive transfusion protocol** (MTP) include:

- Uncontrolled hemorrhage.
- Actual/anticipated use of ≥4 units of RBCs in less than 4 hours or ≥10 units in 24 hours (some may need up to 30 units in 8 hours).
- Hemodynamic instability despite initial management of bleeding and resuscitation efforts that should include avoiding hypothermia and the use of excessive crystalloid.
- Allowing permissive hypotension to 80–100 systolic BP to help control bleeding. Autotransfusion may be used when appropriate.

Protocols may vary somewhat:

- MTPs are activated by a clinician in response to massive bleeding, generally after transfusion of 4–10 units.
- Obtain baseline laboratory tests (CBC, coagulation screen, blood gases, and chemistry panel) and repeat CBC, blood gases, coagulation screen, and ionized calcium test hourly.
- MTP packs have a predetermined ratio (e.g., 1:1:1 or 2:1:1 ratio) of RBCs, FFPs, and platelet units for transfusion, prepared by the blood bank for rapid and timely delivery.

- Targets of resuscitation include:
  - Mean arterial pressure (MAP) around 60 mmHg
  - Core temperature >35 °C
  - Hemoglobin 7–9 g/dL
  - pH 7.35–7.45
  - Lactate <4 mmol/L
  - Calcium >1.1 mmol/L
  - Platelets >50,000
  - PT/aPTT <1.5 times normal
  - INR ≤1.5
  - Fibrinogen >1.5–2.0 g/L

# Gastrointestinal Pathophysiology

## Peritonitis

Peritonitis (inflammation of the peritoneum) may be primary (from infection of blood or lymph) or, more commonly, secondary, related to perforation or trauma of the gastrointestinal tract. Common causes include perforated bowel, ruptured appendix, abdominal trauma, abdominal surgery, peritoneal dialysis or chemotherapy, or leakage of sterile fluids, such as blood, into the peritoneum.

**Symptoms:** Diffuse abdominal pain with rebound tenderness (Blumberg's sign), abdominal rigidity, paralytic ileus, fever (with infection), nausea and vomiting, and sinus tachycardia.

**Diagnosis:** Increased WBC (>15,000), abdominal x-ray/CT, paracentesis, blood and peritoneal fluid culture.

**Treatment** includes:

- Intravenous fluids and electrolytes
- Broad-spectrum antibiotics
- Laparoscopy as indicated to determine cause of peritonitis and effect repair

## Appendicitis

Appendicitis is inflammation of the appendix often caused by luminal obstruction and pressure within the lumen; secretions build up and can eventually perforate the appendix. Diagnosis can be made difficult by the fact that there is some variation in the exact location of the appendix in some patients. Appendicitis can occur in all ages, but children younger than 2 years usually present with peritonitis or sepsis because of difficulty in early diagnosis. **Symptoms** include:

- Acute abdominal pain, which may be epigastric, periumbilical, right lower quadrant, or right flank with rebound tenderness
- Anorexia
- Nausea and vomiting
- Positive psoas and obturator signs
- Fever may develop after 24 hours
- Malaise
- Bowel irregularity and flatulence

**Diagnosis** is based on clinical presentation, CBC (although leukocytosis may not be present), urinalysis, and imaging studies (usually an abdominal CT with contrast).

## Cholecystitis

Cholecystitis can result in obstruction of the bile duct related to calculi as well as pancreatitis from obstruction of the pancreatic duct. In acute cholecystitis, there is fever, leukocytosis, right upper quadrant abdominal pain, and inflammation of the gallbladder. The disease is most common in overweight women 20–40 years of age, but can occur in pregnant women and people of all ages, especially those who are diabetic or elderly. Cholecystitis may develop secondary to cystic fibrosis, obesity, or total parenteral nutrition. Many times, cholecystitis may resolve in about 7–10 days on its own, but acute cholecystitis may need surgical intervention to prevent complications such as gangrene in the gallbladder or perforation. Diagnosis is confirmed by ultrasound of gallbladder showing thickening of gallbladder walls or positive Murphy's sign, or a HIDA scan showing failure to fill.

**Symptoms:**

- Severe right upper quadrant or epigastric pain (ranging from 2–6 hours per episode)
- Nausea and vomiting
- Jaundice
- Altered mental status
- Positive Murphy's sign

**Treatment**:

- Antibiotics for sepsis/ascending cholangitis
- Antispasmodic agents (glycopyrrolate) for biliary colic and vomiting
- Analgesics (note that opioids result in increased sphincter of Oddi pressure)
- Antiemetics
- Surgical consultation for possible laparoscopic or open cholecystectomy

## Erosive vs. Nonerosive Gastritis

Gastritis is inflammation of the epithelium or endothelium of the stomach. Types include:

- **Erosive**: Typically caused by alcohol, NSAIDs, illness, portal hypertension, and/or stress. Risk factors include severe illness, mechanical ventilation, trauma, sepsis, organ failure, and burns. Patients may be essentially asymptomatic but may have hematemesis or "coffee ground" emesis. Treatment depends on cause and severity but often includes a proton pump inhibitor (such as omeprazole 20–40 mg per day). Some may receive an H2-rceptor (such as famotidine). Those with portal hypertension may respond to propranolol or nadolol or portal decompression.
- **Nonerosive**: Typically caused by Helicobacter pylori infection or pernicious anemia. H. pylori infection can lead to gastric and duodenal ulcers. Treatment for H. pylori is per antibiotics and proton pump inhibitors with standard triple or standard quadruple therapy. Pernicious anemia is treated with vitamin B-12. Gastritis may also be caused by a wide range of pathogens, including parasites, so treatment depends on the causative agent.

**Review Video: Pernicious Anemia**
Visit mometrix.com/academy and enter code: 353419

## Gastroenteritis

### Viral Gastroenteritis

Viral gastroenteritis (commonly referred to as stomach flu) is characterized by nausea, vomiting, abdominal cramping, watery (may become bloody) diarrhea, headache, muscle aches, and fever. Viral gastroenteritis is spread through the fecal-oral route. Common **causes** include:

- **Norovirus**: Symptoms generally include diarrhea and vomiting with symptoms persisting for 1–3 days. Most people do not require treatment, but if diarrhea or vomiting is severe, an antiemetic or antidiarrheal may be prescribed if the patient is younger than 65. If severe dehydration occurs, the patient may require intravenous fluids until she is able to resume adequate oral intake.
- **Rotavirus**: Symptoms include watery diarrhea, nausea, vomiting, abdominal pain and cramping, lack of appetite and fever. Patients may become easily dehydrated and require rehydration with Pedialyte or Rice-Lyte or IV fluids. Medications are usually not needed but the rotavirus vaccine prevents severe rotavirus-related diarrhea and is given in 3 doses (2 months, 4 months, and 6 months).

### Bacterial Gastroenteritis

Bacterial gastroenteritis generally results in cramping, nausea, and severe diarrhea. Some bacteria cause gastroenteritis because of enterotoxins that adhere to the mucosa of the intestines and others because of exotoxins that remain in contaminated food. Some bacteria directly invade the intestinal mucosa. Bacterial gastroenteritis is commonly **caused** by:

- ***Salmonella***: Sudden onset of bloody diarrhea, abdominal cramping, nausea, and vomiting, leading to dehydration. Infection may become systemic and life-threatening. Treatment is supportive although antibiotics may be administered to those at risk.
- ***Campylobacter***: Bloody diarrhea, cramping, fever, for up to 7 days that usually resolves but may become systemic in those who are immunocompromised. Treatment is primarily supportive with antibiotics only for those at risk.
- ***Shigella* spp.**: Most common in children <5 and presents with fever, abdominal cramping, and bloody diarrhea, persisting 5–7 days. Treatment is primarily supportive (rehydration) although those at risk (very young, old, immunocompromised) may receive antibiotics because the disease may become systemic.
- ***Escherichia coli***: Different strains are associated with traveler's diarrhea and food-borne illnesses, and severity varies. Most result in diarrhea, nausea, vomiting, and cramping, but some strains (0157) may develop into life-threatening hemolytic uremic syndrome (HUS). Treatment is supportive. Antibiotics increase risk of developing HUS.



### Parasitic Gastroenteritis

Parasitic gastroenteritis is generally caused by infection with protozoa (one-celled pathogens):

- ***Giardia intestinalis***: Common cause of waterborne (drinking and recreational) disease and non-bacterial diarrhea, resulting from fecal contamination. Symptoms include diarrhea, abdominal cramping, flatulence, greasy floating stools, nausea and vomiting as well as weight loss. Symptoms usually persist for up to 3 weeks although some develop chronic disease. Metronidazole is the drug of choice: Adults, 250 mg TID for 5–7 days. Pediatrics, 15 mg/kg/day in 3 doses for 5–7 days.
- ***Cryptosporidium parvum***: About 10,000 cases occur in the US each year, usually from contact with fecal-contaminated water. Symptoms include watery diarrhea, abdominal pain, nausea, vomiting, weight loss, and fever and persist for up to 2 weeks although a severe chronic infection may occur in those who are immunocompromised. Treatment for non-HIV-infected patients (medications ineffective for HIV patients): Adults and children >11, Nitazoxanide 500 mg BID for 3 days. Pediatrics, 1–3 years 100 mg BID for 3 days; 4–11 years 200 mg BID for 3 days.

## Constipation and Impaction

**Constipation** is a condition with bowel movements less frequent than normal for a person, or hard, small stool that is evacuated fewer than 3 times weekly. Food moves through the GI from the small intestine to the colon in semi-liquid form. Constipation results from the colon, where fluid is absorbed. If too much fluid is absorbed, the stool can become too dry. People may have abdominal distension and cramps and need to strain for defecation.

**Fecal impaction** occurs when the hard stool moves into the rectum and becomes a large, dense, immovable mass that cannot be evacuated even with straining, usually as a result of chronic constipation. In addition to abdominal cramps and distention, the person may feel intense rectal pressure and pain accompanied by a sense of urgency to defecate. Nausea and vomiting may also occur. Hemorrhoids will often become engorged. Fecal incontinence, with liquid stool leaking about the impaction, is common.

### *Medical Procedures to Evaluate Causes of Constipation*

Medical procedures to evaluate causes of constipation should be preceded by a careful history as this may help to define the type and guide the choice of diagnostic procedures. Most tests are necessary only for severe constipation that does not respond to treatment. Medical **diagnostic procedures** may include the following:

- **Physical exam** should include rectal exam and abdominal palpation to assess for obvious hard stool or impaction.
- **Blood tests** can identify hypothyroidism and excess parathyroid hormone.
- **Abdominal x-ray** may show large amounts of stool in the colon.
- **Barium enema** can indicate tumors or strictures causing obstruction.
- **Colonic transit studies** can show defects of the neuromuscular system.
- **Defecography** shows the defecation process and abnormalities of anatomy.
- **Anorectal manometry studies** show malfunction of anorectal muscles.
- **Colonic motility studies** measure the pattern of colonic pressure.
- **Colonoscope** allows direct visualization of the lumen of the rectum and colon.

## Bowel Obstructions

Bowel obstruction occurs when there is a mechanical obstruction of the passage of intestinal contents because of constriction of the lumen, occlusion of the lumen, adhesion formation, or lack of muscular contractions (paralytic ileus). **Symptoms** include abdominal pain, rigidity, and distention, n/v, dehydration, constipation, respiratory distress from the diaphragm pushing against the pleural cavity, sepsis, and shock. **Treatment** includes strict NPO, insertion of naso/orogastric tube, IV fluids and careful monitoring; may correct spontaneously, severe obstruction requires surgery.

## Bowel Infarctions

Bowel infarction is ischemia of the intestines related to severely restricted blood supply. It can be the result of a number of different conditions, such as strangulated bowel or occlusion of arteries of the mesentery, and may follow untreated bowel obstruction. Patients present with acute abdomen and shock, and mortality rates are very high even with resection of infarcted bowel. **Treatment** includes replacing volume, correcting the underlying issue, improving blood flow to the mesentery, insertion of NGT, and/or surgery.

## Intestinal Perforation

Intestinal perforation is a partial or complete tear in the intestinal wall, leaking intestinal contents into the peritoneum. Causes include trauma, NSAIDs (elderly, patients with diverticulitis), acute appendicitis, PUD, iatrogenic (laparoscopy, endoscopy, colonoscopy, radiotherapy), bacterial infections, IBS, and ingestion of toxic substances (acids) or foreign bodies (toothpicks). The danger posed by infection after perforation varies depending upon the site. The stomach and proximal portions of the small intestine have little bacteria, but the distal portion of the small intestine contains aerobic bacteria, such as *E. coli,* as well as anaerobic bacteria.

**Signs/symptoms:** (appear within 24–48 hours): Abdominal pain and distention and rigidity, fever, guarding and rebound tenderness, tachycardia, dyspnea, absent bowel sounds/paralytic ileus with nausea and vomiting; Sepsis and abscess or fistula formation can occur.

**Diagnosis:** Labs: elevated WBC; lactic acid and pH change as late signs. X-ray and CT will show free air in abdominal cavity.

**Treatment** includes:

- Prompt antibiotic therapy and surgical repair with peritoneal lavage
- The abdominal wound may be left open to heal by secondary intention and to prevent compartment syndrome

## Gastroesophageal Reflux Disease

Gastroesophageal reflux occurs when the lower esophageal sphincter fails to remain closed, allowing the contents of the stomach to back into the esophagus. This reflux of the acid containing contents of the stomach may cause irritation of the lining of the esophagus. When experienced chronically, as in gastroesophageal reflux disease (GERD), damage to the lining of the esophagus can occur. In some patients, this may lead to the formation of Barrett's esophagus. In Barrett's esophagus, the lining of the esophagus begins to resemble the tissue lining the intestine. Patients with Barrett's esophagus have an increased risk of developing esophageal adenocarcinoma.

**Signs/symptoms**: Heartburn, dysphagia, belching, water brash, sore throat, hoarseness, and chest pain.

**Diagnosis**: Clinical signs/symptoms, ambulatory esophageal reflux monitoring (this test uses a thin pH probe that is placed in the esophagus). Data is collected on the amount of acid entering the esophagus along with the presence of clinical symptoms. Endoscopy may be used in the diagnosis of GERD in patients with persistent or progressive symptoms.

**Treatment**: GERD is often treated with proton pump inhibitors (inhibit gastric acid secretion). Surgical therapy may be utilized if medical management is unsuccessful. Patients are taught to eliminate foods that trigger symptoms (chocolate, caffeine, alcohol, and highly acidic foods). In addition, patients with GERD should avoid meals 2–3 hours before bed and may find it helpful to sleep with the head of the bed elevated to alleviate symptoms.

**Review Video: GERD**
Visit mometrix.com/academy and enter code: 294757

## Peptic Ulcer Disease

Peptic ulcer disease (PUD) includes both ulcerations of the duodenum and stomach. They may be primary (usually duodenal) or secondary (usually gastric). Gastric ulcers are commonly associated with ***H. pylori*** infections (80%) but may be caused by aspirin and NSAIDs. *H. pylori* are spread in the fecal-oral route from person to person or contaminated water and cause a chronic inflammation and ulcerations of the gastric mucosa. PUD is 2–3 times more common in males and is associated with poor economic status that results in a crowded, unhygienic environment, although it can occur in others. Usually, other family members have a history of ulcers as well.

**Symptoms** include abdominal pain, nausea, vomiting, and GI bleeding in children younger than 6 years with epigastric and postprandial pain and indigestion in older children and adults.

**Treatment** includes:

- Antibiotics for *H. pylori*: amoxicillin, clarithromycin, metronidazole
- Proton pump inhibitors: lansoprazole or omeprazole
- Bismuth
- Histamine-receptor antagonists: cimetidine or famotidine

**Review Video: Peptic Ulcers and GERD**
Visit mometrix.com/academy and enter code: 184332

## Inflammatory Bowel Disease

### *Ulcerative Colitis*

Ulcerative colitis is superficial inflammation of the mucosa of the colon and rectum, causing ulcerations in the areas where inflammation has destroyed cells. These ulcerations, ranging from pinpoint to extensive, may bleed and produce purulent material. The mucosa of the bowel becomes swollen, erythematous, and granular. Patients may present emergently with **severe ulcerative colitis** (having >6 blood stools a day, fever, tachycardia, anemia) or with **fulminant colitis** (>10 blood stools per day, severe bleeding, and toxic symptoms) These patients are at high risk for megacolon and perforation. For patients with severe and fulminant ulcerative colitis:

**Symptoms:**

- Abdominal pain
- Anemia
- F&E depletion
- Bloody diarrhea/rectal bleeding
- Diarrhea
- Fecal urgency
- Tenesmus
- Anorexia
- Weight loss
- Fatigue
- Systemic disorders: Eye inflammation, arthritis, liver disease, and osteoporosis as immune system triggers generalized inflammation

**Treatment:**

- Glucocorticoids
- Aminosalicylates
- Antibiotics if signs/symptoms of toxicity
- D/C anticholinergics, NSAIDS, and antidiarrheals
- If fulminant: Admitted & monitored for deterioration. Kept NPO, and given IV F&E replacement. NGT for decompression if intestinal dilation is present. Knee-elbow position to reposition gas in bowel. Colectomy for those with megacolon or who are unresponsive to therapy.

**Review Video: Ulcerative Colitis**
Visit mometrix.com/academy and enter code: 584881

### *Crohn's Disease*

Crohn's disease manifests with inflammation of the GI system. Inflammation is transmural (often leading to intestinal stenosis and fistulas), focal, and discontinuous with aphthous ulcerations progressing to linear and irregular-shaped ulcerations. Granulomas may be present. Common sites of inflammation are the terminal ileum and cecum. The condition is chronic, but patients with severe or fulminant disease (fevers, persistent vomiting, abscess, obstruction) often present emergently for treatment.

**Symptoms:**

- Perirectal abscess/fistula in advanced disease
- Diarrhea
- Watery stools
- Rectal hemorrhage
- Anemia
- Abdominal pain (commonly RLQ)
- Cramping
- Weight loss
- Nausea and vomiting
- Fever
- Night sweats

**Treatment:**

- Triamcinolone for oral lesions, aminosalicylates, glucocorticoids, antidiarrheals, probiotics, avoid lactose, and identify and eliminate food triggers.
- For patients who present with toxic symptoms: hospitalization for careful monitoring, IV glucocorticoids, aminosalicylates, antibiotics, and bowel rest. Parenteral nutrition for the malnourished.
- For repeated relapses (refractory):
    - Immunomodulatory agents (azathioprine, mercaptopurine, methotrexate) or Biologic therapies (infliximab). Bowel resection if unresponsive to all treatment or with ischemic bowel.



## Diverticular Disease

Diverticular disease is a condition in which diverticula (saclike pouchings of the bowel lining that extend through a defect in the muscle layer) occur anywhere within the GI tract. About 20% of patients with diverticular disease will develop acute diverticulitis, which occurs as diverticula become inflamed when food or bacteria are retained within the diverticula. This may result in abscess, obstruction, perforation, bleeding, or fistula. Diagnosis is best confirmed by abdominal CT with contrast (showing a localized thickening of the bowel wall, increased density of soft tissue, and diverticula in the colon). Many patients have normal lab studies, but some present with leukocytosis, elevated serum amylase, and pyuria on urinalysis.

**Symptoms** (similar to appendicitis):

- Steady pain in left lower quadrant
- Change in bowel habits
- Tenesmus
- Dysuria from irritation
- Recurrent urinary infections from fistula
- Paralytic ileus from peritonitis or intra-abdominal irritation
- Toxic reactions: fever, severe pain, leukocytosis

**Treatment**:

- Rehydration and electrolytes per IV fluids
- Nothing by mouth initially
- Antibiotics, broad spectrum (IV if toxic reactions)
- NG suction if necessary, for obstruction
- Careful observation for signs of perforation or obstruction

## ACUTE GASTROINTESTINAL HEMORRHAGE

Gastrointestinal (GI) hemorrhage may occur in the upper or lower gastrointestinal track. The primary cause (50–70%) of GI hemorrhage is gastric and duodenal ulcers, generally caused by stress, NSAIDs or infection with *Helicobacter pylori.*

**Symptoms:** Abdominal pain and distention, coffee-ground emesis/hematemesis, bloody or tarry stools, hypotension with tachycardia.

**Diagnosis:** Stool occult blood (Guaiac test), EGD, colonoscopy, GI Bleed scan.

**Treatment** includes:

- Medications: Fluid replacement with blood transfusions if necessary, antibiotic therapy for *Helicobacter pylori,* continuous pantoprazole IV to prevent further irritation
- Endoscopic thermal therapy to cauterize or injection therapy (hypertonic saline, epinephrine, ethanol) to cause vasoconstriction
- Arteriography with intra-arterial infusion of vasopressin and/or embolizing agents, such as stainless-steel coils, platinum microcoils, or Gelfoam pledgets
- Vagotomy and pyloroplasty if bleeding persists

**Prevention**: Prophylactic medications (pantoprazole [Protonix] IV is common).

## HEPATIC CIRRHOSIS

### *COMPENSATED*

Cirrhosis is a chronic hepatic disease in which normal liver tissue is replaced by the fibrotic tissue that impairs liver function. There are three **types**:

- **Alcoholic** (from chronic alcoholism) is the most common type and results in fibrosis about the portal areas. The liver cells become necrotic, replaced by fibrotic tissue, with areas of normal tissue projecting in between, giving the liver a hobnail appearance.
- **Post-necrotic** with broad bands of fibrotic tissue is the result of acute viral hepatitis.
- **Biliary**, the least common type, is caused by chronic biliary obstruction and cholangitis, with resulting fibrotic tissue about the bile ducts.

Cirrhosis may be either compensated or decompensated. **Compensated** cirrhosis usually involves non-specific symptoms, such as intermittent fever, epistaxis, ankle edema, indigestion, abdominal pain, and palmar erythema. Hepatomegaly and splenomegaly may also be present.

### *DECOMPENSATED*

Decompensated cirrhosis occurs when the liver can no longer adequately synthesize proteins, clotting factors, and other substances so that portal hypertension occurs.

**Symptoms:**

- Hepatomegaly
- Chronic elevated temperature
- Clubbing of fingers
- Purpura resulting from thrombocytopenia, with bruising and epistaxis
- Portal obstruction resulting in jaundice and ascites
- Bacterial peritonitis with ascites
- Esophageal varices
- Edema of extremities and presacral area resulting from reduced albumin in the plasma. Vitamin deficiency from interference with formation, use, and storage of vitamins, such as A, C, and K
- Anemia from chronic gastritis and decreased dietary intake
- Hepatic encephalopathy with alterations in mentation
- Hypotension
- Atrophy of gonads

**Treatment** varies according to the symptoms and is supportive rather than curative as the fibrotic changes in the liver cannot be reversed:

- Dietary supplements and vitamins
- Diuretics (potassium sparing), such as Aldactone and Dyrenium, to decrease ascites
- Colchicine to reduce fibrotic changes
- Liver transplant (the definitive treatment)



## FULMINANT HEPATITIS

Fulminant hepatitis is a severe acute infection of the liver that can result in hepatic necrosis, encephalopathy, and death within 1–2 weeks. Most hepatitis is caused by infection with hepatitis viruses A, B, C, D, or E, but it can also be caused by numerous viruses, toxic chemicals (carbon tetrachloride), metabolic diseases (Wilson disease), and drugs, such as acetaminophen. Fulminant hepatitis can result from any of these factors. Fulminant hepatitis can be divided into three stages according to the duration from jaundice to encephalopathy:

$$\begin{aligned} 0-7 \text{ days} &= \text{Hyperacute liver failure} \\ 7-28 \text{ days} &= \text{Acute liver failure} \\ 28-72 \text{ days} &= \text{Subacute liver failure} \end{aligned}$$

**Symptoms**:

- Poor feeding/anorexia
- Increased intracranial pressure with cerebral edema and encephalopathy
- Coagulopathies
- Renal failure
- Electrolyte imbalances

**Treatment**:

- Identify and treat underlying cause
- Intracranial pressure monitoring and treatment
- Diuresis; liver transplantation may be necessary
- Survival rates vary from 50–85%

## Portal Hypertension

Portal hypertension occurs when obstructed blood flow increases blood pressure throughout the portal venous system, preventing the liver from filtering blood and causing the development of collateral blood vessels that return unfiltered blood to the systemic circulation. Increasing serum aldosterone levels cause sodium and fluid retention in the kidneys, resulting in hypervolemia, ascites and esophageal varices. Portal hypertension can be caused by any liver disease, especially cirrhosis and inherited or acquired coagulopathies that cause thrombosis of the portal vein.

**Symptoms:** Ascites with distended abdomen, esophageal varices with bleeding, dyspnea, abdominal discomfort, fluid/electrolyte imbalances.

**Diagnosis:** Labs (CBC, BMP, liver panel, Hep B &C), abdominal ultrasound or CT/MRI, EGD, Hemodynamic measurement of the hepatic venous pressure gradient (HVPG)

**Treatment** includes:

- Restricted sodium intake & use diuretics as needed
- Endoscopic treatment of obstruction
- Portal vein shunting redirecting blood from the portal vein to the vena cava
- Liver transplant in severe cases
- These patients are at high risk for esophageal varices, which, if they rupture, can cause instantaneous hemorrhage and death

## Esophageal Varices

Esophageal varices are torturous, dilated veins in the submucosa of the esophagus (usually the distal portion). They are a complication of cirrhosis of the liver, in which obstruction of the portal vein causes an increase in collateral vessels and resulting decrease in circulation to the liver, increasing the pressure in the collateral vessels. This causes the vessels to dilate. Because they tend to be fragile and inelastic, they tear easily, causing sudden, massive esophageal hemorrhage.

**Signs/symptoms:** Usually asymptomatic until rupture; projectile vomiting bright red blood, dark stools, and shock.

**Diagnosis:** EGD, capsule endoscopy, CT, and MRI.

**Treatment** (in the case of rupture) includes:

- Emergent fluid and blood replacement
- IV vasopressin, somatostatin, and octreotide to decrease venous pressure and provide vasoconstriction/clotting
- Endoscopic injection with sclerosing agents and band ligation
- Esophagogastric balloon tamponade using Sengstaken-Blakemore and Minnesota tubes (Note: always inflate gastric balloon first, keep scissors nearby in case of balloon migration, do not use longer than 24 hrs as there is increased risk of ulceration from pressure.)
- Transjugular intrahepatic portosystemic shunting (TIPS) creates a channel between systemic and portal venous systems to reduce portal hypertension

## HEPATIC COMA

Hepatic coma or hepatic encephalopathy occurs when the liver's inability to remove ammonia and other toxins from the bloodstream causes a decrease in neurologic function. Hepatic encephalopathy often occurs in patients with severe liver disease, most commonly in patients diagnosed with cirrhosis of the liver. The fibrous tissue that forms in cirrhosis affects the liver structure and impedes the blood flow to the liver, ultimately causing the liver to fail. There are four stages of hepatic encephalopathy ranging from grade 0 to grade 4. Grade 4 encephalopathy is defined as hepatic coma. Neurologic alterations may progress slowly and if left untreated may result in irreversible neurologic damage.

**Signs/symptoms**: Altered mental status, personality or mood changes, poor judgment, and poor concentration. As symptoms progress, patients may experience agitation, disorientation, drowsiness, increasing confusion, lethargy, slurred speech, tremors, and seizures. In grade 4 encephalopathy, patients become unresponsive and ultimately comatose.

**Diagnosis**: Physical assessment, lab tests including a complete blood count, liver function tests, serum ammonia levels, BUN, creatinine and electrolyte levels, CT or MRI of the brain, and electroencephalogram may be used to diagnose hepatic encephalopathy.

**Treatment**: Address precipitating factors such as infection, gastrointestinal bleeding, dehydration, hypotension, or alcohol use. Other treatment options may include limiting protein intake, administration of lactulose to prevent the absorption of ammonia, and the administration of an antibiotic such as neomycin, rifaximin, or metronidazole (Flagyl) to reduce the serum ammonia level.

## ACUTE PANCREATITIS

Acute pancreatitis is related to chronic alcoholism or cholelithiasis in 90% of patients, but may have unknown etiology. It may also be triggered by a variety of drugs (tetracycline, thiazides, acetaminophen, and oral contraceptives). Complications may include shock, acute respiratory distress syndrome, and MODs.

**Signs/symptoms:** acute pain (mid-epigastric, LUQ, or generalized), nausea and vomiting, Abdominal distension.

**Diagnosis:** Serum lipase (>2x normal), amylase (less accurate), CT with contrast, abdominal U/S, MRI cholangiopancreatography, ERCP.

**Treatment** (supportive) includes:

- **Medications**: IV fluids, antiemetics, antibiotics (if necrosis is secondary to infection), and analgesia. NOTE: do not give morphine, can cause spasms in sphincter of Oddi, making pain worse.
- **TPN, NPO, or restricted to clear liquids** may help manage vomiting, ileus, and aspiration.
- **Surgical**: may remove gallbladder and biliary duct obstructions if cause of recurrent pancreatitis.

**Prevention**: Avoid smoking and alcohol consumption; limit fat intake and increase fresh fruits/vegetables and water.

## HERNIAS

Hernias are protrusions into or through the abdominal wall and may occur in children and adults. Hernias may contain fat, tissue, or bowel. There are a number of **types**:

- **Direct inguinal hernias** occur primarily in adults and rarely incarcerate.
- **Indirect inguinal hernias** related to congenital defect is most common on the right in males and can incarcerate, especially during the first year and in females.
- **Femoral hernias** occur primarily in women and may incarcerate.
- **Umbilical hernias** occur in children, especially those of African-American descent, and rarely incarcerate. They may also occur in adults, primarily women, and may incarcerate.
- **Incisional hernias** are usually related to obesity or wound infections, and may incarcerate.

Hernias are evident on clinical examination.

**Symptoms** of incarceration include:

- Severe pain
- Nausea and vomiting
- Soft mass at hernia site
- Tachycardia
- Temperature

**Treatment** for hernias includes:

- Reduction if incarceration is very recent with patient in Trendelenburg position and gentle compression
- Surgical excision and fixation
- Broad-spectrum antibiotics

## BILIARY ATRESIA

Biliary atresia is a rare life-threatening condition that occurs in infancy of unknown cause. Bile ducts are tubes that transport bile from the liver to the gallbladder (where it is stored) and the small intestine (where it aids in digestion). Biliary atresia occurs when the bile ducts (either inside or outside of the liver) become inflamed, causing damage to the ducts and an impedance of bile flow. Without treatment, the trapped bile causes damage to the liver eventually causing it to fail. The life expectancy for infants with untreated biliary atresia is approximately 2 years.

**Signs/symptoms**: Early identification is key in successfully treating biliary atresia. Signs and symptoms include dark urine, gray or white stools, slow weight gain and delayed growth, jaundice, abdominal swelling, and itching.

**Diagnosis**: Physical assessment, abdominal films, ultrasound, lab tests including bilirubin levels, and liver biopsy.

**Treatment**: The only treatment options for biliary atresia are liver transplant or the Kasai procedure. Named after the surgeon who invented it, the Kasai procedure involves using a loop of intestine to act as a new bile duct and removing the damaged ducts. Flow of bile is then restored to the small intestine. The Kasai procedure is most successful when performed on younger infants (less than 3 months old).

# Gastrointestinal Procedures and Interventions

## NG Tubes, Sump Tubes, and Levin Tubes

Nasogastric **(NG) tubes** are plastic or vinyl tubes inserted through the nose, down the esophagus, and into the stomach. **Sump tubes** are radiopaque with a vent lumen to prevent a vacuum from forming with high suction. **Levin tubes** have no vent lumen and are used only with low suction. NG tubes drain gastric secretions, allow sampling of secretions, or provide access to the stomach and upper GI tract. They are used for lavage after medication overdose, for decompression, and for instillation of medications or fluids. NG tubes are contraindicated with obstruction proximal to the stomach or gastric pathology, such as hemorrhage.

**Levin Tube**

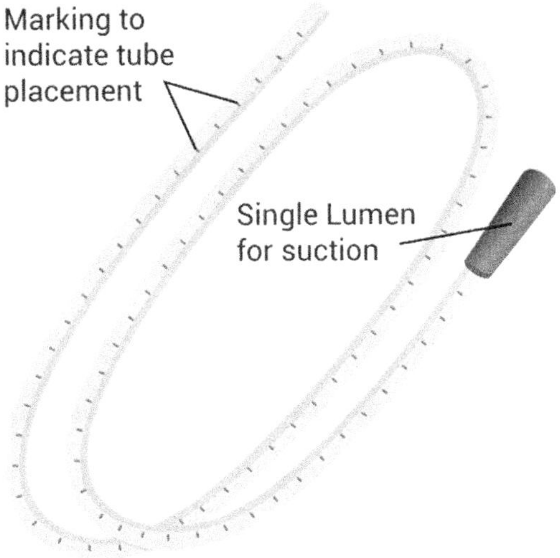


### *NG Tube Insertion*

Insertion of a nasogastric tube includes:

- **Examination**: Review the patient's medical history for possible contraindications. Assess the size and patency of the nares and select the most patent side. Assess mental status.
- **Select and measure tube**: For decompression, 14–16 Fr is most common; for enteral feeding, 8–12 Fr. Adult insertion length is about 55 cm. To estimate, measure from the tip of the nose to the earlobe and then to the xiphoid process; mark the desired length (permanent marker, tape).
- **Preparation**: Drape the patient's chest and provide an emesis basin. Prepare tape and an anchoring device. Inject 10 mL of water into the tube to check patency. Lubricate 2–3 inches of the tube (with a water-soluble lubricant). For decompression, connect the tube to the suction machine to prevent aspiration of emesis, but leave the machine off.
- **Insertion**: Place the patient in high Fowler's position (at least 60°). Gently insert the tube posteriorly into the nasopharynx, which usually triggers gag reflex. Ask the patient to flex their head forward and take sips of water or suck on ice chips so swallowing will help guide tube. At 25–30 cm, listen for air exchange at distal end of tube and watch carefully for signs of pulmonary placement (cough, cyanosis, abnormal breathing). Continue inserting tube to desired length. Anchor tube. Verify correct placement (x-ray, pH testing).

## PEG Tube

**Percutaneous endoscopic gastrostomy** (PEG), used for tube feedings, involves intubation of the esophagus with the endoscope and insertion of a sheathed needle with a guidewire through the abdomen and stomach wall so that a catheter can be fed down the esophagus, snared, and pulled out through the opening where the needle was inserted and secured. The PEG tube should not be secured to the abdomen until the PEG is fully healed, which usually takes 2–4 weeks, because tension caused by taping the tube against the abdomen may cause the tract to change shape and direction. The tract should be straight to facilitate insertion and removal of catheters. Once the tract has healed, the original PEG tube can generally be replaced with a balloon gastrostomy tube. External stabilizing devices can be applied to the skin to hold the tube in place but should be placed 1–2 cm above the skin surface to prevent excessive tension that may result in buried bumper syndrome (BBS) in which the internal fixation device becomes lodged in the mucosal lining of the gastric wall, resulting in ulceration.

## Drains

The following are different types of drains a patient may have, including pertinent nursing considerations:

- **Simple drains** are latex or vinyl tubes of varying sizes/lengths. They are usually placed through a stab wound near the area of involvement.
- **Penrose drains** are flat, soft rubber/latex tubes placed in surgical wounds to drain fluid by gravity and capillary action.

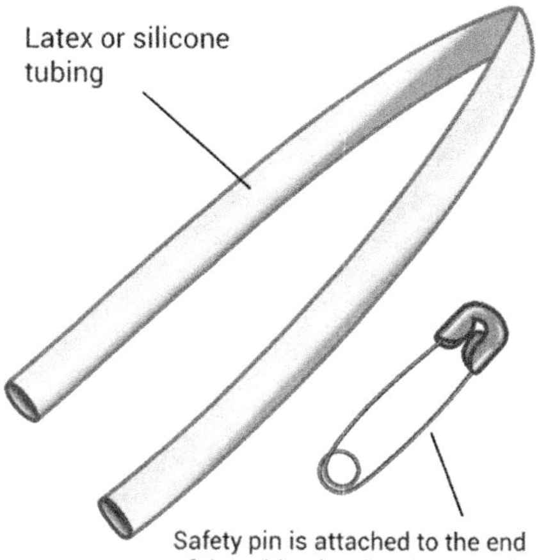


- **Sump drains** are double-lumen or tri-lumen tubes (with a third lumen for infusions). The multiple lumens produce venting when air enters the inflow lumen and forces drainage out of the large lumen.

- **A percutaneous drainage catheter** is inserted into the wound to provide continuous drainage for infection/fluid collection. Irrigation of the catheter may be required to maintain patency. Skin barriers and pouching systems may also be necessary.

SAFE PERCUTANEOUS DRAINAGE KIT

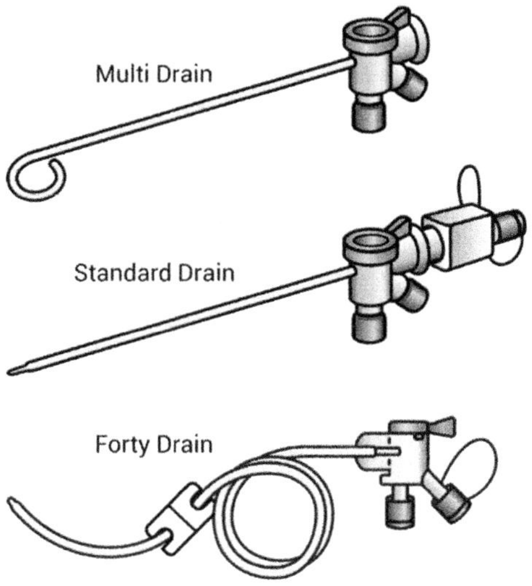


- **Closed drainage systems** use low-pressure suction to provide continuous gravity drainage of wounds. Drains are attached to collapsible suction reservoirs that provide negative pressure. The nurse must remember to always re-establish negative pressure after emptying these drains. There are two types in frequent use:
    - *Jackson-Pratt is* a bulb-type drain that is about the size of a lemon. A thin plastic drain from the wound extends to a squeeze bulb that can hold about 100 mL of drainage.

JACKSON PRATT DRAIN

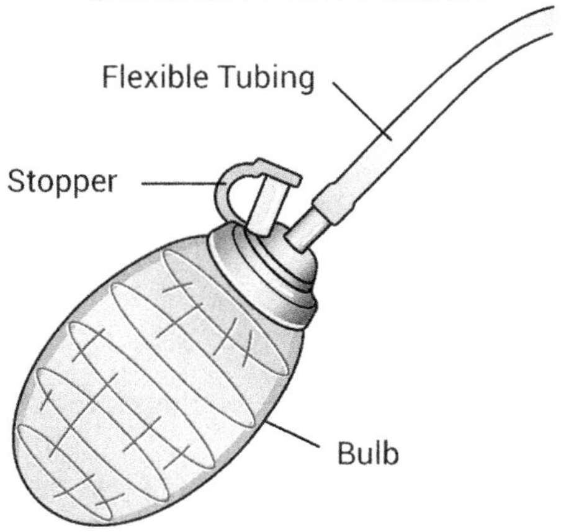


    - *Hemovac* is a round drain with coiled springs inside that are compressed after emptying to create suction. The device can hold up to 500 mL of drainage.

## Enteral Support and Parenteral Support

**Enteral nutrition** is a method of providing nutrition to a patient through a tube; the tube may be placed in either the nose (a nasogastric tube), the stomach (a percutaneous endoscopic gastrostomy [PEG] tube), or the small bowel (a percutaneous endoscopic jejunal [J] tube). When the tube has been placed, nutrition can be administered through the tube and absorbed by the patient's digestive system. Various **enteric formulas** exist, and the choice is dependent on the nutritional requirements of the patient.

**Parenteral nutrition** (also called total parenteral nutrition [**TPN**]) is a method of providing nutrition that completely bypasses the digestive system by administering nutrition through an intravenous line. Enteral support is the preferred method of providing nutrition, although in patients suffering from some compromise of the gastrointestinal tract, parenteral nutrition is the only option.

## Trouble-Shooting Problems Related to Enteral Feedings

**Feeding tubes** are commonly found in the critical care setting, as many patients are intubated and unable to take oral nutrition or medication. General maintenance involves checking placement before flushing anything into the tube (prevents aspiration), flushing the tubes with at least 30 mL of water before and after use, and every 4 hours. Never crush enteric-coated medications, and keep the HOB inclined at least 30° at all times during feeding. **Complications** include:

- **Vomiting/aspiration:** Caused by incorrect placement, gastric emptying, and/or formula intolerance.
  - Treatment: Confirm placement by checking pH (preferred to air bolus); delay feeding one hour and check residual volume before resuming. Refrigerate formula, check expiration, and use only for 24 hours.
- **Diarrhea:** Caused by rapid feeding, antibiotics/medications, intolerance of formula or hypertonic formula, and/or tube migration.
  - Treatment: Reduce rate of feeding, evaluate medications, avoid hanging feedings longer than 8 hours, and add fiber or decrease sodium in the feed.
- **Displacement of tube:**
  - Treatment: For NG tube, replace using the other nostril, only if not surgically placed. For G-tube or J-tube, cover the site and notify the physician.
  - Prevention: secure all tubes with the appropriate device and mark placement to identify migration.
- **Tube occlusion:**
  - Treatment: Check for kinks and obvious problems. Aspirate fluid, instill warm water, and aspirate to loosen occlusion. The physician may order an enzyme or sodium bicarb solution.

# TPN

**Total parenteral nutrition** (TPN) is an intravenous hypertonic solution containing glucose, fat emulsion, protein, minerals, and vitamins. TPN is generally given through a central line (PICC if short-term), and used only when other methods of nutrition are not feasible.

**Nursing considerations:**

- **Infection prevention**: Use aseptic technique for feedings and dressing changes; change solution, filter, and tubing every 24 hours, discard cloudy solutions, and monitor the site for signs of infection.
- **Risk of embolus/contamination**: Use micropore filter (TPN without fat emulsion) or 1.2-micron filter (TPN with fat emulsion); heparin can be added to the solution. Never infuse any medication or product in the same line as the TPN; blood cannot be drawn from this line either.
- **Malnutrition and electrolytes**: Check daily weight and check BMP and CBC 3x a week until stable, then weekly. Check the label and ingredients before administration and watch for signs of fluid overload. A cloudy blood specimen could indicate hyperlipidemia. Patients on TPN are also at risk for hyperammonemia (demonstrated by asterixis and altered mental status) and azotemia (demonstrated by dehydration and elevated BUN).

- **Hyper/hypoglycemia**: Initiate slowly, increasing rate over 24–48 hours. NEVER try to "catch-up" at a higher rate if there is a delay/pause in feeding; only administer with a pump and do not change the rate without order. If the bag runs out, hang a bag of D10W until a new bag can be obtained. Monitor BG every 4–6 hours; sliding scale insulin may be used.

## Gastrointestinal Surgery

### *Whipple*

The Whipple (pancreaticoduodenectomy) procedure is used to surgically remove the head of the pancreas, the gallbladder, part of the bile duct, the duodenum, and sometimes the distal portion of the stomach. After excision, the remaining pancreas, bile duct, and intestinal stump are sutured to the intestine so that secretions empty into the intestine. The Whipple procedure may be done as an open procedure or laparoscopically. This procedure is used primarily for malignant or benign tumors of the head of the pancreas but can also be used for chronic pancreatitis, duodenal cancer, cancer of the ampulla, and cholangiocarcinoma. Whipple is recommended only if the cancer has not spread beyond the pancreas and has not invaded major vessels. Usually, the pancreas is still able to produce adequate insulin, but the production of pancreatic enzymes may be impaired. A pylorus-preserving variation preserves the stomach and part of the pylorus to decrease nutritional deficiencies and weight loss associated with the standard Whipple.

Post-op treatment includes monitoring fluid/electrolyte balance and monitoring drains. These patients have a very high risk of developing numerous complications, including peritonitis, bowel obstruction, sepsis, and acute abdomen, along with others.

### *Esophagectomy and Esophagogastrectomy*

**Esophageal cancer** starts in the inner layer of the esophagus and spreads. It may develop after long-term reflux because of cell changes brought about by gastric acid. Symptoms include throat or epigastric discomfort, increasing dysphagia and inability to swallow solids, unexplained weight loss, hoarseness, hiccups, hematemesis, and the feeling of something in the throat. *Treatment* for esophageal cancer involves surgical removal of the affected portion of the esophagus. Two common procedures include:

- **Esophagectomy** is the removal of all or part of the esophagus with the distal end resutured to the stomach or an intestinal graft used to replace the excised portion of the esophagus.
- **Esophagogastrectomy** is the removal of the distal portion of the esophagus, lymph nodes, and the upper portion of the stomach, after which the remaining esophagus and stomach are reattached.

#### Postoperative Management

Postoperative management for esophagectomy/gastrectomy includes the following:

- Monitor intubation and ventilation (increased risk for ARDS), encourage pulmonary hygiene, and monitor chest tubes (change in color or sudden increase in drainage could indicate leak; notify physician).
- Subcutaneous emphysema in the chest/neck could indicate a leak in the anastomosis and should be reported immediately.
- Manage pain, which is often severe; a PCA or epidural may be used initially.
- Hemodynamics: IV fluids, 100–200 mL/hr, bolus PRN; however, be cautious as there is an increased risk of pulmonary edema.
- Monitor the NG tube; **NEVER replace or irrigate the NG tube**, as it could damage the anastomosis. Notify MD if complications arise.
- Maintain NPO for 5–7 days; nutrition should be provided via J-tube or TPN.

- Drains: Penrose, Jackson-Pratt, possible drainage collection bag at the base of the cervical incision for saliva if >250 mL in 8 hr.
  *NOTE*: Patients often have history of alcohol abuse; observe for signs of DTs/withdrawal.
- Prior to initiating oral intake, a fluoroscopic examination with water-soluble contrast will be done to check for leaks. If no leaks, patients begin with clear liquids and progress to 6–8 small meals per day.

### *Bariatric Gastrointestinal Surgery*

Bariatric surgery is used to promote weight loss in the morbidly obese (100 pounds over normal weight or BMI of 35–40). Surgery is done to restrict intake and/or prevent the absorption of calories. Procedures are open surgical or laparoscopic and include:

- **Banding** places a band around the upper portion of the stomach, creating a small pouch with a small distal opening to slow gastric emptying.
- **Sleeve gastrectomy** removes about 2/3 of the stomach, and a distal part of the small intestine is attached, bypassing part of the small intestine, reducing absorption.
- **Roux-en-Y** uses staples and a vertical band to decrease the size of the stomach, creating a small pouch. Then, a section of the small intestine is attached to the pouch, bypassing the first and second segments of the intestine to reduce absorption.
- **Gastric ballooning** places a balloon in the stomach and fills it with liquid to decrease stomach capacity; this is used primarily in Europe.

**Nursing considerations:** Use extreme caution with post-bariatric NG/PEG tubes – generally do not check placement/irrigate with normal amounts (risk of rupturing stomach); ensure patient maintains strict NPO. There is an increased risk of respiratory complications post-surgery.

## Indwelling Fecal Management Systems

Indwelling fecal management systems are used for incontinent clients with loose or watery stools in order to prevent skin breakdown, discomfort, odor, and contamination of wounds, and to control the spread of organisms, such as *Clostridioides difficile,* in bedridden or immobile clients. A number of different devices, such as the Flexi-Seal FMS, are available and work similarly. A typical management system includes:

- A silicone catheter
- A silicone retention balloon at end of the catheter
- A 45-mL syringe
- Charcoal filter collection bags

The application of the fecal management system is relatively simple: The catheter is inserted into the rectum and the balloon is inflated with water or saline (using the 45-mL syringe) to hold it in place and to block fecal leakage. Some systems, such as Flexi-Seal FMS, have a pop-up button to indicate when the balloon is adequately filled for the size of the rectum. The catheter contains an irrigation port so that irrigating fluid can be instilled if necessary. The charcoal filter collection bag is attached to the end of the silicone catheter to contain fecal material.

# Genitourinary Pathophysiology

## Urinary Incontinence

Urinary incontinence occurs more commonly in women than men and can range from an intermittent leaking of urine to a full loss of bladder control. Causes of urinary incontinence may include neurologic injury (including cerebral vascular accidents), infections, weakness of the muscles of the bladder, and certain medications, including diuretics, antihistamines, and antidepressants. **Stress incontinence** is defined as an involuntary leakage of urine with sneezing, coughing, laughing, lifting, or exercising. **Urge incontinence** is defined as an uncontrollable need to urinate on a frequent basis. **Total incontinence** is the full loss of bladder control.

**Signs/symptoms**: Urinary frequency and urgency may accompany the inability to control urine. If urinary incontinence is severe, incontinence-associated dermatitis may occur, predisposing the patient to skin breakdown and the development of pressure injuries.

**Diagnosis**: Physical assessment and presence of symptoms. Ultrasound, urinalysis, urodynamic testing, and cystoscopy may be used to determine the underlying cause.

**Treatment**: Treatment options are dependent on the type of urinary incontinence and the severity. Bladder training and pelvic muscle exercises may be utilized to strengthen muscles to control leakage of urine. In female patients with stress incontinence, a vaginal pessary may be inserted into the vagina to help support the bladder. Suburethral slings may also be surgically implanted to support the urethra. Anticholinergics, antispasmodics, and tricyclic antidepressants may also be used in the treatment of urinary incontinence.

## Hydronephrosis

Hydronephrosis is a symptom of a disease involving swelling of the kidney pelvises and calyces because of an obstruction that causes urine to be retained in the kidney. In chronic conditions, symptoms may be delayed until severe kidney damage has occurred. Over time, the kidney begins to atrophy. The primary conditions that predispose to hydronephrosis include:

- Vesicoureteral reflux
- Obstruction at the ureteropelvic junction
- Renal edema (non-obstructive)
- Any condition that impairs drainage of the ureters can cause backup of the urine

**Symptoms** vary widely depending upon cause and whether the condition is acute or chronic.

- Acute episodes are usually characterized by flank pain, abnormal creatinine and electrolyte levels, and increased pH.
- The enlarged kidney may be palpable as a soft mass.

**Treatment** includes:

- Identifying the cause of obstruction and correcting it to ensure adequate drainage.
- A nephrostomy tube, ureteral stent or pyeloplasty may be done surgically in some cases.
- A urinary catheter may be inserted if there is outflow obstruction from the bladder.

## Acute Tubular Necrosis

Acute tubular necrosis (ATN) occurs when a hypoxic condition causes renal ischemia that damages tubular cells of the glomeruli so they are unable to adequately filter the urine, leading to acute renal failure. Causes include hypotension, hyperbilirubinemia, sepsis, surgery (especially cardiac or vascular), and birth complications. ATN may result from nephrotoxic injury related to obstruction or drugs, such as chemotherapy, acyclovir, and antibiotics, such as sulfonamides and streptomycin. Symptoms may be non-specific initially and can include life-threatening complications.

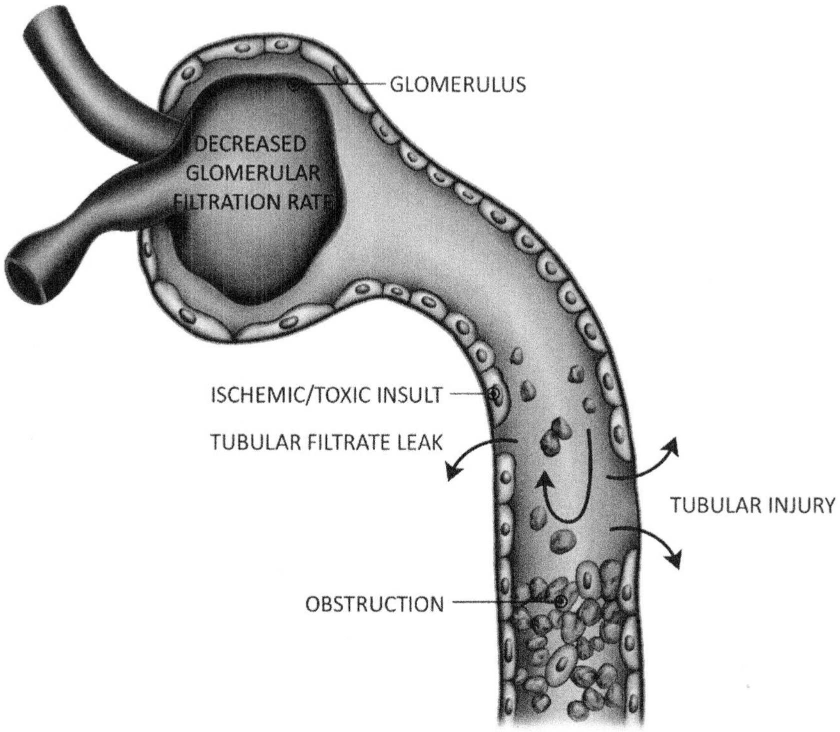


**Symptoms** include:

- Lethargy
- Nausea and vomiting
- Hypovolemia with low cardiac output and generalized vasodilation
- Fluid and electrolyte imbalance leading to hypertension, CNS abnormalities, metabolic acidosis, arrhythmias, edema, and congestive heart failure
- Uremia leading to destruction of platelets and bleeding, neurological deficits, and disseminated intravascular coagulopathy (DIC)
- Infections, including pericarditis and sepsis

**Treatment** includes:

- Identifying and treating underlying cause, discontinuing nephrotoxic agents
- Supportive care
- Loop diuretics (in some cases), such as Lasix
- Antibiotics for infection (can include pericarditis and sepsis)
- Dialysis

## ACUTE KIDNEY INJURY

Acute kidney injury (AKI), previously known as acute renal failure, is an acute disruption of kidney function that results in decreased renal perfusion, a decrease in glomerular filtration rate and a buildup of metabolic waste products (azotemia). Azotemia is the accumulation of urea, creatinine and other nitrogen containing end products into the bloodstream. The regulation of fluid volume, electrolyte balance and acid base balance is also affected. The causes of acute kidney injury are divided into pre-renal (caused by a decrease in perfusion), intrarenal or intrinsic (occurring within the kidney) and post-renal (caused by the inadequate drainage of urine). Acute kidney injury is common in hospitalized patients and even more common in critically ill patients, carrying a mortality rate of 50–80%. Risk factors for acute kidney injury include advanced age, the presence of co-morbid conditions, pre-existing kidney disease and a diagnosis of sepsis.

**Signs/symptoms**: Malaise, fatigue, lethargy, confusion, weakness, change in urine color, change in urine volume, and flank pain.

**Diagnosis**: Urinalysis, serum BUN and creatinine levels, renal ultrasound, CT or MRI and renal biopsy.

**Treatment**: The treatment of acute kidney injury is based on the underlying cause. Treatment options may include fluid and electrolyte replacement, diuretic therapy, fluid restriction, renal diet, and low dose dopamine to increase renal perfusion. Hemodialysis may also be necessary in patients with acute kidney injury.

**Review Video: Acute Kidney Injury (AKI)**
Visit mometrix.com/academy and enter code: 780321

## RENAL AND URETERAL CALCULI

Renal and urinary calculi occur frequently, more commonly in males, and can relate to diseases (hyperparathyroidism, renal tubular acidosis, gout) and lifestyle factors, such as sedentary work. Calculi can form at any age, most composed of calcium, and can range in size from very tiny to larger than 6 mm. Those smaller than 4 mm can usually pass in the urine easily.

**Diagnostic** studies include clinical findings, UA, pregnancy test to rule out ectopic pregnancy, BUN and creatinine if indicated, ultrasound (for pregnant women and children), IV urography. Helical CT (non-contrast) is diagnostic.

**Symptoms** occur with obstruction and are usually of sudden onset and acute:

- Severe flank pain radiating to abdomen and ipsilateral testicle or labium majus, abdominal or pelvic pain (young children)
- Nausea and vomiting
- Diaphoresis
- Hematuria

**Treatment** includes:

- Instructions and equipment for straining urine
- Antibiotics if concurrent infection
- Extracorporeal shock-wave lithotripsy
- Surgical removal: percutaneous/standard nephrolithotomy
- Analgesia: opiates and NSAIDs

## Chronic Kidney Disease

Chronic kidney disease (CKD) occurs when the kidneys are unable to filter and excrete wastes, concentrate urine, and maintain electrolyte balance because of hypoxic conditions, kidney disease, or obstruction in the urinary tract. It results first in azotemia (increase in nitrogenous waste in the blood) and then in uremia (nitrogenous wastes cause toxic symptoms). When >50% of the functional renal capacity is destroyed, the kidneys can no longer carry out necessary functions, and progressive deterioration begins over months or years. Symptoms are often non-specific in the beginning, with loss of appetite and energy.

**Symptoms and complications** are as follows:

- Weight loss
- Headaches, muscle cramping, general malaise
- Increased bruising and dry or itchy skin
- Increased BUN and creatinine
- Sodium and fluid retention with edema
- Hyperkalemia
- Metabolic acidosis
- Calcium and phosphorus depletion, resulting in altered bone metabolism, pain, and retarded growth
- Anemia with decreased production on RBCs. Increased risk of infection
- Uremic syndrome

**Treatment** includes:

- Supportive/symptomatic therapy
- Dialysis and transplantation
- Diet control: low protein, salt, potassium, and phosphorus
- Fluid limitations
- Calcium and vitamin supplementation
- Phosphate binders

## Uremic Syndrome

Uremic syndrome is a number of disorders that can occur with end-stage renal disease and renal failure, usually after multiple metabolic failures and decrease in creatinine clearance to <10 mL/min. There is compromise of all normal functions of the kidney: fluid balance, electrolyte balance, acid-base homeostasis, hormone production, and elimination of wastes. Metabolic abnormalities related to uremia include:

- **Decreased RBC production**: The kidney is unable to produce adequate erythropoietin in the peritubular cells, resulting in anemia, which is usually normocytic and normochromic. Parathyroid hormone levels may increase, causing calcification of the bone marrow, causing hypoproliferative anemia as RBC production is suppressed.
- **Platelet abnormalities**: Decreased platelet count, increased turnover, and reduced adhesion leads to bleeding disorders.
- **Metabolic acidosis**: The tubular cells are unable to regulate acid-base metabolism, and phosphate, sulfuric, hippuric, and lactic acids increase, leading to congestive heart failure and weakness.
- **Hyperkalemia**: The nephrons cannot excrete adequate amounts of potassium. Some drugs, such as diuretics that spare potassium may aggravate the condition.
- **Renal bone disease**: Decreased calcium, elevated phosphate, elevated parathyroid hormone, decreased utilization of vitamin D lead to demineralization. In some cases, calcium and phosphate are deposited in other tissues (metastatic calcification).

- **Multiple endocrine disorders**: Thyroid hormone production is decreased and abnormalities in reproductive hormones may result in infertility/impotence. Males have decreased testosterone but elevated estrogen and LH. Females experience irregular cycles, lack of ovulation and menses. Insulin production may increase but with decreased clearance, resulting in episodes of hypoglycemia or decreased hyperglycemia in those who are diabetic.
- **Cardiovascular disorders**: Left ventricular hypertrophy is most common, but fluid retention may cause congestive heart failure and electrolyte imbalances, dysrhythmias. Pericarditis, exacerbation of valvular disorders, and pericardial effusions may occur.
- **Anorexia and malnutrition**: Nausea and poor appetite contribute to hypoalbuminemia, sometimes exacerbated by restrictive diets.

**Review Video: End Stage Renal Disease**
Visit mometrix.com/academy and enter code: 869617

## PYELONEPHRITIS

Pyelonephritis is a potentially organ-damaging bacterial infection of the parenchyma of the kidney. Pyelonephritis can result in abscess formation, sepsis, and kidney failure. Pyelonephritis is especially dangerous for those who are immunocompromised, pregnant, or diabetic. Most infections are caused by *Escherichia coli.* **Diagnostic studies** include urinalysis, and blood and urine cultures. Patients may require hospitalization or careful follow-up.

**Symptoms** vary widely but can include:

- Dysuria and frequency, hematuria, flank and/or low back pain
- Fever and chills
- Costovertebral angle tenderness
- Change in feeding habits (infants)
- Change in mental status (geriatric)
- Young women often exhibit symptoms more associated with lower urinary infection, so the condition may be overlooked.

**Treatment** includes:

- Analgesia
- Antipyretics
- Intravenous fluids
- Antibiotics: started but may be changed based on cultures
  - IV ceftriaxone with fluoroquinolone orally for 14 days
  - Monitor BUN. Normal 7–8 mg/dL (8–20 mg/dL >age 60). Increase indicates impaired renal function, as urea is end product of protein metabolism.

## Cystitis

Cystitis is a common and often-chronic low-grade kidney infection that develops over time, so observing for symptoms of urinary infections and treating promptly are very important.

Changes in **character of urine**:

- **Appearance**: The urine may become cloudy from mucus or purulent material. Hematuria may be present.
- **Color**: Urine usually becomes concentrated and may be dark yellow/orange or brownish in color.
- **Odor**: Urine may have a very strong or foul odor.
- **Output**: Urinary output may decrease markedly.

**Pain**: There may be lower back or flank pain from inflammation of the kidneys.

**Symptoms**: Fever, chills, headache, and general malaise often accompany urine infections. Some people suffer a lack of appetite as well as nausea and vomiting. Fever usually indicates that the infection has affected the kidneys. Children may develop incontinence or loose stools and cry excessively.

**Treatment:**

- Increased fluid intake
- Antibiotics

## Nephrotoxic Agents

Medications are a common cause of renal damage, especially among older patients. The **nephrotoxic effects** may be reversible if the drug is discontinued before permanent damage occurs. Those at increased risk include patients who are older than 60, have a history of renal insufficiency, suffer from volume depletion, or have diabetes mellitus, sepsis, or heart failure. Initial signs may be quite subtle. Preventive measures include baseline renal function tests and monitoring of renal function and vital signs during treatment. The following are some common effects, and the drugs that may cause them:

- **Chronic interstitial nephritis**: Acetaminophen, lithium, carmustine, cisplatin, cyclosporine.
- **Acute interstitial nephritis**: NSAIDs, acyclovir, beta-lactams, rifampin, quinolones, sulfonamides, vancomycin, indinavir, loop/thiazide diuretics, lansoprazole, allopurinol, phenytoin.
- **Rhabdomyolysis**: Amitriptyline, diphenhydramine, doxylamine, benzodiazepines, haloperidol, lithium, ketamine, methadone, methamphetamine, statins.
- **Crystal nephropathy**: Acyclovir, foscarnet, ganciclovir, quinolones, sulfonamides, indinavir, methotrexate, triamterene.
- **Tubular cell toxicity**: Aminoglycosides, amphotericin B, pentamidine, adefovir, tenofovir, contrast dye, zoledronate.
- **Thrombotic microangiopathy**: Cyclosporine, clopidogrel, mitomycin-C, quinine.
- **Impaired intraglomerular hemodynamics**: NSAIDs, cyclosporine, tacrolimus, ACE inhibitors.
- **Glomerulonephritis**: NSAIDs, lithium, beta-lactams, interferon-alpha, gold therapy, pamidronate.

## Phimosis and Paraphimosis

Phimosis and paraphimosis are both restrictive disorders of the penis that occur in males who are uncircumcised or incorrectly circumcised. **Phimosis** is the inability to retract the foreskin proximal to the glans penis, sometimes resulting in urinary retention or hematuria. **Treatments** include:

- Dilating the foreskin with a hemostat (temporary solution)
- Circumcision
- Application of topical steroids (triamcinolone 0.025% twice daily) from end of foreskin to glans corona for 4–6 weeks

**Paraphimosis** occurs when the foreskin tightens above the glans penis and cannot be extended to normal positioning. This results in edema of the foreskin and circulatory impairment of the glans penis, sometimes progressing to gangrene, so immediate treatment is critical. **Symptoms** include pain, swelling, and inability to urinate. **Treatments** include:

- Compression of the glans to reduce edema (wrapping tightly with 2-inch elastic bandage for 5 minutes)
- Reducing edema by making several puncture wounds with 22- to 25-gauge needle
- Local anesthetic and dorsal incision to relieve pressure

## Testicular Torsion

Testicular torsion is a twisting of the spermatic cord within or below the inguinal canal, causing constriction of blood supply to the testis. Testicular torsion is most common at puberty but can occur at any age, sometimes precipitated by strenuous athletic participation or trauma, but it can also occur during sleep.

**Symptoms** include acute onset of severe testicular pain and edema, although children may present with nonspecific abdominal discomfort initially.

**Diagnosis** is based on clinical examination that demonstrates a firm scrotal mass. Color-flow duplex Doppler ultrasound may be helpful if diagnosis is not clear.

**Treatment** includes:

- **Manual detorsion** (usually 1.5 rotations) with elective surgical repair. Right testicle is usually rotated counterclockwise and left, clockwise. Reduction of pain should occur. If pain increases with rotation, then rotation should be done in the opposite direction.
- **Emergency surgical repair** (if manual detorsion not successful)

## Epididymitis and Orchitis

**Epididymitis**, infection of the epididymis, is often associated with infection in a testis (epididymo-orchitis). In children, infection may be related to congenital anomalies that allow reflux of urine. In sexually active males 35 years or younger, it is usually related to STDs. In men older than 40, it is often related to urinary infections or benign prostatic hypertrophy with urethral obstruction.

**Symptoms** include progressive pain in lower abdomen, scrotum, and/or testicle. Late symptoms include large tender scrotal mass.

**Diagnosis** includes: Clinical examination. Pyuria. Urethral culture for STDs. Sonography.

**Orchitis** alone is rare but occurs with mumps, other viral infections, and epididymitis. Ultrasound may be needed to rule out testicular torsion.

**Treatment** for both conditions depends upon the cause, but epididymitis usually resolves with antibiotics:

- Younger than 40, associated with STDs:
  - Ceftriaxone 500 mg IM and doxycycline 100 mg twice daily for 10 days
- Older than 35, associated with other bacteria:
  - Levofloxacin 500 mg daily for 10–14 days
  - TMP/SMS DS twice daily for 10–14 days

## Prostatitis

Prostatitis is an acute infection of the prostate gland, commonly caused by *Escherichia coli, Pseudomonas aeruginosa, Staphylococcus aureus,* or other bacteria. *Symptoms* include fever, chills, lower back pain, urinary frequency, dysuria, painful ejaculation, and perineal discomfort. PSA will often be elevated in this patient population, unrelated to prostate cancer. *Diagnosis* is based on clinical findings of perineal tenderness and spasm of rectal sphincter. *Treatments* include Ciprofloxacin 500 mg orally twice daily for 1 month **or** TMP/SMX DS twice daily for 1 month. Most patients also have a urethral culture to check for STDs. Patients with suspected bacteremia should be admitted for monitoring.

## Benign Prostatic Hypertrophy

Benign prostatic hypertrophy/hyperplasia usually develops after age 40. The prostate may slowly enlarge, but the surrounding tissue restrains outward growth, so the gland compresses the urethra. The bladder wall also goes through changes, becoming thicker and irritated, so that it begins to spasm, causing frequent urinations. The bladder muscle eventually weakens and the bladder fails to empty completely.

**Symptoms** include urgency, dribbling, frequency, nocturia, incontinence, retention, and bladder distention.

**Diagnosis** may include IVP, cystogram, and PSA.

**Treatment** includes: Catheterization for urinary retention/bladder distention. Surgical excision. Avoid fluids close to bedtime, double void, avoid caffeine and alcohol, alpha-adrenergic antagonists, and 5-alpha-reductase inhibitors.

## PID

Pelvic inflammatory disease (PID) comprises infections of the upper reproductive system, often ascending from vagina and cervix, and includes salpingitis, endometritis, tubo-ovarian abscess, peritonitis, and perihepatitis. *Neisseria gonorrhoeae* and *Chlamydia trachomatis* are implicated in most cases but some infections are polymicrobial. Complications include increase in ectopic pregnancy and tubal factor infertility. *Symptoms* include lower abdominal pain, vaginal pain, discharge, or bleeding, dyspareunia, dysuria, fever, and nausea and vomiting.

**Diagnostic studies** include:

- Pregnancy test
- Vaginal secretion testing, endocervical culture
- CBC
- Syphilis, HIV, and hepatitis testing
- Transvaginal pelvic ultrasound
- Endometrial biopsy
- Laparoscopy for definitive diagnosis

**Treatments** include:

- Broad spectrum antibiotics:
  - (Inpatient) Cefotetan 2 g IV every 12 hours or cefoxitin 2 g IV every 6 hours with doxycycline 100 mg every 12 hours
  - (Outpatient) Ceftriaxone 250 mg IM x 1 dose with doxycycline 100 mg orally every 12 hours for 14 days with metronidazole 500 mg twice daily for 2 weeks for patients who had gynecological procedures recently
- Laparoscopy to drain abscesses if symptoms do not improve in 72 hours or less
- Treatment specific to associated disorders (such as HIV or hepatitis)

## Vulvovaginitis

Vulvovaginitis is inflammation of vulvar and vaginal tissues:

- **Bacterial vaginosis** (Gardnerella vaginalis or other bacteria)
- **Fungal infections** (usually Candida albicans)
- **Parasitic infections** (Trichomonas vaginalis)
- **Allergic contact vaginitis** (from soaps or other irritants)
- **Atrophic vaginitis** (postmenopause)

**Symptoms** include vaginal odor, swelling, discharge, or bleeding, pain and discomfort, or severe itching (common with *C. albicans).*

**Diagnostic studies** include:

- Physical exam and culture of discharge, pH testing with nitrazine paper: Greater than 4.5 is typical of bacterial and trichomonas infections. Less than 4.5 is typical of fungal infections.

**Treatment** includes:

- **Bacterial infections**: Metronidazole 500 mg orally twice daily for 7 days AND Metronidazole 0.75% gel intravaginally twice daily for 5 days AND Clindamycin 2% cream intravaginally at bedtime for 7 days
- **Fungal infections**: Fluconazole 150 mg tablet in 1 dose OR vaginal creams, tablets, or suppositories, such as butoconazole 2% cream for 3 days or tioconazole 6.5% ointment for 1 dose
- **Parasitic (trichomonas)**: Metronidazole 2 g orally in 1 dose

## Ovarian Cysts

Ovarian cysts can grow within or on the ovaries. When a normal monthly follicle continues to grow, this is known as a functional cyst, of which there are two types:

- A follicular cyst begins when the follicle doesn't rupture or release its egg, but continues to grow.
- A corpus luteum cyst develops when fluid accumulates inside the follicle after it releases its egg.

Functional cysts are usually harmless, rarely cause pain, and often resolve on their own within 2–3 months. Other types of ovarian cyst include the following:

- **Cystadenomas** form on the exterior of an ovary and may enlarge and cause pain.
- **Endometriomas** develop as a result of endometriosis, where some of the tissue attaches to the ovary and causes pain during menses and sexual activity.
- **Dermoid cysts**, also called teratomas, can contain tissue, such as skin or teeth, because they from embryonic cells. They may enlarge and cause pain but are rarely cancerous.

**Polycystic ovaries** have multiple cysts. Ovarian cysts may cause problems if they rupture or hemorrhage and if they twist or become infected. Presenting symptoms include **hypotension** and **hypovolemia** if hemorrhage occurs, pain (often acute) and tenderness in the lower abdomen on the affected side, lower back pain, dysuria, and weight gain.

**Diagnostic** studies include a pregnancy test to rule out ectopic pregnancy, ultrasound with Doppler flow.

**Treatment** depends upon the type of cyst and complications:

- Emergency surgery for torsion
- Antibiotics for infection
- Hormone therapy may be useful for endometrioma

### Bartholin Cysts

The Bartholin glands are small glands located on both sides of the vagina in the lips of the *labia minora*. The glands help to lubricate the vulvar area. A Bartholin cyst occurs when a duct to one gland becomes obstructed, usually because of infection or trauma, resulting in swelling and formation of a cyst (usually 1–3 cm but may be much larger with infection). Bartholin cyst is most common in women in their 20s. Blockage may result from tumors as well, but usually in women older than 40.

**Symptoms** of a Bartholin cyst include:

- Palpable mass on one side of the vagina (usually painless)
- Pain and tenderness and increasing size of lesion if infection and abscess occurs

**Treatment** includes:

- Warm, moist compresses or sitz baths
- Antibiotics for infection
- Surgical incision and drainage may be necessary in some cases

## Genitourinary Procedures and Interventions

### Procedures for Insertion and Removal of Urinary Catheter

Procedure for inserting and removing a urinary catheter:

1. Gather supplies (included in a urinary catheter insertion kit), perform hand hygiene, place a waterproof pad under the patient, and ensure that the light source is adequate to view the urinary meatus.
2. Place females in supine position with knees flexed and males in supine position.
3. Apply gloves and wash the perineal area with facility provided cleanser (sometimes included in the outside of the urinary catheter kit) and allow to dry.
4. Remove gloves and wash hands.
5. Using aseptic technique, place the catheter kit between the patient's legs, open the kit touching only the corners of the drape that wraps around the kit.
6. Apply sterile gloves.
7. Apply sterile drapes to the patient.
8. Following the steps provided with the kit, place the lubricant into the appropriate section of tray, remove the catheter from its plastic and place the tip into the lubricant, and pour iodine over the three cleansing swabs (if they do not come impregnated with iodine already). Attach the 10-cc syringe (filled with sterile water) to the appropriate port of the catheter.
9. Cleanse the urethral meatus with the iodine impregnated swabs.

10. Using the nondominant hand, hold the penis or open the labia to observe the urethral meatus. This hand now becomes "dirty" and cannot be used to touch the catheter.
11. Using the dominant hand, insert catheter with the drainage end attached to the collection bag. Insert until urine flows freely, advancing a little further after that point.
12. Inflate the balloon using the 10-cc sterile water syringe, and ensure the catheter is secure.
13. Secure the catheter to the patient's leg and hang the collection bag below the level of the patient. Secure any tubing to the bed and ensure no kinking is present.

**Removal**: Straight catheter—remove by pulling out slowly. To remove indwelling catheter, deflate the balloon using the appropriate port and gently pull the catheter out.

## Reducing Infection Risks Associated with Urinary Catheters

Strategies for reducing infection risks associated with urinary catheters include:

- Using **aseptic technique** for both the straight and indwelling catheter insertion
- **Limiting catheter use** by establishing protocols for use, duration, and removal; training staff; issuing reminders to physicians; using straight catheterizations rather than indwelling; using ultrasound to scan the bladder; and using condom catheters
- Utilizing **closed-drainage systems** for indwelling catheters
- **Avoiding irrigation** unless required for diagnosis or treatment
- Using **sampling port** for specimens rather than disconnecting catheter and tubing
- Maintaining **proper urinary flow** by proper positioning, securing of tubing and drainage bag, and keeping the drainage bag below the level of the bladder
- **Changing catheters** only when medically needed
- **Cleansing external meatal area** gently each day, manipulating the catheter as little as possible
- Avoiding placing catheterized patients adjacent to those infected or colonized with antibiotic-resistant bacteria to reduce **cross-contamination**

## Renal Dialysis

### *Peritoneal Dialysis*

**Renal dialysis** is used primarily for those who have progressed from renal insufficiency to uremia with end-stage renal disease (ESRD). It may also be temporarily for acute conditions. People can be maintained on dialysis, but there are many complications associated with dialysis, so many people are considered for renal transplantation. There are a number of different approaches to **peritoneal dialysis:**

- **Peritoneal dialysis:** An indwelling catheter is inserted surgically into the peritoneal cavity with a subcutaneous tunnel and a Dacron cuff to prevent infection. Sterile dialysate solution is slowly instilled through gravity, remains for a prescribed length of time, and is then drained and discarded.
- **Continuous ambulatory peritoneal dialysis:** a series of exchange cycles is repeated 24 hours a day.
- **Continuous cyclic peritoneal dialysis:** a prolonged period of retaining fluid occurs during the day with drainage at night.

Peritoneal dialysis may be used for those who want to be more independent, don't live near a dialysis center, or want fewer dietary restrictions.

**Review Video: End-Stage Renal Disease**
Visit mometrix.com/academy and enter code: 869617

### *Hemodialysis*

Hemodialysis, the most common type of dialysis, is used for both short-term dialysis and long-term for those with ESRD. Treatments are usually done three times weekly for 3–4 hours or daily dialysis with treatment either during the night or in short daily periods. **Hemodialysis** is often done for those who can't manage peritoneal dialysis or who live near a dialysis center, but it does interfere with work or school attendance and requires strict dietary and fluid restrictions between treatments. Short daily dialysis allows more independence, and increased costs may be offset by lower morbidity. A vascular access device, such as a catheter, fistula, or graft, must be established for hemodialysis, and heparin is used to prevent clotting. With hemodialysis, blood is circulated outside of the body through a dialyzer (a synthetic semipermeable membrane), which filters the blood. There are many different types of dialyzers. High flux dialyzers use a highly permeable membrane that shortens the duration of treatment and decreases the need for heparin.

### *Dialysis Complications*

There are many complications associated with dialysis, especially when used for long-term treatment:

- **Hemodialysis**: Long-term use promotes atherosclerosis and cardiovascular disease. Anemia and fatigue are common, as are infections related to access devices or contamination of equipment. Some experience hypotension and muscle cramping during treatment. Dysrhythmias may occur. Some may exhibit dialysis disequilibrium from cerebral fluid shifts, causing headaches, nausea and vomiting, and alterations of consciousness.
- **Peritoneal dialysis:** Most complications are minor, but it can lead to peritonitis, which requires removal of the catheter if antibiotic therapy is not successful in clearing the infection within 4 days. There may be leakage of the dialysate around the catheter. Bleeding may occur, especially in females who are menstruating as blood is pulled from the uterus through the fallopian tubes. Abdominal hernias may occur with long use. Some may have anorexia from the feeling of fullness or a sweet taste in the mouth from the absorption of glucose.

# Musculoskeletal Pathophysiology

## Immobility

Critical care patients are often **immobile** for extended periods of time, thereby increasing their risk of skin breakdown and the development of pressure-related injuries, deep vein thrombosis, functional decline, decreased muscle mass, impaired coordination and gait, cardiovascular deconditioning, depression, and constipation. Immobility leads to impaired physical functioning in which muscle mass is lost and weakness develops. Intensive care unit acquired weakness can develop during hospitalization and is associated with an increased hospital length of stay as well as an increased mortality rate. ICU acquired weakness may last years after discharge with residual effects often affecting the patient's quality of life. Progressive mobility is defined as the gradual progression of positioning and mobility techniques and should be utilized to improve muscle strength and provide the patient a greater ability to resume activities of daily living. Patients should be assessed daily for their readiness to progress in their mobility goals in order to prevent the adverse effects of immobility.

## Muscular Deconditioning

Muscular deconditioning is reversible changes in musculature (i.e., a loss of muscle mass) and strength that occur as the result of inactivity. Symptoms of muscular deconditioning include impaired balance and mobility (increasing the risk of falls), dyspnea on exertion (from weakened cardiac muscles), loss of strength and endurance (1–3% per day and 20–30% after 1 week of bed rest), and muscle atrophy. Deconditioning begins within 72 hours of inactivity, and obvious decreases in strength occur within 3 weeks, although older adults undergo muscular deconditioning at a more rapid rate. Common complaints include feeling weak, tiring rapidly, having difficulty climbing stairs, or standing from a sitting position as well as increased back pain and dyspnea on even mild exertion.

**Preventive measures** include bed exercises, early and frequent ambulation, encouraging independence, and using assistive devices. Reconditioning typically takes twice as long as deconditioning.

**Reconditioning** includes beginning with low-intensity activities (including range-of-motion and sitting exercises), progressing to strength training (e.g., using resistance bands or light weights), aerobic activities (e.g., walking), and balance and coordination training. Adequate nutrition (≥1.0 g/kg of protein per day for older adults) is essential, along with adequate hydration.

## Gait Disorders

**Functional movement disorders** are defined as an involuntary, abnormal movement of part of the body in which pathophysiology is not fully understood. Functional tremors are the most frequent type of functional movement disorder. Dystonia, myoclonus, and Parkinsonism are other types of functional movement disorders. Functional gait disorders are another type of functional movement disorder and are common in the elderly. Gait disorders can manifest as a dragging gait, knee buckling, small slow steps or "walking on ice," swaying gait, fluctuating gait, hesitant gait, and hyperkinetic gait in which there is excessive movement of the arms, trunk, and legs when ambulating. Patients with gait disorders are at an increased risk of falling. Gait disorders are diagnosed by a thorough clinical examination (including a neurologic assessment) and health history. Treatment for functional gait disorders includes strength and balance training. Assistive devices such as walkers and canes may also be utilized.

## Falls

Falls are the most commonly occurring adverse event in the hospital setting. Confusion and agitation are factors that contribute to an increased risk for falling. In addition, impaired balance or gait, orthostatic hypotension, altered mobility, a history of falling, advanced age and the use of certain medications are additional risk factors. Approximately 30% of patient falls result in injury, some of which can significantly contribute to an increase in morbidity and mortality including fractures and subdural hematomas. Both physical and environmental factors contribute to patient falls, some of which are preventable. Fall prevention strategies include utilization of a standardized fall risk assessment to determine the patient's level of risk and subsequent care planning and interventions individualized to the patient. Fall prevention should also be balanced with progressive mobility. Many falls are related to toileting needs, and nurses often utilize scheduled rounding to address such needs.

**Review Video: Fall Prevention**
Visit mometrix.com/academy and enter code: 972452

## Carpal Tunnel Syndrome

Carpal tunnel syndrome is a type of entrapment neuropathy in which the median nerve is compressed by thickening of the flexor tendon sheath, skeletal encroachment, or mass in the soft tissue. Carpal tunnel syndrome is often associated with repetitive hand activities, arthritis, hypothyroidism, diabetes, and pregnancy. Patients complain of pain in wrist, radiating to forearm, and numbness and tingling in the first 2–3 fingers, especially during the night.

**Diagnosis** is based on symptoms and tests such as:

- **Positive Tinel test**: Gentle percussion over medial nerve in inner aspect of wrist elicits numbness and pain.
- **Positive Phalen test**: The backs of the hands are pressed together and the wrists sharply flexed for 1 minute to elicit pain and numbness.

**Treatment** includes identifying and treating the underlying cause:

- Steroid injection may relieve symptoms
- Splint during the night or during repetitive activities
- Modification of activities
- Referral for decompression surgery in recalcitrant cases or those with severe loss of sensation

## Infectious Arthritis

Infectious arthritis may be bacterial, viral (rubella, parvovirus, and hepatitis B), parasitic, or fungal, with bacterial arthritis causing the most rapid destruction to the joint. *Neisseria gonorrhoeae* (most common), *Staphylococcus*, *Streptococcus*, and *Escherichia coli* are the most common bacterial agents. The infection may be bloodborne or spread from an infection near the joint or from direct implantation or postoperative contamination of the wound. Usually, the infection involves just one joint.

**Symptoms** include acute edema, erythema, and pain in a joint. Systemic reactions, such as fever and polyarthralgia, may occur, especially with gonorrhea.

**Diagnosis** requires a complete history and physical examination, arthrocentesis and synovial fluid culture, and WBC.

**Treatment** includes:

- Antibiotics as indicated by organism
- Arthrocentesis to drain fluid accumulation in joint (may need to be repeated)
- Analgesia

## Bursitis and Tendinitis

**Bursitis** is inflammation of the bursa, fluid-filled spaces or sacs that form in tissues to reduce friction, causing thickening of the lining of the bursal walls. This can be the result of infection, trauma, crystal deposits, or chronic friction from trauma.

**Tendinitis** is inflammation of the long, tubular tendons and tendon sheaths adjacent to the bursa. Causes of tendinitis are similar to bursitis but tendinitis may also be caused by quinolone antibiotics. Frequently, both bursa and tendons are inflamed. Common types of bursitis include shoulder, olecranon (elbow), trochanteric (hip), and prepatellar (front of knee). Common types of tendinitis include wrist, Achilles, patellar, and rotator cuff.

**Symptoms** include pain with movement, edema, dysfunction, and decreased range of motion.

**Diagnosis** is by clinical examination, although x-rays may rule out fractures. The bursa may be aspirated diagnostically to aid in ruling out other diagnosis, like gout or infection.

**Treatment** for bursitis and tendinitis includes:

- Rest and immobilization
- NSAIDs
- Application of cold packs to affected area
- Steroid injections

## Joint Effusion and Arthrocentesis

Joint effusion is the accumulation of fluid (clear, bloody, or purulent) within a joint capsule. Joint effusion can cause pressure on the joint and severe pain. Arthrocentesis relieves the pressure and the fluid aspirated can be examined to aid in diagnosis. Arthrocentesis is usually contraindicated in the presence of overlying infection, prosthetic joint, and coagulopathy without referral to an orthopedic specialist.

**Procedure**:

1. Patient is **positioned** according to joint to be aspirated and encouraged to relax muscles.
2. **Overlying area** is cleansed with povidone-iodine solution, air-dried a few minutes, and cleansed of iodine with alcohol wipe.

3. **Local anesthetic** is given to the area (but not into the joint) with 25- to 30-gauge needle (lidocaine 1–2%) or a regional nerve block for severe pain.
4. The joint is **aspirated** with insertion in a straight line, using a 30–60 mL syringe (depending upon expected amount of fluid) and an 18- to 22-gauge needle or IV catheter.
5. The joint is completely **drained** of fluid.
6. Observe for **complications**: bleeding, infection, or allergic reaction.

## Lumbosacral Pain

Lumbosacral (low back) pain may be related to strain, muscular weakness, osteoarthritis, spinal stenosis, herniated disks, vertebral fractures, bony metastasis, infection, or other musculoskeletal disorders. Disk herniation or other joint changes put pressure on nerves leaving the spinal cord, causing pain to radiate along the nerve. Pain may be acute or chronic (more than 3 months).

**Symptoms** include local or pain radiating down the leg (radiculopathy), impaired gait and reflexes, difference in leg lengths, decreased motor strength, and alteration of sensation, including numbness.

**Diagnosis** is by careful clinical examination and history as well as x-ray (fractures, scoliosis, dislocations), CT (identifies underlying problems), MRI (spinal pathology), and/or EMG and nerve conduction studies. Diagnostic studies may be deferred in many cases for 4–6 weeks as symptoms may resolve over time. **Treatments** for nonspecific back pain include:

- Analgesia: acetaminophen, NSAIDS, opiates
- Encourage activity to tolerance but not bed rest
- Muscle relaxants: diazepam 5–10 mg every 6–8 hours
- Cold and heat compresses



## Strains and Sprains

A **strain** is an overstretching of a part of the musculature ("pulled muscle") that causes microscopic tears in the muscle, usually resulting from excess stress or overuse of the muscle. Onset of pain is usually sudden with local tenderness on use of the muscle. A **sprain** is damage to a joint, with a partial rupture of the supporting ligaments, usually caused by wrenching or twisting that may occur with a fall. The rupture can damage blood vessels, resulting in edema, tenderness at the joint, and pain on movement with pain increasing over 2–3 hours after injury. An avulsion fracture (bone fragment pulled away by a ligament) may occur with strain, so x-rays rule out fractures.

**Treatment** for both strains and sprains includes:

- **PRICE protocol**: protection, rest, ice, compression, and elevation
- **Ice compresses** (wet or dry) applied 20–30 minutes intermittently for 48 hours and then intermittent heat 15–20 minutes 3–4 times daily
- Monitor **neurovascular status** (especially for sprain)
- **Immobilization** as indicated for sprains for 1–3 weeks

## High Energy Joint Injuries

Low energy injuries include those that occur as a result of a fall from standing position or less than one-meter height, but **high energy injuries** include those with greater impact, such as from an automobile accident, falls from greater height, and sports accidents (downhill skiing, ice hockey) as well as gunshot wounds, stab wounds, and blast injuries. High energy injuries are likely to be more severe and may include:

- Fractures, both open and closed
- Compression fractures
- Dislocations and fracture-dislocations

- Comminution
- Strains and sprains, injury to ligaments and tendons
- Lacerations, bleeding
- Soft tissue trauma, edema, and ecchymosis
- Shock

Patients typically have severe pain, and the affected joint may be very unstable with obvious misalignment if fractures or dislocations are present. Older adults are particularly at risk for fractures because of osteoporosis, and healing may be impaired because of chronic disease. With high energy injuries, patients also have greater risk of complications, such as fat embolism, hemorrhage, pulmonary embolism, compartment syndrome, infection, neurological damage, avascular necrosis, and mal-union, delayed union, or non-union.

## FRACTURES AND DISLOCATIONS

### *TYPES OF FRACTURES*

Fractures and dislocations usually occur as the result of trauma, such as from falls and auto accidents, but *pathologic* fractures can result from minor force to diseased bones such as those with osteoporosis or metastatic lesions. *Stress* fractures are caused by repetitive trauma, such as from forced marching. *Salter* fractures involve the cartilaginous epiphyseal plate near the ends of long bones in children who are growing. Damage to this area can impair bone growth. Orthopedic injuries that are of special concern include:

- **Open fractures** with soft tissue injury overlying the fracture, including puncture wounds from external forces or bone fragments, can result in osteomyelitis.
- **Subluxation, partial dislocation of a joint, and luxation** (complete dislocation) can cause neurovascular compromise, which can be permanent if reduction is delayed. Dislocation of the hip can result in avascular necrosis of the femoral head.

### *DIAGNOSIS AND TREATMENT*

Fractures and dislocations are commonly **diagnosed** by clinical examination, history, and radiographs. Careful inspection and observation of range of motion, palpation, and observation of abnormalities is important because pain may be referred. Neurovascular assessment should be done immediately to prevent vascular compromise. Radiographs should usually precede reduction of dislocations to ensure there are no fractures and follow reduction to ensure the dislocation is reduced.

**Treatment** includes:

- Analgesia and sedation as indicated
- Application of cold compresses and elevation of fractured area to reduce edema
- Reduction of fracture: steady and gradual longitudinal traction to realign bone
- Immobilization with brace, cast, sling, or splint indicated
- Reduction of dislocation: Varies according to area of dislocation
- Open fracture: Wound irrigation with NS
- Tetanus prophylaxis
- Antibiotic prophylaxis
- Referral to orthopedic specialist for open fractures, irreducible dislocations, and complications such as compartment syndrome or circulatory impairment

### PELVIC FRACTURES

Pelvic fractures may be fairly benign or seriously life threatening, depending on the degree and type of fracture. They most often result from high-speed trauma related to vehicular accidents or skiing accidents:

- **Open book**: Pelvis is pulled apart, usually from frontal injury (may cause severe hemorrhage)
- **Closed book**: Lateral compression occurs from side injury
- **Vertical shear**: Injury occurs from fall

Indications of pelvic fracture include localized edema, tenderness, obvious pelvic deformity, abnormal pelvic movement, and abdominal bruising. Associated intra-abdominal injuries and complications are common, including paralytic ileus, hemorrhage, urethral, colon, or bladder laceration. Patients may develop sepsis, peritonitis, fat embolism syndrome, or DVT. Displaced fractures may require open reduction and internal fixation. Treatment usually includes bedrest (up to 6 weeks) with care in handling to prevent further injury. Patients should be turned and moved in accordance with specific physician's orders. Ambulation using walker or crutches may be allowed for non-displaced fractures.

### ACETABULAR FRACTURES

Acetabular (hip-socket) fractures occur primarily in young adults with motor vehicle accidents or falls from a height, resulting in impact pressure from the head of the femur to the joint and frequently associated (up to 50% of cases) with other severe injuries, including dislocation (which can lead to avascular necrosis if not promptly reduced). Up to 20% of those with acetabular fractures also have pelvic fractures. The degree of displacement that occurs depends on the amount of force as well as the position of the femur during impact. Acetabular fracture may be classified as posterior-wall, posterior-column, anterior-column, or transverse. Acetabular fractures in children less than 12 years may result in growth arrest. Complications may include sepsis, chondrolysis, and injury to vessels and/or nerves. Post-traumatic arthritis of the joint may develop. **Diagnosis** is per examination, radiograph, and/or CT with Doppler ultrasound with suspected DVT. Treatment includes emergent closed reduction if necessary, longitudinal skeletal traction, and open reduction and internal fixation (ORIF) for displaced fractures and serious injury (usually delayed for 2–3 days because of initial bleeding).



### CLOSED FRACTURES AND OPEN FRACTURES

**Closed fractures** are those in which the damage to the bone and tissue (bleeding, swelling) remains enclosed within intact skin and does not invade any internal cavity. The bone segments are more likely to be aligned, although some comminution may have occurred from splintering when the bone breaks. It may be difficult to differentiate a closed fracture from an open fracture if there are abrasions and lacerations over the area of the fractures, but it is closed if there is no continuity between the fracture and the external injury.

**Open fractures**, on the other hand, cause an external wound and may result from fragments of the fractured bone penetrating the skin or an external force penetrating the skin and bone. Open fractures may also appear closed on the surface but invade a body cavity. Open fractures carry a much higher risk of contamination and infection as well as severe bleeding. The external wounds associated with open fractures may vary in size, but even small wounds are considered emergent because of risk of infection.

### FAT EMBOLISM AS COMPLICATION OF TRAUMATIC FRACTURE

In instances of **traumatic fracture**, the possibility of **fat embolism** should be considered; this is especially true in fractures involving the long bones (femur, humerus). When the bone is fractured, this allows for some of the fatty marrow contained within the bone to escape. Because the fracture and subsequent trauma to the area surrounding the fracture results in broken vessels, it is possible that the fatty marrow can be introduced into the bloodstream. When this happens, the events are similar to that of a deep venous thrombosis; the fat embolus dislodges from the lumen of the vessel and travels to the lung. When the embolus enters the pulmonary circulation, it eventually blocks blood flow as the caliber of the vessel through which it travels decreases, keeping blood from flowing to the lung tissue. The disruption in blood flow results in inflammation and necrosis of the lung, and eventually pulmonary failure ensues.

## Osteomyelitis

**Musculoskeletal infections** encompass a variety of different disorders with differing pathologies. Osteomyelitis, cellulitis, and septic arthritis are examples of musculoskeletal infections that can be both serious and debilitating in nature.

**Osteomyelitis** is an infection of the bone that can occur from an open fracture or an infection that has occurred somewhere else in the body. Osteomyelitis can also be caused by wounds or soft tissue infections that have progressed and extended to the bone. Signs and symptoms of osteomyelitis include pain, swelling, erythema and possible drainage at the site. The patient may also experience fever and chills. Diagnosis includes lab work including a complete blood count, erythrocyte sedimentation rate (ESR), C-reactive protein (CRP), and blood cultures, as well as radiologic testing that may include CT, MRI, x-ray, bone scan, or a bone biopsy. Treatment includes the administration of IV antibiotics. A needle aspiration may be performed to determine the organism and drain the area. Surgical irrigation and debridement may also be indicated.

## Compartment Syndrome

Compartment syndrome occurs when there is an increase in the amount of pressure within a grouping of muscles, nerves, and blood vessels resulting in compromised blood flow to muscles and nerves. This is a medical emergency. If left untreated, tissue ischemia and eventual tissue death will occur. **Compartment syndrome** most often occurs after a fracture, particularly a long bone fracture, but can also occur with crushing syndrome and rhabdomyolysis. Risk factors include lower extremity trauma, massive tissue injury, venous obstruction, the use of certain medications (anticoagulants), burns and compressive dressings or casts. Compartment syndrome can affect the hand, forearm, upper arm, abdomen, and lower extremities. It can be acute or chronic in nature with acute compartment syndrome requiring immediate intervention.

**Signs/symptoms**: Intense pain, decreased sensation and paresthesia, firmness at the affected site, swelling and tightness at the affected site, pallor and pulselessness (late signs).

**Diagnosis**: Physical assessment and the measurement of intra-compartmental pressures.

**Treatment**: The goal of treatment in compartment syndrome is decompression and the restoration of perfusion to the affected area. Surgical fasciotomy is often indicated to relieve pressure and prevent tissue death. Fasciotomy involves the opening of the skin and muscle fascia to release the pressure within the compartment and restore blood flow to the area.

**Prevention**: Leave large abdominal wounds open to drain, delay casting on affected extremities, and use flexible casts. Watch circumferential burns closely and perform frequent neurovascular checks on those at risk.

## Rhabdomyolysis

Rhabdomyolysis occurs when damage of the cells of the skeletal muscles causes the release of toxins from injured cells into the bloodstream. Rhabdomyolysis may be caused by trauma, tissue ischemia, infection, certain medications (statins, selective serotonin reuptake inhibitors, lithium, and antihistamines), sepsis, immobilization, extraordinary physical exertion, myopathies and cocaine or alcohol abuse. Additionally, rhabdomyolysis may occur with exposure to certain toxins such as snake/insect venoms or mushroom poisoning. In rare circumstances, the identifiable cause cannot be determined. The most serious complication of rhabdomyolysis is renal failure. Rhabdomyolysis may be life threatening. Early recognition and treatment are critical to avoid serious complications and for patients to make a full recovery.

**Signs/symptoms**: Electrolyte imbalance, muscle pain and weakness, fever, tachycardia, dehydration, fatigue, lethargy, hypotension, and metabolic acidosis. Dark, reddish-brown urine may occur due to the presence of myoglobin released from the muscles and excreted into the urine.

**Diagnosis**: Laboratory studies such as creatinine kinase (CK) level, metabolic panel, urinalysis, and blood gases.

**Treatment**: The treatment of rhabdomyolysis includes fluid administration to eliminate toxins and prevent renal failure. Bicarbonate may be administered to correct metabolic acidosis. Mannitol or dopamine may be administered to increase renal perfusion. Electrolyte replacement may also be indicated. In severe cases, emergency dialysis may be necessary.

# Musculoskeletal Procedures and Interventions

## Monitoring Devices for Extremity Compartment Syndrome

Signs of extremity compartment syndrome include the 5 P's:

- Pain that is severe and out of proportion to injury
- Paresthesia
- Pallor
- Paresis
- Pulse deficit

Pressure is typically measured with a device specially intended for measurement although it can also be measured by attaching a manometer to a needle and syringe. The supplies for pressure monitoring generally include a 3 mL syringe, a chamber and needle that connect to the syringe, and a pressure monitor into which the syringe is placed. The procedure with the **Stryker intercompartmental pressure monitor device** includes:

1. The skin is cleansed with antiseptic and a local anesthetic administered.
2. Air is purged from the chamber and needle with the saline.
3. The syringe is placed into the pressure monitoring device.
4. The device is turned on, zeroed automatically by pressing the "zero" button.
5. The needle is inserted into the compartment.
6. Once the needle is inserted, about 0.3 mL of NS is injected and the device automatically records the compartment pressure. If the compartment pressure is over 30 mmHg, a fasciotomy is usually needed.



## Pelvic Stabilizer

Pelvic stabilizers are used to prevent excessive bleeding associated with pelvic fractures, to maintain the bones in the correct position, and to prevent further damage. Maintaining pressure and reducing the fracture often reduces bleeding. Various methods of stabilizing the pelvis may be employed, including the sheet wrap method in which a sheet is folded, center under the patient, wrapped tightly about the pelvis, and secured. The pneumatic anti-shock garment (PASG) is indicated for hypovolemic shock, and hypotension associated with and for stabilization of pelvic and bilateral femur fractures. PASG is contraindicated with respiratory distress, pulmonary edema, pregnancy (after the first trimester), heart failure, myocardial infarction, stroke, evisceration, abdominal or leg impalement, head injuries, and uncontrolled bleeding above the garment. Another device is the SAM pelvic sling, which has a wide band that fits under and about the pelvis and lateral hips and a belt anteriorly that allows adjustment.

## Immobilization Devices

Immobilization devices include:

- **Cervical collar**: Support the head to prevent spinal cord injury with suspected injury to cervical vertebrae.
- **Cervical extrication splints**: Short board used to immobilize and protect the head and neck during extrication.

- **Backboards**: Used to immobilize the spine to prevent further injury to spinal cord. Both long and short spine boards are available in a number of different shapes and sizes.
- **Full-body splints** (such as vacuum mattress splint): Provide cushioned support to maintain body alignment.
- **Various types of splints for extremities**: Include rigid (should be padded), non-rigid (moldable), traction, and air (pneumatic devices) as well as the use of blankets, rolled towels, sheets, and pillows to maintain position. Traction splints are used for fractured femurs to keep bones in position.
- **Pneumatic anti-shock garment** (PASG): Provides pressure on lower extremities and abdomen and is used to control hemorrhage and shock to prevent pooling of blood in extremities and return blood to general circulation. Often used for pelvic fractures, but may increase risk of internal hemorrhage.

## Spinal Immobilization

Spinal immobilization, once a standard for trauma patients, has been shown to have little effect and in some cases may cause harm. Because of these findings, spinal immobilization with backboard is now recommended only for patients with neurological complaints, such as numbness, tingling, weakness, paralysis, pain or tenderness in the spine, spinal deformity, blunt trauma associated with alterations of consciousness, and high energy injuries associated with drugs/alcohol, inability of the patient to communicate, and/or distracting injury. Cervical collars for cervical spine immobilization are to be utilized for trauma based on the NEXUS criteria or Canadian C-spine rules (CCR). According to **NEXUS criteria**, a patient who exhibits <u>all</u> of the following does <u>not</u> require a cervical collar:

- Alert and stable
- No intoxication
- No midline tenderness of the spine
- No distracting injury
- No neurological deficit

Spinal immobilization should be continued for the shortest time possible, so imaging, such as CT, should be carried out upon admission. Cervical collars are applied while the head is supported in neutral position, and the patient is logrolled onto a backboard and strapped in place.

## Immobilization of Fractures and Dislocations

Immobilization techniques for fractures and dislocations include:

- **Cast**: Plaster and fiberglass casts are applied after reduction to ensure that the bone is correctly aligned. Cast should be placed over several layers of padding that extends slightly beyond the cast ends. Cast material, such as plaster, should NOT be immersed in hot water but water slightly above room temperature (70 °F).
- **Splint**: Plaster splints use 12 or more layers of plaster measured to the correct length and then several layers of padding (longer and wider than splint should be measured and cut). The plaster splint is submerged in water to saturate, removed, laid on a flat surface, and massaged to fuse the layers. The padding is laid on top, and the splint is positioned and wrapped with gauze to hold it in place. While setting the splint, position can be maintained by holding it in place with the palm of the hand (not the fingers). After setting, the splint may be wrapped by elastic compression bandages.

## Amputation Care

### *Immediate Interventions for Traumatic Amputation*

**Amputations** may be partial or complete. The amputated limb should be treated initially as though it could be reattached or revascularized. Single digits, except the thumb, are often not reattached. Initial treatment includes stabilizing patient and stopping bleeding by applying a proximal blood pressure cuff proximal to injury 30 mmHg above systolic for <30 minutes. Instruments, such as clamps and hemostats, should be avoided. Other treatment includes:

- Tetanus prophylaxis
- Analgesia
- Prophylactic antibiotics may be needed
- Irrigation of stump with NS (not antiseptics) if contaminated
- Splint and elevate stump, with saline-moistened sterile dressing in place
- Neurovascular examinations of stump

The Allen test should be done to determine arterial injury if digits are amputated. In the Allen test, both the radial and ulnar artery are compressed and the patient is asked to clench the hand repeatedly until it blanches, and then one artery is released, and the tissue on that side should flush. Then the test is repeated again, releasing the other artery.

### *Care of Amputated Part Prior to Reattachment or Revascularization*

The amputated part should be cooled to 4 °C to extend the time of viability and decrease damage from ischemia. (Single digits and lower limbs are not usually reattached, but the limbs should be treated as though they will until determination is made, especially for children.) The part should be reattached within 6 hours if possible but up to 24 hours if properly cooled. **Initial care of amputated part** includes:

- Removal of jewelry
- Irrigation with NS to remove debris or contamination
- Part stored wrapped in saline moistened dressing but NOT immersed in saline or hypotonic solution
- Minimal handling to prevent tissue damage
- Cool by placing wrapped part in sealed plastic bag and immersing the bag in ice water (1:1 ice to water), but avoid freezing the part

If the amputation is partial, treatment is similar but NS wrapped part is splinted and ice packs or commercial cold packs are applied over area that is devascularized.

## Tourniquets

Tourniquets are used to control hemorrhage in an extremity and should be applied immediately with arterial bleeds or if pressure does not stop bleeding. Commonly used **tourniquets** include adjustable bands that are tightened and secured and then include a windlass handle twisted until blood flow stops and the handle is secured. Another type is a wide elastic band that is stretched, wrapped about the extremity tightly a number of times and secured. Blood pressure cuffs may also be used to apply pressure if standard tourniquets are not available. Regardless of the type, the tourniquet should be placed as high on the extremity as possible (avoiding joints), and the date and time of placement should be documented (on the tourniquet if possible). Tourniquets may be contraindicated with DVT, Reynaud's disease, crushing injuries, sickle cell disease, severe peripheral arterial disease, and open lower extremity fractures. Risks include damage to muscles, nerves, and vessels as well as increased risk of amputation. However, the first priority is always to prevent exsanguination.

## Teaching Patients How to Walk with Crutches

**Crutches** should be properly fitted before a patient attempts ambulation. Correct height is one hand-width below axillae. The handgrips should be adjusted so the patient supports the body weight comfortably with elbows slightly flexed rather than locked in place. The patient should be cautioned not to bear weight under the axillae as this can cause nerve damage but to hold the crutches tightly against the side of the chest wall. The type of gait that the patient uses depends on the type of injury. Typical gaits include:

- **Two-point** in which each crutch is advanced in tandem with the opposite side leg (i.e., the left crutch is advanced at the same time as the right leg, and the right crutch is advanced at the same time as the left leg).
- **Three-point** in which the injured extremity and both crutches are advanced together and then the well leg advances to (or past) the crutches.

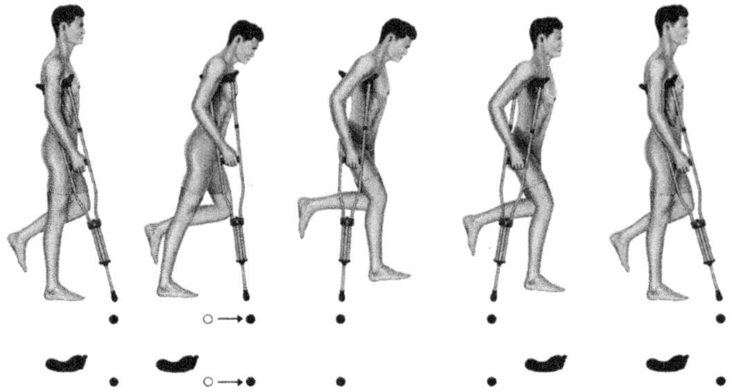

- **Four-point** in which the injured side crutch is advanced, followed by the non-injured leg, followed by the non-injured side crutch, followed by the injured leg.

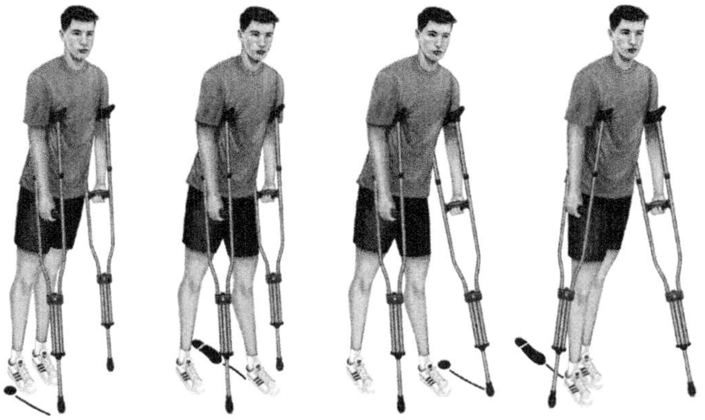

The patient should be advised whether there is partial or no weightbearing and a demonstration should be provided. Stair climbing should be practiced:

- **Ascending**: well foot goes first and then crutches and injured extremity.
- **Descending**: crutches go first and then the well foot.

# Integumentary Pathophysiology

## Cellulitis

Cellulitis occurs when an area of the skin becomes infected, usually following injury or trauma to the skin. Cellulitis is most likely to be caused by staphylococcus or streptococcus bacteria. Patients with peripheral vascular disease, diabetes mellitus, and immunosuppression are at a higher risk for the development of cellulitis. **Signs and symptoms** include pain, erythema, and warmth at the affected site that progresses rapidly. In addition, the patient may experience fever, chills, fatigue, and malaise. **Diagnosis** is made by physical exam. Labs include complete blood count, culture of the involved area and blood. **Treatment** for cellulitis is the administration of antibiotics. Surgical irrigation and debridement may be indicated in severe cases.

## Extravasation

Extravasation occurs when an intravenously infused vesicant medication or fluid leaks from the vein and into the subcutaneous space. Vesicant medications are those that cause tissue injury if extravasated and that may ultimately lead to tissue necrosis. Extravasation and infiltration are similar in nature, with infiltration occurring when the infusate is a non-vesicant solution or medication. Extravasation occurs more commonly in peripheral IVs; however, it can also occur with central venous catheters. Common vesicant agents include several chemotherapeutic agents, vancomycin, electrolytes, dobutamine, norepinephrine, phenytoin, promethazine, propofol, and vasopressin.

**Signs/symptoms**: Pain, burning, erythema, and edema at the site of the extravasation. Oftentimes, a blood return from the peripheral IV or central venous catheter is not present. Long term complications include complex regional pain syndrome, tissue necrosis, and nerve or tendon damage.

**Diagnosis**: Physical assessment and review of patient symptoms and medications/infusions administered.

**Treatment**: Early recognition is key to the successful treatment of an extravasation. When an extravasation is suspected, the IV infusion should be immediately stopped and the infusion site assessed. For some medications, antidotes may be available to minimize the damage caused by the extravasation. Heat or cold therapy may also be utilized depending on the medication. In cases of severe damage, debridement, skin grafting, and even amputation may result.

## Septic Arthritis

Septic arthritis is defined as an invasion of the joint space by bacteria, virus, or fungi. Elderly patients, immunosuppressed patients, and those with prosthetic joints are at an increased risk for septic arthritis. The most commonly affected joints include the knee, hip, shoulder, ankle, and wrist. **Signs and symptoms** include joint pain, fever, impaired range of motion, chills, edema, erythema, warmth, and the abnormal presence of fluid (effusion) surrounding the joint. **Diagnosis** is made by aspiration of the fluid with stain and culture, x-ray, and blood tests including CBC and cultures. **Treatment** is the administration of antibiotics. Surgical irrigation and debridement may also be indicated. The patient will likely undergo physical therapy as part of their recovery to improve and restore mobility and range of motion.

## Tissue Damage Related to Allergic Contact Dermatitis

**Contact dermatitis** is a localized response to contact with an allergen, resulting in a rash that may blister and itch. Common allergens include poison oak, poison ivy, latex, benzocaine, nickel, and preservatives, but there is a wide range of items, preparations, and products to which people may react.

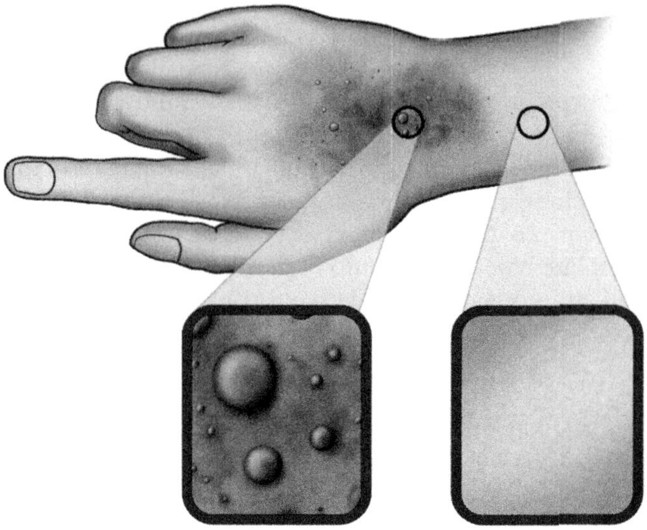


**Treatment** includes:

- Identifying the causative agent through evaluating the area of the body affected, careful history, or skin patch testing to determine allergic responses
- Corticosteroids to control inflammation and itching
- Soothing oatmeal baths
- Pramoxine lotion to relieve itching
- Antihistamines to reduce allergic response
- Lesions should be gently cleansed and observed for signs of secondary infection
- Antibiotics are used only for secondary infections as indicated
- Rash is usually left open to dry
- Avoidance of allergen to prevent recurrence

### Infectious Wounds

All types of wounds have the potential to become infected. Infectious wounds are commonly health care acquired. Wound infections increase a patient's risk of sepsis, multisystem organ failure and death. Trauma patients are at an increased risk of developing an infected wound due to exposure to various contaminants that they may have encountered during their injury (e.g., dirt from a motor vehicle accident).

**Signs/symptoms**: Erythema, edema, induration, drainage, increasing pain and tenderness, fever, leukocytosis, and lymphangitis.

**Diagnosis**: Wound infections are diagnosed by wound cultures (anaerobic and aerobic). Fluid or tissue biopsy may also be performed.

**Treatment**: Wound infections are treated with antibiotics and a wound care regimen that includes routine cleaning and dressing of the wound. Wound care treatment is based on the type and severity of the wound. Surgical irrigation and debridement may also be indicated. For deep, complex wounds, a wound-care consult is often indicated.

**Review Video: Treating Wound Infections**
Visit mometrix.com/academy and enter code: 761736

## Necrotizing Fasciitis

Necrotizing fasciitis is an infection that develops deep within the fascia, causing a rapidly developing tissue necrosis resulting in destruction and death of the soft tissue and nerves. Complications of necrotizing fasciitis may include the loss of the affected limb, sepsis, and death. Group A *Streptococcus*, *Klebsiella*, *Clostridioides*, *Escherichia coli*, *Staphylococcus aureus*, and *Aeromonas hydrophila* are organisms that have the potential to cause necrotizing fasciitis.

**Signs/symptoms**: Edema, erythema, and pain at the affected site. Nausea, vomiting, fatigue, malaise, fever, and chills may also occur.

**Diagnosis**: Diagnosis is based on physical assessment and patient history. In addition, excisional deep skin biopsy and gram staining may be performed to determine the causative organism. CT/MRI may also be utilized to assess the extent of the infection.

**Treatment**: Treatment options for necrotizing fasciitis include antibiotics and fasciotomy with radical debridement. Hyperbaric oxygen therapy may also be utilized.

## Surgical Wounds

Surgical wounds or incisions are made during a surgical procedure in a sterile, controlled environment. The American College of Surgeons has defined four classes of surgical wound types. This classification can help to predict how the wound will heal and the risk of infection.

- **Class I** is defined as clean (e.g., laparoscopic surgeries and biopsies).
- **Class II** is defined as clean contaminated (e.g., GI and GU surgeries).
- **Class III** is defined as contaminated (e.g., traumatic wounds such as a gunshot wound).
- **Class IV** is defined as dirty (e.g., traumatic wound from a dirty source).

Surgical wounds should be assessed for signs and symptoms of infection including erythema, edema, fever, increasing pain, and drainage. Surgical drains are commonly placed near the surgical incision to promote drainage—inspect drains for patency, amount, and characteristics of drainage. Patients are often treated with antibiotics prophylactically to help prevent a surgical site infection. Wound vacuum assisted closure devices may also be utilized to remove blood or serous fluid from the surgical wound/incision site.



## Management of Inflammation Resulting from Tattoos and Piercing

Tattoos and piercing have both been implicated in **MRSA infections**. Tattooing uses needles that inject dye, sometimes resulting in local infection with erythema, edema, and purulent discharge. Body piercing for insertion of jewelry carries similar risks. Piercings of concern include the upper ear cartilage, nipples, navel, tongue, lip, penis, and nose. Some people who do piercings use reusable piercing equipment that is difficult to adequately clean and sterilize. Infections resulting from piercing in cartilage are often resistant to antibiotics because of lack of blood supply.

**Treatment** includes:

- **Cleansing wounds**. Jewelry may need to be removed in some cases.
- **Antibiotics**: Culture should be obtained, but medications for community-acquired MRSA should be started immediately:
  - **Mupirocin** may be used topically 3 times daily for 7–10 days with or without systemic antimicrobials.
  - **Trimethoprim-sulfamethoxazole DS** (TMP 160 mg/SMX 800 mg), 1–2 tablets twice daily. Children, dose based on TMP: 8–12 mg/kg/day in 2 doses.

## Tissue Damage

**Abrasion** is damage to superficial layers of skin, such as with road burn or ligature marks.

**Contusion** occurs when friction or pressure causes damage to underlying vessels, resulting in bruising. Contusions that are bright red/purple with clear margins have occurred within 48 hours and those with receding edges or yellow-brown discoloration are older than 48 hours.

**Laceration** is a tear in the skin resulting from blunt force, often from falls on protuberances, such as elbows, or other blunt trauma. Lacerations may be partial to full-thickness.

**Avulsion** is tissue that is separated from its base and lost or without adequate base for attachment.

**Treatments** include:

- Local anesthetic if needed
- Low pressure, high volume irrigation with 35–50 mL syringe of open wound with normal saline, water, or non-antiseptic nonionic surfactants, and mechanical scrubbing of surrounding tissue with disinfectant
- Topical antibiotics as indicated
- Prophylactic antibiotics or antibiotic irrigation if wound contaminated
- Suturing/debridement as needed
- Hydrocolloids, Steri-Strips, and transparent dressings to stabilize flaps

## Perfusion Injuries

Skin failure occurs when the integrity of the skin has been compromised so that it no longer serves as an effective barrier. Skin failure can occur as the result of pressure, such as over bony prominences, or from injuries, such as burns or moisture-associated skin injury; however, it may also result from hypoperfusion. With perfusion injuries, skin failure may occur despite adequate pressure-prevention methods. Perfusion injuries can occur with multiorgan failure, hemodynamic instability, and shock when the blood supply is shunted to protect the internal organs. For example, Kennedy terminal ulcers, which often occur as a patient nears death, may result from generalized ischemia and are often not preventable. Perfusion injuries may occur over bony prominences, but perfusion is often lower in those areas than in other body parts, so the primary cause may be hypoperfusion rather than pressure. Patients especially at risk include those who are critically ill (with sepsis, multiorgan failure, prolonged surgery, high-dose vasopressors), those at the end of life, and those in intensive care units (due to mechanical ventilation, edema, hypoxia). Distinguishing perfusion injuries from pressure injuries is critical to enforce appropriate prevention measures, which include optimizing hemodynamics and perfusion.

## Traumatic Wounds

Traumatic wounds include cuts, punctures, lacerations, force trauma, gunshot wounds, bites, abrasions, crush injuries, degloving injuries, and contusions. Trauma wounds can vary in severity and may be associated with serious underlying injuries. Once the patient is stabilized, wound management is initiated and should include thorough wound cleansing and debridement with removal of any foreign objects or materials. Irrigation and debridement are critical steps in minimizing the risk of infection. **Signs and symptoms** include bleeding, pain, erythema, and edema. With severe traumatic injury patients may experience signs of hemorrhagic shock including heavy bleeding, loss of consciousness, tachypnea, tachycardia, hypotension, decreased urinary output, and pallor.

**Treatment** of traumatic wounds is dependent on the location and severity of the wound. Treatment options may include irrigation and debridement, foreign body removal, wound closure including sutures, staples or fibrin glue, antibiotics, prophylactic tetanus injection, and fasciotomy.

### *Mechanical Trauma*

Mechanical trauma may result in stripping of the epidermis and sometimes the dermis of the skin or lacerations. Mechanical trauma may occur from tape removal or blunt trauma, such as colliding with furniture. Skin tears are categorized with the **Payne-Martin Classification System**:

- Skin tear leaves avulsed skin adequate to cover wound; tears may be linear or flap-type
- Skin tear with loss of partial thickness, involving either scant (less than 25% of epidermal flap over tear is lost) to moderate-large (more than 25% of dermis in tear is lost)
- Skin tear with complete loss of tissue, involving a partial-thickness wound with no epidermal flap

**Treatment** includes:

- Recognizing fragile skin and treating carefully
- Applying emollients, skin sealants, and skin barriers as indicated
- Applying and removing tape appropriately
- Avoiding adhesives when possible
- Using hydrocolloids, Steri-Strips, and transparent dressings to stabilize flaps

## Foreign Bodies in Subcutaneous Tissue

Foreign bodies (FB) imbedded in subcutaneous tissue can include metal, glass, plastic, and wood.

**Symptoms** may include pain, infection, or inflammatory response, pseudotumor, sinus tracts, or osteomyelitis. Patients often sense presence of FB.

**Treatment** includes careful history and examination to determine if the trauma of removing the foreign object is worse than leaving the object in place. Inert objects, such as metal and sometimes plastic or glass may be left in place, but wood always causes infection and must be removed. **Diagnosis** includes:

- Radiographs of soft tissue (metal and glass)
- Ultrasound (wood or thorns)
- CT for dangerous FB only

**MRIs** are usually only done if the initial attempt to remove the FB was unsuccessful and infection has developed, but metal fragments may move during an MRI so it is contraindicated for intraorbital or intracranial FBs.

### *Removal of Foreign Bodies in Subcutaneous Tissue*

Treatment to remove a foreign body (FB) should not exceed 30 minutes in the ED. Open tissue should not be probed with a gloved finger to locate the FB because of the danger of tearing a glove:

- Palpate tissue and use **metal instrument** to search for glass fragments rather than gloved finger
- **Local anesthetic**: lidocaine with epinephrine
- Use **radiographs or ultrasound** for guidance, using metal markers or inserting 2 needles to isolate location
- **BP cuff or tourniquet** may be needed to slow arterial flow to extremity
- **Incise** tissue adequately and use hemostat to remove the FB
- **Irrigate** wound with normal saline
- Wound is usually left **opened and bandaged**; large wounds may be sutured closed in 3–5 days
- **Antibiotics** as indicated

- FBs under **nails** may require removing all or part of nail:
  - **Digital block**
  - Sterile **hypodermic needle** (straight or bent) slid under nail to capture the FB
  - **$CO_2$ laser vaporization** may be used to vaporize nail above foreign object

## High-Pressure Injection Injuries

High-pressure injection injuries involve injection of materials (such as nails) or substances (water, air, oil, paint) into the tissue under high pressure. The severity of the injury depends on the location of the injury, the material or substance, and the size or amount of the injection. High-pressure injection injuries may result in ischemia, tissue destruction, open wounds, and inflammatory response even though the external injury may appear small.

**Signs/symptoms** include pain and swelling. Crepitus may be present with air injection. Ischemia may occur. These injuries may result in fractures, contractures, amputations, fibrosis, and fistulae. Common substances involved in high-pressure injection injuries include grease (over half of injuries) and diesel fuel. Injuries often occur on fingers of the non-dominant hand.

**Diagnosis** includes clinical symptoms and may include CBC (as some substances may cause increase WBC count) and electrolytes (some substances cause imbalance).

**Treatment** depends on the extent of the injury and includes supportive care, tetanus prophylaxis, and broad-spectrum antibiotic. Surgical repair may be required.

## Management of Missile Injuries

Missile injuries include arrow, gunshot, paint gun, nail gun, and shrapnel wounds. These injuries are usually circular, oval, or triangular, and may have both an entry (with abrasion at periphery) and exit site. Other residue, such as gunpowder, may be evident at the entry. Careful documentation should be done and clothes retained for evidence in gunshot wounds. Puncture wounds are difficult to properly cleanse and become easily infected, even with treatment.

**Treatment** varies according to the site, type, and degree of injury and may include:

- Tetanus prophylaxis
- Irrigation of wound with NS if both entry and exit
- Incision over puncture wound to create a linear incision that can be irrigated and cleansed adequately
- Removal of foreign body if in place
- Antibiotics as indicated
- Follow-up care to check for infection

# Integumentary Procedures and Interventions

## Wound VACs

**Wound vacuum-assisted closure (wound VAC)** (i.e., negative pressure wound therapy) uses subatmospheric (negative) pressure with a suction unit and a semi-occlusion vapor-permeable dressing. The suction reduces periwound and interstitial edema, decompressing vessels, improving circulation, stimulating production of new cells, and decreasing colonization of bacteria. Wound VAC also increases the rate of granulation and re-epithelialization to hasten healing. The wound must be debrided of necrotic tissue prior to treatment. Wound VAC is used for a variety of difficult-to-heal wounds, especially those that show less than 30% healing in 4 weeks of post-debridement treatment or those with excessive exudate, including chronic stage II and IV pressure injuries, skin flaps, diabetic ulcer, acute wounds, burns, surgical wound, and those with dehiscence and nonresponsive arterial and venous ulcers. Contraindications include:

- Wound malignancy
- Untreated osteomyelitis
- Exposed blood vessels or organs
- Non-enteric, unexplored fistulas.

Nonadherent porous foam is cut to fit and cover the wound and is secured with occlusive transparent film with an opening cut to accommodate the drainage tube, which is attached to a suction canister in a closed system. The pressure should be set at 75–125 psi and the dressing changed 2–3 times weekly.

## Pressure Reduction Surfaces

Pressure reduction surfaces redistribute pressure to prevent pressure injuries and reduce shear and friction. There are various types of support surfaces for beds, examining tables, operating tables, and chairs. Functions of pressure reduction surfaces include temperature control, moisture control, and friction/shear control. **General use guidelines** include:

- Pressure redistribution support surfaces should be used for patients with stage II, III, and IV pressure injuries, as well as for those that are at risk for developing pressure injuries.
- Chairs should have gel or air support surfaces to redistribute pressure for chair-bound patients, critically ill patients, or those who cannot move independently.
- Support surface material should provide at least an inch of support under areas to be protected when in use to prevent bottoming out. (Check by placing hand palm-up under the overlay below the pressure point.)
- Static support surfaces are appropriate for patients who can change position without increasing pressure to a preexisting pressure injury.
- Dynamic support surfaces are needed for those who need assistance to move or when static pressure devices provide less than an inch of support.

# Ear, Nose, and Throat Pathophysiology

## Recurrent Epistaxis

Recurrent epistaxis is common in young children (2 to 10 years), especially boys, and is often related to nose picking, dry climate, or central heating in the winter. Incidence also increases between 50 and 80 years of age, and may be caused by NSAIDs and anticoagulants. Kiesselbach plexus in the anterior nares has plentiful vessels and bleeds easily. Bleeding in the posterior nares is more dangerous and can result in considerable blood loss. Bleeding from the anterior nares is usually confined to one nostril, but from the posterior nares, blood may flow through both nostrils or backward into the throat and the person may be observed swallowing. People abusing cocaine may suffer nosebleeds because of damage to the mucosa. Hematocrit and hemoglobin should be done to determine if blood loss is significant. Bleeding should stop within 20 minutes. Treatment:

- Upright position, leaning forward so blood does not flow down throat.
- Applying pressure below the nares or by pinching the nostrils firmly for 10 minutes.
- Severe bleeding: packing and/or topical vasoconstrictors.
- Humidifiers may decrease irritation.

## Bell's Palsy

Bell's palsy is a temporary paralysis/weakness of muscles of the face due to dysfunction of the facial nerve (cranial nerve VII), usually associated with herpes simplex I or II infection (although idiopathic in nature). It generally affects only one side of the paired nerves, so the paralysis is seen only on one side of the face. Onset is generally sudden, and symptoms peak by 48 hours with a wide range of presentation. **Symptoms** usually subside within two to six months but may persist one year:

- Mild weakness on one side of face to complete paralysis with distortion of features
- Drooping of eyelid and mouth
- Tearing in affected eye
- Taste impairment

**Diagnosis** includes:

- Neurological, eye, parotid gland, and ear exam to rule out other cranial nerve involvement or conditions.

**Treatment** includes:

- Artificial tears during daytime with lubricating ophthalmic ointment and patch at night to protect eye
- Prednisone 60 mg daily for 5 days with tapering over 5 days.
- For severe cases use prednisone AND valacyclovir 1000 mg 3 times daily for 7 days, with acyclovir as an alternative.

## Temporal Arteritis

Temporal arteritis (TA), also called giant cell arteritis, is inflammation of the blood vessels of the head, especially the temporal artery, and the thoracic aorta and branches. TA is commonly associated with polymyalgia rheumatica (30% or less of patients) but can occur with other systemic disorders such as lupus erythematous, Sjögren syndrome, and rheumatoid arthritis. TA is a progressive disorder that can result in blindness and is most common in those older than 50. **Symptoms** include:

- New onset of headaches
- Vision fluctuations, including decreased visual acuity and loss of vision
- Intermittent claudicating pain in jaw, tongue, and upper extremities
- Fever

**Diagnosis** includes:

- Temporal artery biopsy (definitive)
- ESR greater than 50 mm/hr (may be normal in about 20%)
- CRP greater than 2.45 mg/dL

**Treatment** should begin immediately if the diagnosis is suspected to prevent blindness:

- Prednisone 60 mg daily

## Trigeminal Neuralgia

Trigeminal neuralgia (tic douloureux) is a neurological condition in which blood vessels press on the trigeminal nerve as it leaves the brainstem causing severe pain on one side of the face or jaw. The shock-like pains may involve a small area or half the face and in rare cases both sides of the face at different times. The pain lasts from seconds to two minutes and is extremely debilitating and may be precipitated by movement, vibration, or contact with the face or mouth. Trigeminal neuralgia is most common in women older than 50. Patients may go through periods of remission and recurrences. Diagnosis is by history and neurological exam.

**Treatment** is focused on symptom management and includes:

- **Carbamazepine** is the drug of choice and usually controls pain initially, but the effects may decrease over time.
- **Oxcarbazepine** may be used in place of carbamazepine.
- **Baclofen** (muscle relaxant) potentiates other drugs.
- **Surgical procedures** may be done if no response to medications.

## Foreign Bodies

### *Foreign Bodies in the Ear*

Foreign bodies in the ear (most often in children) can be organic or inorganic materials or insects. Careful history should be done to determine the type of foreign body before attempting removal. Children may require conscious sedation or general anesthesia for deep insertions. Irrigations should not be done if tympanic membrane is ruptured or cannot be visualized. Procedure:

1. Examine ear to determine if tympanic membrane is intact.
2. Drown insects with lidocaine 2% solution and then suction.
3. Irrigate small nonorganic particles with pulsatile flow aimed at wall of the canal.
4. Use cerumen loops, right-angle hooks, and/or alligator forceps to grasp and remove item.
5. Carefully examine the ear canal after removal of the item for lacerations or abrasions.
6. Topical antibiotic if extensive cutaneous abrasion or laceration or for organic material.

### *Foreign Bodies in the Eye*

Foreign bodies in the eye should be assessed carefully with slit lamp with corneal examination using optical sectioning before attempting removal of the foreign body. Foreign bodies that penetrate the cornea full-thickness should not be removed in the ED, but superficial foreign bodies can safely be removed. Procedure:

1. Apply topical anesthetic to both eyes (to suppress blinking in the unaffected eye).
2. Eye held open by hand or with wire eyelid speculum.
3. Foreign body is carefully removed with small gauge needle or moistened cotton swab.
4. Rust ring from metallic objects should be removed with ophthalmic burr (if not over pupil), and patient referred to ophthalmologist for further rust ring removal within 24 hours.
5. Eyelid everted and examined carefully for further foreign bodies.
6. Abrasions treated as indicated.

### *Foreign Bodies in the Nares*

Children may insert various organic and inorganic foreign bodies in the nose. In most cases, this is observed, but persistent unilateral obstruction of nose, foul discharge, or epistaxis is suggestive of foreign body. Small or uncooperative children may need to be restrained with conscious sedation or papoose board.

**Procedure**:

1. Vasoconstrictor/topical anesthetic applied: 1 mL of phenylephrine with 3 mL of lidocaine 4%.
2. Aerosolized racemic epinephrine may be used for decongestion, to loosen foreign body.
3. Examine nares with speculum.

**Removal techniques**:

- Positive pressure: Blowing nose on command. For small children, block opposite nares and have caregiver blow puff of air in mouth, forcing item out of nares.
- Suction with catheter.
- Use alligator or bayonet forceps to grasp item.
- Pass a curette behind item, rotate, and the use to pull item out.
- Pass Fogarty vascular catheter past item, inflate balloon, pull catheter back out.

## Ludwig Angina

Ludwig angina is cellulitis, usually caused by *Streptococcus* or *Staphylococcus,* of the submandibular spaces and lingual space that can result in obstruction of the airway as the swelling in the mouth floor pushes the tongue superior and posterior.

**Symptoms** include:

- Evidence of poor dental hygiene and odontogenic abscess (usually from lower third molars or surrounding gums) that has spread into soft tissue
- Dysphagia
- Odynophagia, trismus, edema of the upper neck (midline)
- Erythema, stridor, and cyanosis (late signs of obstruction)
- Changes in mental status

**Diagnosis** includes:

- Examination of the head and neck to observe for swelling of the upper neck, floor of mouth, and tongue
- CT scan
- Culture (treatment should, however, begin immediately)

**Treatments** include:

- Nasotracheal intubation (with fiberoptic tube if necessary) and ventilation if respiratory obstruction
- IV antibiotics, such as penicillin or clindamycin
- Referral to surgeon for incision and drainage as indicated

## OTITIS EXTERNA

Otitis externa is infection of the external ear canal, either bacterial or mycotic. Common pathogens include bacteria, *Pseudomonas aeruginosa*, *Staphylococcus aureus,* and fungi, *Aspergillus* and *Candida.* OE is often caused by chlorine in swimming pools killing normal flora and allowing other bacteria to multiply. Fungal infections may be associated with immune disorders, diabetes, and steroid use.

**Symptoms** include:

- Pain, swelling, and exudate
- Itching (pronounced with fungal infections)
- Red pustular lesions
- Black spots over tympanic membrane (fungus)

**Diagnosis**: On exam, tenderness when touched on tragus or when the auricle is pulled, erythema, and history.

**Treatment** includes:

- Irrigate ear with Burow's solution or saline to clean and remove debris or foreign objects.
- **Bacteria**: Antibiotic ear drops, such as ciprofloxacin and ofloxacin. If impetigo, flush with hydrogen peroxide 1:1 solution and apply mupirocin twice daily for 5-7 days. Lance pointed furuncles.
- **Fungus**: Solution of boric acid 5% in ethanol; clotrimazole-miconazole solution with/without steroid for 5-7 days.
- Analgesics as needed.

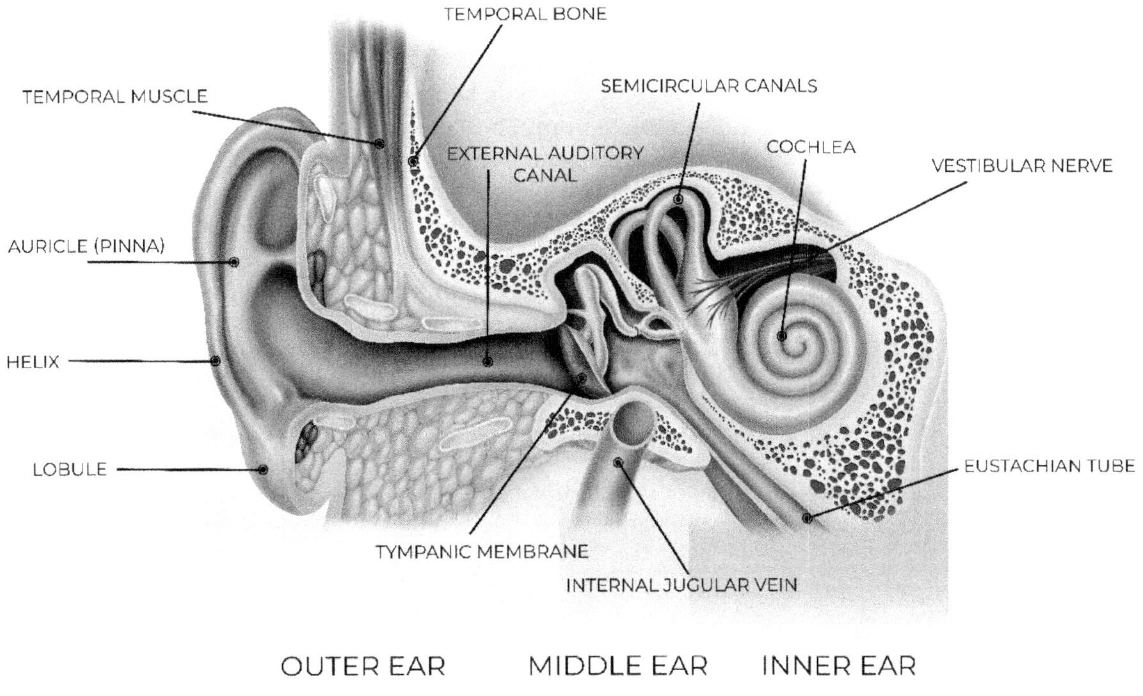


Physiological Adaptation

## Otitis Media

Otitis media, inflammation of the middle ear, usually follows upper respiratory tract infections or allergic rhinitis. The eustachian tube swells and prevents the passage of air. Fluid from the mucous membrane pools in the middle ear, causing infection. Common pathogens include *Streptococcus pneumoniae, Haemophilus influenzae,* and *Moraxella catarrhalis.* Some genetic conditions, such as trisomy 21 and cleft palate, may include abnormalities of the eustachian tube, increasing risk. There are four forms:

- **Acute**: 1-3 weeks with swelling, redness, and possible rupture of the tympanic membrane, fever, pain (ear pulling), and hearing loss.
- **Recurrent**: 3 episodes in 6 six months or 4-6 in 12 months.
- **Bullous**: Acute infection with ear popping pressure in middle ear, pain, hearing loss, and bullae between layers of tympanic membrane, causing bulging.
- **Chronic**: Persists at least 3 months with thick retracted tympanic membrane, hearing loss, and drainage.

**Diagnosis**: Distinguishing features on assessment of acute otitis media include a bulging or perforated tympanic membrane, signs of inflammation, or purulent fluid present.

**Treatment**: 75-90% resolve spontaneously, so antibiotics are **withheld** for 2-3 days. Amoxicillin for 7-10 days. Referral for **tympanostomy and pressure-equalizing tubes** (PET) for severe chronic or recurrent infections.

**Review Video: Otitis Media**
Visit mometrix.com/academy and enter code: 328778

## Mastoiditis

Mastoiditis usually results from extension of acute otitis media because the mucous membranes of the middle ear are continuous with the mastoid air cells in the temporal bone. All patients with otitis media should be considered at risk for mastoiditis. Patients with chronic otitis media also often develop chronic mastoiditis, which can result in formation of benign cholesteatoma. Signs and symptoms of mastoiditis include persistent fever, pain in or behind the ear (especially during the night), and hearing loss. Differential diagnoses may include Bell's palsy, otitis externa, and otitis media. **Diagnosis** is based on symptoms, CBC, audiometry, tympanocentesis or myringotomy with culture and sensitivities, and CT scan (definitive). Acute mastoiditis is treated with antibiotics, usually beginning with a 3rd generation cephalosporin or penicillin/aminoglycoside combination until culture and sensitivity results return. If spreading empyema or osteitis is present, then surgical mastoidectomy is required.

## Sinusitis

Sinusitis is inflammation of the nasal sinuses, of which there are two maxillary, two frontal, and one sphenoidal, as ethmoidal air cells. Inflammation causes obstruction of drainage with resultant discomfort.

**Symptoms** include:

- Frontal and maxillary presents with pain over sinuses
- Ethmoidal present with dull aching behind eye
- Tenderness to palpation and percussion of sinuses
- Mucosa of nasal cavity edematous and erythematous
- Purulent exudate

**Diagnosis** includes:

- Transillumination of sinus (diminished with inflammation)
- CT for those who are immunocompromised or if diagnosis is not clear
- Careful examination to rule out spreading infection, especially with signs of fever, altered mental status, or unstable vital signs

**Treatment** includes:

- Symptomatic relief with analgesia
- Topical decongestants and nasal irrigation
- Antimicrobial therapy if symptoms persist at least seven days or are severe (avoid routine use): Amoxicillin or TMP/SMX
- Steroid nasal spray twice daily

## Meniere's Disease

Meniere's disease occurs when a blockage in the endolymphatic duct of the inner ear causes dilation of the endolymphatic space and abnormal fluid balance, which causes pressure or rupture of the inner ear membrane.

**Symptoms** include:

- Progressive fluctuating sensorineural hearing loss
- Tinnitus
- Pressure in the ear
- Severe vertigo that lasts minutes to hours
- Diaphoresis
- Poor balance
- Nausea and vomiting

**Diagnosis** includes:

- Complete physical exam and evaluation of cranial nerves
- Tuning fork sounds may lateralize to unaffected ear
- Assessment of hearing loss

**Treatment**:

- Low sodium diet
- Vestibular suppressant (antihistamine): Meclizine
- Benzodiazepine or SSRI for anxiety
- Antiemetics, such as promethazine suppositories
- Diuretics, such as hydrochlorothiazide
- Referral for surgical repair for persistent vertigo, but this will not correct other symptoms

## Labyrinthitis

Labyrinthitis is a viral or bacterial inflammation of the inner ear, and it may occur secondary to bacterial otitis media. Viral labyrinthitis may be associated with mumps, rubella, rubeola, influenza, or other viral infections, such as upper respiratory tract infections. Because the labyrinth includes the vestibular system that is responsible for sensing head movement, labyrinthitis causes balance disorders. The condition often persists for 1 to 6 weeks with acute symptoms the first week and then decreasing symptoms. **Symptoms** include:

- Sudden onset of severe vertigo
- Hearing loss and sometimes tinnitus
- Nausea and vomiting
- Panic attacks from severe anxiety related to symptoms

**Treatment** includes:

- **Bacterial**: IV antibiotics
- **Viral**: Symptomatic as for bacterial (except for antibiotics)
- Volume replacement
- Antiemetics, such as promethazine suppositories
- Vestibular suppressant (antihistamine): Meclizine
- Benzodiazepine or SSRI for anxiety
- Referral to surgeon for I&D if necessary

## TMD

Temporomandibular disorder (TMD) is jaw pain caused by dysfunction of the temporomandibular joint (TMJ) and the supporting muscles and ligaments. It may be precipitated by injury, such as whiplash, or grinding or clenching of the teeth, stress, or arthritis.

**Symptoms** include:

- Clicking or popping noises on jaw movement
- Limited jaw movement or "locked" jaw
- Acute pain on chewing or moving jaw
- Headaches and dizziness
- Toothaches

**Diagnosis** includes:

- Complete dental exam with x-rays to rule out other disorders
- MRI or CT may be needed

**Treatment** usually begins conservatively:

- Ice pack to jaw area for 10 minutes followed by jaw stretching exercises and warm compress for 5 minutes 3-4 times daily
- Avoidance of heavy chewing by eating soft foods and avoiding hard foods, such as raw carrots and nuts
- NSAIDs to relieve pain and inflammation
- Night mouthguard
- Referral for dental treatments to improve bite as necessary

## TEMPOROMANDIBULAR FRACTURE AND/OR DISLOCATION

Temporomandibular fracture and/or dislocation can occur as a result of trauma, such as a direct blow to the jaw, or chronic disorders. Dislocations may be anterior (most common and often after extreme mouth opening), posterior, lateral, or superior.

**Symptoms**:

- Acute pain
- Dysphagia
- Difficulty speaking
- Edema and rigidity of surrounding muscles
- Inability to open mouth

**Diagnosis** includes:

- Complete head, neck, ear, and dental examination
- Radiography, such as x-rays or CT, with significant trauma
- Tongue blade test: Patient bites hard on tongue blade while examiner twists blade, attempting to break it. If fracture, patient opens mouth to release blade

**Treatment** (dislocation) includes:

- Short-acting muscle relaxant
- Narcotic analgesia/conscious sedation
- Reduction: Patient on chair with head against hard surface
- Examiner in front of patient places gloved thumbs in patient's mouth, posteriorly over the surface of the mandibular molars
- Examiner applies pressure posteriorly and inferiorly
- Alternately, examiner stands behind recumbent patient and applies pressure posteriorly and inferiorly



## NASAL FRACTURE

Nasal fracture can result from any type of blunt trauma to the face. Fracture may be overlooked because of edema, so careful examination of the nose with facial injuries is important. Common causes include altercations and sporting injuries. Septal cartilage is often fractured as well as nasal bones.

**Symptoms** include:

- Edema
- Pain
- Crepitation
- Ecchymosis
- Deformity
- Nasal bleeding

**Diagnosis** is based on clinical examination and otoscope. Radiographic studies are not indicated unless other facial fractures are suspected. Clear nasal discharge following injury to the face may indicate leaking of cerebrospinal fluid from torn meninges resulting from fracture of cribriform plate. A drop of clear drainage should be placed on filter paper and examined for a clear area around a central stain of blood. If CSF drainage is suspected, the patient should be placed upright, and have a CT scan and neurological consult.

**Treatment** for fracture includes:

- Realignment if necessary
- Analgesia
- Nasal decongestant
- Protective covering
- Packing only for persistent epistaxis

## MAXILLARY FRACTURES

Maxillary fractures of the face often are associated with significant other trauma because of the degree of force necessary to fracture the maxilla. Three primary types include:

- **Le Fort I**: Horizontal (low downward force)
- **Le Fort II**: Pyramidal (low or mid maxilla force)
- **Le Fort III**: Transverse (force to bridge of nose or upper maxilla)

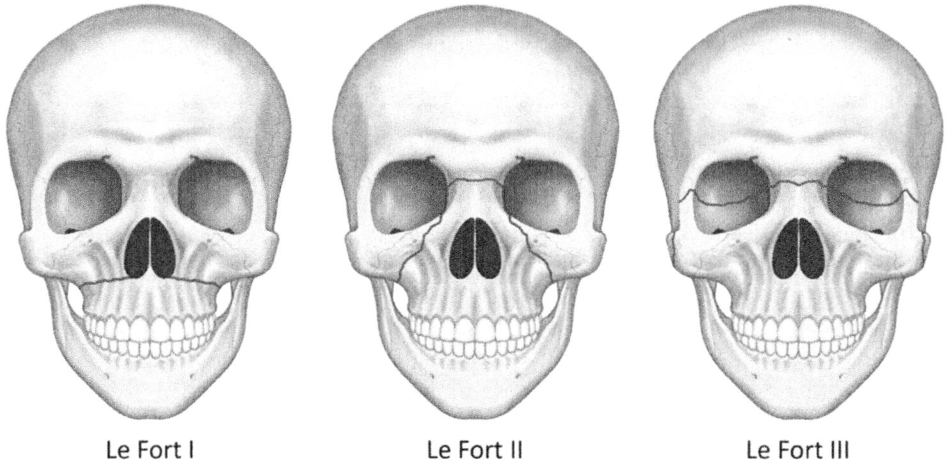


However, many injuries are a combination with more than one type of fracture.

**Symptoms** may include:

- Malocclusion and open bite
- Apparent lengthening of face
- CSF rhinorrhea (clear nasal discharge)
- Periorbital ecchymosis

**Diagnosis**: Grasping and moving the hard palate back and forth may shift the facial bones. Complete head, neck, ear, oral, and nasal examination with slit headlamp, suction as needed, nasal speculum, and otoscope. CT scans of face and brain.

**Treatment**:

- Stabilize patient and ensure patent airway
- Disimpaction of displaced fragments manually
- Obtain pre-injury photograph to guide surgical fixation
- Referral to surgeon for fixation

# Fever and Fibromyalgia

## Febrile Seizure

Febrile seizure is a generalized seizure associated with high fever (usually more than 38°C [100.4°F]) from any type of infection (upper respiratory tract, urinary) but without intracranial infection or other cause, occurring between six months and five years of age. Careful clinical examination must be conducted to rule out more serious disorders. Laboratory tests are conducted in relation to symptoms. Lumbar puncture is not usually indicated unless intracranial infection is suspected. Seizures usually last less than 15 minutes and are without subsequent neurological deficit.

**Treatment** includes:

- Fever control: Acetaminophen 10-15 mg/kg every 4-6 hours OR ibuprofen 10 mg/kg every 6-8 hours. Antipyretics are NOT recommended as prophylaxis for recurrent febrile seizures.
- Tepid water bath.
- Antiepileptic drugs (AEDs) are usually not advised unless seizures are complex or continuous, child is younger than 6 months, or there is a preexisting neurological disorder: IV diazepam 0.1-0.2 mg/kg or IV lorazepam 0.05-0.1 mg/kg. (May cause lethargy.)

## Fibromyalgia

Fibromyalgia is a complex syndrome of disorders that include fatigue, chronic generalized muscle pain, and focal areas of tenderness persisting for at least three months. The cause of fibromyalgia is not clear and has only recently been recognized as a distinct disorder. Diagnosis is by clinical exam and ruling out joint and muscle inflammation that could be cause of the pain. On clinical exam there are specific points of tenderness, usually in multiple areas of the body.

**Symptoms**:

- Fatigue.
- Pain and stiffness unresponsive to treatment, persisting for months.
- Sleep disorders.
- Irritable bowel syndrome.
- Stiffness in neck and shoulders associated with headache and pain in face.
- Sensitivity to odor, noises, and lights.
- Mood disorders, such as depression, anxiety.
- Dysmenorrhea.
- Paresthesia in hands and feet.

**Treatment**:

- **Analgesia**: Acetaminophen, tramadol, or NSAIDs.
- **Antidepressants**, such as amitriptyline, nortriptyline, or fluoxetine. Duloxetine and venlafaxine have been shown to reduce pain.
- **Antiseizure medication**: Pregabalin is the first FDA-approved treatment for the pain of fibromyalgia.
- **Referral** for physical therapy and/or cognitive therapy.

# Electrolyte Imbalances

## Sodium Imbalance

Sodium (**Na**) regulates fluid volume, osmolality, acid-base balance, and activity in the muscles, nerves, and myocardium. It is the primary **cation** (positive ion) in extracellular fluid (ECF), necessary to maintain ECF levels that are needed for tissue perfusion:

- Normal range: 135–145 mEq/L
- Hyponatremia: <135 mEq/L
- Hypernatremia: >145 mEq/L

**Hyponatremia** may result from inadequate sodium intake, excess sodium loss through diarrhea, vomiting, or NG suctioning, or illness, such as severe burns, fever, SIADH, and ketoacidosis.

- **Symptoms**: Irritability to lethargy and alterations in consciousness, cerebral edema with seizures and coma, dyspnea to respiratory failure.
- **Treatment**: Identify and treat the underlying cause and provide Na replacement.

**Hypernatremia** may result from renal disease, diabetes insipidus, and fluid depletion.

- **Symptoms**: Irritability to lethargy to confusion to coma; seizures; flushing; muscle weakness and spasms; thirst.
- **Treatment**: Identify and treat the underlying cause, monitor Na levels carefully, and give IV fluid replacement.

## Potassium Imbalance

Potassium (**K**) is the primary **electrolyte** in intracellular fluid (ICF), with about 98% inside cells and only 2% in ECF, although this small amount is important for neuromuscular activity. Potassium influences activity of the skeletal and cardiac muscles. Its level is dependent upon adequate renal functioning because 80% is excreted through the kidneys and 20% through the bowels and sweat:

- Normal range: 3.5–5.5 mEq/L
- Hypokalemia: <3.5 mEq/L. Critical value: <2.5 mEq/L
- Hyperkalemia: >5.5 mEq/L. Critical value: >6.5 mEq/L

A healthy NPO patient will need about 40 mEq of K per day to maintain serum K levels. Expect alterations in renal disease and other disease processes.

**Hypokalemia** is caused by alkalosis, decreased intake associated with starvation, nephritis, and loss of potassium through diarrhea, vomiting, gastric suction, and diuresis.

- **Symptoms**: Lethargy and weakness; nausea and vomiting; paresthesia and tetany; muscle cramps with hyporeflexia; hypotension; dysrhythmias with EKG changes: PVCs or flattened T-waves.
- **Treatment**: Treatment involves identifying and treating the underlying cause and replacing K. When possible, oral replacement is preferable to IV, as it allows slower adjustment of K levels. When given IV, K should be given no faster than 20 mEq/hour via central line if possible. If given peripherally, 10 mEq/hour is preferable for patient comfort.

**Hyperkalemia** is caused by renal disease, adrenal insufficiency, metabolic acidosis, severe dehydration, burns, hemolysis, and trauma. It rarely occurs without renal disease but may be induced by treatment (such as NSAIDs and potassium-sparing diuretics). Untreated renal failure results in reduced excretion. Those with Addison disease and deficient adrenal hormones suffer sodium loss that results in potassium retention.

- **Symptoms**: The primary symptoms relate to the effect on the cardiac muscle: ventricular arrhythmias with increasing changes in EKG lead to cardiac and respiratory arrest, weakness with ascending paralysis and hyperreflexia, diarrhea, and increasing confusion.
- **Treatment**: Treatment includes identifying the underlying cause and discontinuing sources of increased K. Calcium gluconate to decrease cardiac effects. Sodium bicarbonate, insulin, and hypertonic dextrose shift K into the cells temporarily. Cation exchange resin (Kayexalate) to decrease K. Peritoneal dialysis or hemodialysis to remove excess K.

*Note*: When a tourniquet is on, a patient opening and closing their hand can lead to falsely elevated K levels.

## Calcium Imbalance

More than 99% of calcium (**Ca**) is in the skeletal system with 1% in serum, but it is important for transmitting nerve impulses and regulating muscle contraction and relaxation, including the myocardium. Calcium activates enzymes that stimulate chemical reactions and has a role in the coagulation of blood:

- Normal range: 8.2–10.2 mg/dL
- Hypocalcemia: <8.2. Critical value: <7 mg/dL
- Hypercalcemia: >10.2 mg/dL. Critical value: >12 mg/dL

**Hypercalcemia** may be caused by acidosis, kidney disease, hyperparathyroidism, prolonged immobilization, and malignancies. Crisis carries a 50% mortality rate.

- **Symptoms**: Increasing muscle weakness with hypotonicity; anorexia; nausea and vomiting; constipation; bradycardia and cardiac arrest.
- **Treatment**: Identify and treat underlying cause, loop diuretics, IV fluids, phosphate.

**Hypocalcemia** may be caused by damage to the parathyroid resulting in hypoparathyroidism (directly decreasing calcium production), vitamin D resistance or inadequacy, or liver/kidney disease.

- **Symptoms**: Muscle cramping or spasms; seizures; numbness or tingling of the feet, hands, or lips; tetany if severe.
- **Treatment**: Identify and treat underlying cause, replace calcium by administering IV calcium gluconate in acute circumstances or increasing oral Vitamin D and calcium in chronic cases.

## Phosphorus Imbalance

Phosphorus, or phosphate, **($PO_4$)** is necessary for neuromuscular and red blood cell function, the maintenance of acid-base balance, and provides structure for teeth and bones. About 85% is in the bones, 14% in soft tissue, and <1% in ECF.

- Normal range: 2.4–4.5 mEq/L
- Hypophosphatemia: <2.4mEq/L
- Hyperphosphatemia: >4.5 mEq/L

**Hypophosphatemia** occurs with severe protein-calorie malnutrition, hyperventilation, severe burns, diabetic ketoacidosis, and excess antacids with magnesium, calcium, or aluminum.

- **Symptoms**: Irritability, tremors, seizures to coma; hemolytic anemia; decreased myocardial function; respiratory failure.
- **Treatment***:* Identify and treat underlying cause and replace phosphorus.

**Hyperphosphatemia** occurs with renal failure, hypoparathyroidism, excessive intake, neoplastic disease, diabetic ketoacidosis, muscle necrosis, and chemotherapy.

- **Symptoms**: Tachycardia; muscle cramping; hyperreflexia and tetany; nausea and diarrhea.
- **Treatment**: Identify and treat underlying cause, correct hypocalcemia, and provide antacids and dialysis.

## Magnesium Imbalance

Magnesium (**Mg**) is the second most common intracellular electrolyte (after potassium) and activates many intracellular enzyme systems. Mg is important for carbohydrate and protein metabolism, neuromuscular function, and cardiovascular function, producing vasodilation and directly affecting the peripheral arterial system:

- Normal range: 1.7–2.2 mg/dL
- Hypomagnesemia critical value: <1.2 mg/dL
- Hypermagnesemia critical value: >4.9 mg/dL

**Hypomagnesemia** occurs with chronic diarrhea, chronic renal disease, chronic pancreatitis, excess diuretic or laxative use, hyperthyroidism, hypoparathyroidism, severe burns, and diaphoresis.

- **Symptoms**: Neuromuscular excitability or tetany; confusion, headaches, dizziness; seizure and coma; tachycardia with ventricular arrhythmias; respiratory depression.
- **Treatment**: Identify and treat underlying cause, provide magnesium replacement. IV magnesium is a vasodilator, 2 g over 60 mins.

**Hypermagnesemia** occurs with renal failure or inadequate renal function, diabetic ketoacidosis, hypothyroidism, and Addison disease.

- **Symptoms**: Muscle weakness, seizures, and dysphagia with decreased gag reflex; tachycardia with hypotension.
- **Treatment**: Identify and treat underlying cause, IV hydration with calcium, and dialysis.

**Review Video: Fluid and Electrolyte Balance**
Visit mometrix.com/academy and enter code: 384389

# Acid Base Imbalances

## Invasive Blood Gas Monitoring

Invasive blood gas monitoring options include the following:

- **Arterial blood gas (ABG)** is the most informative measurement of blood gas status. If an arterial catheter is in place, it is easily obtained by aspirating 1–2 mL of blood.
- **Venous blood gas (VBG)** is easier to obtain if an arterial catheter is not in place. In order to compare the values in the VBG with an ABG, make the following calculations:
    - Add 0.05 to the pH of the VBG.
    - Subtract 5–10 mmHg from the $PCO_2$ of the VBG.
- **Capillary blood gas (CBG)** can be obtained with a heel stick, without a venous or arterial line, but the values obtained in a CBG are the least accurate and are rarely useful. This is used most often in neonates.

### *Components of a Blood Gas Reading*

The following are components of a blood gas reading:

- **pH** measures the circulating acid and base levels. Neutral pH for humans is 7.4. A value below 7.35 indicates acidosis and a value greater than 7.45 indicates alkalosis.
- **$pCO_2$** is the partial pressure of carbon dioxide and it determines the respiratory component of pH. An elevated $pCO_2$ lowers the pH. A low $pCO_2$ raises the pH. The $pCO_2$ value is dependent on adequate pulmonary ventilation and respiration. Changes in respiratory status quickly alter this value. Normal value range for $pCO_2$ is 35–45 mmHg.
- **$pO_2$** is the partial pressure of oxygen, which indicates how well the individual is transporting oxygen from the lungs into the bloodstream. Normal value is 75–100 mmHg.
- **$HCO_3^-$** is bicarbonate, the metabolic component of pH. This value may slowly change in response to abnormal pH, or a disease process may cause an elevation or depression. Low values decrease the pH and high values raise the pH. Normal value for bicarbonate is 22–26 mEq/L.

**Review Video: Acid-Base Balance & Blood Gas Interpretation**
Visit mometrix.com/academy and enter code: 611909

## Metabolic and Respiratory Acidosis

### *Pathophysiology*

- Metabolic acidosis
    - Increase in fixed acid and inability to excrete acid, or loss of base, with compensatory increase of $CO_2$ excretion by lungs
- Respiratory acidosis
    - Hypoventilation and $CO_2$ retention with renal compensatory retention of bicarbonate ($HCO_3$) and increased excretion of hydrogen

### *Laboratory*

- Metabolic acidosis
    - Decreased serum pH (<7.35) and $PCO_2$ normal if uncompensated and decreased if compensated
    - Decreased $HCO_3$
- Respiratory acidosis
    - Decreased serum pH (< 7.35) and increased $PCO_2$
    - Increased $HCO_3$ if compensated and normal if uncompensated

### *Causes*

- Metabolic acidosis
  - DKA, lactic acidosis, diarrhea, starvation, renal failure, shock, renal tubular acidosis, starvation
- Respiratory acidosis
  - COPD, overdose of sedative or barbiturate (leading to hypoventilation), obesity, severe pneumonia/atelectasis, muscle weakness (Guillain-Barré), mechanical hypoventilation

### *Symptoms*

- Metabolic acidosis
  - Neuro/muscular: Drowsiness, confusion, headache, coma
  - Cardiac: Decreased BP, arrhythmias, flushed skin
  - GI: Nausea, vomiting, abdominal pain, diarrhea
  - Respiratory: Deep inspired tachypnea
- Respiratory acidosis
  - Neuro/muscular: Drowsiness, dizziness, headache, coma, disorientation, seizures
  - Cardiac: Flushed skin, VF, ↓BP
  - GI: Absent
  - Respiratory: Hypoventilation with hypoxia

## Metabolic and Respiratory Alkalosis

### *Pathophysiology*

- Metabolic alkalosis
  - Decreased strong acid or increased base with possible compensatory $CO_2$ retention by lungs
- Respiratory alkalosis
  - Hyperventilation and increased excretion of $CO_2$ with compensatory $HCO_3$ excretion by kidneys

### *Laboratory*

- Metabolic alkalosis
  - Increased serum pH (>7.45)
  - $PCO_2$ normal if uncompensated and increased if compensated
  - Increased $HCO_3$
- Respiratory alkalosis
  - Increased serum pH (>7.45)
  - Decreased $PCO_2$
  - $HCO_3$ normal if uncompensated and decreased if compensated

### *Causes*

- Metabolic alkalosis
  - Excessive vomiting, gastric suctioning, diuretics, potassium deficit, excessive mineralocorticoids and $NaHCO_3$ intake
- Respiratory alkalosis
  - Hyperventilation associated with hypoxia, pulmonary embolus, exercise, anxiety, pain, and fever
  - Encephalopathy, septicemia, brain injury, salicylate overdose, and mechanical hyperventilation

### *Symptoms*

- Metabolic alkalosis
    - Neuromuscular: Dizziness, confusion, nervousness, anxiety, tremors, muscle cramping, tetany, tingling, seizures
    - Cardiac: Tachycardia and arrhythmias
    - GI: Nausea, vomiting, anorexia
    - Respiratory: Compensatory hypoventilation
- Respiratory alkalosis
    - Neuro/muscular: Light-headedness, confusion, lethargy
    - Cardiac: Tachycardia and arrhythmias
    - GI: Epigastric pain, nausea, and vomiting
    - Respiratory: Hyperventilation

# Multisystem Pathophysiology

## Range of Severe Infection

There are a number of terms used to refer to severe infections which are often used interchangeably. It is important to know these terms to properly perform the continuum of care.

- **Bacteremia** is the presence of bacteria in the blood without systemic infection.
- **Septicemia** is a systemic infection caused by pathogens (usually bacteria or fungi) present in the blood.
- **Systemic inflammatory response syndrome** (SIRS) is a generalized inflammatory response affecting many organ systems. It may be caused by infectious or non-infectious agents, such as trauma, burns, adrenal insufficiency, pulmonary embolism, and drug overdose. If an infectious agent is identified or suspected, SIRS is an aspect of sepsis. Infective agents include a wide range of bacteria and fungi, including *Streptococcus pneumoniae* and *Staphylococcus aureus.* SIRS includes 2 of the following:
    - Elevated (>38 °C) or subnormal rectal temperature (<36 °C)
    - Tachypnea or $PaCO_2$ <32 mmHg
    - Tachycardia
    - Leukocytosis (>12,000) or leukopenia (<4000)
- **Sepsis** is the presence of infection either locally or systemically in which there is a generalized life-threatening inflammatory response (SIRS). It includes all the indications for SIRS as well as one of the following:
    - Changes in mental status
    - Hypoxemia without preexisting pulmonary disease
    - Elevation in plasma lactate
    - Decreased urinary output <5 mL/kg/hr for ≥1 hour
- **Severe sepsis** includes both indications of SIRS and sepsis as well as indications of increasing organ dysfunction with inadequate perfusion and/or hypotension.
- **Septic shock** is a progression from severe sepsis in which refractory hypotension occurs despite treatment. There may be indications of lactic acidosis.
- **Multi-organ dysfunction syndrome** (MODS) is the most common cause of sepsis-related death. Cardiac function becomes depressed, acute respiratory distress syndrome (ARDS) may develop, and renal failure may follow acute tubular necrosis or cortical necrosis. Thrombocytopenia appears in about 30% of those affected and may result in disseminated intravascular coagulation (DIC). Liver damage and bowel necrosis may occur.

**Review Video: Multiple Organ Dysfunction Syndrome**
Visit mometrix.com/academy and enter code: 394302

## Shock

There are a number of different types of shock, but there are general characteristics that they have in common. In all types of shock, there is a marked decrease in tissue perfusion related to hypotension, so that there is insufficient oxygen delivered to the tissues and inadequate removal of cellular waste products, causing injury to tissue:

- Hypotension (systolic below 90 mmHg); this may be somewhat higher (110 mmHg) in those who are initially hypertensive
- Decreased urinary output (<0.5 mL/kg/hr), especially marked in hypovolemic shock
- Metabolic acidosis
- Peripheral/cutaneous vasoconstriction/vasodilation resulting in cool, clammy skin
- Alterations in level of consciousness

**Types of shock** are as follows:

- **Distributive:** Preload decreased, CO increased, SVR decreased. Examples include septic shock, neurogenic shock, and anaphylactic shock.
- **Hypovolemic:** Preload decreased, CO decreased, SVR increased. Hypovolemic shock can be hemorrhagic or nonhemorrhagic.
- **Cardiogenic:** Preload increased, CO decreased, SVR increased. This form of shock is secondary to cardiovascular dysfunction.
- **Obstructive:** Preload decreased, CO decreased, SVR increased. Obstructive shock is rare and usually secondary to a pulmonary obstruction (pulmonary embolism), tension pneumothorax, or cardiac tamponade.

## Distributive Shock

Distributive shock occurs with adequate blood volume but inadequate intravascular volume because of arterial/venous dilation that results in decreased vascular tone and hypoperfusion of internal organs. Cardiac output may be normal or blood may pool, decreasing cardiac output. **Distributive shock** may result from anaphylactic shock, septic shock, neurogenic shock, and drug ingestions.

**Symptoms** include:

- Hypotension (systolic <90 mmHg or <40 mmHg below normal), tachypnea, tachycardia (>90) (may be lower if patient receiving β-blockers)
- Hypoxemia
- Skin initially warm, later hypoperfused
- Hyper- or hypothermia (>38 °C or <36 °C)
- Alterations in mentation
- Decreased urinary output
- Symptoms related to underlying cause

**Treatment** includes:

- Treating underlying cause while stabilizing hemodynamics
- Oxygen with endotracheal intubation if necessary

- Rapid fluid administration at 0.25–0.5 L NS or isotonic crystalloid every 5–10 minutes as needed to 2–3 L
- Vasoconstrictive and inotropic agents (dopamine, dobutamine, norepinephrine) if necessary, for patients with profound hypotension

### *Septic Shock*

Septic shock is a form of distributive shock caused by toxins produced by bacteria and cytokines that the body produces in response to severe infection, resulting in a complex syndrome of disorders. **Symptoms** are wide-ranging:

- **Initial**: Hyper- or hypothermia, increased temperature (>38 °C) with chills, tachycardia with increased pulse pressure, tachypnea, alterations in mental status (dullness), hypotension, hyperventilation with respiratory alkalosis ($PaCO_2 \leq 30$ mmHg), increased lactic acid, unstable BP, and dehydration with increased urinary output
- **Cardiovascular**: Myocardial depression and dysrhythmias
- **Respiratory**: Acute respiratory distress syndrome (ARDS)
- **Renal**: Acute kidney injury (AKI) with decreased urinary output and increased BUN
- **Hepatic**: Jaundice and liver dysfunction with an increase in transaminase, alkaline phosphatase, and bilirubin
- **Hematologic**: Mild or severe blood loss (from mucosal ulcerations), neutropenia or neutrophilia, decreased platelets, and DIC
- **Endocrine**: Hyperglycemia, hypoglycemia (rare)
- **Skin**: Cellulitis, erysipelas, and fasciitis, acrocyanotic and necrotic peripheral lesions

Septic shock is most common in newborns, those >50, and those who are immunocompromised. There is no specific test to confirm a diagnosis of septic shock, so **diagnosis** is based on clinical findings and tests that evaluate hematologic, infectious, and metabolic states: Lactic acid, CBC, DIC panel, electrolytes, liver function tests, BUN, creatinine, blood glucose, ABGs, urinalysis, ECG, radiographs, blood and urine cultures.

**Treatment** must be aggressive and includes:

- Oxygen and endotracheal intubation as necessary
- IV access with 2-large bore catheters and central venous line
- Rapid fluid administration at 0.5L NS or isotonic crystalloid every 5–10 minutes as needed (to 4–6 L)
- Monitoring urinary output to optimal >30 mL/hr (>1 mL/kg/hr)
- Inotropic or vasoconstrictive agents (dopamine, dobutamine, norepinephrine) if no response to fluids or fluid overload
- Empiric IV antibiotic therapy (usually with 2 broad spectrum antibiotics for both gram-positive and gram-negative bacteria) until cultures return and antibiotics may be changed
- Hemodynamic and laboratory monitoring
- Removing source of infection (abscess, catheter)

### *Neurogenic Shock*

Neurogenic shock is a type of distributive shock that occurs when injury to the CNS from trauma resulting in acute spinal cord injury (from both blunt and penetrating injuries), neurological diseases, drugs, or anesthesia, impairs the autonomic nervous system that controls the cardiovascular system. The degree of symptoms relates to the level of injury with injuries above T1 capable of causing disruption of the entire sympathetic nervous system and lower injuries causing various degrees of disruption. Even incomplete spinal cord injury can cause neurogenic shock.

**Symptoms** include:

- Hypotension and warm dry skin related to lack of vascular tone that results in hypothermia from loss of cutaneous heat
- Bradycardia (common but not universal)

**Treatment** includes:

- ABCDE (airway, breathing, circulation, disability evaluation, exposure)
- Rapid fluid administration with crystalloid to keep mean arterial pressure at 85–90 mmHg
- Placement of pulmonary artery catheter to monitor fluid overload
- Inotropic agents (dopamine, dobutamine) if fluids don't correct hypotension

## Hypovolemic Shock/Volume Deficit

Hypovolemic shock occurs when there is inadequate intravascular fluid. The loss may be *absolute* because of an internal shifting of fluid or an external loss of fluid, as occurs with massive hemorrhage, thermal injuries, severe vomiting or diarrhea, and internal injuries (such as ruptured spleen or dissecting arteries) that interfere with intravascular integrity. Hypovolemia may also be *relative* and related to vasodilation, increased capillary membrane permeability from sepsis or injuries, and decreased colloidal osmotic pressure that may occur with loss of sodium and some disorders, such as hypopituitarism and cirrhosis.

Hypovolemic shock is **classified** according to the degree of fluid loss:

- **Class I:** <750 mL or ≤15% of total circulating volume (TCV)
- **Class II:** 750–1500 mL or 15–30% of TCV
- **Class III:** 1500–2000 mL or 30–40% of TCV
- **Class IV:** >2000 mL or >40% of TCV

### *Symptoms and Treatment*

Hypovolemic shock occurs when the total circulating volume of fluid decreases, leading to a fall in venous return that in turn causes a decrease in ventricular filling and preload, indicated by ↓ in right atrial pressure (RAP) and pulmonary artery occlusion pressure (PAOP). This results in a decrease in stroke volume and cardiac output. This in turn causes generalized arterial vasoconstriction, increasing afterload (↑ systemic vascular resistance), causing decreased tissue perfusion.

**Symptoms**: Anxiety, pallor, cool and clammy skin, delayed capillary refill, cyanosis, hypotension, increasing respirations, weak, thready pulse.

**Treatment** is aimed at identifying and treating the cause:

- Administration of blood, blood products, autotransfusion, colloids (such as plasma protein fraction), and/or crystalloids (such as normal saline)
- Oxygen—intubation and ventilation may be necessary
- Medications may include vasopressors, such as dopamine. **Note: Fluids must be given before starting vasopressors**!

### *Anaphylactic Shock*

Anaphylactic reaction or anaphylactic shock, another form of distributive shock, may present with a few symptoms or a wide range of potentially lethal effects.

**Symptoms** may recur after the initial treatment (biphasic anaphylaxis), so careful monitoring is essential:

- Sudden onset of weakness, dizziness, confusion
- Severe generalized edema and angioedema; lips and tongue may swell
- Urticaria
- Increased permeability of vascular system and loss of vascular tone leading to severe hypotension and shock
- Laryngospasm/bronchospasm with obstruction of airway causing dyspnea and wheezing
- Nausea, vomiting, and diarrhea
- Seizures, coma, and death

**Treatments**:

- Establish patent airway and intubate if necessary, for ventilation
- Provide oxygen at 100% high flow
- Monitor VS
- Administer epinephrine (Epi-pen or solution)
- Albuterol per nebulizer for bronchospasm
- Intravenous fluids to provide bolus of fluids for hypotension
- Diphenhydramine if shock persists
- Methylprednisolone if no response to other drugs

## Burn Injuries

### *Types and Classifications*

Burn injuries may be chemical, electrical, or thermal, and are assessed by the area, percentage of the body burned, and depth:

- **First-degree burns** are superficial and affect the epidermis, causing erythema and pain.
- **Second-degree burns** extend through the dermis (partial thickness), resulting in blistering and sloughing of epidermis.
- **Third-degree burns** affect underlying tissue, including vasculature, muscles, and nerves (full thickness).

Burns are also classified according to the **American Burn Association's classification**:

- **Superficial**: red, dry, and easily blanching
- **Superficial partial thickness**: red and moist with blisters and severe pain
- **Deep partial thickness**: drier and paler with less blanching and pain
- **Full thickness**: dry and leathery in nature; may be white, brown, or black; no sensation

### *Systemic Complications*

Burn injuries begin with the skin but can affect all organs and body systems, especially with a major burn:

- **Cardiovascular**: Cardiac output may fall by 50% as capillary permeability increases with vasodilation and fluid leaks from the tissues.
- **Urinary**: Decreased blood flow causes kidneys to increase ADH, which increases oliguria. BUN and creatinine levels increase. Cell destruction may block tubules, and hematuria may result from hemolysis.

- **Pulmonary**: Injury may result from smoke inhalation or (rarely) aspiration of hot liquid. Pulmonary injury is a leading cause of death from burns and is classified according to the degree of damage:
  - *First*: Singed eyebrows and nasal hairs with possible soot in airways and slight edema
  - *Second*: (At 24 hours) Stridor, dyspnea, and tachypnea with edema and erythema of upper airway, including area of vocal cords and epiglottis
  - *Third*: (At 72 hours) Worsening symptoms if not intubated and if intubated, bronchorrhea and tachypnea with edematous, secreting tissue
- **Neurological**: Encephalopathy may develop from lack of oxygen, decreased blood volume and sepsis. Hallucinations, alterations in consciousness, seizures, and coma may result.
- **Gastrointestinal**: Ileus and ulcerations of mucosa often result from poor circulation. Ileus usually clears within 48–72 hours, but if it returns it is often indicative of sepsis.
- **Endocrine/metabolic**: The sympathetic nervous system stimulates the adrenals to release epinephrine and norepinephrine to increase cardiac output and cortisol for wound healing. The metabolic rate increases markedly. Electrolyte imbalance occurs with fluid loss from exposed tissue, resulting in decreased phosphorus, calcium, and sodium, and increased potassium. Electrolyte imbalance can be life-threatening if burns cover >20% of BSA. Glycogen depletion occurs within 12–24 hours and protein breakdown and muscle wasting occur without sufficient intake of protein.

### *Management*

Management of burn injuries must include both wound care and systemic care to avoid complications that can be life threatening. **Treatment** includes:

- Establishment of airway and treatment for inhalation injury as indicated:
  - Supplemental oxygen, incentive spirometry, nasotracheal suctioning
  - Humidification
  - Bronchoscopy as needed to evaluate bronchospasm and edema
  - β-Agonists for bronchospasm, followed by aminophylline if ineffective
  - Intubation and ventilation if there are indications of respiratory failure (This should be done prior to failure. Tracheostomy may be done if ventilation >14 days.)
- Intravenous fluids and electrolytes, based on weight and extent of burn. Parkland formula: Fluid replacement (mL) in first 24 hours = (mass in kg) × (body % burned) × 400
- Enteral feedings, usually with small lumen feeding tube into the duodenum
- NG tube for gastric decompression to prevent aspiration
- Indwelling catheter to monitor urinary output. Urinary output should be 0.5–2.0 mL/kg/hr
- Analgesia for reduction of pain and anxiety
- Topical and systemic antibiotics
- Wound care with removal of eschar and dressings as indicated

## Chemical Burns

Chemical burns may result from contact with acid or alkali substances. The pH scale ranges from 0–14 with 7 being neutral, 0 being extremely acidic, and 14 being extremely alkaline. Alkali burns tend to be more severe because acid burns denature proteins, resulting in formation of eschar that prevents deeper penetration of the acid. Alkaline burns, however, both denature proteins and hydrolyze fats, allowing for deeper penetration and tissue damage because of liquefaction necrosis. Hydrofluoric acid is similar to alkaline substances in that it also causes liquefaction necrosis. Symptoms vary depending on the substance, strength, and site of injury but often includes severe pain, tissue blistering and sloughing, and bleeding. Initial treatment includes removal of contaminated clothing and copious wound irrigation with water. If substances contain Na, K, Mg, or metallic lithium, then the burn area should be covered with mineral oil rather than irrigated. If hydrofluoric acid, copious water irrigations and soft-tissue injection or IV infusion of calcium gluconate may help reduce pain and tissue destruction. Patients may need fluid resuscitation and skin grafting. Complications include disfigurement, infection, and electrolyte imbalance.

## Electrical Burns

Electrical injuries result from electricity passing through the body from contact with live wires, lighting strikes, and short-circuiting equipment. Injuries may be high voltage (≥1000 volts) or low voltage (<1000 volts). Electrical injuries can result in extensive subdermal burns. The injury severity correlates with resistance of tissue and current amperage (AC usually causes more damage than DC). Tissue with the highest degree of resistance tends to suffer the most damage with low voltage injury, but high voltage injury can destroy all tissue. Tissue resistance (highest to lowest) include bone >fat >tendons >skin >muscles >vessels > nerves.

- **Low voltage** injuries may cause cardiac dysrhythmias (VF), external burns, tissue damage, fractures and dislocations from muscle contractions, respiratory arrest, or oral burns (children particularly). Treatment includes monitoring and cardiac care as needed, topical antimicrobials, and excision and grafting if necessary.
- **High voltage** injuries may result in additional symptoms of myonecrosis, thrombosis, compartment syndrome, nerve entrapment syndrome. Treatment may include fluid resuscitation, wound debridement, fasciotomy, and amputation, topical antibiotics, systemic antibiotics, and analgesia.

## Thermal Burns

Thermal burns are caused by heat (hot iron, stove, sun exposure) or fire. Burn injuries begin with the skin but can affect all organs and body systems, especially with a major burn. Management of burn injuries must include both wound care and systemic care to avoid complications that can be life threatening. Patients may experience open blistering wounds and severe pain. **Treatment** varies according to severity and may include:

- Establishment of airway and treatment for inhalation injury if necessary
- Cleansing of burned areas, flushing
- Debridement of open blisters (no needle aspiration)
- Tetanus immunization if needed
- Intravenous fluids and electrolytes, based on weight and extent of burn
- Enteral feedings, usually with small lumen feeding tube into the duodenum
- NG tube for gastric decompression to prevent aspiration
- Indwelling catheter to monitor urinary output. Urinary output should be 0.5–2.0 mL/kg/hr
- Analgesia for reduction of pain and anxiety
- Topical (usually silver sulfadiazine) and systemic antibiotics
- Wound care with removal of eschar and dressings as indicated
- Skin grafting

**Complications** include scarring, disfigurement, contractures, and infection.

## Radiation Injuries

Radiation injuries may be caused by direct radiation in which waves pass through the body (locally or to the entire body), which can result in acute radiation illness and genetic damage. **Contamination** usually occurs from radioactive dust or liquid contacting the skin. It can be absorbed into the tissues (eventually causing chronic illnesses, such as cancer) or contaminate others who contact it. Contaminated material may also be ingested. The lethal dose of 50% of those exposed within 60 days (LD50/60) is 4.5 Gy with immediate intensive treatment.

**Diagnosis** for direct radiation is symptomatic as there is no specific test; however, laboratory studies may reflect secondary effects of radiation injury, such as lymphocyte depletion, and should be done serially. Contamination can be measured by Geiger-Mueller counter to identify individuals who have been in contact with a radioactive material and are at risk for injury.

Syndromes of **acute radiation sickness** vary according to exposure:

- **Hematopoietic**: (at least 2 Gy exposure) affects blood cell production. 2–12 hours after exposure: anorexia, nausea, vomiting, lethargy. Symptom-free week during which blood cell production decreases causing decreased WBC and platelet count, resulting in infection and hemorrhage with weakness and dyspnea. Recovery begins in 4–5 weeks if patient survives.
- **GI**: (at least 4 Gy exposure)
  - 2–12 hours after exposure: nausea, vomiting, diarrhea, dehydration. 4–5 days, fewer symptoms but lining of GI tract sheds, leaving ulcerated tissue.
  - Severe diarrhea (bloody) and dehydration and systemic infections
- **Cerebrovascular**: (20–30 Gy exposure) always fatal
  - Alterations in mental status, nausea, vomiting, and diarrhea (bloody), progressing to shock, seizures, coma, and death

**Treatment** includes:

- Decontamination if contamination irradiation or if source of irradiation not clear
- Complete history of event, including source of radiation
- Protocol for decontamination and securing of area should be followed, including use of individual dosimeters and protective coverings
- **Localized**: burn care and analgesia
- **Internal**: gastric decontamination, collection of urine and feces for 4 days to monitor rate of radioisotopes excretion, and collection of body fluids for bioassay
- **Whole body irradiation**: supportive treatment and prophylactic measures to combat opportunistic infections, hematopoietic growth factor for bone marrow depression

## Heat-Related Illness

Children and the elderly are particularly vulnerable to heat-related illness, especially when heat is combined with humidity. Heat-related illnesses occur when heat accumulation in the body outpaces dissipation, resulting in increased temperature and dehydration, which can then lead to thermoregulatory failure and multiple organ dysfunction syndromes. Each year in the United States, about 29 children die from heat stroke after being left in automobiles. At temperatures of 72–96 °F, the temperature in a car rises 3.2 °F every 5 minutes, with 80% of rise within 30 minutes. Temperatures can reach 117 °F even on cool days. There are three **types of heat-related illness**:

- **Heat stress**: Increased temperature causes dehydration. Patient may develop swelling of hands and feet, itching of skin, sunburn, heat syncope (pale moist skin, hypotension), heat cramps, and heat tetany (respiratory alkalosis). Treatment includes removing from heat, cooling, hydrating, and replacing sodium.
- **Heat exhaustion**: Involves water or sodium depletion, with sodium depletion common in patients who are not acclimated to heat. Heat exhaustion can result in flu-like aching, nausea and vomiting, headaches, dizziness, and hypotension with cold, clammy skin and diaphoresis. Temperature may be normal or elevated to less than 106 °F. Treatment to cool the body and replace sodium and fluids must be prompt in order to prevent heat stroke. Careful monitoring is important and reactions may be delayed.
- **Heat stroke**: Involves failure of the thermoregulatory system with temperatures that may be more than 106 °F and can result in seizures, neurological damage, multiple organ failures, and death. Exertional heat stroke often occurs in young athletes who engage in strenuous activities in high heat. Young children are susceptible to nonexertional heat stroke from exposure to high heat. Treatment includes evaporative cooling, rehydration, and supportive treatment according to organ involvement.

## HYPOTHERMIA

Hypothermia occurs with exposure to low temperatures that cause the core body temperature to fall below 95 °F (35 °C). Hypothermia may be associated with immersion in cold water, exposure to cold temperature, metabolic disorders (hypothyroidism, hypoglycemia, hypoadrenalism), or CNS abnormalities (head trauma, Wernicke disease). Many patients with hypothermia are intoxicated with alcohol or drugs.

**Symptoms** of hypothermia include pallor, cold skin, drowsiness, alterations in mental status, confusion, and severe shivering. The patient can progress to shock, coma, dysrhythmias (T-wave inversion and prolongation of PR, QRS, and QT) including atrial fibrillation and AV block, and cardiac arrest.

**Diagnosis** requires low-reading thermometers to verify temperature.

**Treatment** includes:

- Passive rewarming if cardiac status stable
- Active rewarming (external) with immersion in warm water or heating blankets at 40 °C, radiant heat
- Active rewarming (internal) with warm humidified oxygen or air inhalation, heated IV fluids, and internal (bladder, peritoneal, pleural, or GI) lavage
- Warming with extracorporeal circuit, such as arteriovenous or venovenous shunt that warms the blood
- Supportive treatment as indicated

## LOCALIZED COLD INJURIES

Frostnip is a superficial freeze injury that is reversible. Frostbite is damage to tissue caused by exposure to freezing temperatures, most often affecting the nose, ears, and distal extremities. As frostbite develops, the affected part feels numb and aches or throbs, becoming hard and insensate as the tissue freezes, resulting in circulatory impairment, necrosis of tissue, and gangrene. There are **three zones of injury:**

- **Coagulation** (usually distal): severe, irreversible cellular damage
- **Hyperemia** (usually proximal): minimal cellular damage
- **Stasis** (between other 2 zones): severe but sometimes reversible damage

**Symptoms** vary according to the degree of freezing:

- **Partial freezing** with erythema and mild edema, stinging, burning, throbbing pain
- **Full-thickness freezing** with increased edema in 3–4 hours, edema and clear blisters in 6–24 hours, desquamation with eschar formation, numbness, and then aching and throbbing pain
- Prognosis is very good for **first-degree** and good for **second-degree** frostbite
- Full-thickness and into **subdermal tissue** freezing with cyanosis, hemorrhagic blisters, skin necrosis, and "wooden" feeling, severe burning, throbbing, and shooting pains
- Freezing extends into **subcutaneous tissue**, including muscles, tendons, and bones with mottled appearance, non-blanching cyanosis, and eventual deep black eschar

Prognosis is poor for **third-degree** and **fourth-degree** freeze injuries. Determining the degree of injury can be difficult because some degree of thawing may have occurred prior to admission to the hospital.

**Treatment** includes:

- Rapid rewarming with warm water bath (40–42 °C [104–107.6 °F]) 10–30 minutes or until the frostbitten area is erythematous and pliable
- Treatment for generalized hypothermia

Treatment **after warming**:

- Debridement of clear blisters but not hemorrhagic blisters
- Aloe vera cream every 6 hours to blistered areas
- Dressings, separating digits
- Tetanus prophylaxis
- Ibuprofen 12 mg/kg daily in divided doses
- Antibiotic prophylaxis if indicated (penicillin G 500,000 units IV every 6 hours for 24–72 hours)

## Toxic Exposures

### *Carbon Monoxide Poisoning*

Carbon monoxide (CO) poisoning occurs with inhalation of fossil fuel exhausts from engines, emission of gas or coal heaters, indoor use of charcoal, and smoke and fumes. The CO binds with hemoglobin, preventing oxygen carriage and impairing oxygen delivery to tissue.

**Diagnosis** includes history, on-site oximetry reports, neurological examination, and CO neuropsychological screening battery (CONSB) done with patient breathing room air, CBC, electrolytes, ABGs, ECG, chest radiograph (for dyspnea); *pulse oximetry is not a reliable measure of CO poisoning, and may show normal findings because of it capturing carboxyhemoglobin and interpreting it as oxyhemoglobin.*

**Symptoms:**

- Cardiac: chest pain, palpitations, decreased capillary refill, hypotension, and cardiac arrest
- CNS: malaise, nausea, vomiting, lethargy, stroke, coma, and seizure
- Secondary injuries: Rhabdomyolysis, AKI, non-cardiogenic pulmonary edema, multiple organ failure (MOF), DIC, and encephalopathy

**Treatment** includes:

- Immediate support of airway, breathing, and circulation
- Non-barometric oxygen (100%) by non-breathing mask with reservoir or ETT if necessary
- Mild: Continue oxygen for 4 hours with reassessment
- Severe: hyperbaric oxygen therapy (usually 3 treatments) to improve oxygen delivery

### *Cyanide Poisoning*

Cyanide poisoning, from hydrogen cyanide (HCN) or cyanide salts, can result from sodium nitroprusside infusions, inhalation of burning plastics, intentional or accidental ingestion or dermal exposure, occupation exposure, ingestion of some plant products, and the manufacture of PCP. Inhalation of HCN causes immediate symptoms, and the ingestion of cyanide salts causes symptoms within minutes.

**Diagnosis** is by history, clinical examination, normal $PaO_2$ accompanied by elevated $SvO_2$, and metabolic acidosis.

**Symptoms:** Increase in severity and alter with the amount of exposure: tachycardia, hypertension, leading to bradycardia, hypotension, and cardiac arrest. Pink or cherry-colored skin because of oxygen remaining in the blood. Other symptoms include headaches, lethargy, seizures, coma, dyspnea, tachypnea, and respiratory arrest.

**Treatment** includes:

- Supportive care as indicated
- Removal of contaminated clothes
- Gastric decontamination
- Copious irrigation for topical exposure
- Antidotes:
    - Amyl nitrate ampule cracked and inhaled 30 seconds
    - Sodium nitrite (3%) 10 mL IV
    - Sodium thiosulfate (25%) 50 mL IV

### *Caustic Ingestions*

Caustic ingestions of acids (pH <7) such as sulfuric, acetic, hydrochloric, and hydrofluoric found in many cleaning agents and alkalis (pH >7) such as sodium hydroxide, potassium hydroxide, sodium tripolyphosphate (in detergents) and sodium hypochlorite (bleach) can result in severe injury and death. Acids cause coagulation necrosis in the esophagus and stomach and may result in metabolic acidosis, hemolysis, and renal failure if systemically absorbed. Alkali injuries cause liquefaction necrosis, resulting in deeper ulcerations, often of the esophagus, but may involve perforation and abdominal necrosis with multi-organ damage.

**Diagnosis** is by detailed history, airway examination (oral intubation if possible), arterial blood gas, electrolytes, CBC, hepatic and coagulation tests, radiograph, and CT for perforations.

**Symptoms** may vary but can include pain, dyspnea, oral burns, dysphonia, and vomiting.

**Treatment** includes:

- Supportive and symptomatic therapy
- **No ipecac, charcoal, neutralization, or dilution**
- NG tube for acids only to aspirate residual
- Endoscopy in first few hours to evaluate injury/perforations
- Prednisolone (alkali injuries)



### *Allergic Reactions*

Exposure to certain toxins, medications, illegal substances, and allergens can cause life threatening effects in some patients. The physiologic response of the patient is dependent on the agent and the degree of exposure. Tissue hypoperfusion and lactic acidosis often occur as a result of the exposure. This can lead to metabolic acidosis, shock, organ failure, and death.

**Signs/symptoms**: In allergic type reactions, urticaria, pruritus, chest, back or abdominal pain, facial flushing, shortness of breath, wheezing and stridor may occur. Beta- and alpha-adrenergic responses may occur with exposure to amphetamines, cocaine, ephedrine, and pseudoephedrine. This response is manifested by diaphoresis, hypertension, tachycardia, and mydriasis. Diarrhea, nausea, and vomiting can occur with exposure to certain toxins.

**Diagnosis**: Physical assessment and testing to discover the toxin, drug, or allergen the patient was exposed to. Labs—blood gases, BMP, complete blood count, toxicology screen, urinalysis, and allergy testing.

**Treatment**: Priority is to eliminate exposure to the drug/toxin/allergen. Antidotes (if available) may be administered in the case of toxin exposure. Activated charcoal may be administered in the case of medication/drug overdose. For allergic reactions, antihistamines and corticosteroids may be administered. Severe allergic reactions may need to be treated with epinephrine. Dialysis may be indicated in some patients. Sodium bicarbonate may be administered for the treatment of metabolic acidosis caused by many toxic reactions.

### Acetaminophen Toxicity

Acetaminophen toxicity from accidental or intentional overdose has high rates of morbidity and mortality unless promptly treated. **Diagnosis** is by history and acetaminophen level, which should be completed within 8 hours of ingestion if possible. Toxicity occurs with dosage >140 mg/kg in one dose or >7.5g in 24 hours.

**Symptoms** occur in stages:

- (Initial) Minor gastrointestinal upset
- (Days 2–3) Hepatotoxicity with RUQ pain and increased AST, ALT, and bilirubin
- (Days 3–4) Hepatic failure with metabolic acidosis, coagulopathy, renal failure, encephalopathy, nausea, vomiting, and possible death
- (Days 5–12) Recovery period for survivors

**Treatment** includes:

- GI decontamination with activated charcoal (orally or NG); this is most effective when administered within 4 hours of ingestion
- Toxicity is plotted on the Rumack-Matthew nomogram with serum levels >150 requiring antidote. The antidote is most effective ≤8 hours of ingestion but decreases hepatotoxicity even >24 hours.
- Antidote: 72-hour N-acetylcysteine (NAC) protocol includes 140 mg/kg initially and 70 mg/kg every 4 hours for 17 more doses (orally or IV)
- Supportive therapy: Continuous dialysis, fluids, blood pressure medications

### Amphetamine and Cocaine Toxicity

Amphetamine toxicity may be caused by intravenous use, inhalation, or insufflation of various substances that include methamphetamine (MDA or "ecstasy"), methylphenidate (Ritalin), methylenedioxymethamphetamine (MDMA), and ephedrine and phenylpropanolamine. Cocaine may be ingested orally, intravenously, or by insufflation while crack cocaine may be smoked. Amphetamines and cocaine are CNS stimulants that can cause multi-system abnormalities.

**Symptoms** may include chest pain, dysrhythmias, myocardial ischemia, myocardial infarction, seizures, intracranial infarctions, hypertension, dystonia, repetitive movements, unilateral blindness, lethargy, rhabdomyolysis with acute kidney failure, perforated nasal septum (cocaine), and paranoid psychosis (amphetamines). Crack cocaine use may cause pulmonary hemorrhage, asthma, pulmonary edema, barotrauma, and pneumothorax. Swallowing packs of cocaine can cause intestinal ischemia, colitis, necrosis, and perforation. **Diagnosis** includes clinical findings, CBC, chemistry panel, toxicology screening, ECG, and radiography.

**Treatment** includes:

- Gastric emptying (<1 hour), often via charcoal administration
- IV access in anticipation of fluids and medication administration
- Supplemental oxygen
- Sedation for seizures: Lorazepam 2 mg, diazepam 5 mg IV; titrated in repeated doses
- Agitation treatment: Haloperidol
- Hypertension management: Nitroprusside/nicardipine, phentolamine IV
- Management of cocaine quinidine-like effects: Sodium bicarbonate

### Salicylate Toxicity

Salicylate toxicity may be acute or chronic and is caused by ingestion of OTC drugs containing salicylates, such as ASA, Pepto-Bismol, and products used in hot inhalers.

**Diagnosis** is confirmed by serum salicylate concentration but due to the delay in an increase in serum level after ingestion, treatment should be based on history and acid-base balance. Salicylate toxicity initially causes respiratory alkalosis secondary to hyperventilation, which can then cause a compensatory metabolic acidosis. Co-ingestion of sedatives may alter symptoms.

**Symptoms** include:

- <150 mg/kg: Nausea and vomiting
- 150–300 mg/kg: Vomiting, hyperpnea, diaphoresis, tinnitus, and alterations in acid-base balance
- >300 mg/kg (usually intentional overdose): Nausea, vomiting, diaphoresis, tinnitus, hyperventilation, respiratory alkalosis, and metabolic acidosis
- Chronic toxicity results in hyperventilation, tremor, and papilledema, alterations in mental status, pulmonary edema, seizures, and coma

**Treatment** includes:

- Gastric decontamination with lavage (≤1 hour) and charcoal
- Volume replacement (D5W)
- Sodium bicarbonate 1–2 mEq/kg
- Monitoring of salicylate concentration, acid-base, and electrolytes every hour
- Whole-bowel irrigation (sustained release tablets)

### *Benzodiazepine Toxicity*

Benzodiazepine toxicity may result from accidental or intentional overdose with such drugs as Xanax, Librium, Valium, Ativan, Serax, Versed, and Restoril. Mortality is usually the result of co-ingestion of other drugs.

**Diagnosis** is based on history and clinical exam, as benzodiazepine level does not correlate well with toxicity.

**Symptoms:** Non-specific neurological changes: Lethargy, dizziness, alterations in consciousness, and ataxia. Respiratory depression and hypotension are rare complications. Coma and severe central nervous depression are usually caused by co-ingestions.

**Treatment** includes:

- Gastric emptying (<1 hour)
- Charcoal
- Concentrated dextrose, thiamine, and naloxone if co-ingestions suspected, especially with altered mental status
- Monitoring for CNS/respiratory depression
- Supportive care
- Flumazenil (antagonist) 0.2 mg each minute to total 3 mg may be used in some cases but not routinely advised because of complications related to benzodiazepine dependency or co-ingestion of cyclic antidepressants. Flumazenil is contraindicated in patients with increased ICP.

### *Ethanol Overdose*

Ethanol overdose affects the central nervous system as well as other organs in the body. Alcohol is an inhibitory neurotransmitter that depresses the central nervous system. In most states, the legal intoxication blood alcohol level is defined as 80 mg/dL. Blood alcohol levels of **500 mg/dL or greater** are associated with a high mortality rate. The central nervous system depressant effect is further enhanced when alcohol is mixed with other agents.

Ethanol is absorbed through the mucosa of the mouth, stomach, and intestines, with concentrations peaking about 30–60 minutes after ingestion. If people are easily aroused, they can usually safely sleep off the effects of ingesting too much alcohol, but if the person is semi-conscious or unconscious, emergency medical treatment should be initiated.

**Symptoms** include:

- Altered mental status with slurred speech and stupor
- Nausea and vomiting
- Hypotension
- Bradycardia with arrhythmias
- Respiratory depression and hypoxia
- Cold, clammy skin or flushed skin (from vasodilation)
- Acute pancreatitis with abdominal pain
- Lack of consciousness
- Circulatory collapse

**Treatment** includes:

- Careful monitoring of arterial blood gases and oxygen saturation
- Ensure patent airway with intubation and ventilation if necessary
- Intravenous fluids
- Dextrose to correct hypoglycemia if indicated
- Maintain body temperature (warming blanket)
- Dialysis may be necessary in severe cases

### *Gastric Emptying for Toxic Substance Ingestion*

Gastric emptying for toxic substance ingestion should be done ≤60 minutes of ingestion for large life-threatening amounts of poison. The patient requires IV access, oximetry, and cardiac monitoring. Sedation (1–2 mg IV midazolam) or rapid sequence induction and endotracheal intubation may be necessary. Patients should be positioned in left lateral decubitus position with head down at 20° to prevent passage of stomach contents into duodenum, although intubated patients may be lavaged in the supine position. With a bite block in place, an orogastric Y-tube (36–40 Fr. for adults) should be inserted after estimating length. Placement should be confirmed with injection of 50 mL of air confirmed under auscultation and aspiration of gastric contents, as well as abdominal x-ray (pH may not be reliable depending on substance ingested). Irrigation is done by gravity instillation of about 200–300 mL warmed (45 °C) tap water or NS. The instillation side is clamped and drainage side opened. This is repeated until fluid returns clear. A slurry of charcoal is then instilled, and the tube is clamped and removed when procedures completed.

## Thermoregulation in Critically Ill Patients

The hypothalamus, limbic system, lower brainstem, reticular formation, spinal cord, and sympathetic ganglia all play a role in the regulation of core temperature. The normal core body temperature of 35.5–37.5 °C is a narrow range which is frequently disrupted in the critically ill patient. **Impaired thermoregulation** can occur in patients with sepsis, brain or spinal cord trauma, stroke, and tumors of the central nervous system. Mild hypothermia is common during deep sedation. Hypothermia (core temperature of <35 °C) is associated with an increased risk of postoperative wound infections, blood loss, and adverse cardiovascular events. Hypothermia may occur in trauma patients, patients with sepsis, postoperative patients, and patients with severe burns. Hyperthermia (core temperature of >38 °C) may occur in systemic inflammatory response syndrome, malignant hyperthermia, heatstroke, neuroleptic malignant syndrome, and serotonin syndrome. Hyperpyrexia occurs when the core temperature exceeds 40 °C. Core temperatures exceeding 41.5 °C may be life-threatening.

# Multisystem Procedures and Interventions

## Targeted Temperature Management

Targeted temperature management (previously referred to as therapeutic hypothermia) is used to reduce ischemic tissue damage associated with cardiac arrest, ischemic stroke, traumatic brain/spinal cord injury, neurogenic fever, and subsequent coma (3 on Glasgow scale). Reducing the body's temperature to below normal range has a neuroprotective effect by making cell membranes less permeable, thus reducing neurologic edema and damage. Hypothermia should be initiated immediately after an ischemic event if possible, but some benefit remains up to 6 hours. Hypothermia to 33 °C may be induced by cooled saline through a femoral catheter, reducing temperature 1.5–2.0 °C/hr by an electronic control unit. Hypothermic water blankets covering ≥80% of the body's surface can also lower body temperature. In some cases, both a femoral cooling catheter and a water blanket are used for rapid reduction of temperature. Rectal probes are used to measure core temperature, but Foley temperature catheters are more common. Desflurane or meperidine is given to reduce the shivering response. Hypothermia increases risk of bleeding (decreased clotting time), infection (due to impairing leukocyte function and introducing catheters), arrhythmias, hyperglycemia, and DVT. Rewarming is done slowly at 0.5–1.0 °C/hr. through warmed intravenous fluids, warm humidified air, and/or warming blanket. The warming process is a critical time, as it causes potassium to be moved from extracellular to intracellular spaces and the patient's electrolyte levels must be monitored regularly.

## Continuous Temperature Monitoring

Continuous temperature monitoring may be carried out through various means:

- Pulmonary artery catheter (most accurate but generally not recommended because of invasiveness and potential for complications)
- Rectal or Foley temperature probes
- Skin probes
- Wearable Bluetooth monitors (patch applied to the skin), which transmit information to an external monitor or the patient's electronic health record. (For external temperature monitoring, the device must be applied properly and for the correct duration of time [e.g., the TempTraQ wearable patch is applied in the underarm area and measures temperature for 72 hours].)



**Indications** for continuous temperature monitoring include:

- Skin flap transplantation—to assess perfusion
- Brain injury—to assess thermoregulation
- Therapeutic hypothermia—for cardiac arrest or post-cardiac surgery
- Malignant hyperthermia
- Immunocompromised patients—to assess for signs of infection
- Critically ill patients—at risk for temperature dysregulation

## Fluid Resuscitation for Burn Injuries

Burn victims are at risk for hypovolemia and electrolyte imbalances because of loss of body fluids through burned areas. **Fluid resuscitation** is indicated with burns of 20% or more of total body surface area (TBSA) burned. Lactated Ringers IV solution is used instead of NS, which can lead to hypernatremia and hyperchloremia. The Parkland/Baxter formula is used to calculate the volume of LR solution needed:

$$24 \text{ hour volume} = (\text{body weight [kg]}) \times (\text{TBSA burned [\%]}) \times (4 \text{ mL})$$

Example—70 kg adult with 36% TBSA burned:

$$24 \text{ hour volume} = 70 \times 36 \times 4 \text{ mL} = 10{,}080 \text{ mL}$$

Half of the volume is administered over the first 8 hours and half over the next 16 hours. Using the preceding example, this patient will receive 5,040 mL each over the first 8 hours (rate = (5040/8) = 630 mL/hr), and over the following 16 hours (rate = (5040/16) = 315 mL/hr). Fluid intake should be sufficient to produce 30–50 mL of urine per hour. In the second 24 hours, fluid volume should be 1.5–2.0 times the normal maintenance values with crystalloid with appropriate electrolyte balance.

## Permissive Hypotension

Permissive hypotension procedures allow the systolic blood pressure to fall low enough to prevent or control hemorrhage while still high enough to maintain perfusion. With trauma patients, this means restricting fluid resuscitation when active bleeding is occurring. While protocols vary, permissive hypotension usually includes systolic blood pressure no higher than 80 mmHg, although this may vary. For example, permissive hypotension with systolic blood pressure maintained at 80–100 mmHg may be indicated when massive transfusion protocols are activated. Permissive hypotension helps decrease some of the adverse effects associated with rapid and high-dose fluid resuscitation (emboli, coagulopathy, and hypothermia). However, the patient does remain at risk of hypoperfusion and must be monitored carefully. Permissive hypotension is generally contraindicated with brain or spinal cord injury, although studies are ongoing (and mostly conducted with animals) and some controversy remains about the use of permissive hypotension.

## Sedation

### *Minimal Sedation*

Minimal sedation includes local/topical anesthesia, peripheral nerve blocks, administration of <50% nitrogen oxide in oxygen by itself, or administration of one sedative or analgesic medication in a dosage that does not typically require supervision. The patient should be fully aware, able to respond appropriately to verbal and tactile stimulation, and able to maintain an airway independently, as these medications should not have cardiovascular or respiratory effects. The purpose of minimal sedation is to decrease perception of pain, relax the patient, and reduce fear. The patient's level of consciousness, sedation, and pain should be monitored throughout the procedure to ensure the dosage is adequate and the patient is not excessively sedated. Medications may include benzodiazepines (diazepam, lorazepam) and opioids (fentanyl, morphine, meperidine). Reversal agents (flumazenil, naloxone) should be available. Minimal sedation is often used during labor and delivery and for minor procedures, such as skin biopsies and removal of skin lesions.

### *Continuous vs. Intermittent Sedation*

Sedation for critically ill patients may include:

- **Intermittent sedation** is that administered through IV push, so the expected duration is relatively short. Typical agents include benzodiazepines and opioids. Intermittent sedation is most often used for endoscopic procedures but is also sometimes used for patients who are on mechanical ventilation, especially if they have regular trials of weaning. Also, intermittent sedation is less likely to result in oversedation.
- **Continuous sedation** is that administered through a steady intravenous infusion to ensure longer-lasting sedation. Typical agents include opioids, midazolam, and propofol. Continuous sedation is more commonly used for patients on mechanical ventilation because it requires less intervention and maintains a steady blood level. Daily interruptions of continuous sedation may be carried out as a trial for weaning patients on mechanical ventilation.

With both intermittent sedation and continuous sedation, the patient's vital signs, respiratory status, temperature, and oxygen saturation should be monitored. Arousal scales (Richmond or Riker Agitation/Sedation Scales) should be utilized to assess arousal and to adjust sedation dosages.

### Neuromuscular Blockade Agents

Neuromuscular blocker agents are used for induced paralysis of those who have not responded adequately to sedation, especially for intubation and mechanical ventilation. NMBAs do not produce unconsciousness, amnesia, or analgesia, therefore it is critical that they are administered *after* the patient has been adequately sedated. NMBAs include:

- **Depolarizing agents**: Succinylcholine. Risk for severe hyperkalemia after denervation injury persists for 7–10 days. Post-operative myalgia is common, and succinylcholine may trigger malignant hyperthermia and severe anaphylactic/anaphylactoid reactions.
- **Non-depolarizing agents**: Aminosteroid compounds (rocuronium, vecuronium, and pancuronium) and benzylisoquinolinium compounds (atracurium, cisatracurium). Should be given for ≤2 days for those on ventilators because they may develop persistent quadriparesis. Most are not associated with malignant hyperthermia.

Eye lubricant should be applied every 2 hours and the eyes kept closed. Range of motion exercises should not extend beyond normal range because of the potential to damage joints. The patient must be repositioned frequently while paralyzed and on an adequate support surface. Pupil reactivity should be assessed every 1–4 hours to evaluate neurological status. Temperature should be monitored hourly if <36 °C or if placed under a cooling blanket because heat production is depressed. After cessation, the patient should be closely monitored to ensure that muscle function has returned to normal.

### Moderate (Conscious) Sedation

The ASA sedation guidelines (2018) are intended for **moderate (conscious) sedation** used for procedures, such as colonoscopy. Steps include:

- **Pre-procedure evaluation**: Includes review of health records, physical examination and laboratory testing as indicated a few days or weeks prior to the procedure, and re-evaluating the patient again before the procedure.
- **Patient preparation**: Consult with a specialist if indicated, ensure the patient has informed consent and has been compliant with pre-procedure fasting, and insert intravenous line.
- **Patient monitoring**: LOC (every 5 minutes), oxygenation/ventilation (capnography, pulse oximetry), and hemodynamic with a designated person responsible for monitoring and recording.
- **Supplemental oxygen:** Use unless contraindicated by condition.
- **Emergency interventions**: Resuscitative equipment and reversal agents for opioids (naloxone) and benzodiazepines (Romazicon) must be present with a person trained in assessment and use available.
- **Sedatives**: Analgesics (opioids) and combinations of drugs as appropriate may be used (benzodiazepines and dexmedetomidine).
- **Sedative (propofol, ketamine, etomidate) and analgesics (local anesthetics, NSAIDs, and opioids) intended for general anesthesia**: Care must be consistent with that of general anesthesia and IV medications administered incrementally.
- **Recovery care**: Monitor oxygenation, ventilation, and circulation every 5–15 minutes.

### Sedation Using Propofol

Sedation used for a drug-induced coma often includes **propofol**. Propofol is an IV non-opioid hypnotic anesthetic, the most common used for induction. It is also used for maintenance and postoperative sedation. Onset of action is rapid because of high lipid solubility, and propofol has a short distribution half-life and rapid clearance, so recovery is also fast. Propofol is metabolized by the liver, as well as through the lungs. Propofol decreases cerebral blood flow, metabolic rate of oxygen consumption, and ICP. Propofol causes vasodilation with resultant hypotension, but with bradycardia rather than tachycardia. Propofol is a respiratory depressant, resulting in apnea after induction and decreased tidal volume, respiratory rate, and hypoxic drive during maintenance. Propofol has antiemetic properties as well but does not produce analgesia.

### *Delayed Emergence*

Delayed emergence (failure to emerge for 30–60 minutes after anesthesia ends) is more common in the elderly because of slowed metabolism of anesthetic agents but may have a variety of causes, such as drug overdose during surgery, overdose related to preinduction use of drugs or alcohol that potentiates intraoperative drugs. In this case, naloxone or flumazenil may be indicated if opioids or benzodiazepines are implicated. Physostigmine may also be used to reverse effects of some anesthetic agents. Hypothermia may also cause delay in emergence, especially core temperatures <33 °C, and may require forced-air warming blankets to increase the temperature. Other metabolic conditions, such as hypoglycemia or hyperglycemia, may also affect emergence. Patients suffering from delayed emergence must be evaluated for perioperative stroke, especially after neurological, cardiovascular, or cerebrovascular surgery. Metabolic disturbance may also delay emergence.

## Postanesthetic Respiratory Complications

Postoperative respiratory complications are most common in the postanesthesia period, so monitoring of oxygen levels is critical to preventing hypoxemia:

- **Airway obstruction** may be partial or total. Partial obstruction is indicated by sonorous or wheezing respirations, and total by absence of breath sounds. Treatment includes supplemental oxygen, airway insertion, repositioning (jaw thrust), or succinylcholine and positive-pressure ventilation for laryngospasm. If edema of the glottis is causing obstruction, IV corticosteroids may be used.
- **Hypoventilation** ($PaCO_2$ >45 mmHg) is often mild but may cause respiratory acidosis. It is usually related to depression caused by anesthetic agents. A number of factors may slow emergence (hypothermia, overdose, metabolism) and cause hypoventilation. It may also be related to splinting because of pain, requiring additional pain management.
- **Hypoxemia** (mild is $PaO_2$ 50–60 mmHg) is usually related to hypoventilation and/or increased right to left shunting and is usually treated with supplementary oxygen (30–60%) with or without positive airway pressure.

## Postanesthetic Cardiovascular Complications

Cardiovascular complications after surgery are sometimes related to respiratory complications, which may need to be addressed as well. Complications include:

- **Hypotension** is most often mild and requires no specific treatment. It is most commonly caused by hypovolemia and is significant if BP falls 20–30% below the normal baseline. A bolus (100–250 mL IV colloid) is used to confirm hypovolemia. If severe, then medications such as vasopressors may be indicated. Hypotension may occur with pneumothorax, so careful respiratory assessment must be done.
- **Hypertension** usually occurs ≤30 minutes after surgery and is common in those with a history of hypertension. It may be secondary to hypoxemia or metabolic acidosis. Mild increases usually don't require treatment but medications may be used for moderate (β-adrenergic blockers) or severe (nitroprusside) increases.
- **Arrhythmias** usually relate to respiratory complications or effects of anesthetic agents. Bradycardia may relate to cholinesterase inhibitors, opioids, or propranolol. Tachycardia may relate to anticholinergics, β-agonists, and vagolytic drugs. Hypokalemia and hypomagnesemia may cause premature atrial and ventricular beats.

# Obstetrical and Gynecologic Emergencies

## Abruptio Placentae

Abruptio placenta occurs when the placenta separates prematurely from the wall of the uterus. **Symptoms** include:

- Vaginal bleeding
- Tender uterus with increased resting tone
- Uterine contractions (hypertonic or hyperactive)
- Nausea and vomiting (in some patients)
- Dizziness

Complications include fetal distress, hypotension, and disseminated intravascular coagulopathy (DIC), as well as fetal and/or maternal death. Fetal death is common with at least 50% separation.

**Diagnosis** includes:

- Ultrasound
- Blood work: CBC, type and crossmatch, coagulation studies (50% have coagulopathy)

**Treatment** includes:

- Gynecological consultation
- Crystalloids to increase blood volume
- Fresh frozen plasma for coagulopathy

## Placenta Previa

Placenta previa occurs when the placenta implants over the cervical opening. Implantation may be complete (covering the entire opening), partial, or marginal (to the edge of the cervical opening). Symptoms include painless bleeding after the 20th week of gestation.

**Diagnosis** is per ultrasound. Vaginal examination with digit or speculum should be avoided. The condition may correct itself as the uterus expands, but bed rest may be needed. Emergency cesarean section is done for uncontrolled bleeding.

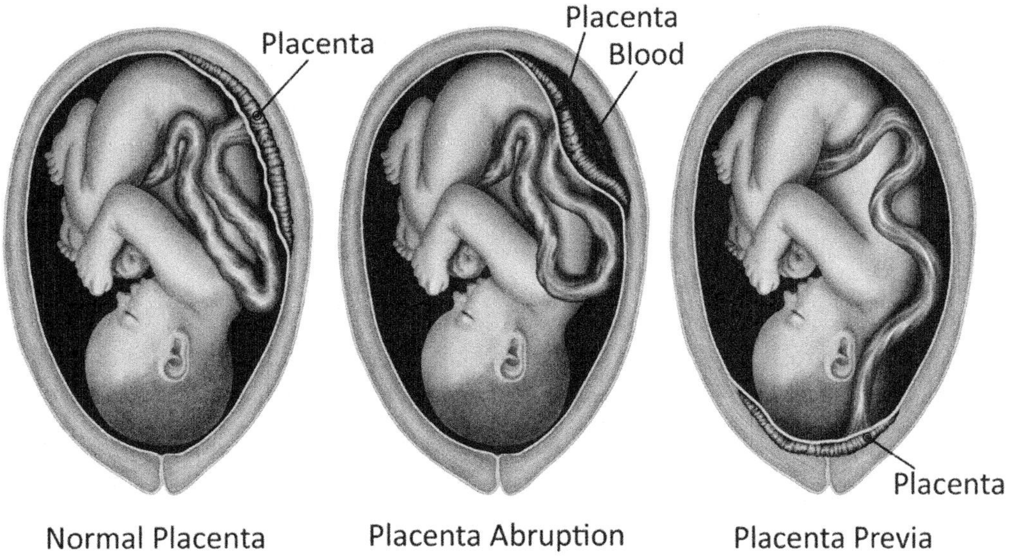

## Ectopic Pregnancy

Ectopic pregnancy occurs when the fertilized ovum implants outside the uterus in an ovary, fallopian tube (the most common site), peritoneal cavity, or cervix.

- **Early symptoms** may include: Indications of pregnancy such as amenorrhea, breast tenderness, nausea, and vomiting. Positive Chadwick's sign (blue discoloration of cervix). Positive Hegar's sign (softening of isthmus). Bleeding may be the first indication as hormones fluctuate. Hormone hCG present in blood and urine.
- **Symptoms of rupture** include: One-sided or generalized abdominal pain. Decreased hemoglobin and hematocrit. Hypotension with hemorrhage. Right shoulder pain because of irritation of the subdiaphragmatic phrenic nerve.
- **Diagnostic studies** include: Vaginal exam. Pregnancy test. Transvaginal sonography (TVS) to rule out intrauterine pregnancy. hCG titers (increase more slowly with ectopic pregnancy).

**Treatments** include:

- Methotrexate IM or IV if unruptured and 3.5 cm or less in size to inhibit growth and allow body to expel
- Laparoscopic linear salpingostomy or salpingectomy

## Nausea and Vomiting and Hyperemesis Gravidarum Related to Pregnancy

About 60–80% of pregnant woman suffer from nausea and vomiting (NV), especially during the first trimester, but only about 2% suffer severe (sometimes intractable) nausea and vomiting, known as **hyperemesis gravidarum (HG)**, associated with weight loss, dehydration, hypokalemia, or ketonemia. Nausea and vomiting may be associated with numerous disorders, including cholelithiasis, pancreatitis, hepatitis, and ectopic pregnancy, especially when accompanied by abdominal pain. **Diagnosis** includes:

- Physical examination to rule out other disorders
- CBC with serum electrolytes, BUN, creatinine, and urinalysis
- Ketonuria is an indication of inadequate nutrition

**Treatment** includes:

- IV fluids with glucose 5% in normal saline or Ringer's lactate
- Oral fluids after nausea and vomiting controlled
- Antiemetic drugs
- Acute treatment for NV and HG: promethazine, prochlorperazine, or chlorpromazine
- Maintenance for NV: Doxylamine with pyridoxine, diphenhydramine, or cisapride
- Maintenance for HG: Metoclopramide, trimethobenzamide, or ondansetron

## Hypertensive Disorders of Pregnancy During the Second Half of Pregnancy

Hypertensive disorders of pregnancy comprise a continuum ranging from mild to severe:

- **Hypertension**: BP increased to at least 140/90, or 20 mmHg increase in systolic or 10 mmHg diastolic. May be chronic or transient without signs of preeclampsia or eclampsia.
- **Preeclampsia**: Hypertension, often associated with proteinuria (300 mg per 24 hours), and edema (peripheral or generalized) or increase of at least 5 pounds of weight in 1 week after 20th week of gestation. Severe preeclampsia is BP at least 160/110. Symptoms include headache, abdominal pain, and visual disturbances.
- **Eclampsia**: Preeclampsia with seizures occurring at 20th week of gestation to 1 month after delivery.
- **HELLP syndrome**: Hemolysis, elevated liver enzymes [AST and ALT], and low platelets [less than 100,000]. Usually accompanied by epigastric or right upper quadrant pain.

**Treatments** include:

- **Chronic hypertension**: Methyldopa beginning with 250 mg every 6 hours.
- **Preeclampsia, eclampsia, HELLP:** Delivery of fetus (may be delayed with mild preeclampsia if fewer than 37 weeks gestation). Magnesium sulfate 4–6 g IV over 15 minutes initially and then 1–2 g/hr. Antihypertensive drugs.

## Vaginal Bleeding and Types of Abortion

Vaginal bleeding during the first trimester of pregnancy may indicate spontaneous abortion, ectopic pregnancy, gestational trophoblastic disease, or infection. All women of childbearing age with an intact uterus presenting with abdominal pain or vaginal bleeding should be assessed for pregnancy.

Abortion **classifications**:

- **Threatened**: Vaginal bleeding during first half of pregnancy without cervical dilatation
- **Inevitable**: Vaginal bleeding with cervical dilatation
- **Incomplete**: Incomplete loss of products of conception, usually at 6–14 weeks
- **Complete**: Complete loss of products of conception, before 20 weeks
- **Missed**: Death of fetus before 20 weeks without loss of products of conception within 4 weeks
- **Septic**: Infection with abortion

**Diagnostic** tests include:

- Pelvic examination. CBC, Rh factor, antibody screen, urinalysis, quantitative serum beta-hCG level
- Ultrasound to rule out ectopic pregnancy

**Treatment** includes:

- Suctioning of vaginal vault with Yankauer suction tip with pathologic examination of tissue
- Evacuation of uterus for incomplete abortion
- RhoGAM (50–150 mcg) for bleeding in unsensitized Rh-negative women



## Emergency Delivery

### *Prolapsed Umbilical Cord*

Prolapsed umbilical cord occurs when the umbilical cord precedes the presenting fetal part or, in some cases, presents at the same time, so that pressure is applied to the cord, decreasing circulation to the fetus. Decelerations in fetal pulse less than 110 may indicate prolapse. Pulsations may be felt in the cord or may be absent, but relieving pressure on the cord by holding back the presenting part is critical for fetal survival. Oxygen should be administered and fetal heart rate monitored. Infusing the bladder with 350–500 mL of fluid (warm normal saline) while pressure is held against the presenting part may lift the fetal head and relieve pressure on the cord. Other methods include placing the woman in the Trendelenburg position or with knees to chest as medical personnel apply continued pressure to the presenting part while awaiting Cesarean section for delivery.

### *Breech Presentation*

Emergency delivery may occur when there are complications of pregnancy or a woman is in advanced labor with birth imminent. The delivery may proceed normally, but complications may require immediate intervention. **Breech presentation** (common in premature births) is when the buttocks or lower extremities are the presenting part during delivery. Types include:

- **Complete**: knees and hips both flexed with buttocks and feet presenting
- **Frank**: hips flexed and knees extended with buttocks presenting
- **Footling** or **incomplete**: hips and legs extended and one or both feet presenting (In some incomplete cases, the knees may present.)

Complete and frank breech presentations may often be delivered vaginally as enough pressure is applied to adequately dilate the vagina, but the delivery should be spontaneous with medical staff keeping hands off until the umbilicus presents, then assisting with delivery of the legs and rotating the fetus to the sacrum anterior position and then gently turning to deliver the arms. Incomplete or footling presentations require Cesarean sections.

## *PROM*

**Preterm or premature labor** occurs between weeks 20 and 37. PROM occurs when the membranes rupture before the onset of labor, and may lead to premature labor. There are numerous causes for PROM, including infections and digital pelvic exams. When a woman presents in labor, the estimated date of delivery should be obtained by questioning the date of the last menstrual period (LMP) and using a gestation calculator wheel or estimating with **Naegele's rule**:

*First day LMP minus 3 months plus 7 days = estimated date of delivery*

Fetal viability is very low before 23 weeks of gestation but by 25 weeks, delaying delivery for 2 days can increase survival rates by 10%. Tocolytic drugs, which have many negative side effects, may be used to delay delivery in order to administer glucocorticoids, such as betamethasone or dexamethasone, to improve fetal lung maturity between weeks 24 and 36. **Tocolytics** include:

- Beta-adrenergic agonists
- Magnesium sulfates
- Calcium channel blockers
- Prostaglandin synthetase inhibitors

### *Preterm Infants*

Emergency delivery often involves **preterm infants**, whose gestational age may not be clear upon delivery, so initial resuscitative efforts should be carried out until viability is determined. The infant should be dried and warmed immediately, such as by placing in a double-walled heated incubator or under a Plexiglas heat shield in a single-walled incubator to prevent heat loss. Radiant warmers and plastic wrap over the infant may also be used. The head and neck must be well supported to prevent blockage of the trachea. A small roll should be placed under the shoulders and the head slightly elevated if child is in supine position, but the prone position splints the chest and decreases respiratory effort. Gentle nasopharyngeal suctioning may be needed to clear secretions. The infant should be evaluated with the Apgar scale and transferred to the neonatal ICU as necessary for further interventions. Apgar score below 4 requires resuscitations (8–10 is normal range).

## Postpartum Hemorrhage

Most postpartum hemorrhage is excessive vaginal bleeding (greater than 500 mL for vaginal and greater than 1,000 mL for Cesarean section) occurring within 24 hours of delivery, related to uterine atony caused by failure of the uterus to contract adequately, uterine rupture or inversion, lacerations, or coagulopathies. It is more common after Cesarean section than vaginal delivery. Hemorrhage may be delayed in some cases, related to retained products of conception, uterine polyps, or coagulopathies. Careful history and examination to determine the cause of bleeding is necessary. **Symptoms** include:

- Excessive bleeding
- Hypotension and tachycardia
- Decreased hematocrit
- Pain and/or edema in vagina/perineum

**Treatment** includes:

- Stabilizing patient
- Two IV lines (large bore) inserted
- Laboratory testing for CBC, clotting, and type and crossmatch
- Vaginal exam with speculum to identify and repair lacerations
- Oxytocin or methylergonovine maleate for uterine atony
- Ultrasound to check for retained products of conception
- Obstetric consultation for uterine inversion (observed as mass in vagina)
- Fresh frozen plasma for coagulopathies

### TRAUMA DURING PREGNANCY

Trauma during pregnancy is one of the leading causes of death and injury to pregnant women. Automobile accidents, falls, and assault (often related to domestic abuse) can all result in death of the fetus. Complications of trauma may be uterine rupture, abruption, or uterine irritability, and the onset of premature labor. Fetal-maternal hemorrhage may also occur. Direct injury to the fetus is common only in the late stages of pregnancy when blunt abdominal trauma with pelvic fracture may cause fetal skull fracture or with gunshot wounds. Because fetal survival depends on maternal survival, initial resuscitation efforts are for the mother. After the airway is secured and IV (large bore) access is obtained, volume replacement is provided and any bleeding controlled. When the mother is stabilized, the gestational age of the fetus should be estimated and pelvic exam done. Radiologic exams should be done as indicated. All unsensitized Rh-negative (D-negative) women should receive **RhoGAM**. Tetanus prophylaxis should be given. Fetal assessment should include ultrasound and monitoring of fetal heart rate.



## Geriatric Pathophysiology

### GERIATRIC SYNDROMES

Geriatric syndromes represent a category of illnesses that is comprised of the most common non-disease conditions that are seen amongst the geriatric community. It is the responsibility of the nurse to be competent in these critical areas:

- **Falls**: As individuals age, their senses dull, leaving them vulnerable to falls due to a combination of sensory decline and chronic disease. Patients and caregivers should be provided with recommendations for fall prevention, and health care providers should create safe inpatient environments with proper fall prevention protocols.
- **Frailty**: A syndrome characterized by decreased stamina, strength, weight, and speed. This combination of issues results from the natural decline of aging and presents specific risks (falls, confusion, and depression) that must be assessed amongst the geriatric population.
- **Incontinence**: Urinary incontinence is an especially common ailment amongst the elderly population due to neurological conditions, physical limitations, and cognitive decline. This particular ailment is not only physically limiting and introduces risks for skin breakdown and infection, but it is socially limiting and can lead to psychological issues as well.

- **Delirium**: Confusion is the most common manifestation of any physical ailment amongst the elderly, along with the prevalence of dementia amongst the elderly. Delirium should never be cast aside in an elderly individual. Though common, it may be an indication of other more serious issues.
- **Functional Decline**: Functional decline is the diminished ability of an individual to carry out the activities of daily living to sustain independence and perform self-care. With this, comes the consideration for additional support, be it live-in care, nursing homes, or assisted living communities.

## Additional Health Issues for the Elderly

The following are additional health issues for the elderly:

- **Antibodies and Immunity**: An elderly patient can react to an infection with antibodies that have been created by the body before, but if the infection is new, it is more difficult for the body to respond appropriately. Cells in the immune system cannot proliferate as easily in an older patient as in a younger one. The number of T-cells is stable, but they do not work as well and can have less cytotoxicity. Additionally, there is not as much thymus-gained immunity because the thymus gland is smaller. This also means it is harder for an older patient to make antibodies.
- **Allergies**: Identify the type of allergic response the patient has and to what allergens, especially when getting the patient history. Determine if the response is actually an allergy to a medication or an adverse effect of it.
- **Driving**: An elderly patient senses change with age. A decreased ability to hear does not mean a patient cannot drive, but sight is very important, including binocular sight, ability to see color, and ability to see in the dark.
- **REM**: Rapid eye movement starts approximately 120 minutes after going to sleep, and happens again in 3–4 evenly spread out increments that last 10–15 minutes. It is linked to skeletal muscle atonia, rapid eye movements, and dreaming. REM sleep occurs less frequently as one gets older. With aging, the patient is more likely to wake up, which affects their sleep quality.

## Urinary Incontinence

Urinary incontinence (UI) is the involuntary loss of urine. Incidence increases with age and is more common in women. There are several **types of urinary incontinence**:

- **Transient**: Adverse medication reaction, urinary tract infection, severe constipation, immobility, mental disorders.
- **Urge or Reflex**: Detrusor muscle spasms cause an urgent desire to urinate because of neurological impairment in Parkinson's, stroke, Alzheimer's, and sitting. Can be triggered by drinking, or hearing or seeing running water.
- **Stress (SUI)**: Increased intra-abdominal pressure from sneezing, coughing, laughing, pregnancy, childbirth damage to the detrusor muscle and pelvic floor fascia, and menopausal hormone changes. Twice as common in women as men.
- **Enuresis**: Bedwetting while asleep.

Decreased bladder strength, diminished ability to concentrate urine, and decreased urethral closing pressure following menopause are common causes of incontinence in the elderly. Incontinence is also influenced by depression, less mobility, decreased vision, and less awareness of feeling a full bladder. Voiding routines are helpful in managing incontinence among the elderly. The typical voiding routine for a fully-grown adult patient is as follows: The initial urge to go to the bathroom happens at the point of the bladder having 200-300 mL in it. Grown patients generally void 4-6 times daily, and most will not need to go during the night except when there is a condition that makes it so or if the patient is using diuretic medication. The sensation of the bladder beginning to fill up begins at 90-150 mL, and the need to go starts at 200-300 mL. Usually, an hour or two will elapse between the first feeling of needing to go and the bladder being at full capacity. Full, easy capacity is around 300-600 mL. There should not be any leaking if going to the bathroom has to be postponed.

## AGE-RELATED CHANGES IN RESPIRATORY SYSTEM

As a patient ages, the respiratory system changes in the following ways:

- **Rib cage becomes more rigid**. There will be more width measured across the anteroposterior chest. When a patient gets old, the number of alveoli decreases. They get inflexible and can no longer draw back. This means that the patient cannot breathe out as well, leading to more residual volume. There is less basilar inflation and the patient cannot get foreign bodies out as well. This condition also happens to someone who has kyphosis.
- **Decreased ability for the chest wall to work** so that it is harder to take a deep inhalation.
- **Trachea and bronchi increase in measurement** so that there is more unused area and lessened air volume that gets to the alveoli. Small airway shutting means there is less vital capacity and more residual volume.
- **Lung parenchyma is not as elastic** so that the alveoli do not function as effectively.
- **Breaths are not as deep and coughs are not as forceful** because the muscles are not as strong.

## CHRONIC DIARRHEA

Chronic diarrhea is more than three bowel movements per day, with watery stools lasting more than two weeks. It is more common and potentially more serious for the elderly population. The most common cause is infectious, but **chronic diarrhea** in the elderly population can also be caused by inflammatory bowel disease, diverticulitis, colon cancer, medication side effects, and irritable bowel syndrome. Take a careful history, including a list of travel destinations. Look for these signs and **symptoms of dehydration** in the physical exam:

- Flushed, dry skin
- Dark, scanty urine
- Fast pulse and respiration
- Fever
- Vomiting or nausea
- Head rushes
- Thirst
- Dry mouth
- Anorexia
- Chills
- Tingling
- Cramps
- Exhaustion
- Confusion
- Seizures
- Unconsciousness

Send stools to the lab for culture, ova and parasites, occult blood, fecal leukocytes, and *C. difficile* toxin, especially if the patient was recently hospitalized. Collect blood for a CBC and electrolytes. Order an abdominal x-ray, and follow up with a barium enema or colonoscopy, if indicated. Treat the underlying cause. Significantly dehydrated patients require hospital admission for IV therapy.

## FRACTURES

Fractures are a common cause of disability in the elderly population. The elderly population is at higher risk for sustaining **fractures** due to decreased bone mass and strength, and increased risk for falls due to poor vision and balance. The most common locations for fractures in the elderly are the distal radius, proximal humerus, proximal femur and tibia, vertebrae, hip, and pubic ramus. Most fractures are the result of minor trauma. Fractures are slightly more common in women. Make the diagnosis based on the history, physical exam, and x-ray results. Immobilize the fracture above and below the break. Administer analgesics. Refer the patient to a physiotherapist, an orthopedic surgeon, and a PSW. The goal of treatment is as rapid a return to normal activity as is possible. The elderly population is more vulnerable to complications, such as permanent functional impairment, bedsores, and pulmonary embolism. The aide, nurse, or caregiver must turn the patient every two hours to minimize complications.

## Age-Related Cataracts

The lens is the clear part of the eye behind the pupil that focuses light on the retina. **Cataracts** are categorized by gradual clouding or opacification of the lens. One or both eyes can be affected, and cataracts can be congenital. Incidence increases with age and affects 70% of people over the age of 75. Risk factors include trauma, radiation, diabetes, family history, smoking, alcoholism, sun exposure, steroid use, and previous eye surgery. Signs and symptoms for cataracts include gradual lens clouding; blurry vision; decreased night vision; brown tint or color fading; halo or glare around lights; diplopia (double vision); trouble distinguishing blue and purple. An ophthalmologist makes the diagnosis by slit lamp exam and retinal exam. Cataracts are followed until they cause significant visual loss and then are treated by surgical removal of the clouded lens and replacement with a permanent intraocular or removable external lens.

**Review Video: Glaucoma vs. Cataracts**
Visit mometrix.com/academy and enter code: 279024

## Hearing Loss

Approximately 25% of adults over the age of 65 have varying degrees of hearing loss. Risk factors for hearing loss include:

- A positive family history
- Chronic exposure to loud noises, especially if hearing protection was not worn
- Use of ototoxic drugs, like Gentamicin, NSAIDs, loop diuretics, or cancer chemotherapy

Hearing loss can be either peripheral or central. **Peripheral hearing loss** results when the ear canal is obstructed by impacted wax, a foreign object, or damage to the middle or inner ear. **Central hearing loss** is the result of damage to the portions of the brain that are needed for hearing: Vestibulocochlear nerve, brain stem, contralateral inferior colliculus, superior olivary nucleus, inferior colliculi, ipsilateral medial geniculate nucleus of the thalamus, and primary auditory cortex below the superior temporal gyrus in the temporal lobe.

## Common Comorbidities Seen Amongst the Elderly Population

**Geriatric comorbidities** are combinations of chronic or acute illnesses that significantly increase the mortality rate amongst this population and are also associated with faster rates of disability exacerbation and functional decline. Understanding these comorbidities not only help the nurse manage these specific comorbidities, but also aid in the guidance of health promotion and disease prevention efforts to decrease the rates of comorbidity amongst their elderly patients. A 2010 study clustered comorbidities most commonly found in the elderly population into 3 groups (Ross, 2010). The three most common comorbidity patterns amongst the geriatric population include:

- **Cardiovascular/metabolic disorders**: Heart disease, MI, coronary artery disease and congestive heart failure often coincide with metabolic issues such as hypertension, diabetes, obesity, and gout.
- **Anxiety/depression/somatoform disorders and pain**: Pain (systemic, localized, or joint related) often coincide with psychological conditions such as anxiety, depression, and cognitive decline. Gastrointestinal issues also seem to coincide with these psychological conditions.
- **Neuropsychiatric disorders**: Psychiatric conditions such as Parkinson's and dementia, are often tied to neurological issues such as incontinence, vascular issues, and/or nerve pain.

## Common Psychological Responses to Chronic Illness

Chronic illness not only effects the physical health of individuals, but often has many **psychological manifestations** as well. This psychological stress is tied to the most basic needs that are engrained in individuals as children, and therefore can cause the regression of the patient to adapt more childlike responses to chronic illness over time. Often these psychological responses to chronic illnesses are based on general concepts of fear, self-esteem, and loss of control.

- **Fear**: Chronic illness, when debilitating with possibly severe consequences, forces patients to face common fears of death, loss, and pain. Remaining in a constant state of fear (stress) can lead to depression, anxiety, and anger.
- **Self-esteem**: While in the early stages of chronic illness many patients find strength and determination to conquer the disease. But, after time, the inability to do so wears on the individual's sense of strength and capability. With a loss of self-esteem, can come feelings of despair and hopelessness, which often result in an increasing rate of decline. Patients with strong support systems and positive outlooks often fare better with chronic disease.
- **Loss of control**: When chronic disease dictates an individual's life and abilities, the patient loses a sense of control over their own life. Losing one's independence can be extremely difficult mentally and emotionally, especially when the patient was previously active and healthy. By providing the patient with treatment options and educating the patient on self-care the nurse can attempt to return some elements of control to the patient, which can motivate them to own their fight against disease and find a new normal in their life that is manageable and fulfilling.

# Chapter Quiz

Ready to see how well you retained what you just read? Scan the QR code to go directly to the chapter quiz interface for this study guide. If you're using a computer, simply visit the online resources page at **mometrix.com/resources719/nclexrn-31183** and click the Chapter Quizzes link.

# NCLEX-RN Practice Test #1

## Case Study 1

The nurse is caring for a 52-year-old male in the emergency department.

NURSES' NOTES (EMERGENCY DEPARTMENT)

**1415:** The client reports nausea, vomiting, and intermittent abdominal pain that started this morning. Abdominal pain is rated at 7/10 on the numerical pain rating scale, and it is cramp-like in nature. The client reports having loose stools yesterday, and he denies having a bowel movement or flatus today. The client's abdomen is mildly distended and tender to the touch on the right side; bowel sounds are hyperactive. The client reports infrequent urination that was amber in color when he last voided. The client has a past medical history of gastroesophageal reflux disease, benign prostatic hypertrophy, and hypertension; he has a surgical history of abdominal inguinal hernia repair 6 months ago and hip arthroplasty 2 years ago.

**1425:** The client voided 120 mL of amber-colored urine. A bladder scan was performed, and postvoid residual testing showed less than 30 mL of urine volume remaining in the bladder. The client vomited 450 mL of clear bile. I notified the primary health provider regarding the client's assessment and status.

VITAL SIGNS

| | **1425** |
|---|---|
| **Temp** | 98.9 °F |
| **P** | 105 |
| **BP** | 145/89 |
| **RR** | 24 |
| **Pulse oximetry** | 95% on room air |

LABORATORY RESULTS

| Laboratory Test and Reference Range | Result |
|---|---|
| **Hemoglobin**<br>Male: 14–18 g/dL | 16.5 g/dL |
| **White blood cell (WBC) count**<br>Adult/child > 2 years: 5,000–10,000/mm$^3$ | 13,000/mm$^3$ |
| **Creatinine**<br>Adult male: 0.6–1.2 mg/dL | 1.4 mg/dL |
| **Blood urea nitrogen (BUN)**<br>Adult: 6–20 mg/dL | 32 mg/dL |
| **Aspartate transaminase (AST)**<br>Adult: 0–35 U/L | 18 U/L |
| **Alanine transaminase (ALT)**<br>Adult: 7–56 U/L | 37 U/L |

**1. The nurse reviews the collected data and recognizes that follow-up is <u>immediately</u> required on which aspects of the patient's condition? (Select all that apply)**

1. Medical history
2. Surgical history
3. Abdominal assessment
4. Reports of nausea and vomiting
5. Vital signs
6. Bowel and bladder reports
7. Laboratory results

**2. Based on the notes, laboratory values, and vital signs, the nurse understands that the client is most likely experiencing _______________.**

1. cholecystitis
2. nephrolithiasis
3. a small bowel obstruction

NURSES' NOTES (EMERGENCY DEPARTMENT)

**1440:** Obtained new orders from the primary care provider for STAT computed tomography (CT) scan of the abdomen. Client is prepared and transported to radiology.

**1500:** Client returned from radiology.

**1515:** Obtained orders from the primary care provider to admit to the medical-surgical unit for conservative management. Patient is prepared for transfer.

DIAGNOSTIC RESULTS

**1450:** Abdominal CT scan results: Increased diameter of the proximal small bowel indicating likely partial obstruction.

**3. The nurse on the medical-surgical unit reviews the collected data. The nurse is monitoring the client closely for complications and recognizes that the client is at the most immediate risk for _______________ and _______________. (Select two answers.)**

1. urinary retention
2. infection
3. dehydration
4. respiratory distress

**4. The nurse anticipates receiving orders from the primary care provider. For each potential order, specify whether each potential order is indicated or not indicated for the client's condition by marking in the corresponding column.**

| Potential Orders | Indicated | Not Indicated |
|---|---|---|
| Initiate a clear liquid diet. | ○ | ○ |
| Insert a nasogastric tube, and set it to low intermittent suction. | ○ | ○ |
| Start a normal saline (0.9% NaCl) IV at 125 mL/hr. | ○ | ○ |
| Administer morphine sulfate 5 mg IV every 4 hours as needed for pain. | ○ | ○ |
| Insert a rectal tube. | ○ | ○ |
| Administer metoclopramide 10 mg IV three times daily for constipation. | ○ | ○ |

**5. The nurse is preparing to insert the nasogastric tube. Of the following options, which two actions should the nurse take? (Select 2 answers)**

1. Determine the appropriate insertion length of the nasogastric tube by measuring from the tip of the client's chin to his earlobe and from his earlobe to his xiphoid process.
2. Instruct the client to swallow and place his chin to his chest while inserting the tube through the client's left nostril and down his pharynx.
3. Once the nasogastric tube is inserted, use bedside ultrasound to confirm that the tube is located in the correct position in the stomach.
4. Following insertion of the nasogastric tube, have the client lie flat in bed to aid with gastric decompression.
5. Provide water-soluble lubricant to the client, or assist in administering it to his lips or inside his nares in case of dryness or irritation.

Nurses' Notes (Medical-Surgical Unit)

**1700:** Nasogastric tube is inserted. Client reports feeling comfortable. There is no further emesis, and pain is currently 3/10 in the abdomen. Client reports toleration of his current pain level.

**1830:** Client voided 500 mL of clear amber urine. There was 250 mL of clear bile gastric output via suction.

**2230:** Client requested assistance with reaching the television remote; he was observed lying very still in bed and was unwilling to lean forward to reach for the remote due to the pain in his abdomen. Client reports that his pain is 9/10 on the right side of his abdomen. Client has hyperactive bowel sounds; the abdomen is board-like upon palpation. The primary care physician was notified of these findings.

**6. Highlight the findings in the nurses' notes that are the most concerning indicators that the patient's condition is declining.**

1700: Nasogastric tube is inserted. Client reports feeling comfortable. There is no further emesis, and pain is currently 3/10 in the abdomen. Client reports toleration of his current pain level.

1830: Client voided 500 mL of clear amber urine. There was 250 mL of clear bile gastric output via suction.

2230: Client requested assistance with reaching the television remote; he was observed lying very still in bed and was unwilling to lean forward to reach for the remote due to the pain in his abdomen. Client reports that his pain is 9/10 on the right side of his abdomen. Client has hyperactive bowel sounds; the abdomen is board-like upon palpation. The primary care physician was notified of these findings.

## Case Study 2

A 26-year-old female presents to the emergency department, driven by her spouse, expressing complaints of a severe headache. The client is 37 weeks pregnant.

NURSES' NOTES

**0900:** A 26-year-old at 37 weeks into her first pregnancy presented to triage with complaints of a severe headache that was unrelieved by 1,000 mg of Tylenol 2 hours before and severe epigastric pain for the past 4 hours. She rates her pain at 9/10. The client states that she has had an uncomplicated pregnancy so far. The client endorses only slightly less fetal movement and denies any vaginal bleeding, leaking of fluid, or contractions. Also notable upon exam: Client has 3+ pitting edema bilaterally on lower extremities and 3+ brisk reflexes.

VITAL SIGNS

| Vital Signs | 0900 |
|---|---|
| HR | 110 |
| RR | 23 |
| BP | 190/110 |
| Temp | 97.8 °F |
| Pulse oximetry | 98% on room air |

**1. Which of the following findings require immediate follow-up? (Select all that apply)**

1. Heart rate
2. Headache
3. Fetal movement
4. Maternal blood pressure
5. Brisk reflexes
6. Epigastric pain
7. Respiratory rate

**2. For the list of client findings below, specify for each whether it is consistent with the disease processes of placental abruption, preeclampsia, and maternal heart failure. Select all supported disease processes for each finding.**

| Client Findings | Placental Abruption | Preeclampsia | Maternal Heart Failure |
|---|---|---|---|
| Blood pressure | ☐ | ☐ | ☐ |
| Headache | ☐ | ☐ | ☐ |
| Lower extremity swelling | ☐ | ☐ | ☐ |
| Epigastric pain | ☐ | ☐ | ☐ |
| Temperature | ☐ | ☐ | ☐ |
| Respiratory rate | ☐ | ☐ | ☐ |

NURSES' NOTES

**0945:** The client now has an 18-gauge IV in her left forearm with lactated Ringer's running at 125 mL/hr. Fetal monitoring is initiated, and the fetal heart rate tracing shows a reassuring category 1 tracing. The client's current blood pressure is 192/112. The nurse refers to the physician orders at this time.

PHYSICIAN ORDERS

- Start magnesium sulfate IV 4 g bolus over 20 minutes, followed by 2 g/hr continuous infusion.
- Measure magnesium levels every 6 hours.
- Continuous fetal monitoring.
- Maintain nothing by mouth status.

PHYSICAL ASSESSMENT

| Body system | 0945 |
|---|---|
| Neurological | The client reports having a severe headache. Client is alert and oriented ×3. Client denies any visual disturbances. Deep tendon reflexes are brisk at 3+ with no clonus. Client denies any dizziness. |
| Pulmonary | Lung sounds are clear bilaterally. Client denies any shortness of breath. |
| Gastrointestinal | Client has complaints of severe heartburn but denies any nausea or vomiting. Abdomen palpates as a soft, gravid uterus. |
| Musculoskeletal | Within normal limits. |
| Genitourinary | Client reports minimal urine output for the past 12 hours, and client states that her urine appears very dark. Client is complaining of urinary urgency. |
| Cardiovascular | Regular heart rhythm and rate. |
| Integumentary | 3+ bilateral edema to both lower extremities. Capillary refill within normal limits. Skin is warm and dry to the touch. |

**3. For the following list of potential nursing interventions, specify whether each one is indicated or not indicated for the care of the client while she is on the magnesium sulfate drip.**

| Potential Nursing Interventions | Indicated | Not Indicated |
|---|---|---|
| Assess headache every 2 hours. | ○ | ○ |
| Assess deep tendon reflexes every hour. | ○ | ○ |
| Auscultate lung sounds every 1-2 hours. | ○ | ○ |
| Monitor blood pressure every hour. | ○ | ○ |
| Evaluate lower extremity edema every 1-2 hours. | ○ | ○ |
| Monitor magnesium levels. | ○ | ○ |
| Strict input and output monitoring. | ○ | ○ |

**4. The nurse has reviewed the history and physical and the physician orders. According to the new orders, the nurse should first _______________.**

1. start the magnesium sulfate drip
2. insert a Foley catheter
3. administer an antacid
4. draw blood for a baseline magnesium level

NURSES' NOTES

**1030:** The magnesium sulfate infusion is currently running. The client is on continuous fetal monitoring, and her lab work is now back. Vital signs are rerun.

VITAL SIGNS

| Vital Signs | 0900 | 1030 |
|---|---|---|
| HR | 110 | 82 |
| RR | 23 | 17 |
| BP | 190/110 | 150/90 |
| Temp | 97.8 °F | 98 °F |
| Pulse oximetry | 98% on room air | 98% on room air |

LAB RESULTS

| Laboratory Test and Reference Range | 1030 |
|---|---|
| **Hemoglobin**<br>Male: 14–18 g/dL | 16.5 g/dL |
| **White blood cell count**<br>Adult/child > 2 years: 5,000–10,000/mm$^3$ | 13,000/mm$^3$ |
| **Creatinine**<br>Adult female: 0.5–1.1 mg/dL | 1.4 mg/dL |
| **Blood urea nitrogen**<br>Adult: 6–20 mg/dL | 32 mg/dL |
| **Aspartate transaminase**<br>Adult: 0–35 U/L | 18 U/L |
| **Alanine transaminase**<br>Adult: 7–56 U/L | 37 U/L |

NURSES' NOTES

**1600:** The client is now complaining of feeling very lethargic and having difficulty keeping her eyes open. The magnesium drip is continuing to infuse at 2 g/hr. The doctor is notified of the client's complaint, and a STAT magnesium level is ordered and drawn.

**1610:** The magnesium level result is 8.9 mg/dL.

VITAL SIGNS

| Vital Signs | 0900 | 1030 | 1600 |
|---|---|---|---|
| HR | 110 | 82 | 79 |
| RR | 23 | 17 | 14 |
| BP | 190/110 | 150/90 | 120/75 |
| Temp | 97.8 °F | 98 °F | 97 °F |
| Pulse oximetry | 98% on room air | 98% on room air | 97% on room air |

**5. Based on the most recent information, the nurse should recognize that the client is experiencing ____________ and the magnesium should be ____________. (Select the appropriate term to fill in each blank)**

**Blank 1:**

1. eclampsia
2. lethargy
3. magnesium toxicity

**Blank 2:**

1. increased
2. maintained
3. decreased
4. discontinued

NURSES' NOTES

**1800:** The client is now alert and states that she is feeling more like herself. The fetal heart rate continues to be reassuring. The client's labor is now being induced, and the client is progressing as expected. The physician ordered a new magnesium level to be drawn, which has returned at 4.1 mg/dL. The client's urine output has been averaging 15 mL/hr for the past several hours. The client is resting comfortably with an epidural currently infusing.

VITAL SIGNS

| Vital Signs | 0900 | 1030 | 1600 | 1800 |
|---|---|---|---|---|
| HR | 110 | 82 | 79 | 75 |
| RR | 23 | 17 | 14 | 18 |
| BP | 190/110 | 150/90 | 120/75 | 170/80 |
| Temp | 97.8 °F | 98 °F | 97 °F | 98.3 °F |
| Pulse oximetry | 98% on room air | 98% on room air | 97% on room air | 97% on room air |

**6. Highlight any client findings below that require follow-up.**

The client is now alert and states that she is feeling more like herself. The fetal heart rate continues to be reassuring. The client's labor is now being induced, and the client is progressing as expected. The physician ordered a new magnesium level, which has returned at 4.1 mg/dL. The client's urine output has been averaging 15 mL/hr for the past several hours. The client is resting comfortably with an epidural currently infusing.

| Vital Signs | 1800 |
|---|---|
| HR | 75 |
| RR | 18 |
| BP | 170/80 |
| Temp | 98.3 °F |
| Pulse oximetry | 97% on room air |

# Case Study 3

The nurse is caring for a 75-year-old man on the medical-surgical unit following a right hip arthroplasty.

## Nurses' Notes

**Day 1, 0930:** The client arrived on the unit following successful completion of right hip arthroplasty. He has a past medical history of gastroesophageal reflux disease and depression. He is alert and oriented to self, time, place, and situation. His heart rate is regular, and his radial pulses are 2+ bilaterally. His respirations are regular. He reports mild pain rated at 2/10 at the surgical site, but he says it feels tolerable with the current pain medication regimen. The client has a new rash of red wheals on his torso and on his legs bilaterally and reports having uncomfortable itching. It appears to be an allergic reaction to the skin preparation used prior to surgery. The primary physician was notified and ordered diphenhydramine 25 mg every 6 hours due to the concern of an allergic reaction.

**Day 1, 1900:** The rash has decreased, and the client denies itchiness. The client ambulated to the bathroom using a walker and stand-by assistance. He reports mild pain to the right hip surgical site at 3/10. Tylenol 650 mg was given as needed, and the client reported adequate pain relief.

**Day 1, 2300:** The client called the nurse into his room, and he requested help catching a train to go to his office. He was reoriented to the time of day and location and was encouraged to try to go back to sleep.

**Day 2, 0400:** The client appears very anxious and was using the nursing call bell many times per hour throughout the night. He is still worried that he will miss work, and he insists that the train station is next door in another client's room. He made multiple attempts throughout the night to leave his bed to get to the train station, saying he could see some of his coworkers in the hallway and wanted to catch up with them. He would get out of bed without calling for help or using his walker. The nursing assistant stayed in the room with the patient and provided reassurance.

**Day 2, 0630:** The client has been sleeping for the past 2 hours and currently appears calm.

**Day 2, 0900:** The client's adult son is visiting and he says that he is concerned about his father: "My father is very upset, and he told me he thinks that he will be fired from his job. My dad has been retired for 20 years. This is not like him—he has never been confused like this." The client is easily distracted and unable to follow directions. He is oriented to himself only. The client is still able to ambulate with a walker and stand-by assistance, and equal strength is present in the bilateral extremities. The client's pupils are equal, round, and reactive to light and accommodation. The primary care physician was notified of the client's condition.

## Vital Signs

| | Day 2, 0900 |
|---|---|
| Temp | 97.9 °F |
| HR | 92 |
| BP | 136/85 |
| RR | 20 |
| Pulse oximetry | 95% on room air |

**1. The nurse reviews the assessment data. From the following list, select the findings that require <u>immediate</u> follow-up. (Select all that apply)**

1. Heart rate (HR)
2. Pulse oximetry level
3. Conversation with his son
4. Medication administration record
5. Activity in room
6. Client report of seeing coworkers in the hallway
7. Pain in his hip

**2. Based on the assessment data, the nurse suspects that the client is most likely experiencing ____________.**

1. a transient ischemic attack
2. vascular dementia
3. hyperactive delirium
4. sundowning

NURSES' NOTES

**Day 2, 1030:** The primary physician diagnosed the client with acute delirium.

**3. The nurse recognizes that if the client's condition is not addressed, the client is at the most <u>immediate</u> risk for developing __________ and __________. (Select 2 answers)**

1. injury to self
2. aspiration pneumonia
3. persistent altered mental status
4. one-sided weakness

**4. For the following list of potential nursing interventions, specify whether each one is indicated or not indicated for the care of the client.**

| Potential Nursing Interventions | Indicated | Not Indicated |
|---|---|---|
| Remove the clock and calendar from the client's room. | ○ | ○ |
| Request that the client's adult son remain in the room with him at his bedside. | ○ | ○ |
| Open the blinds each morning promptly at the beginning of the shift. | ○ | ○ |
| Remove the client's eyeglasses and hearing aids so that they are not broken or lost. | ○ | ○ |
| Monitor the client closely for pain, and treat it promptly. | ○ | ○ |
| Place the client's walker within reach at his bedside. | ○ | ○ |

**5. The nurse should anticipate that the provider will place which of the following orders as a <u>priority</u>? (Select all that apply)**

1. Start normal saline (0.9% NaCl) at 125 mL/hr via intravenous (IV) line for hydration.
2. Discontinue the diphenhydramine.
3. Apply four-point restraints to prevent the client from getting out of bed.
4. Collect blood for complete blood count and basic metabolic panel laboratory tests.
5. Complete a clean catch urine sample for urinary analysis and bacterial culture.
6. Give haloperidol 5 mg intramuscularly now for agitation.

NURSES' NOTES

**Day 3, 0700:** The client used his call light multiple times overnight, he was frequently unsure of what time of day it was, and he required frequent reorientation. Multiple times, he requested help to go to the bathroom. He ambulated with a walker and the assistance of one helper to go to the bathroom three times overnight.

**Day 3, 1000:** The client's son has stayed at the client's bedside overnight. He reported that the client was asking about his hip surgery, wondering how it went and how long he would have to stay in the hospital. The nurse reviewed the lab results from the day before and provided education that the client does not have signs of any underlying infection or metabolic disorder at this time.

**Day 3, 1700:** The client has been sleeping in bed since this morning. He is arousing briefly for sips of water, but he is not engaging in conversation. He appears calm and comfortable.

VITAL SIGNS

| | Day 2, 0900 | Day 3, 1700 |
|---|---|---|
| **Temp** | 97.9 °F | 98.2 °F |
| **HR** | 92 | 80 |
| **BP** | 136/85 | 130/89 |
| **RR** | 20 | 18 |
| **Pulse oximetry** | 95% on room air | 94% on room air |

**6. For the following list of assessment findings, specify whether each one indicates that the client's condition has improved, is unchanged, or has worsened.**

| Assessment Findings | Improved | Unchanged | Worsened |
|---|---|---|---|
| HR, 80 | ○ | ○ | ○ |
| Oxygen level, 94% | ○ | ○ | ○ |
| Client's conversation with his son | ○ | ○ | ○ |
| Client's sleep pattern | ○ | ○ | ○ |
| Client's mobility status | ○ | ○ | ○ |

## Standalone Questions

**1. A client is to receive 1,000 mL of 0.15% potassium chloride in 5% dextrose injection (D5W) intravenously over 3 hours and 20 minutes using a drop factor of 15 drops/mL. What is the required flow rate (drops) per minute?** ***Record your answer as a whole number.***

_________ drops/min

**2. A client develops mastitis in the postpartum period. Which of the following instructions should the nurse anticipate when notifying the physician?** ***Select all that apply.***

1. Antibiotics for 7–14 days
2. Opioid analgesia
3. Alternating hot and cold compresses to relieve the pain
4. Discontinuation of breastfeeding
5. Continuation of breastfeeding

**3. The nurse is teaching a new parent about the use of car seats for infants. Which of the following information should the nurse include?** ***Select all that apply.***

1. The shoulder straps should be fed through slots at or below the infant's shoulders.
2. Infants should always be in rear-facing car seats.
3. The mother should place padding on the car seat underneath the infant.
4. The harness clip should be positioned at the infant's abdomen.
5. The car seat should be positioned so that the infant's head does not fall forward.

**4. An irregular ECG characterized by closely spaced premature ventricular contractions (PVCs), a lack of P waves, and distorted QRS complexes indicates:**

1. Atrial fibrillation
2. Paroxysmal atrial tachycardia
3. Ventricular tachycardia
4. Ventricular fibrillation

**5. A client requires insertion of a nasogastric tube. When preparing the client for the procedure, the nurse should place the client in which of the following positions?**

1. High Fowler's position with the head tilted forward
2. High Fowler's position with the head tilted backward
3. Semi-Fowler's position with the head in a neutral position
4. Semi-Fowler's position with the head tilted backward

**6. A client returns to his room after a liver biopsy. The nurse should place the client in which of the following positions?**

1. Left side-lying with a folded towel under the biopsy site
2. Right side-lying with a folded towel under the biopsy site
3. Supine with a pressure dressing over the biopsy site
4. Prone with a small pillow under the biopsy site

**7. What is the approximate duration of the PR interval on the following ECG tracing?**

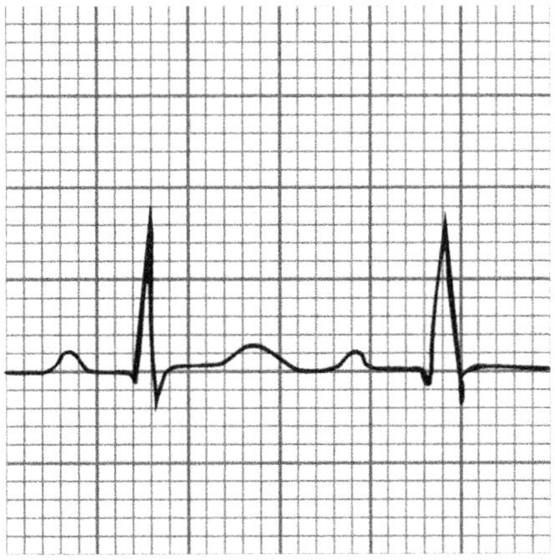

1. 0.24 s
2. 0.20 s
3. 0.16 s
4. 0.12 s

**8. A client with a tracheostomy is exhibiting difficulty breathing. Respirations are increasingly noisy, and secretions are very thick. Which of the following initial interventions is <u>most</u> indicated?**

1. Increase humidification, and suction the tracheostomy tube.
2. Notify the physician.
3. Sit the client upright and encourage them to breathe deeply and cough.
4. Gently irrigate and suction the tracheostomy tube.

**9. A client has a chest tube in place with a three-chamber chest drainage system. The nurse notes continuous bubbling in the water seal chamber. This indicates which of the following?**

1. Pneumothorax
2. Adequate suction
3. System air leak
4. Tube positioned incorrectly

**10. The following pattern on an ECG tracing is characteristic of:**

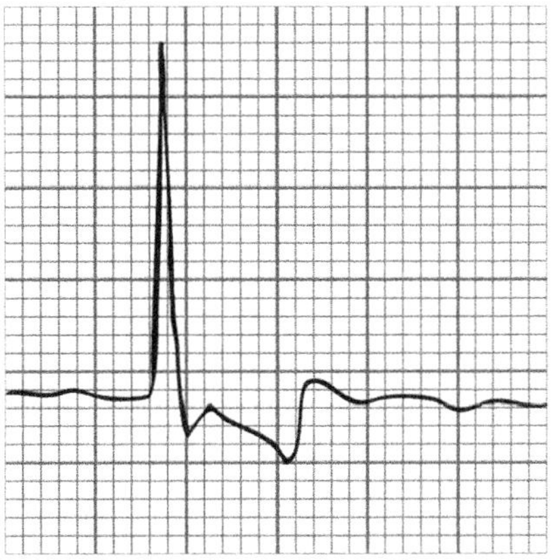

1. Digoxin therapy
2. Hypokalemia
3. Ischemia
4. Myocardial infarction

**11. The nurse is reviewing medications with a client who is to be scheduled for outpatient rotator cuff repair. Which of the following medications does the nurse anticipate the client will be advised to avoid on the morning of the surgery?**

1. Metoprolol
2. Levothyroxine
3. Aspirin
4. Fluoxetine

**12. A patient with hypothyroidism states that she takes levothyroxine 0.112 mg daily, but the pharmacy has issued the drug labeled in micrograms. How many micrograms of levothyroxine is equivalent to 0.112 mg?** ***Record your answer as a whole number.***

_________ mcg

**13. The nurse is caring for an unvaccinated child who developed complications related to German measles (rubella). Which of the following infection control protocols is appropriate?**

1. Standard only
2. Standard and contact
3. Standard and droplet
4. Standard and airborne

**14. A client is scheduled for knee replacement surgery, and the nurse is reviewing preoperative laboratory results. The nurse should notify the physician about which of the following abnormal laboratory results?**

1. Platelets: 119,000
2. Glucose: 83
3. Hemoglobin: 13.7
4. Sodium: 141

**15. The nurse is caring for a client with diabetes mellitus, type 1. Which of the following signs and symptoms are indicative of diabetic ketoacidosis?** ***Select all that apply.***

1. Dehydration
2. Polyuria
3. Hyperventilation
4. Polydipsia
5. Blurred vision
6. Abdominal pain

**16. A 15-year-old client was involved in an auto accident and requires emergency surgery to control bleeding, but both parents are out of town and unable to sign the consent form. Which of the following is the <u>most</u> appropriate action?**

1. The client signs the consent form.
2. The parents give telephone consent with two witnesses listening.
3. The parents give email consent.
4. The physician operates without consent because of the emergency situation.

**17. The nurse is administering an intermittent tube feeding to a client through a nasogastric tube. Which of the following positions is optimal for tube feedings?**

1. The head of the bed is elevated to at least 45°.
2. The head of the bed is elevated to at least 90°.
3. The head of the bed is elevated to at least 30°.
4. The head of the bed is flat with the client supine.

**18. When considering fluid balance, if 60% of an adult's body is composed of water, approximately what percentage of this is found in intracellular fluid?**

1. 33%
2. 25%
3. 67%
4. 8%

**19. Whole blood is primarily indicated for which of the following purposes?**

1. To treat extreme loss of blood volume
2. To increase clotting factors
3. To increase oxygen-carrying capacity for those with anemia
4. To control acute bleeding

**20. A client who has undergone a thyroidectomy complains of numbness, tingling, and stiffness in her hands, feet, and face as well as muscle tremors, spasmodic muscle contractions, and anxiety during the postoperative period. Which laboratory tests does the nurse anticipate that the physician will request?**

1. Hemoglobin
2. Sodium
3. Thyroid-stimulating hormone (TSH)
4. Calcium

**21. A client receiving chemotherapy and opioids for renal cancer has had no bowel movement for five days and no results from two doses of laxatives in the past 48 hours. The client is passing no flatus and complains of increasing abdominal pain and nausea. Which of the following should the nurse anticipate?**

1. Abdominal examination and abdominal x-ray
2. Oil retention enema and manual removal of impaction
3. Oil retention enema followed by a soapsuds enema
4. Another dose of laxative followed by a soapsuds enema if there are no results in 24 hours

**22. An 82-year-old female complains of generalized fatigue and has new onset of urinary incontinence as well as anorexia, hyperventilation, and low-grade fever. The nurse anticipates that the client will be evaluated for which of the following?**

1. Diabetes mellitus
2. Bladder cancer
3. Urinary tract infection
4. Influenza

**23. The nurse administers a dose of acetaminophen to the wrong client. Which of the following actions is the most appropriate after notifying the physician?**

1. Notify her supervisor and complete an incident report.
2. Ask the physician for an order of acetaminophen to cover the inadvertent administration.
3. Take no further action because acetaminophen is relatively benign.
4. Document in the client's record that an error in drug administration occurred.

**24. What is the rhythm in the following ECG strip?**

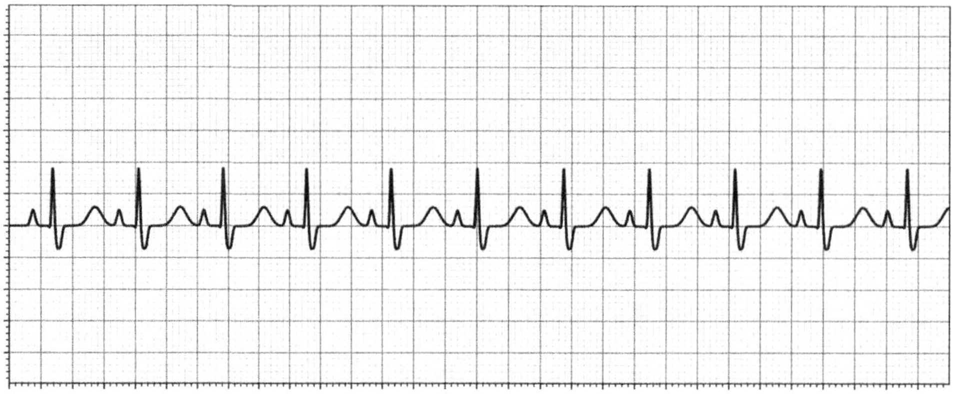

1. Sinus tachycardia
2. Normal sinus rhythm
3. Atrial tachycardia
4. Junctional escape rhythm

**25. What is the rhythm in the following ECG tracing?**

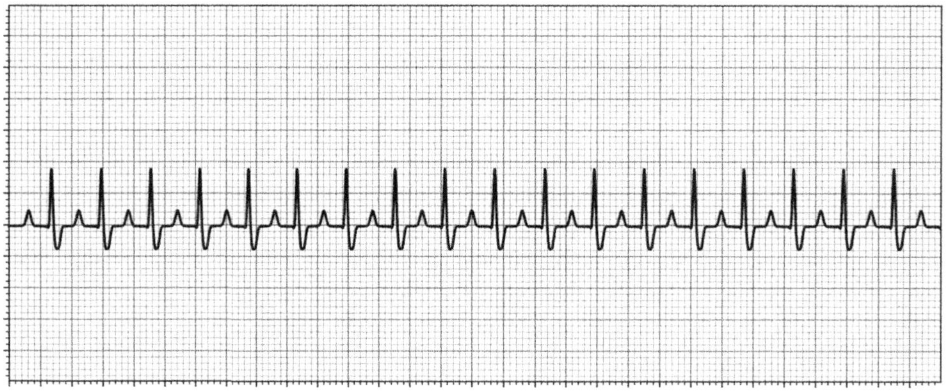

1. Normal sinus rhythm
2. Ventricular tachycardia
3. Atrial fibrillation
4. Atrial tachycardia

**26. A client's wife states that her elderly husband has begun to slightly slur his words and drop word endings. He has become increasingly withdrawn socially and irritable. He has also accused her of talking behind his back and whispering at him. The nurse suspects that the client should be <u>initially</u> evaluated for which of the following?**

1. Depression
2. Alzheimer's disease
3. Hearing loss
4. Stroke

**27. Which of the following tasks are appropriate for the nurse to delegate to unlicensed assistive personnel? *Select all that apply.***

1. Checking temperature and vital signs for a client acutely ill with sepsis
2. Checking routine temperature and vital signs for clients at the beginning of the shift
3. Emptying catheter bags and measuring the urinary output from Foley catheters
4. Monitoring the transfusion of red blood cells
5. Assisting an ambulatory client with walking to the bathroom

**28. Two days postpartum, a nursing mother develops swollen, taut, and very painful breasts. Which of the following is the most likely cause?**

1. Engorgement
2. Insufficient milk
3. Blocked milk ducts
4. Mastitis

**29. Following surgical repair of a fractured femur, a client's hemoglobin falls to 7.4, and the physician orders one unit of packed red blood cells (250 mL) to be administered over two hours with a drop factor of 10 drops/mL. What flow rate (drops per minute) is needed? *Record your answer as a whole number.***

_______ drops/min

**30. Place the following metric capacity measures (in Roman numerals) in the correct position in the table below.**

I. Deciliter
II. Milliliter
III. Dekaliter
IV. Kiloliter
V. Hectoliter

| | | | | | | |
|---|---|---|---|---|---|---|
| 1. _____ | Centiliter | 2. _____ | Liter | 3. _____ | 4. _____ | 5. _____ |

**31. A client with recurrent episodes of gout has been advised to eat a low-purine diet. Which of the following foods should the nurse advise him to limit or avoid? *Select all that apply.***

1. Liver
2. Sardines
3. Wine
4. Low-fat yogurt
5. Beef broth
6. Potatoes

**32. A client develops anaphylaxis syndrome and loses consciousness after eating fruit salad containing kiwi fruit, which the client is severely allergic to. The nurse is aware that the initial intervention is which of the following?**

1. Establish a patent airway.
2. Administer intravenous fluids.
3. Administer oxygen at 100% high flow.
4. Administer epinephrine.

**33. An infant is to receive 250 mL of 5% dextrose/0.45 normal saline (D5/0.45 NS) in five hours. The pediatric IV system has a drop factor of 60 drops per mL. What is the flow rate (in drops per minute)? *Record your answer as a whole number.***

_______ drops/min

**34. A client states that he takes five grains of aspirin daily, but the hospital issues aspirin in milligrams. How many milligrams are approximately equivalent to five grains of aspirin?**

1. 81 mg
2. 120 mg
3. 325 mg
4. 500 mg

**35. A child who weighs 40 kg is prescribed clarithromycin at 15 mg/kg per day for 10 days in two divided doses for acute strep throat. If the medication is provided in suspension with 250 mg/5 mL, how many total milliliters of medication are required to complete the treatment? *Record your answer as a whole number.***

________ mL

**36. The physician had prescribed 10 mL of oral suspension twice daily for a child, but the mother is confused about the metric system and wants to know how many teaspoons of medication to give the child. How many teaspoons are equivalent to 10 mL of oral suspension? *Record your answer as a whole number.***

________ teaspoons

**37. An electrical fire occurs in a client's room shortly after the client returns from the recovery room after repair of a hip fracture with insertion of a prosthesis. What is the <u>best</u> method of removing the client from the room?**

1. Place the client in a wheelchair.
2. Transfer the client to a gurney.
3. Move the bed with the client on it.
4. Do a two-person carry.

**38. A client is confused after receiving morphine for analgesia and repeatedly tries to pull out the intravenous (IV) line in her left arm. Which of the following actions is the best <u>initial</u> solution?**

1. Attempt to camouflage the IV and tie a piece of tubing to the bedrail so the client can pull on that safely.
2. Apply wrist restraints.
3. Apply wrist and vest restraints.
4. Discontinue the IV line and reinsert at a more distant site.

**39. A patient appears cyanotic and apneic during an ECG, and no palpable pulse can be detected. The ECG strip shows the following:**

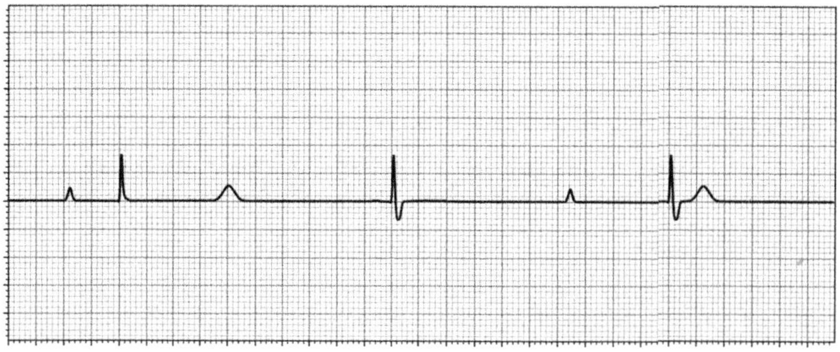

**What condition should be suspected?**

1. Pulseless electrical activity
2. Pulseless ventricular tachycardia
3. Normal sinus rhythm
4. Severe bradycardia

**40. A client is prescribed 0.25 mg terbutaline subcutaneously, but the medication is provided as 1 mg/mL. How many mL of medication are needed to provide the correct dosage?** ***Round your answer to two decimal places.***

_________ mL

**41. A client has returned from surgery after removal of a tumor of the colon and creation of a temporary colostomy. She refuses to take a deep breath and cough then refuses to turn. Which of the following should the nurse assess <u>first</u> in trying to understand her lack of cooperation?**

1. Delirium status
2. Vital signs
3. Oxygen saturation
4. Level of pain

**42. When assisting a client with range-of-motion exercises, which movements should be carried out on the client's elbows?** ***Select all that apply.***

1. Supination
2. Flexion
3. Circumduction
4. Pronation
5. Rotation
6. Hyperextension

**43. What is the duration of the QRS complex on this ECG strip?**

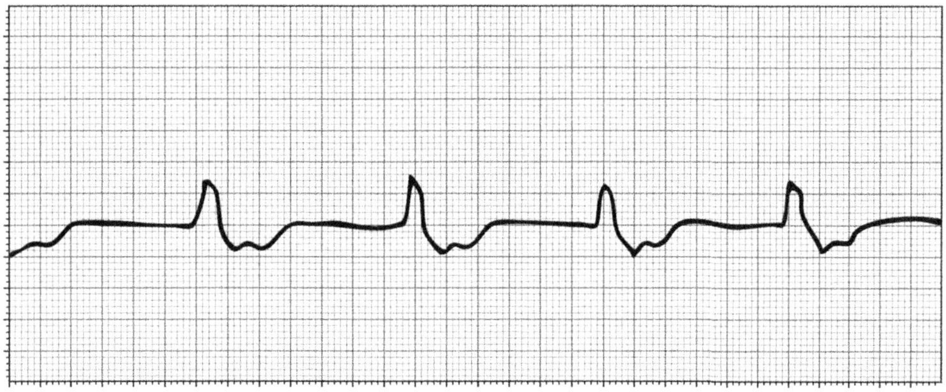

1. 0.12 s
2. 0.14 s
3. 0.18 s
4. 0.22 s

**44. What abnormality is evident on the following ECG tracing?**

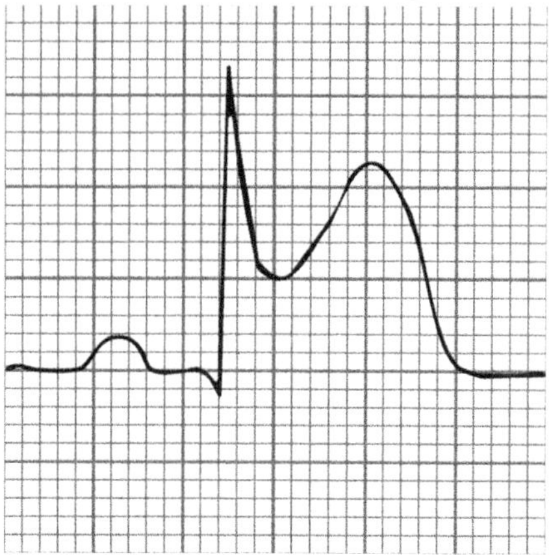

1. Tented T waves
2. QRS slurring
3. U waves
4. Elevated ST segment

**45. What is the duration of the QT interval in the following tracing?**

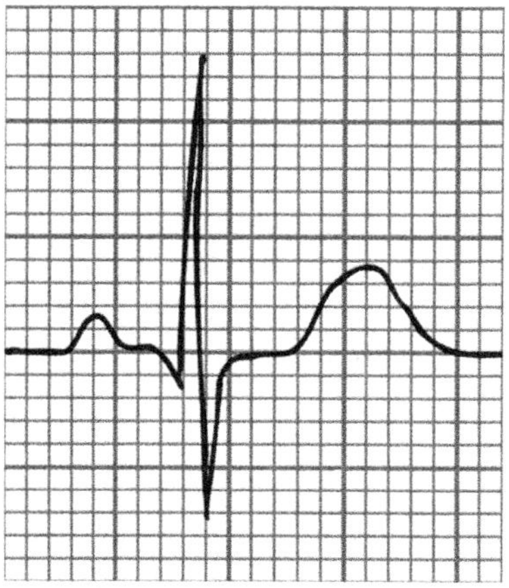

1. 0.60 s
2. 0.48 s
3. 0.52 s
4. 0.40 s

**46. For which of the following reasons would the nurse use the Braden Scale to assess a client?**

1. To determine if the client is suffering from delirium
2. To determine if the client is at risk for developing pressure sores
3. To determine if the client is at risk for falls
4. To determine if the client is at risk for substance abuse

**47. Following a disaster with multiple victims and danger to those present, which group should have priority for protection from injury?**

1. The victims
2. The firefighters and police officers
3. The bystanders and news reporters
4. The healthcare providers

**48. Which of the following statements by the client suggests that the client has given made informed consent for a craniotomy?**

1. "I know that surgery could cause a stroke, and I'm scared."
2. "I told the doctor I didn't want to know anything about the surgery, and she agreed."
3. "I have one more question before I sign the consent form."
4. "This is a really complicated procedure. So many things could go wrong."

**49. The computers for documenting client care and treatment are located at the nursing station. Which of the following is the <u>most</u> important consideration regarding the computers?**

1. The height of the computer stations
2. The ratio of computers to staff
3. The positioning of the computer screens away from the line of sight of unauthorized persons
4. The brand of computer and operating system

**50. The physician has ordered that a serum trough level be drawn for a medication. Which of the following is the correct time to draw blood for a trough level?**

1. At the midpoint in time between two scheduled doses of the drug
2. At the time the drug peaks
3. Immediately after a scheduled dose is administered
4. Immediately before a scheduled dose is due

**51. A client tells the nurse that she is on a high-protein diet and averages 75 g of protein daily, 120 g of carbohydrates, and 40 g of fat. If fat is equal to 9 calories per gram and protein and carbohydrates are equal to 4 calories per gram, how many total calories is the client averaging each day? *Record your answer as a whole number.***

_________ calories

**52. An elderly preoperative client seems very anxious but denies concerns when the nurse asks; however, the client's son confides that the client is very superstitious and believes it is bad luck that he is in room 113. Which of the following actions is the <u>best</u> response?**

1. Reassure the client that the room number will not affect his surgery outcome.
2. Contact the admissions department and request that the client be reassigned to a different room.
3. Ask the physician for medication to relax the client.
4. Ask the son to stay with the client to reassure him.

**53. A client experiencing transient homelessness with a history of mental illness and substance abuse is to be discharged. Which of the following support systems are most likely to provide social support for the client? *Select all that apply.***

1. Self-help programs
2. Internet-based programs
3. Community agencies
4. Governmental agencies
5. Friends
6. Family

**54. A client is receiving oxygen therapy at 3 L/min per nasal cannula. Which of the following fraction of inspired oxygen ($FiO_2$) measurements does the nurse expect that the client is receiving?**

1. 24%
2. 60%
3. 32%
4. 100%

**55. A 43-year-old client has developed progressive frontotemporal dementia and is exhibiting inappropriate and compulsive behaviors, difficulty with language, and impaired judgment. Which statement by the client's wife suggests that she has not accepted a permanent role change in their relationship?**

1. "I need my husband to take care of financial matters."
2. "It's so frustrating that my husband refuses to bathe."
3. "My husband doesn't pay attention to anything I try to tell him."
4. "I want my husband to do the things that he can still manage independently."

**56. A client undergoing "cold-turkey" withdrawal from years of substance abuse is most at risk of serious life-threatening complications with which of the following substances?**

1. Heroin
2. Cocaine
3. Alcohol
4. Marijuana

**57. The nurse finds a client smoking marijuana in the hospital and tells her that no smoking or use of drugs is allowed in the facility. The client responds by shouting, "What business is it of yours? Leave me alone!" Which of the following <u>initial</u> responses is the best for the nurse to use to defuse the situation?**

1. "It's my business because I'm your nurse."
2. "If you don't put that out immediately, I will call security."
3. "You are violating the facility policies and the law!"
4. "I'm sorry, but I have to ask you again to put out your marijuana cigarette."

**58. A client who served three tours of duty in Afghanistan has been diagnosed with post-traumatic stress disorder (PTSD). Which of the following signs and symptoms should the nurse expect the client to exhibit? *Select all that apply.***

1. Recurring flashbacks
2. Detachment from others
3. Anger
4. Hyperacute memory regarding the events associated with the trauma
5. Nightmares
6. Excessive sleeping

**59. A diabetic client self-administers insulin four times daily. Which of the following statements by the client indicates the need for further education?**

1. "I flush the used needles down the toilet."
2. "I carry glucose tablets with me at all times."
3. "I eat a little dessert occasionally."
4. "I avoid wearing sandals."

**60. A hospice client is to receive 4 mg of morphine sulfate (MS) subcutaneously from a vial that contains 10 mg/mL. How many milliliters of MS should the patient receive to equal a dose of 4 mg? *Round your answer to one decimal place.***

_________ mL

**61. Which of the following findings are indicative of peripheral arterial insufficiency?** ***Select all that apply.***

1. Throbbing, cramping pain that increases with exercise
2. Aching pain that increases with dependency
3. Capillary refill time of less than two seconds
4. Shiny skin with decreased hair
5. Brown pigment about the ankles and lower legs
6. Pale color on elevation and redness on dependency

**62. The nurse is assisting a client with a colostomy irrigation. The client is positioned on the toilet and has removed the colostomy pouch, and the irrigation bag is filled with 1000 mL of warm water. Place the following actions (in Roman numerals) in the correct order from first to last.**

I. Allow 15–20 minutes for evacuation and then fold the sleeve, secure it, and leave it in place for 30–45 minutes before removing it.
II. Allow the solution to flow in for 5–10 minutes and then clamp the tubing and close the top of the irrigation sleeve.
III. Apply gloves, lubricate the cone tip, and insert it into the stoma, holding it securely.
IV. Apply the irrigation sleeve over the stoma.
V. Hang the irrigation solution bag with the bottom 20 inches above the stoma.

1. ____
2. ____
3. ____
4. ____
5. ____

**63. A client complains of sleeping poorly, arousing many times during the night, awakening with a headache, and feeling tired and sluggish in the morning and throughout the day. For which of the following tests does the nurse anticipate that the client will be scheduled?**

1. Electroencephalogram
2. Electrocardiogram
3. Nocturnal polysomnogram
4. Magnetic resonance imaging (MRI) of the brain

**64. A pregnant woman undergoes a 40-minute nonstress test for evaluation of fetal heart rate (FHR) accelerations. Which of the following test results is normal (reactive)?**

1. One acceleration of the FHR of 10 beats per minute (bpm) above the baseline for 10 seconds
2. Two accelerations of the FHR of 10 bpm above the baseline for 15 seconds
3. No accelerations of the FHR
4. Three accelerations of the FHR of 15 bpm above the baseline for 20 seconds

**65. The nurse is conducting an aphasia assessment of a client who has suffered a stroke. Which of the following observations should the nurse include in the assessment?** ***Select all that apply.***

1. Spontaneous speech
2. Comprehension of the spoken and written word
3. Ability to name objects
4. Ability to describe objects
5. Ability to write
6. Ability to recall four named items after five minutes

**66. A client is receiving end-of-life care and tells the nurse that he has not always lived the way he should have or treated his children well. Which of the following responses is the <u>most</u> appropriate?**

1. "What kinds of things have you done?"
2. "There are things that you regret."
3. "I'm sure those things don't matter anymore."
4. "It's not too late to ask for forgiveness."

**67. A nurse is at a local swimming pool, and a man collapses with a cardiac arrest after exiting the pool. The man is still wet when the nurse begins cardiopulmonary resuscitation (CPR), and another person brings the automated external defibrillator (AED). Which of the following should the nurse do next?**

1. Apply the AED pads and deliver a shock.
2. Wipe the chest dry with an available cloth or towel.
3. Continue CPR because a client who is wet cannot receive a shock.
4. Wipe the chest with an alcohol hand wipe to speed the evaporation of the water.

**68. The client's intravenous (IV) line has a gauze pad wrapped around the IV catheter at the insertion site and a transparent dressing over the gauze dressing. How long after application should the nurse change the dressing?**

1. At the normal rotation time for the IV
2. When the transparent dressing loosens
3. In 48 hours
4. In 24 hours

**69. Which of the following groups of neonates should be screened for hearing loss?**

1. Premature neonates
2. Neonates with risk factors for hearing loss
3. Neonates with abnormal Apgar scores
4. All neonates

**70. A child weighing 20 kg is to receive 45 mg/kg of amoxicillin per day in a divided dose every 12 hours. The oral suspension contains 250 mg/5 mL. How many milliliters should the child receive in each dose? *Record your answer as a whole number.***

_________ mL

**71. A client has a rate-responsive permanent pacemaker in his upper chest. The nurse understands rate-responsive to mean which of the following?**

1. A pacemaker function prevents excessive changes in the pacing rate.
2. The pacing rate increases above the normal pacing rate with sudden bradycardia.
3. The pacemaker switches from atrial tracking mode to non-tracking mode with atrial fibrillation.
4. The pacing rate increases when the sensors note increased activity.

**72. The "5 A's" of smoking cessation intervention begin with which of the following?**

1. Advise all clients who smoke to stop smoking.
2. Ask all clients about tobacco use at every visit.
3. Assess the client's willingness to stop smoking.
4. Assist the client to stop smoking.

**73. The nurse is educating a client about lifestyle modifications to manage hypertension. Which of the following modifications should the nurse recommend? *Select all that apply.***

1. Limit fluid intake to 2,000 mL daily.
2. Engage in regular aerobic exercise (30 minutes most days).
3. Adopt the dietary approaches to stop hypertension (DASH) eating plan.
4. Lose weight.
5. Eliminate all alcoholic beverages.
6. Stop smoking.

**74. The nurse is caring for a Muslim client who is recovering from an automobile accident and is unable to cleanse herself after a bowel movement. Which of the following should the nurse attempt to do whenever possible to show respect for the woman's cultural and religious beliefs?**

1. Use the left hand to cleanse the client's rectal area.
2. Ask a female family member to assist the client.
3. Wear gloves when cleansing the client's rectal area.
4. Ask the client's husband to assist the client.

**75. A client is upset that the physician has refused to order a stronger pain medication for the client and berates the nurse, calling the nurse "worthless and stupid" when the nurse brings the prescribed medication. Which of the following ego defense mechanisms is the client exhibiting?**

1. Compensation
2. Reaction formation
3. Displacement
4. Regression

**76. The mother of a 24-month-old child tells the nurse that she is concerned that her child's language abilities are delayed. Which of the following language milestones does the nurse expect the child to exhibit?**

1. The child understands 300 words and uses two- and three-word sentences.
2. The child says and understands a few words, such as "Mama" and "Dada," and can imitate animal sounds, such as "moo" and "woof."
3. The child says and understands four to six words but understands more and can point to items he wants.
4. The child says and understands up to 20 words and can point to his body parts.



**77. A client who experienced a cardiac arrest and resuscitation is exhibiting characteristics of mild anoxic brain injury. Which of the following characteristics does the nurse expect her to exhibit? *Select all that apply.***

1. Decreased ability to concentrate
2. Seizures
3. Memory impairment
4. Semicomatose state
5. Decreased balance
6. Restlessness

**78. A client has developed osteomyelitis of the bones of the left foot following the infection of a diabetic ulcer. The nurse anticipates which of the following treatments to be the <u>primary</u> focus?**

1. Warm wet soaks
2. Analgesia
3. Surgical debridement
4. Intravenous (IV) antibiotic therapy

**79. When determining whether or not a client is a candidate for restraints, which of the following would be considered an appropriate reason for a restraint?**

1. Current dangerous behavior
2. A history of falls
3. A recent violent attack on a staff member
4. Refusal to cooperate with treatment

**80. A client with rheumatoid arthritis tells the nurse that she is having increasing difficulty cooking, cleaning, and attending to activities of daily living. Which of the following referrals is the most appropriate?**

1. An occupational therapist
2. A physical therapist
3. A home health agency
4. An assisted-living facility

**81. If the nurse is teaching a group of clients about risk factors for diabetes mellitus, type 2, the nurse should include which of the following? *Select all that apply.***

1. Obesity
2. Hypertension and/or heart disease
3. 45 years or older
4. Caucasian race
5. Family history of diabetes mellitus, type 2

**82. The nurse is assessing an older adult. The client does not appear to always understand the questions, sometimes answering incorrectly, and stares at the nurse's mouth rather than the nurse's eyes when the nurse is speaking. The client answers in an unusually loud voice. Which of the following impairments should the nurse suspect?**

1. Hearing impairment
2. Cognitive impairment
3. Vision impairment
4. Anxiety

**83. A client is to be discharged 48 hours after a normal vaginal delivery of an infant with no laceration or episiotomy. Which of the following danger signs should the client be advised to report to her physician? *Select all that apply.***

1. Temperature higher than 38 °C (100.4 °F)
2. Difficulty urinating
3. Swelling, redness, or pain in one or both legs
4. Fatigue
5. Foul-smelling vaginal discharge

**84. An ECG tracing shows persistent artifacts because the patient is diaphoretic and the electrodes are not securely attaching. The best solution is to:**

1. Apply the 60 Hz notch filter.
2. Replace the electrodes.
3. Apply the electrodes only to the limbs.
4. Cleanse and dry the skin and use an adhesive enhancer.

**85. If a client is to have a nasogastric (NG) tube inserted for intermittent feedings, which of the following is an appropriate task to delegate to unlicensed assistive personnel?**

1. Inserting the NG tube
2. Verifying tube position
3. Administering tube feedings
4. Reposition a displaced NG tube

**86. A client has had a recent below-knee (BK) amputation of the right leg because of a traumatic injury. After removing the elastic wrap, which the client had applied, the nurse notes an unusual pattern of swelling. Which of the following is the <u>most</u> likely reason for this observation?**

1. Wound infection
2. Impaired circulation to the stump
3. Incorrect wrap technique
4. Bleeding into the tissues

**87. A client with prostate cancer has been given the option of various treatments and asks the nurse for advice. Which of the following is the <u>most</u> appropriate response?**

1. "Let's discuss the different options and how you feel about them."
2. "I can't help you to make a decision about your treatment."
3. "You need to discuss this decision with your physician."
4. "I would choose surgery if I were in your position."

**88. A heart rate of 125 beats per minute with absent or irregular P waves best describes which of the following arrhythmias?**

1. Supraventricular tachycardia
2. Asystole
3. Atrial fibrillation
4. First-degree heart block

**89. A client has increasing pain in both hands. On examination, the nurse notes that the metacarpophalangeal and proximal interphalangeal joints are enlarged and swollen, swan-neck deformity is evident, and the fingers on both hands show ulnar deviation. These findings are consistent with which of the following disorders?**

1. Osteoarthritis
2. Rheumatoid arthritis
3. Gouty arthritis
4. Psoriatic arthritis

**90. A neonate has severe congenital abnormalities that make death imminent. The NICU team believes that further attempts at treatment or feeding are not warranted and that palliative care only should be provided. When speaking with the parents about this, which of the following is the <u>best</u> approach?**

1. Tell the parents that the team suggests that all food and treatment will be withheld.
2. Tell the parents that the team suggests a change in care plan to focus on comfort measures.
3. Tell the parents that any further efforts at treatment are futile, as the infant is dying.
4. Tell the parents that the best thing is to let nature take its course.

**91. If a client weighs 132 lb and has a caloric requirement of 28 calories per kg of body weight per day, what is the number of calories that the client needs each day to maintain body weight? *Record your answer as a whole number.***

________ calories

**92. A client has an open draining wound infected with MRSA and is on contact precautions. If the nurse is entering the room to care for the client, when are gloving and gowning necessary?**

1. When the nurse has direct contact with the wound or drainage
2. When the nurse has direct contact with the client's body, wound, or drainage
3. When the nurse enters the room for any type of patient or environmental contact
4. When drainage is not contained by a dressing

**93. If a six-year-old child has influenza with a fever and cough, which statements by the child's caregiver suggest a need for education? *Select all that apply.***

1. "If his fever gets too high, I'll give him a bath in cold water."
2. "I try to offer him plenty of liquids."
3. "Sipping hot lemonade seems to help relieve his cough."
4. "I've been giving him baby aspirin to lower his fever."
5. "I alternate giving him acetaminophen and ibuprofen for this fever."

**94. Following procurement of organs from a standard criteria donor (donor younger than 50 years who suffered brain death), within what time period should the heart and lungs be transplanted?**

1. 4–6 hours
2. 8–12 hours
3. 24 hours
4. 36 hours

**95. The nurse must administer in one syringe a combined dose of two different insulins from two vials. The procedure includes:**

I. Cleanse the tops of the vials.
II. Inject air into vial 1.
III. Withdraw medication from vial 1.
IV. Change needles.
V. Withdraw medication from vial 2.
VI. Inject air into vial 2.

**Place the steps (Roman numerals) in the correct order.**

1. _____
2. _____
3. _____
4. _____
5. _____
6. _____

**96. If teaching a client to use a metered-dose inhaler (MDI) without a spacer, how far away from the mouth should the nurse advise the client that the inhaler be positioned when administering a dose of inhaled medication?**

1. The inhaler should be enclosed within the client's lips.
2. The inhaler should be immediately outside of the client's lips.
3. The inhaler should be 1–2 inches away from the client's lips.
4. The inhaler should be 3–4 inches away from the client's lips.

**97. A client is receiving an opioid per patient-controlled analgesia (PCA) pump to control postoperative pain; however, when the nurse assesses the client, she finds the client is pale and hypotensive with a respiratory rate of 6 breaths per minute. The PCA pump record shows that the limit for maximum dosage was set far too high, resulting in an overdose. The client is very somnolent and barely responsive. What interventions should the nurse anticipate? *Select all that apply.***

1. Immediately stop the infusion.
2. Discontinue the PCA pump.
3. Administer naloxone per standing orders.
4. Administer supplementary oxygen.
5. File an incident report.

**98. A client is hospitalized in a long-term care facility because of Alzheimer's disease. The client is incontinent of urine and feces. The nurse has delegated incontinent care to unlicensed assistive personnel (UAP). How frequently should the nurse advise that the UAP check the client for dryness?**

1. Every 2 hours
2. Every hour
3. When the client appears restless
4. Before meals and at bedtime

**99. A client with epilepsy is taking phenytoin. What long-term effects should the nurse advise the client can occur with prolonged administration of phenytoin? *Select all that apply.***

1. Gingival hypertrophy
2. Hirsutism
3. Hypertrophy of facial subcutaneous tissue
4. Dementia
5. Anemia

**100. A 60-year-old client has undergone a nerve-sparing prostatectomy and has been advised by his physician that he may not recover normal sexual functioning. The client is very concerned about this and asks the nurse for more information. Which of the following information should the nurse include? *Select all that apply.***

1. Retrograde ejaculation may occur.
2. Recovery rates vary but can take up to a year or more.
3. If sexual functioning is going to return, it will do so within a month.
4. Attempts at sexual intercourse are usually avoided for 1 month after surgery.
5. Anxiety can interfere with sexual functioning.
6. Other forms of sexual intimacy are more important than sexual intercourse.

# Answer Key and Explanations for Test #1

## Case Study 1

**1. 2, 3, 4, 6, and 7:** The client is showing some of the primary signs of a small bowel obstruction (i.e., abdominal pain and distension, vomiting, and possible constipation). The client also has a history of recent abdominal surgery—one of the most significant risk factors of small bowel obstruction. The client's laboratory results indicate possible inflammation consistent with small bowel obstruction (i.e., elevated WBC count) as well as possible dehydration (i.e., elevated creatinine and BUN values). Amber-colored urine could also indicate dehydration. It is essential for the nurse to alert the client's primary care provider about these findings as soon as possible. The patient's medical history is not concerning for any disease process related to the client's current symptoms, especially because urinary retention has been ruled out with the completion of the bladder scan and finding a postvoid residual measurement that is within normal limits. The patient's vital signs are stable at this point. Although the client's heart rate and respiration rate are slightly elevated, that is to be expected in the setting of acute pain. Elevated blood pressure is consistent with the patient's history of hypertension.

**2. 3:** The client is showing some of the primary signs of small bowel obstruction, including colicky abdominal pain and distension, vomiting, and constipation. Hyperactive bowel sounds, elevated WBCs, and signs of dehydration (i.e., elevated creatinine, elevated BUN) are also consistent with small bowel obstruction. Although cholecystitis (i.e., inflammation of the gallbladder) can present as abdominal pain in the right upper quadrant, the pain often radiates to the back or shoulders and is usually accompanied by an increase in bloating or gas, rather than no flatus. Cholecystitis is also often associated with an elevation in AST and ALT indicating liver damage. These laboratory values are within the normal range for this client. Although nephrolithiasis (i.e., kidney stones) could also cause acute pain and nausea/vomiting, the pain is typically located in the flank area and is often described as sharp or shooting and is not associated with distension.

**3. 2 and 3:** The client is at risk for infection due to the possibility of the bowel obstruction leading to a bowel perforation and subsequent peritonitis. The client is also directly at risk for dehydration because the small intestine is unable to properly absorb fluids due to the obstruction and due to the nothing-by-mouth (NPO) status needed to rest the bowel. Although the client is not at direct risk for urinary retention, his urine output should be monitored closely as an indication of hydration status and due to the client's medical history of benign prostatic hypertrophy. The client is also not at direct risk for respiratory distress as a result of the small bowel obstruction, and the client's respirations will likely normalize once his pain is under control.

**4.**

| Potential Orders | Indicated | Not Indicated |
|---|---|---|
| Initiate a clear liquid diet. | ○ | ● |
| Insert a nasogastric tube, and set it to low intermittent suction. | ● | ○ |
| Start a normal saline (0.9% NaCl) IV at 125 mL/hr. | ● | ○ |
| Administer morphine sulfate 5 mg IV every 4 hours as needed for pain. | ● | ○ |
| Insert a rectal tube. | ○ | ● |
| Administer metoclopramide 10 mg IV three times daily for constipation. | ○ | ● |

With a bowel obstruction, bowel rest is indicated, and the patient would be placed on strict NPO status, rather than on a clear liquid diet. A nasogastric tube set to suction is indicated because this aids in bowel decompression and promotes comfort by removing the stomach contents and reducing emesis. Fluid replacement via normal saline IV is indicated because this patient is at risk for dehydration due to his NPO status and due to the bowel being unable to optimally absorb fluids due to the obstruction. Pain management, such as with IV morphine, is a nursing priority because the client may be in acute pain with the obstruction. A rectal tube would not be helpful in the case of small bowel obstruction. Metoclopramide, although it is a treatment for constipation, is directly contraindicated in bowel obstructions because it induces peristalsis of the intestines.

**5. 2 and 5:** Giving the client instructions to tilt his chin and swallow during the insertion process helps guide the nasogastric tube into his stomach, rather than into his lungs. Providing proper oral care and skin care is a priority nursing intervention following nasogastric tube placement and NPO status because the client's mucous membranes are at risk for becoming dry and the nares are at risk for irritation from the nasogastric tube. The nurse should not measure from the tip of the *chin* to the earlobe to the xiphoid process in order to find the appropriate length but should instead measure from the tip of the *nose* to the earlobe to the xiphoid process. Ultrasound is not used to determine correct tube placement; instead, x-ray would be used if imaging were necessary. Finally, it is contraindicated to have the client lie flat following nasogastric tube insertion due to the risk of aspiration of his gastric contents. The client should instead be kept in a semi-Fowler's or upright position.

**6.**

> 1700: Nasogastric tube is inserted. Client reports feeling comfortable. There is no further emesis, and pain is currently 3/10 in the abdomen. Client reports toleration of his current pain level.
>
> 1830: Client voided 500 mL of clear amber urine. There was 250 mL of clear bile gastric output via suction.
>
> 2230: Client requested assistance with reaching the television remote; he was observed lying very still in bed and was unwilling to lean forward to reach for the remote due to the pain in his abdomen. Client reports that his pain is 9/10 on the right side of his abdomen. Client has hyperactive bowel sounds; the abdomen is board-like upon palpation. The primary care physician was notified of these findings.

The client is demonstrating signs of peritonitis, a very serious complication of small bowel obstruction that can result if the bowel perforates and the contents infect the abdominal cavity. Peritonitis should be suspected in patients demonstrating increased or severe abdominal pain, muscle guarding or unwillingness to move due to pain, and a board-like abdomen. The provider should be notified immediately because this development often requires emergency surgery. Although the patient's urine is amber in color and should continue to be monitored, this is not a change from when the patient was admitted and is not a sign of declining condition at this time.

## Case Study 2

**1. 3 and 4:** Fetal well-being should be assessed to ensure that adequate oxygenation and blood flow are being delivered through the placenta. The severely elevated blood pressure puts the client at risk for seizures and placental abruption and should be managed immediately. All other abnormal findings can be addressed after immediately initiating fetal monitoring and maternal blood pressure management measures.

2.

| Client Findings | Placental Abruption | Preeclampsia | Maternal Heart Failure |
|---|---|---|---|
| Blood pressure | □ | ■ | □ |
| Headache | □ | ■ | □ |
| Lower extremity swelling | □ | ■ | ■ |
| Epigastric pain | □ | ■ | □ |
| Temperature | ■ | ■ | ■ |
| Respiratory rate | ■ | □ | ■ |

Preeclampsia symptoms include elevated blood pressure, severe headache, epigastric pain, and overactive reflexes. Preeclampsia can affect multiple organs throughout the body secondary to decreased blood flow throughout the blood vessels to important organs. Placental abruption is an emergency in and of itself, but it can also be caused by preeclampsia. Signs of placental abruption can include severe abdominal pain, tachycardia, vaginal bleeding, and in worst cases absent fetal movement. Maternal heart failure presents with symptoms of chest pain, difficulty breathing, increased edema, and low oxygen saturation. For all three conditions, the client would present as normothermic.

3.

| Potential Nursing Interventions | Indicated | Not Indicated |
|---|---|---|
| Assess headache every 2 hours. | ○ | ● |
| Assess deep tendon reflexes every hour. | ● | ○ |
| Auscultate lung sounds every 1–2 hours. | ● | ○ |
| Monitor blood pressure every hour. | ● | ○ |
| Evaluate lower extremity edema every 1–2 hours. | ○ | ● |
| Monitor magnesium levels. | ● | ○ |
| Strict input and output monitoring. | ● | ○ |

The client's deep tendon reflexes should be monitored hourly to assess for magnesium toxicity. Auscultating lung sounds every 1–2 hours is necessary to ensure that the client does not develop fluid overload or pulmonary edema. Monitoring blood pressure readings hourly is indicated to assure that the client's blood pressure is well controlled. Monitoring magnesium levels is indicated in order to maintain a therapeutic level. Strict input and output monitoring is indicated to further ensure that fluid overload is avoided.

**4. 1**: The nurse's first priority should be to initiate the magnesium infusion to prevent the progression of preeclampsia and the onset of seizure activity. Magnesium induces vasodilation of the blood vessels, including the cerebral vascular system, which helps decrease the risk of seizures. Magnesium is also a calcium antagonist, which causes a decrease in cerebral and vascular resistance. Additionally, magnesium provides neuroprotection for the fetus.

**5. 3 and 4:** The client is experiencing magnesium toxicity, and the magnesium infusion should be discontinued. Signs and symptoms of magnesium toxicity include lethargy, overactive reflexes, decreased heart rate, confusion, and breathing problems. Reversal of magnesium toxicity requires the immediate discontinuation of the infusion and administration of the antidote, which is calcium gluconate.

6.

The client is now alert and states that she is feeling more like herself. The fetal heart rate continues to be reassuring. The client's labor is now being induced, and the client is progressing as expected. The physician ordered a new magnesium level, which has returned at 4.1 mg/dL. The client's urine output has been averaging 15 mL/hr for the past several hours. The client is resting comfortably with an epidural currently infusing.

| Vital Signs | 1800 |
|---|---|
| HR | 75 |
| RR | 18 |
| BP | 170/80 |
| Temp | 98.3 °F |
| Pulse oximetry | 97% on room air |

It is important to notify the physician of the client's sustained high blood pressure reading because additional blood pressure management may be required in the form of pharmacological approaches. The magnesium level is not in a therapeutic range and supplementation may need to be restarted. The kidneys may have been affected with regard to the decrease in urine output (the acceptable rate in an adult is at least 30 mL/hr), which would require further investigation (in the form of laboratory measures) and interventions based on the lab results.

## Case Study 3

**1. 3, 4, 5, and 6:** The client is demonstrating new-onset acute confusion, hyperactivity that fluctuated throughout the night, and hallucinations. The nurse should follow up on these findings immediately because they are of concern for mental status changes. The nurse should keep in mind the client's increased risk factors for delirium, such as advanced age, recent surgery, and taking medication that can cause delirium. The client's vital signs are within normal limits at this time and do not require immediate follow-up. Mild to moderate pain is expected following hip surgery, and, although it should be monitored and treated, it does not require immediate follow-up.

**2. 3:** The client is manifesting several signs of hyperactive delirium, including a sudden onset of confusion, inattention, and disorientation. Delirium is distinct from dementia in that its onset is usually rapid, over hours to days, whereas dementia develops and progresses at a more gradual pace. Although a transient ischemic attack can also result in confusion and disorientation, the symptoms typically last for just a few minutes and resolve independently. In comparison, delirium often persists until the underlying cause is addressed, sometimes for days or weeks. Sundowning can manifest with similar symptoms to delirium; however, the behaviors are typically limited to the afternoon and evening hours, whereas delirium lasts throughout the day and can fluctuate in severity.

**3. 1 and 3:** The most immediate risk to a client with delirium, especially an elderly client with mobility impairments, is risk for injury due to falls because the client is often unaware of his surroundings or abilities. The client is also at risk for persistent altered mental status because delirium can persist for days to weeks if the underlying cause is not identified and addressed. With delirium, the client is not at an immediate risk for aspiration pneumonia or one-sided weakness as he would be if he were having a stroke or demonstrating other neurological changes.

**4.**

| Potential Nursing Interventions | Indicated | Not Indicated |
|---|---|---|
| Remove the clock and calendar from the client's room. | ○ | ● |
| Request that the client's adult son remain in the room with him at his bedside. | ● | ○ |

| Potential Nursing Interventions | Indicated | Not Indicated |
|---|---|---|
| Open the blinds each morning promptly at the beginning of the shift. | ● | ○ |
| Remove the client's eyeglasses and hearing aids so that they are not broken or lost. | ○ | ● |
| Monitor the client closely for pain, and treat it promptly. | ● | ○ |
| Place the client's walker within reach at his bedside. | ● | ○ |

A key nursing intervention for clients with delirium is to reorient them to reality. Clocks and calendars can be helpful with this and should remain in the room. The nurse should also encourage family members to stay at his bedside because familiar faces can help with the client with reorientation and can help promote safety by encouraging the client to stay in bed. Nurses should also help orient the client to the correct time of day and should prevent disruptions to his circadian rhythm by opening the blinds in the morning promptly to allow for natural sunlight to enter the room and turning off lights and keeping noise levels low in the evenings to promote sleep. The client should be encouraged to wear his eyeglasses and hearing aids as he normally would because altered sensory perception can cause confusion and increase delirium. Pain management is another important aspect of delirium management: If the patient's pain is not addressed, it can increase his agitation. The nurse should leave the client's walker near the bed in case he attempts to get out of bed on his own to reduce his risk for falls.

**5. 2, 4, and 5:** Diphenhydramine can increase the risk of delirium in elderly clients, and it should be discontinued. With delirium, it is important to identify any underlying causes such as electrolyte imbalances or infection, so blood work and urine samples would be indicated. IV fluids would be avoided for stable clients who are able to drink adequate amounts of fluids independently, especially in the case of delirium in which additional lines and tubes may increase the client's agitation. Restraints are not typically indicated for clients with delirium except as a last resort if other interventions have failed and the client is at great risk for harming him- or herself or others; in this case, other interventions would be attempted first prior to using restraints. Although haloperidol can be used to calm clients with delirium, it would not be a first-line intervention due to its risk for side effects, including dizziness, drowsiness, and extrapyramidal symptoms.

**6.**

| Assessment Findings | Improved | Unchanged | Worsened |
|---|---|---|---|
| HR, 80 | ○ | ● | ○ |
| Oxygen level, 94% | ○ | ● | ○ |
| Client's conversation with his son | ● | ○ | ○ |
| Client's sleep pattern | ○ | ○ | ● |
| Client's mobility status | ○ | ● | ○ |

The client's vital signs remain stable and within normal limits and do not indicate any changes. The client's conversation with his son indicates that he was at least temporarily oriented to his current reality, which is an improvement. However, the client's excessive daytime sleepiness is of concern for hypoactive delirium and may be a sign that the client has mixed delirium with fluctuating elements of hyperactivity and hypoactivity. The nurse should continue to monitor this closely. The client's mobility status continues to be stable and does not indicate any changes.

## Standalone Questions

**1. 75:** Calculation:

$$\text{Volume (mL)} \times \text{drop factor/total minutes} = \text{flow rate}$$
$$3 \text{ hours and } 20 \text{ minutes} = 200 \text{ minutes}$$
$$1{,}000 \times 15/200 = 75 \text{ drops/min}$$

**2. 1, 3, 5:** Mastitis is a bacterial infection of the breast, most often caused by *Staphylococcus aureus* from the infant, so the mother can continue to breastfeed. The usual treatment includes antibiotics (such as penicillin G or erythromycin). Pain control is achieved with ibuprofen or acetaminophen and alternating hot and cold compresses. The mother should be encouraged to massage her breasts in a hot shower and to pump or express milk on the infected side to prevent an abscess from forming.

**3. 1, 2, 5:** Parents should be advised to follow the manufacturer's directions for securing a car seat. Infants should be placed in rear-facing car seats with no padding underneath them. The shoulder straps should be fed through slots at or below the infant's shoulders and the harness positioned with the clasp at the middle of the chest. The car seat should be positioned so that the infant's head does not fall forward. For neonates, bolsters (such as a rolled infant blanket or diaper) should be placed beside the infant's head to maintain it in a neutral position.

**4. 3:** This pattern of arrhythmias is seen in ventricular tachycardia, which is a very fast heart rate originating in the ventricles. Both ventricular tachycardia and ventricular fibrillation, which looks like an irregular up-and-down pattern on an ECG, can indicate myocardial infarction and other life-threatening situations. Atrial fibrillation can be associated with conditions like mitral valve prolapse, and is indicated on an ECG by irregularly spaced patterns without distinguishable P waves. Paroxysmal atrial tachycardia is a sudden pattern of more rapid heartbeats that lasts for a brief time; it can be seen in cardiac patients but often occurs in healthy people as well.

**5. 1:** For insertion of a nasogastric tube, the client should be placed in the high Fowler's position with the head tilted forward because this position helps to close the trachea and open the esophagus, facilitating correct insertion. The nurse should examine the nasal passages by occluding one naris and then the other while the client is breathing through the nose and should use the side with the best airflow. The length of the tube should be estimated by measuring the distance from the tip of the nose, around the ear, and down to just below the left coastal margin. The end of the tube is lubricated, and then the tube is inserted slowly. The client may suck on ice cubes or swallow small sips of water during the procedure.

**6. 2:** Because the liver is located on the right side, the client should be positioned in the right side-lying position with a folded towel or small pillow under the biopsy site to apply pressure for at least three hours after the procedure is completed. The client should avoid straining or coughing. If this procedure is done on an outpatient basis, upon discharge the client should be advised to avoid any heavy lifting, strenuous exercise, or straining for one week.

**7. 2:** The PR interval is the duration between atrial polarization (i.e., the beginning of the P wave) and ventricular depolarization (i.e., the beginning of the QRS complex, or the beginning of the R wave if no Q wave deflection is present). In this tracing, there are approximately five small boxes comprising the PR interval, which is a duration of approximately 0.20 s (5 × 0.04 s). The normal range for the PR interval is 0.12–0.20 s.

**8. 1:** The client is exhibiting signs of obstruction. Because the secretions are very thick, the best action is to increase the humidification to help loosen the secretions and suction the tracheostomy tube. Suction should not be used during insertion of the suction catheter because this removes oxygen and may traumatize the tracheal tissue, but suction should be used for 5–10 seconds while the catheter is removed. Suctioning for longer periods should be avoided because it may result in hypoxia.

**9. 3:** Continuous bubbling in the water seal chamber indicates a system air leak. Intermittent bubbling occurs with pneumothorax as the air flows from the chest cavity into the chamber. The water level in the water seal chamber should fluctuate. If the fluctuation stops, this is generally an indication of a problem, such as obstruction of the chest tube or inadequate suction. However, it may also indicate reexpansion of the lung. The collection chamber is monitored for drainage. The suction control chamber should exhibit gentle bubbling.

**10. 1:** Digoxin is a medication used to treat heart failure, atrial flutter, and atrial fibrillation. It slows the heart rate and the rate of conduction through the AV node. Patients who are receiving digoxin therapy may have the following ECG changes:

- Sloping ST depression (i.e., the appearance of a reverse checkmark)
- T wave changes: flattened, inverted, or biphasic, peaking of the terminal part of the T wave
- Prominent U waves
- J point depression
- Prolonged PR interval (up to 0.24 s)

**11. 3:** Medications with antithrombotic properties, such as aspirin or nonsteroidal anti-inflammatory drugs (NSAIDs), are usually avoided the morning of a surgery, although other routine medications may generally be taken with a sip of water a few hours before scheduled surgery. Some medications, such as warfarin, may be discontinued for a few days prior to surgery because of the increased risk of bleeding. All medications (prescription and over the counter [OTC]) should be reviewed with the client, and instructions about use of the medication in relation to the surgery should be provided.

**12. 112:** One milligram contains 1,000 micrograms, and 1 gram contains one million micrograms. Although the symbol μg is used to represent micrograms, the Food and Drug Administration (FDA) and the Institute for Safe Medication Practices (ISMP) recommend against using this symbol because it may easily be confused with the abbreviation for milligrams (mg). The abbreviation mcg is sometimes used. Calculation:

$$0.112 \text{ mg} \times 1{,}000 \frac{\text{mcg}}{\text{mg}} = 112 \text{ mcg}$$

**13. 3:** Clients with rubella (German measles) must be maintained on droplet precautions. Standard precautions apply to all clients regardless of other precautions.

| | |
|---|---|
| **Contact** | Use personal protective equipment (PPE), including gown and gloves, for all contact with the client or the client's immediate environment. Clients should be in private rooms or >3 feet from other clients. |
| **Droplet** | Use a mask while caring for the client. Clients should be in a private room or >3 feet away from other clients with a curtain separating them. The patient must be masked for transport. |
| **Airborne** | Place the client in an airborne infection isolation room, and use ≥N95 respirators (or masks) for client care. |

**14. 1:** All of the laboratory results are within the normal range except for the platelet count. The normal range for platelets is 150,000–450,000, so 119,000 is low. This indicates thrombocytopenia, which may increase the risk of bleeding and bruising. A decrease in platelets may indicate aplastic anemia, alcohol toxicity, prolonged hypoxia, iron-deficiency anemia, megaloblastic anemia, or a viral infection. Severe infection may also suppress platelets. The risk of bleeding with invasive procedures is usually minimal until the count drops below 50,000, and the risk is most severe with counts below 20,000.

**15. 1, 2, 3, 4, 5, 6:** Diabetic ketoacidosis (DKA) occurs when the amount of insulin is insufficient, resulting in hyperglycemia. Indications include polyuria and polydipsia, hyperventilation (Kussmaul respirations), blurred vision, weakness, headache, abdominal pain, orthostatic hypotension, and mental status changes. Clinically, the primary indications are hyperglycemia, dehydration, electrolyte imbalance, and acidosis. The primary causes of DKA are missing a dose of insulin, illness or infection, and untreated diabetes mellitus. Illness and infection can increase the need for insulin even if food intake is decreased.

**16. 2:** A minor cannot sign a surgical consent unless she is emancipated. Although a surgeon may, in an emergency, perform surgery on a minor without parental or legal guardian consent, every effort should be made to locate a parent or guardian. If reached by telephone, the parent or guardian can give consent verbally, but two witnesses should listen to the conversation and document that consent was given for the procedure, noting the name of the person granting consent.

**17. 3:** For intermittent tube feedings, the client should be positioned with the head of the bed elevated to 30° to prevent aspiration. The client should remain in this position for at least an hour after each feeding, and the head of the bed should stay elevated to at least 30° at all times if he is receiving continuous feedings. Placement of the tube should be verified through aspiration and assessing the pH of the aspirant prior to every intermittent feeding and at least every 12 hours for continuous feeding.

**18. 3:** Although 60% of the adult's body is composed of water, 67% of this amount is intracellular fluid (ICF), 25% is interstitial fluid (ISF) (found in the spaces between cells, tissues, and organs), and 8% is plasma volume (PV). ISF and PV are classified as extracellular fluids. Fluid balance is extremely important for life because death usually occurs when 20–25% of the total body water is lost, such as through dehydration.

**19. 1:** Whole blood is rarely administered, although it may be given for extreme loss of blood volume when the red blood cells and the plasma need replacement. The most commonly used blood products are packed red blood cells and fresh frozen plasma, so whole blood is usually separated into these components. Red blood cells are preferred for most indications because the extra plasma found in whole blood may result in transfusion-associated circulatory overload.

**20. 4:** These symptoms are consistent with hypoparathyroidism and hypocalcemia, so the physician is likely to monitor the calcium level. One complication of thyroidectomies is trauma to or inadvertent removal of the parathyroid glands. This can result in hyperphosphatemia and hypocalcemia because of decreased intestinal absorption of dietary calcium and decreased resorption from bone related to inadequate parathyroid hormone. Hypocalcemia causes tetany, which may manifest as numbness, tingling, and stiffness in the hands, feet, and face and muscle spasms and contractions. Clients may experience anxiety, depression, and hypotension.

**21. 1:** Constipation and fecal impaction are common with chemotherapy and opioids. Chemotherapeutic agents may cause dysfunction of the autonomic nerves, resulting in abdominal discomfort, and rectal emptying may be slowed. Opioids slow the intestinal motility, so the combination increases the risk of obstruction. The client should have an abdominal examination and abdominal x-ray to evaluate for an obstruction before further treatments because the client has not been passing flatus and has increasing pain and nausea.

**22. 3:** Although difficulty with urination, frequency, and urgency are the usual signs of a urinary tract infection (UTI), these may be absent in elderly clients who frequently exhibit nonspecific symptoms, such as anorexia, hyperventilation, low-grade fever, and new onset of urinary incontinence. General fatigue or malaise is the most common presenting symptom in older adults. Cognitive function may also be impaired, and those with dementia may show a sudden cognitive decline. The most common causative agent for UTI in elderly clients is *Escherichia coli.*

**23. 1:** Although protocols for dealing with medication errors may vary from one institution to another, in most cases, the correct response is to notify the physician, notify the supervisor, and complete an incident report. The nurse should not attempt to cover the mistake by obtaining a physician's order after the fact. Usually, documenting an error on the client's record consists only of documenting the actual treatment given—in this case the acetaminophen—but omitting further information about the error and documenting that only in the incident report.

**24. 1:** This ECG strip represents sinus tachycardia, which is characterized by regular atrial and ventricular rhythms and a heart rate between 100 and 160 bpm. The P wave is usually normal in size and shape and occurs before each QRS complex, although the amplitude may be increased. If the heart rate is too rapid, the P wave may be difficult to identify or may be superimposed on the preceding T wave. While the QT interval usually shortens, the PR interval, QRS complex, and T wave are typically normal.

**25. 4:** In atrial tachycardia, a type of SVT, electrical impulses are generated from a single area of the right or left atrium at a rate that is so rapid that it overrides the SA node. On the ECG, atrial tachycardia is characterized by a rapid atrial rate (100–250 bpm). P waves are typically abnormal in shape or may be hidden in the preceding T wave. The rhythm is regular, and the QRS complex is normal.

**26. 3:** These are indications that the client may be experiencing hearing loss. Hearing loss may be insidious, with the client not being fully aware that his hearing is impaired. Because hearing loss may impair the person's ability to hear his own voice as well as others' voices, he may begin slurring his words or dropping word endings. Clients may react to hearing loss by becoming depressed, withdrawn, and irritable, and they may believe that people are whispering or talking behind their backs because they cannot hear what people are saying.

**27. 2, 3, 5:** Although unlicensed assistive personnel (UAP) can check routine temperatures and vital signs, they should not be responsible for assessing the condition of a client who is acutely ill. UAP may empty catheter bags and measure urinary output as long as they have been trained in the proper techniques, and they may assist ambulatory clients with walking to the bathroom or help clients with a bedpan. The nurse who delegates the task is always responsible for supervising the UAP and ensuring that the task is completed appropriately.

**28. 1:** Engorgement often occurs in the first two to three days after delivery as the mother begins to produce milk and nurse the infant. Because the infant's intake the first few days is usually very small, the production of milk may exceed demand, resulting in breasts that are swollen, taut, and painful. The mother should be encouraged to continue to nurse and gently massage the breast toward the nipple. Application of cold compresses for 15–20 minutes in between feedings may relieve swelling and discomfort. The mother may take acetaminophen for pain. Engorgement usually lasts only 24–48 hours.

**29. 21:** Calculation:

$$\text{Volume (mL)} \times \text{drop factor/total minutes} = \text{flow rate}$$
$$250 \times 10 = 2{,}500$$
$$2 \text{ hours} = 120 \text{ minutes}$$
$$2{,}500/120 = 20.83 \approx 21 \text{ drops per minute}$$

**30. Correct order:**

| | | | | | | |
|---|---|---|---|---|---|---|
| Milliliter | Centiliter | Deciliter | Liter | Dekaliter | Hectoliter | Kiloliter |

1: II. Milliliter
2: I. Deciliter
3: III. Dekaliter
4: V. Hectoliter
5: IV. Kiloliter

**31. 1, 2, 3, 5:** Organ meats, such as liver, and some seafood, such as sardines, mackerels, and scallops, are high in purines and should be avoided. All meats contain purines, so their intake should be limited to 4–6 ounces per day. Broth made from meats should be avoided. Because alcohol impairs the elimination of uric acid, wine intake should not exceed 10 ounces daily. Foods high in fat also impair elimination, so high-fat foods, such as avocados and ice cream, should be limited.

**32. 1:** Although all of these are important, histamine is released in response to the antigen, causing erythema and edema, which can result in airway obstruction, so the primary concern is to ensure patency of the airway. This may require intubation. Epinephrine should be administered as soon as possible, and oxygen is provided at 100% high flow. Intravenous fluids are provided to combat hypotension. Albuterol may be given to relieve bronchospasm. If shock continues, diphenhydramine and methylprednisolone may be required.

**33. 50:** Calculation:

$$\text{Volume (mL)} \times \text{drop factor/total minutes} = \text{flow rate}$$
$$250 \times 60/5 \times 60 = 15{,}000/300$$
$$15{,}000/300 = 50 \text{ drops per minute}$$

**34. 3:** One grain is equal to 60–65 mg (the calculation depends on the manufacturer), so 325 mg is approximately equivalent to five grains of aspirin. Grains are used in the apothecary method of measurement, but only a few medications are still provided using this measurement because most are now provided using metric measurements, such as milligrams. Household measurements, such as ounces and teaspoons, are also used for medications, so nurses should be familiar with conversions among the different measurement systems.

**35. 120:** Calculation:

$$40 \text{ (kg)} \times 15 \text{ (mg per kg)} = 600 \text{ mg per day}$$
$$600 \text{ (mg per day)} \times 10 \text{ (total days)} = 6{,}000 \text{ mg total}$$
$$250/5 = 6{,}000/x$$
$$250x = 30{,}000$$
$$30{,}000/250 = 120 \text{ mL}$$

**36. 2:** Milliliters are metric measurements, and teaspoons are household measurements. Five milliliters is approximately equivalent to one teaspoon, so the child will require two teaspoons for 10 mL of oral suspension. Oral suspensions are often prescribed in household measurements to reduce the chance of medication errors for those unfamiliar with the metric system.

**37. 3:** In the event of a fire, the client must be evacuated as quickly as possible. Because the client has not yet ambulated and the repaired hip must remain abducted, transferring the client to a wheelchair or attempting to carry the client is precluded. Transferring the client to a gurney is too time-consuming. The best solution to moving a client to a safe area as quickly as possible is to move the client in the bed.

**38. 1:** Restraints cannot be applied as the first intervention, so the nurse must attempt other interventions first, such as trying to camouflage the IV with clothing or dressings. Tying a length of IV tubing to the bedrail and allowing the client to pull on it may distract the client. Restraints may result in injuries and should be avoided whenever possible. Vest restraints have resulted in a number of deaths, so many facilities no longer allow their use.

**39. 1:** With pulseless electrical activity, some type of cardiac electrical activity is present but no mechanical activity or contractions are taking place, so there is no palpable pulse and the heart cannot maintain systemic perfusion. Its appearance on the ECG may vary. For example, it may present as a normal sinus rhythm. Pulseless electrical activity does not respond to defibrillation but can be treated with epinephrine.

**40. 0.25:** Calculation:

$$(1 \text{ mg})/(1 \text{ mL}) = (0.25 \text{ mg})/(x \text{ mL})$$
$$1x = 0.25$$
$$x = 0.25 \text{ mL}$$

**41. 4:** The nurse should assess the client's level of pain. Deep breathing, coughing, and turning may be very painful in the first 24–48 hours after major surgery, but they are necessary to prevent atelectasis and other complications. Clients who are in pain are often very reluctant to cooperate, so the nurse should ensure that the client has received adequate analgesia prior to the first time she is asked to deep breathe, cough, and turn.

**42. 2:** The elbow comprises the simplest type of joint: the hinge. The only movements a hinge joint can perform are flexion and extension. Flexion involves the biceps brachii, brachialis, and brachioradialis muscles, and extension uses the triceps brachii. Three bones (the humerus, ulna, and radius) come together at the elbow but in two different joints—the hinged elbow joint and the pivot proximal radioulnar joint, which allows the forearm to supinate and pronate.

**43. 3:** This ECG strip shows an accelerated idioventricular rhythm (AIVR) with a heart rate of 56 bpm. The QRS complex represents ventricular contraction. The QRS complex is generally measured from the first downward deflection of the Q wave, but this downward deflection may be absent, as in this example. The QRS complex is prolonged at 0.18 s (normal QRS duration is 0.06–0.10 s), and the P wave is absent. A wide QRS complex is an indication of abnormal conduction.

**44. 4:** The ECG tracing shown is an example of an elevated ST segment. The ST segment should be within 1 mm of the isoelectric line in the limb leads. In the precordial leads, an elevation of up to 2 mm may be normal in some individuals, but if the elevation is greater than 1 mm in limb leads or greater than 2 mm in precordial leads, this suggests acute myocardial infarction or other cardiac abnormality.

**45. 2:** The QT interval extends from the beginning of the Q deflection to the end of the T wave and represents the total time for ventricular depolarization and repolarization. In the tracing, the QT interval is 0.48 s, or 480 ms.

- Each large box is equal to 0.20 seconds: $0.20 \text{ s} \times 2 = 0.40 \text{ s}$
- Each small box in the remaining box is equal to 0.04 s: $0.04 \text{ s} \times 2 = 0.08 \text{ s}$
- $0.40 \text{ s} + 0.08 \text{ s} = 0.48 \text{ s}$

**46. 2:** The Braden Scale is used to determine if the client is at risk for developing pressure sores. The scale assesses six different areas with scores of 1–4 or 1–3. The lower the total score, the higher the risk. The six areas are sensory perception, moisture, activity, mobility, usual nutrition pattern, and friction and sheer. The Braden Scale is used to help identify the need for a support surface and the type of support surface appropriate for the client's needs.

**47. 4:** Healthcare providers should have priority for protection from injury because if they are injured, then no one will be available to provide care to the others who are injured. Police officers and firefighters are usually the first responders in a disaster, and they must determine when it is safe for healthcare providers to enter the area and provide care. In some cases, this may mean that care for the injured is delayed because of unsafe conditions.

**48. 2:** The statement that indicates the client has not given informed consent is: "I told the doctor I didn't want to know anything about the surgery, and she agreed." The physician has a responsibility to inform the client of the risks and benefits of the treatment and any alternative treatment options even if the client does not want this information. A client who refuses to receive the information may be in denial or may not yet be emotionally prepared to deal with the reality of the treatment.

**49. 3:** Although these are all important considerations, the installed height, the ratio of computers to staff, and the brand of computer are focused on the needs of the staff. However, the positioning of the computer screens away from the line of sight of clients and visitors is essential for maintaining client confidentiality. The screens must be positioned so that others cannot read what is being documented about a client. Computers must be kept in a secure area. In some cases, privacy screens or filters may be used.

**50. 4:** The trough time is when the blood level is at its lowest (in the trough), so the serum trough level should be drawn immediately before a scheduled dose of the medication is due. Blood levels of a drug may also be measured at the peak time. This will vary from drug to drug and should always be checked at the time prescribed. When drawing blood for trough and peak levels, it's important that the medication doses be administered on time.

**51. 1,140:** Calculation:

$$75\ (\text{g protein}) \times 4 = 300\ (\text{calories})$$
$$120\ (\text{g carbohydrate}) \times 4 = 480\ (\text{calories})$$
$$40\ (\text{g fat}) \times 9 = 360\ (\text{calories})$$
$$300 + 480 + 360 = 1{,}140$$

**52. 2:** The nurse should contact the admissions department and ask that the client be reassigned to a different room. Although superstitions may seem irrational at times, fear and anxiety can negatively impact recovery. Anxiety before surgery is common, but severe anxiety can result in an increased induction time and an increased need for analgesia in the postoperative period. Superstitions can compound the fear because the client may feel that the negative outcomes he fears (e.g., pain or disability) are more likely to occur.

**53. 1, 3, 4:** Because this client is transient and homeless, he probably does not have easy access to a computer or friends and family who can help, so he will most likely have to rely on public agencies and services, such as self-help programs, community agencies (including mental health outreach services), and government agencies (such as Medicaid or Social Security). Although the nurse can provide homeless clients with information, follow-up can be poor among homeless and transient populations.

**54. 3:** At 3 L/min per nasal cannula, the client should receive about 32% $FiO_2$. Nasal cannulas deliver low concentrations of oxygen, but they are relatively safe and easily tolerated, although they may cause drying and irritation of nasal passages. The $FiO_2$ measurement may be affected by nasal obstruction and breathing patterns. $FiO_2$ per L/min:

1 L/min: 24%
2 L/min: 28%
3 L/min: 32%
4 L/min: 36%
5 L/min: 40%
6 L/min: 44%

**55. 1:** The statement "I need my husband to take care of financial matters" suggests that the client's wife has not accepted that her husband's condition will continue to deteriorate and, because of behavioral and language difficulties, he will not be able to manage their financial affairs. She will need to assume responsibilities that were previously handled by her husband, who will become increasingly dependent. This change in roles can be very difficult for a spouse, especially as the behaviors worsen and profound personality changes occur.

**56. 3:** Alcohol, benzodiazepines, and barbiturates pose the greatest risk to life if clients attempt to undergo "cold-turkey" withdrawal. Patients may experience seizures, heart attacks, or strokes. Withdrawal from alcohol may result in delirium tremens (DTs). Clients undergoing withdrawal from opiates, such as heroin, may experience severe physical symptoms (nausea, vomiting, pain, muscle cramping, dyspnea, tremors, palpitations, and sweating). However, the symptoms are rarely life threatening. Those withdrawing from cocaine and marijuana have milder withdrawal symptoms (anxiety, insomnia, headaches, and depression).

**57. 4:** In a crisis situation, such as a client shouting at the nurse and refusing to stop smoking marijuana, the best initial response is to remain calm and simply repeat the request. Challenges and threats often cause the client who is angry and belligerent to escalate her behavior. The nurse should not intrude on the client's personal space and should be aware of body language and nonverbal communication so as not to appear to be challenging. If possible, the nurse should try to identify the cause of the client's behavior by asking, "Are you feeling nervous about your upcoming tests?" so the nurse can better understand the whole situation.

**58. 1, 2, 3, 5:** The diagnostic criteria for PTSD includes exposure to actual or threatened death, serious injury, or sexual violation. The disturbance causes clinically significant distress or impairment. Diagnosis is based on behavioral symptoms which include:

- Re-experiencing (flashbacks, spontaneous memories of the traumatic event, nightmares, or other intense psychological distress)
- Avoidance (estrangement from others or diminished interest in activities, to an inability to remember key aspects of the event)
- Negative cognitions and mood (wide range of feelings from a persistent and distorted sense of blame of self or others to distressing memories, feelings, thoughts or external reminders of the event)
- Arousal (aggressive, reckless, or self-destructive behavior; insomnia; hypervigilance or related problems)

Symptoms usually present within three months of a traumatic event, although the reaction may be delayed for many months or years in some individuals.

**59. 1:** Clients should never flush needles or sharps down the toilet but should instead store and dispose of them in accordance with state or local regulations. In some places, needles and sharps must be placed in special sharps containers, but in other places, they may be placed in any secure, puncture-proof container with a lid. People who must dispose of needles and sharps in the community should contact their local refuse disposal service for information about disposal.

**60. 0.4:** Calculation:

$$(10\text{ mg})/(1\text{ mL}) = (4\text{ mg})/(x\text{ mL})$$
$$10x = 4$$
$$4/10 = 0.4\text{ mL}$$

**61. 1, 4, 6:** Peripheral arterial insufficiency is characterized by throbbing, cramping pain that increases with exercise; shiny skin with decreased hair; pale color on elevation; and redness on dependency. The skin is cool to the touch because of impaired circulation. Clients may complain of numbness, tingling, or reduced sensation. Capillary refill is greater than two seconds. Ulcerations tend to occur on the tips of the toes or at the sites of trauma and are deep and well delineated.

**62. Order of actions:**

1. V: Hang the irrigation solution bag with the bottom 20 inches above the stoma.
2. IV: Apply the irrigation sleeve over the stoma.
3. III: Apply gloves, lubricate the cone tip, and insert it into the stoma, holding it securely.
4. II: Allow the solution to flow in for 5–10 minutes and then clamp the tubing and close the top of the irrigation sleeve.
5. I: Allow 15–20 minutes for evacuation and then fold the sleeve, secure it, and leave it in place for 30–45 minutes before removing it.

**63. 3:** Because these signs and symptoms are indicative of obstructive sleep apnea, the client will likely be scheduled for a nocturnal polysomnogram. For the test, which is generally conducted in a sleep center, electrodes are placed on the head, face, and body as well as sensors to evaluate respiratory effort, snoring, airflow, and oxygen saturation. The client spends the night in the sleep center so the different stages of sleep can be observed.

**64. 4:** A nonstress test measures the fetus's heart rate and accelerations during a 20- to 40-minute period. The mother is in the semi-Fowler's position with support placed beneath the right hip so the uterus is displaced to the left. An ultrasound transducer is placed on the abdomen to measure the FHR, and a tocodynamometer is placed over the fundus area of the uterus to monitor uterine contractions and fetal movement. A normal (reactive) result is 2 or more accelerations of the FHR of 15 bpm above baseline for ≥15 seconds. An abnormal (nonreactive) result is less than 2 accelerations of the FHR in a 40-minute period.

**65. 1, 2, 3, 5:** An aphasia assessment includes observations of spontaneous speech (fluent, nonfluent, grammatical errors, and slow or hesitant speech), comprehension of spoken language (ability to follow simple and then more complex commands), comprehension of written language (ability to read and follow written commands), ability to name items (but not describe), ability to recall four named items (immediately, not after five minutes), and the ability to write. The nurse should observe the client carefully during the assessment for signs of frustration or fatigue.

**66. 2:** If a client receiving end-of-life care tells the nurse that he has not always lived the way he should have or treated his children well, the most appropriate response is: "There are things that you regret." This states the point that the client is making without being judgmental or questioning. At the end of life, clients often think back over their lives and consider both positive and negative aspects. They often are not seeking advice but rather an opportunity to verbalize feelings.

**67. 2:** The area of contact for the automated external defibrillator (AED) pads must be dry, so the nurse should wipe the chest dry with an available dry cloth or ask someone else to do it while she continues cardiopulmonary resuscitation (CPR). The chest should not be wiped with alcohol because this could cause a spark and a fire when the AED shocks the heart. The pads should also not be placed over medicine patches, pacemakers, or implanted defibrillators. Different models of AEDs have slightly different directions, but most have audible directions and pictures that are easy to follow.

**68. 3:** Dressings over intravenous (IV) insertion sites are usually left undisturbed for 5–7 days if they are transparent to allow clear visibility and if there is no tenderness. However, gauze dressings must be changed every 48 hours. If a gauze dressing is under a transparent dressing, then the dressing change schedule remains at 48 hours. In any case, the dressing should be changed if it loosens or is compromised or if signs of infection are evident.

**69. 4:** All neonates should be screened for hearing loss, according to the US Preventive Services Task Force. Although those with identifiable risk factors, such as family history, admission to a neonatal intensive care, and craniofacial abnormalities, have up to 20 times the risk of other infants of having hearing loss, about half of infants with hearing loss have no identifiable risk factors. Testing is recommended for all neonates within one month of birth. Those who fail the hearing test should undergo a complete evaluation by three months.

**70. 9:** Calculation:

$$\begin{aligned} 20\ (\text{kg}) \times 45\ (\text{mg}) &= 900 \text{ mg in 24 hours} \\ 900/2 &= 450 \text{ mg each dose (every 12 hours)} \\ 250\ (\text{mg})/5\ (\text{mL}) &= 450\ (\text{mg})/x\ (\text{mL}) \\ 250x &= 2{,}250 \\ 2{,}250/250 &= 9 \text{ mL} \end{aligned}$$

**71. 4:** Rate response refers to the pacing rate increasing when the sensors note increased activity. Rate smoothing is a pacemaker function that prevents excessive changes in the pacing rate. Rate drop response is when the pacing rate increases above the normal pacing rate with sudden bradycardia. Mode switching is when the pacemaker switches from atrial tracking mode to non-tracking mode with atrial fibrillation. Pacemakers may be permanent or temporary and may include single-chamber, dual-chamber, and biventricular pacing. Pacemakers are classified with a five-letter pacemaker code indicating the chamber paced, chamber sensed, response to sensing, programmability, and pacing functions.

**72. 2:** The "5 A's" of the smoking cessation intervention include the following:

Step 1: Ask all clients about tobacco use at every visit. Questions about smoking should be included in all history and physical assessments.
Step 2: Advise all clients who smoke to stop smoking, advising them that smoking is harming their health.
Step 3: Assess the client's willingness to stop smoking. If they are unwilling, ask questions about why.
Step 4: Assist the client to stop smoking. Establish a quit plan with a quit date and a plan for intervention.
Step 5: Arrange for follow-up.

**73. 2, 3, 4, 6:** Those with hypertension should engage in regular aerobic exercise, such as walking, for 30 minutes most days; switch to the dietary approaches to stop hypertension (DASH) diet, which is high in fruits and vegetables and low in saturated fat; and limit alcohol to no more than one drink per day for females and two for males, but they need not completely eliminate alcohol. Smoking cessation is essential as is losing weight for those who are overweight.

**74. 1:** In traditional Muslim culture, the left hand, which is considered unclean, is typically reserved for toileting, so the nurse should use the left hand to cleanse the client's rectal area. For the same reason, the nurse should be careful to always pass food, medications, and other items to the client using the right hand and not the left. Wearing gloves to provide rectal cleansing is required by standard precautions and is unrelated to the woman's cultural and religious beliefs.

**75. 3:** The ego defense mechanism that the client is exhibiting in this scenario is called displacement, which is the transference of feelings from one target to another. Compensation is compensating for a perceived weakness by emphasizing a strength. Reaction formation is covering up unacceptable thoughts/behaviors by emphasizing the opposite. Regression is reverting to an earlier level of development.

**76. 1:** Although children develop at different rates, usually by the age of 24 months a child is able to understand about 300 words and is beginning to use two- and three-word sentences (e.g., "want candy"). At 16–18 months, a child can use and understand 7–20 words and can point to body parts. At 13–15 months, a child can use and understand 4–6 words but understands more and can point to items he wants. At 12 months, a child can use and understand a few words, such as *mama* and *dada*, and can imitate animal sounds, such as *moo* and *woof.*

**77. 1, 3, 5, 6:** Anoxic brain injuries result from insufficient blood flow and oxygen to the brain, resulting from trauma, near-drowning, choking, cardiac arrest, drug overdose, and operative complications. Mild anoxic brain injuries result in a decreased ability to concentrate, memory impairment, decreased balance, and restlessness. Severe anoxic brain injuries have the same symptoms as mild anoxic brain injuries as well as unclear mumbled speech, dysphasia, seizures, and spasticity. Critical anoxic brain injuries result in an impaired ability to communicate, a semicomatose state (still able to open eyes), and an inconsistent response to environmental stimuli.

**78. 4:** The primary focus of treatment for osteomyelitis is intravenous (IV) antibiotic therapy, based on the results of a wound culture. IV antibiotics are administered continuously for three to six weeks, and then oral antibiotics are administered for up to three months. If the wound does not respond adequately to antibiotic therapy, then surgical debridement is indicated, during which time antibiotic-impregnated beads may be inserted into the wound. The infected area is immobilized to reduce pain and to reduce the risk of pathological fractures. Warm, wet soaks may be used to increase circulation, and analgesia may be used to reduce pain.

**79. 1:** When determining whether or not a client is a candidate for restraints, only current behavior should be considered. If the client currently poses a danger to others or to self and no other reasonable alternative exists, then restraints may be considered. Restraints cannot be applied as a preventive measure for such things as a previous violent attack against a staff member or a history of falls. There must be evidence of current risk.

**80. 1:** Because this client faces many challenges in the home environment, the most appropriate referral is to an occupational therapist. The occupational therapist (OT) can meet with the client to determine her goals and may observe her carrying out activities of daily living (ADLs) to evaluate her abilities and deficits. Afterwords, the OT can advise her about modifications needed in the home environment and assistive devices so she can remain independent for as long as possible.

**81. 1, 2, 3, 5:** If the nurse is teaching a group of clients about risk factors for diabetes mellitus, type 2, the nurse should include the following:

- Obesity
- Hypertension and/or heart disease
- 45 years and older (risk increases with age)
- Non-Caucasian race: African American, Asian, Hispanic, Pacific Islander
- History of diabetes mellitus in family
- High level of LDL cholesterol or low level of HDL cholesterol and high level of triglycerides
- History of polycystic ovarian syndrome

**82. 1:** Clients who are hearing impaired often are reluctant to say so but may try to compensate by reading lips. Because their hearing of their own voice may also be impaired, they may speak more loudly than usual. Even clients who are quite adept at lip reading may misunderstand some words, resulting in answering incorrectly. If a client appears to have hearing impairment, the nurse should ask the client directly if he or she is having trouble hearing the nurse and ask how to best communicate.

**83. 1, 2, 3, 5:** When a client is discharged 48 hours after delivery of an infant, the client should be apprised of danger signs that could indicate infection or other complications. Constant fatigue, although debilitating, is usually normal so soon after delivery. Danger signs include:

- Temperature higher than 38 °C (100.4 °F)
- Difficulty urinating
- Swelling, redness, or pain in one or both legs
- Increased vaginal bleeding or foul vaginal discharge
- Swelling, masses, or red streaks in the breasts or bleeding nipples
- Blurred vision, persistent headache
- Depression, overwhelming feeling of sadness

**84. 4:** Skin that remains moist because of diaphoresis, or excessive sweating, can cause the electrodes to adhere poorly or to loosen, which can result in ECG artifacts. The best solution is to wipe the skin with a dry cloth or gauze pad so that it is dry, then wipe the area with an alcohol wipe, which degreases the skin, and allow it to dry. Then, apply an adhesive enhancer, such as tincture of benzoin or Skin Tac. Electrodes may also be secured with transparent dressings or tape.

**85. 3:** If a client is to have a nasogastric tube inserted for intermittent feedings, an appropriate task to delegate to unlicensed assistive personnel (UAP) is the administering of the tube feedings if the person has been trained in doing so. However, an RN or LVN/LPN must verify the tube position first because this cannot be delegated to UAP. UAP cannot insert or reposition a displaced NG tube. UAP can be advised to monitor the client's condition and to report any changes in condition, such as dyspnea or nausea.

**86. 3:** If a client has had a recent BK amputation of the right leg and the nurse notes an unusual pattern of swelling after removing the elastic wrap, which the client had applied, the most likely reason for this observation is incorrect wrap technique in which the pressure from the wrap is uneven. The nurse should point out the swelling and discuss the reasons, demonstrating the correct wrap procedure and then observing the client rewrap the stump.

**87. 1:** If a client with prostate cancer has been given the option of various treatments and asks the nurse for advice, the most appropriate response is: "Let's discuss the different options and how you feel about them." The nurse must avoid trying to directly influence the client's choice; however, since the client asked for advice, this is a good opportunity for the client to express feelings and concerns about the diagnosis and treatment. Additionally, talking through the options may help the client reach an independent decision.

**88. 3:** Atrial fibrillation is an arrhythmia where the atria do not contract in a normal rhythm. The resulting irregular heart rate is often rapid. This can cause palpitations, chest pain, dizziness, and syncope. Long-term, it can result in pulmonary emboli, heart attack, and stroke. On an ECG, the P waves are irregular and not associated with QRS complexes.

**89. 2:** If a client has bilateral pain, enlarged and swollen metacarpophalangeal and proximal interphalangeal joints, swan-neck deformity, and ulnar deviation, these signs and symptoms are consistent with rheumatoid arthritis (RA), an autoimmune disorder that results in inflammation and damage to the joints. RA may also affect other organs of the body. Clients typically experience periods when the disease exacerbates and symptoms worsen. Treatment includes NSAIDs, analgesics, disease-modifying antirheumatic drugs (DMARDs), and biologics.

**90. 2:** If a neonate has severe congenital abnormalities, death is imminent, and the NICU team feels that no further attempts at treatment or feeding are warranted, the best approach is to tell the parents that the team suggests a change in care plan to focus on comfort measures. The nurse should avoid such phrases as "stopping" or "withdrawing" treatment or feeding because these terms may make the parents feel as though they are starving or killing their infant, although the exact plan for care should be explained.

**91. 1680:** In order to calculate a client's necessary caloric intake to maintain body weight, the first step is to convert the client's weight from pounds to kilograms:

$$\frac{132}{2.2} = 60$$

Then, the caloric requirement (usually between 25 and 30 calories per kg) is multiplied by the number of kilograms:

$$60 \times 28 = 1{,}680 \text{ calories}$$

Clients who are exceptionally active, such as athletes, may need to have a higher number of calories, so caloric requirements must be individualized.

**92. 3:** If a client is on contact precautions because of a MRSA infection and has an open, draining wound, the nurse should glove and gown whenever entering the room for any type of patient or environmental contact. MRSA can be spread from the client to surfaces, such as the bedrails or bedside table. Upon leaving the room, the gloves and gown should be removed and placed into a receptacle near the door and inside of the client's room.

**93. 1, 4:** If a 6-year-old child has influenza with a fever and cough, the statements by the child's caregiver that suggest a need for information include:

- "If his fever gets too high, I'll give him a bath in cold water": This could lower the child's fever too quickly. If the child's fever is high (>102 °F or 39 °C), then the child may be bathed with lukewarm water.
- "I've been giving him baby aspirin to lower his fever": Children should not be administered any type of salicylate for viral infections because this places the child at risk for developing Reye syndrome, which can cause progressive encephalopathy, liver failure, and death.

**94. 1:** Following procurement of organs from a standard criteria donor (donor younger than 50 years who suffered brain death), the heart and lungs should be transplanted within 4–6 hours, liver and pancreas within 12 hours, and the kidney within 24 hours. Organ and tissue recovery is carried out in the operating room with members of the recovery team present and transportation to the recipient available. The corneas and skin can be harvested for up to 2 hours after death and bone up to 36 hours. Heart valves can be harvested up to 72 hours after death.

**95.** The steps to combining doses of two different insulins from two vials in one syringe include:

| Step | Procedure |
|---|---|
| 1 | I. Cleanse the tops of the vials. |
| 2 | II. Inject air into vial 1. |
| 3 | VI. Inject air into vial 2. |
| 4 | V. Withdraw medication from vial 2. |
| 5 | IV. Change needles. |
| 6 | III. Withdraw medication from vial 1. |

**96. 3:** If teaching a client to use a metered-dose inhaler without a spacer, the inhaler should be positioned 1–2 inches away from the client's lips for administration of a dose of inhaled medication. The client should be advised to exhale and then to deliver a dose while breathing in slowly for about 5 seconds, followed by holding the breath for 10 seconds before exhaling. If an adult has difficulty with coordinating breathing and delivering of a dosage or holding the inhaler at the correct distance, then a spacer should be used. Children should also use a spacer.

**97. 1, 3, 4, 5:** In this scenario, the nurse should immediately stop the infusion. The nurse should also administer naloxone per standing order (or immediately consult the physician to obtain the order). Because the respirations are so slow, supplementary oxygen will generally be administered. Because an error occurred in setting the parameters of dosage on the PCA, an incident report must be filed.

**98. 1:** If a client with Alzheimer's disease is incontinent of urine and feces and incontinent care has been delegated to UAP, then the UAP should be advised to check the client for dryness on a regular schedule of every 2 hours. Eating and drinking often trigger urination and/or bowel movements, so scheduling checks after meals is advisable. However, if the client appears restless or pulls at their clothing at other times, the UAP should check for dryness then as well.

**99. 1, 2, 3:** The long-term effects of prolonged use of phenytoin include a condition referred to as "Dilantin facies," which is characterized by gingival hypertrophy, hirsutism, and hypertrophy of facial subcutaneous tissue. Clients must be advised to maintain good dental care. Additionally, clients may develop osteoporosis, so supplementary vitamin D is usually advised. Clients with low levels of albumin (usually associated with renal disease or malnutrition) may have more severe effects.

**100. 1, 2, 4, 5:** The nurse should give this patient the following information:

- Retrograde ejaculation may occur.
- Recovery rates vary but can take up to a year or more.
- Attempts at sexual intercourse are usually avoided for 1 month.
- Anxiety can interfere with sexual functioning.
- The client may want to explore other forms of sexual intimacy even though these are not likely as important to the client as sexual intercourse at this time.

# NCLEX-RN Practice Tests #2 and #3

To take these additional NCLEX practice tests, visit our online resources page:
**mometrix.com/resources719/nclexrn-31183**

# Online Resources

Due to our efforts to try to keep this book to a manageable length, we've created a link that will give you access to all of your online resources:

**mometrix.com/resources719/nclexrn-31183**

# It's Your Moment, Let's Celebrate It!

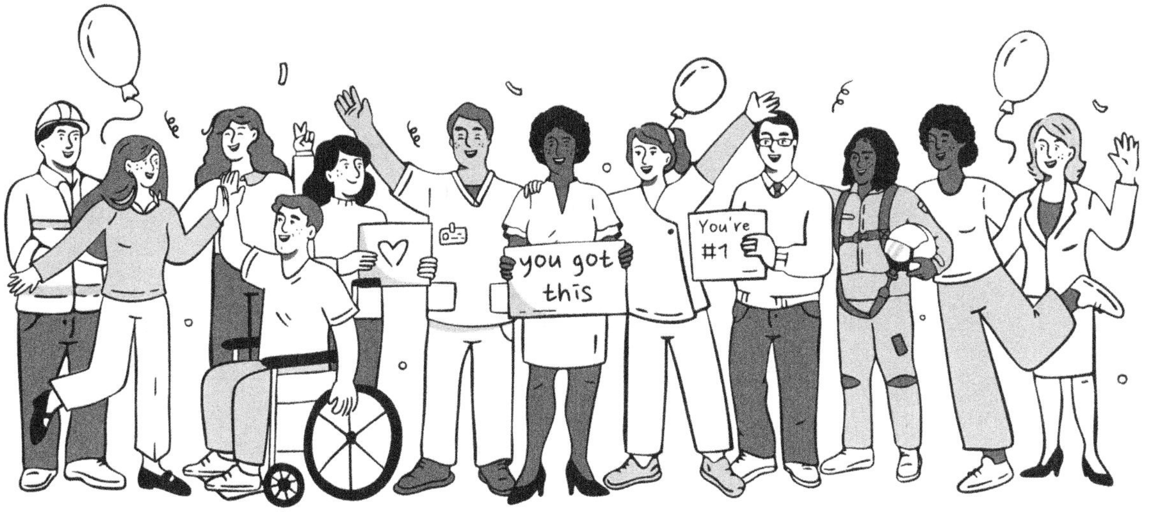


**Share your story @mometrixtestpreparation**

Printed in Dunstable, United Kingdom

91343649R00299